RENEWALS 458-4574

DATE DUE

GAYLORD			PRINTED IN U.S.A.

PRACTICAL ELECTROMYOGRAPHY

SECOND EDITION

This volume is one of the series,
Rehabilitation Medicine Library,
edited by John V. Basmajian.

New books and new editions published, in press or in preparation for this series:

*Originally published as part of the Physical Medicine Library, edited by Sidney Licht.

PRACTICAL
ELECTROMYOGRAPHY
SECOND EDITION

Edited by
Ernest W. Johnson, MD

Professor and Chairman
Department of Physical Medicine
The Ohio State University
Columbus, Ohio

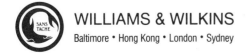

WILLIAMS & WILKINS
Baltimore • Hong Kong • London • Sydney

Editor: John P. Butler
Associate Editor: Linda Napora
Copy Editor: Gail Naron Chalew
Design: Saturn Graphics
Illustration Planning: Wayne Hubbel
Production: Theda Harris

Accurate indications, adverse reactions, and dosage schedules for drugs are provided in this book, but it is possible that they may change. The reader is urged to review the package information data of the manufacturers of the medications mentioned.

Printed in the United States of America
First Edition, 1980
Reprinted, 1981, 1982

Main entry under title:

Library of Congress Cataloging in Publication Data
Practical electromyography.
  (Rehabilitation medicine library)
  Includes index.
  1. Electromyography. 2. Neuromuscular diseases—Diagnosis. I. Johnson, Ernest W., 1924–   . II. Series. [DNLM: 1. Electrodiagnosis. 2. Electromyography. WE 500 P895]
RC77.5.P7 1987   616.7′4′0754   87–10692
ISBN 0-683-04463-X

88 89 90 91 92   10 9 8 7 6 5 4 3 2 1

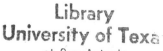

Series Editor's Foreword

To ensure that the first edition of *Practical Electromyography* would be unique among a number of good books on clinical electromyography, I chose Ernest Johnson as its editor. Of course, he and his choice of authors and style became the essential elements of that edition's great success. Nevertheless, my conviction persisted that the success was a measure of the worldwide high regard held by all who have an interest in the work and opinion of Dr. Johnson, his colleagues, and his former students.

Changing times demand positive responses from all new books that hope to receive some measure of acclaim. This is particularly true for second editions of successful books because purchasers of the first edition may be satisfied and so remain passive about checking out (and buying) the new version. Indeed, book reviewers cannot resist comparing and contrasting editions, and sometimes, alas, they do little else. With this new edition, both reviewers and readers can relax: it is as fresh and new as before, and it reflects the opinions and knowledge of the Johnson "Ohio State team" even better than before. The volume happily retains a couple of "non-Ohio" features from the previous editing, but their value is timeless, universal, and irreplacable with the recent deaths of the authors, Stuart Reiner and Joseph Rogoff.

Some critics have become impatient with leaders in the field who, as does Dr. Johnson, continue to use "electromyography or EMG" in a generic sense to include elements of electrodiagnosis or EDX. They feel that EDX should replace EMG. Having once authored a book with the word "Electrodiagnosis" in its title and finding the reading public querulous about its meaning and limits, I do not share this notion. Dr. Johnson and his authors are not confused and neither will their readers be. Although motor unit potentials are featured, this book embraces much more that grew directly out of studies of motor unit potentials— nerve conduction (both motor and sensory) and evoked potentials to sample the central nervous system.

I am pleased and proud to have Dr. Johnson and his "team," past and present, produce this second edition of *Practical Electromyography*. This is a most significant volume in the *Rehabilitation Medicine Library*, and no one will deny that it is truly practical in the best sense of that word.

JOHN V. BASMAJIAN, MD, FACA, FRCP(C)

v

Preface to the Second Edition

The second edition of *Practical Electromyography* is an accurate reflection of my perception of the needs of clinical electromyographers in the United States today. It emphasizes chosen techniques and principles without attempting to be an encyclopedia of clinical neurophysiology. It retains what was good, true, and useful in the first edition and expands areas that have recently emerged. Hence, it is truly a new book to meet the needs of the practical clinician today.

My assessment of those needs is based on 36 courses in practical electromyography given by our group at The Ohio State University in the past 24 years. All attendees at those courses were required to send two EMG reports for my perusal before the course. These reports (over 1000) are an excellent and unique survey of the current practice and problems of these clinical electromyographers and shaped the basic structure of this edition.

If not a textbook—and it is certainly not a reference book—what best describes *Practical Electromyography*? My earnest expectation is that it will be most useful as a monograph . . . but more! Most of the techniques and philosophy are derived from practices at The Ohio State University Department of Physical Medicine. As editor, I am responsible not only for the organization but, more importantly, I stand behind the content as representing the current electrodiagnostic techniques used daily in our clinical practice.

Although most of the current texts and continuing courses on clinical neurophysiology briefly discuss the needle exam, this volume considers that vital area of electromyography more intensively while avoiding the risk of becoming a comprehensive reference volume. My anticipation is that *Practical Electromyography* will fulfill the promise of its title as viewed by me, my associates, and former students.

Working on a second edition is much more difficult than completing the first, both for the contributors and the editor. Chapter authors may not have the same enthusiasm, and updating old material may not be as exciting as writing a new work. Therefore, I owe a special thanks to them for the innovative, fresh approaches they achieved.

ERNEST W. JOHNSON, MD
COLUMBUS, OHIO

Preface to the First Edition

Sidney Licht was pretty proud when he edited the first book solely for physiatrists on electromyography in 1950. Since then, two revised and enlarged editions have been published and now, with the change of publisher from Elizabeth Licht to The Williams & Wilkins Company and the series editor from Sidney Licht to John V. Basmajian, it is meet and right to alter the format and substance as a new edition.

I have chosen to change the title to *Practical Electromyography*. This is for two principal reasons. The first is that clearly the title should reflect the content. Further it is a given that the content must be the responsibility of the editor. For the past 17 years, I have given a continuing education course in electromyography each year (occasionally two). All have been oversubscribed, so I have gradually increased the enrollment from 25 to now 50 students, and the next course will have over 100. I have attempted to restrict the applicants to experienced electromyographers—that is, physicians, usually physiatrists or neurologists, who are doing electromyography everyday in their practice. Each course begins and ends with an examination. This is a mechanism to assess the limitations of the students attending the course and, also, to give some indication of what they have learned during the 3-day intensive course. The experiences gained from these examinations have been a revelation about the common assumptions of those who teach electromyography.

The most serious deficiency is not theoretical knowledge but rather the identified voids, including surface anatomy and certain practical aspects of electrode placement as well as the techniques of needle electromyography. Similarly, understanding and interpretation of subtle abnormalities were invariably lacking in a majority of the physicians enrolled in the courses.

My restriction of enrollees to physicians has been challenged occasionally, but it must remain absolute. The electromyographic examination is an essential extension of the history and physical examination relevant to neuromuscular diseases. It must be planned only after a careful history and physical and it is dynamic—that is, the electromyographic examination must be modified during its actual performance as abnormalities are revealed. Only a practicing physician with both theoretical and clinical knowledge of neuromuscular diseases, including their differential diagnosis, is an appropriate electromyographer.

While an assistant may be helpful in certain instances, I am convinced that the recording of dynamic electromyographic data for later interpretation by the physician-specialist can, and often does, lead to erroneous conclusions.

There are those who would criticize my use of the term "electromyography" as incorrectly describing the contents of the book and would recommend "clinical neurophysiology or electroneuromyography." I accept their semantic implications but reject their suggestion. Historically, traditionally, and practically (if not semantically), the term electromyography has currency when describing the determinations of motor and sensory conduction studies, reflexology and other frequently done data gathering about the electrical phenomenon occurring in the afferent and efferent nervous system.

After all, the phrase motor nerve conduction velocity is technically incorrect—a more appropriate term would be motor nerve impulse propagation rate—but historic and common usage prevails!

Obviously the book editor must be responsible for everything in the book. While the chapter authors properly deserve credit, the concepts presented in this volume are thoroughly and inescapably mine, whether by adoption or conception, and I will stand by them (at least until the next edition)!

The only chapter with which I did not tinker is the one on history by Dr. Sidney Licht, who, I may confess now, provided me some 20 years ago with the initial acceleration for this task of editing. He pointed out that editing is both hard work and low-paying. I can now confirm both of these statements.

To whom it is directed is a universal requisite of all book introductions. Mine, i.e., *Practical Electromyography*, must be considered a book for physicians-specialists who wish to solidify their base of clinical electromyography. The book is specifically directed to raising the level of everyday diagnostic electromyography. Our collective desire is to establish an acceptable level of electrodiagnosis by those physicians who are "into it" and can't seem to find time to polish their techniques with continuing education courses.

Some concepts presented may be authoritarian rather than authoritative, but they represent the distillate of over 20 years of electromyography in a clinical setting where decisions of management were guided by the results!

This is where the scalpel meets the skin or, more appropriately, where the electrode enters the muscle! While theoretical considerations are always necessary as background, one must ascend to practical notions when discussing electromyography with the surgeon who contemplates the potential (no pun intended) of nerve exploration, when and where to take a biopsy, what mode of management is optional, etc. The "practical" assumes primacy when immediate management decisions are beckoning.

My naivete, admittedly profound, does not permit me the musing that only physician-specialists will read the book; not so—hope is that others, perhaps less qualified as electromyographers, will assiduously study the volume and decide that this specialized field of medicine may be more complex than was previously realized.

In any event, the interpretation of electromyography must rest with the performing electromyographer for both effectiveness and correctness. Lacking these two characteristics, the electromyogram is a procedure recorded in the medical chart without substance or value for the patient, and this is the person who is most important in the transaction.

ERNEST W. JOHNSON, M.D.
Book Editor

Contributors

Randall L. Braddom, MD
Clinical Associate Professor
University of Cincinnati
Director
Department of Physical Medicine and Rehabilitation
Providence Hospital
Cincinnati, Ohio

Mohammad Taghi Fatehi, PhD
Assistant Professor
Department of Physical Medicine
The Ohio State University
Columbus, Ohio

Susan L. Hubbell, MD
Clinical Assistant Professor
Department of Physical Medicine
The Ohio State University
Columbus, Ohio

Ernest W. Johnson, MD
Professor and Chairman
Department of Physical Medicine
The Ohio State University
Columbus, Ohio

George H. Kraft, MS, MD
Professor
Department of Rehabilitation Medicine
University of Washington
Seattle, Washington

Ian C. MacLean, MD
Associate Professor of Clinical Rehabilitation Medicine
Director of Medical Education
Department of Rehabilitation Medicine
Northwestern University Medical School
Evanston, Illinois

Stuart Reiner, MEE
Former President of TECA Corporation
Pleasantville, New York
(*Deceased*)

Joseph B. Rogoff, MD
Professor
Rehabilitation Medicine
New York Medical College
Valhalla, New York
(*Deceased*)

Robert J. Weber, MD
Associate Professor and Chairman
Department of Physical Medicine and Rehabilitation
Wright State University
Dayton, Ohio

David O. Wiechers, MD
Clinical Assistant Professor
Department of Physical Medicine
The Ohio State University
Columbus, Ohio

Contents

1

The EMG Examination

ERNEST W. JOHNSON

The electromyographic examination is only a part of the evaluation of a patient with weakness, pain, limp, sensory disturbance, atrophy, and fatigue. This evaluation begins with a detailed history and neuromuscular examination to isolate those areas that should be investigated electrodiagnostically. In a screening function examination the patient walks on heels and toes, squats, and returns and immobilizes the examiner's hands by grasping two fingers of each hand as the examiner attempts to move in four directions. These maneuvers isolate areas that should be checked further with the manual muscle examination.

After those preliminary activities the electrodiagnostic examination is ready for planning. The procedure should be explained to the patient without going into specific details. In most instances it is inadvisable to show the needle electrodes to the patient because patients often equate prospective pain with the length of the needle, rather than its caliber. The discomfort associated with insertion of the needle can be minimized with a concomitant pinch of the skin. In most instances, relaxation can be achieved by having the individual contract the antagonist muscle group slightly.

Most examinations are facilitated, particularly those for radiculopathy, if the patient is placed in the prone position with pillows under the chest for the upper extremity and neck, and pillows under the abdomen and hips for the lower extremity. It is also useful to place a pillow under the ankles so that the knees are slightly flexed.

Generally, the weakest muscle is checked first to identify the specific problem, and then other muscles are examined. Because there are 434 skeletal muscles in the body, it is necessary to be completely familiar with surface and functional anatomy to isolate those areas of investigation that will assist in the diagnosis. Generally, the orderly planning of the examination will facilitate the electrodiagnostic examination by enabling the fewest number of muscles to be examined.

Each muscle should be explored proximally, centrally, and distally. Each needle penetration through the skin should allow 10–20 electrode insertions in a circular pattern. There are five steps to the needle examination.

STEP 1: THE MUSCLE AT REST

For the first step the gain setting should be 50 microvolts (μV) per cm and the sweep speed 5 to 10 msec/cm. Although recommendations of other gain settings have been made, it is necessary in this step to use sufficient gain to ensure the visualization of fibrillation potentials that may be remote or old and therefore quite small. The recommendation of 100 μV/cm is a residual from the use of instruments that were supplied with a 5-inch oscilloscope and the gain setting was 100 μV/inch. Most of the oscilloscopes now use a 10 $\times$ 10 cm face.

The filter setting should be generally 2 Hz to 10 or 20 kilohertz to avoid any distortion of the action potentials that are visualized. The normal muscle is quiet at rest.

Occasionally two types of potentials may be visualized in this step. The first and most frequently seen is a *fasciculation potential*. This is defined as a spontaneous and involuntary discharge of a motor unit or portion of a motor unit. It is recognized by its irregular rate of firing and its generally slow rate of firing—less than 5 Hz—which is the lowest frequency at which a volitional potential motor unit is recruited. In normal individuals fasciculations are frequently seen in the gastrocnemius and often in the orbicularis oculi. This slow and irregular rate of firing differentiates them from a motor unit potential under volitional control.

Although fasciculation potentials are identified by their rate and irregular rhythm, they may be of any size or shape. They are generally classified by their shape as either simple or complex. Simple fasciculations are di- or triphasic, whereas complex fasciculations are polyphasic. Polyphasic fasciculations are further divided into those that are the usual polyphasic potentials—that is, a motor unit potential that crosses the isoelectric line more than four times,—and iterative or repetitive discharge polyphasics. These latter polyphasics may represent a motor unit that fires two or three times. As the relative refractory period is shortened, a single activation results in several discharges of the motor unit, making it a complex motor unit potential. Thus, one visualizes a motor unit potential comprising three, four, or even five discharges.

A special type of repetitive discharge or iterative polyphasic potential is associated with myokymia, alkalotic states, and incipient tetany (Fig. 1.1). Frequently, a hyperventilating patient demonstrates repetitive discharge fasciculations. Early in alkalosis the volitional potentials are iterative, and as the process progresses these volitional iterative

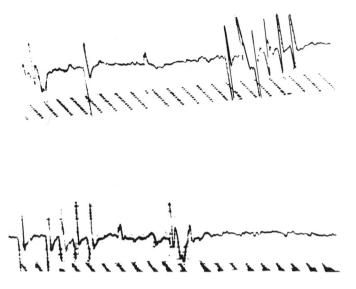

Figure 1.1. Iterative discharges from deltoid m. in patient with radiation myelopathy. (Caliber: Each slanted line = 10 msec. Height = 100μV.)

discharges appear as fasciculation potentials. The first sign of an alkalotic state or incipient tetany, however, is a repetitive discharge motor unit potential under volitional control.

The myokymic discharge is a type of altered excitability (Fig. 1.2). This clinical finding most likely is the result of ephaptic transmission across fragments of injured or diseased nerves, so that a single activation of an axon results in what appears to be a repetitive discharge polyphasic potential at the needle electrode. These can occur in facial myokymia, which is quite recognizable clinically and is seen in brainstem tumors and multiple sclerosis as well. Myokymia is also seen in Guillain-Barré syndrome. It can also be characteristic of ischemic conditions of the spinal cord, such as radiation myelopathy after malignancy.

A motor unit potential that is ragged and has many spikes not crossing the isoelectric line is referred to as a *disintegrative potential* and is described by the number of turns. These are seen in a variety of motor unit diseases.

A number of studies (see Chapter 3) have been made to identify fasciculation potentials that may be seen in motor neuron disease and to differentiate those fasciculations from those that are seen in normal individuals (Fig. 1.3). The rate of firing is not necessarily a characteristic of the type of fasciculation seen in motor neuron disease, how-

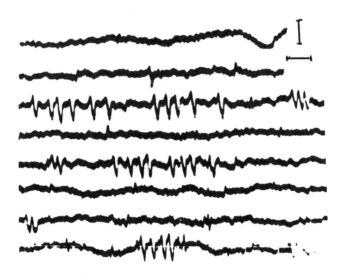

Figure 1.2. Iterative discharges (repetitive discharge fasciculations) recorded in gastroc m. of patient with lumbar stenosis. (Caliber: 50 µV, 20 msec.).

ever; some are reinnervation-type polyphasics where the shape changes as the neuromuscular junctions fail on subsequent discharges of a particular motor unit. Furthermore, the so-called malignant fasciculations seen in motor neuron disease are frequently of very short duration and low amplitude, indicating that the discharge originates in the peripheral portion of the motor unit. Other fasciculations seen in motor neuron disease are of large amplitude and polyphasic.

It is conventional wisdom that fasciculations seen by themselves— that is, without additional electromyographic abnormalities—are not significant or diagnostic. This statement has to be taken in light of some special types of fasciculation potentials that are noted above and also discussed in Chapter 7 on radiculopathies.

Fibrillation Potentials

A single muscle fiber discharge is characterized by a duration of 0.5 to 1.5 msec and an amplitude of 50 to 300 or 400 µV depending on the characteristics of the amplifier and the electrode (Fig. 1.4). Whether that single muscle fiber discharge is the result of a spontaneous activation of the muscle fiber is determined by the rate and rhythm of firing. Generally a spontaneous discharging muscle fiber activates at 2 to 20 Hz and a regular rhythm.

A single muscle fiber discharge can be recorded as a positive sharp wave if the tip of the recording needle electrode is in contact with the

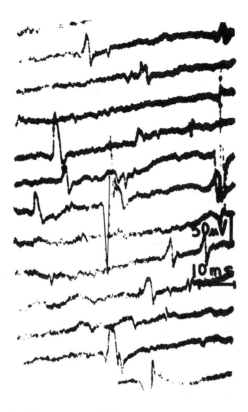

Figure 1.3. Fasciculations recorded from anterior tibial m. of ALS patient. (Caliber: On photo.)

depolarized portion of the muscle fiber (Fig. 1.5). Thus, the positive sharp wave may be recorded either from a fibrillating muscle fiber or an endplate spike because both are single muscle fiber discharges (Fig. 1.6).

The positive sharp waves recorded from a fibrillating muscle fiber are pathologic EDX manifestations, and those recorded from an endplate spike are expected findings with the needle in the endplate zone. Positive waves recorded in the endplate zone should be examined critically to determine whether they are "normal" (i.e., associated with endplate spikes) or pathologic, i.e., associated with fibrillation potentials.

One should note that endplates spikes discussed in the next section, Step 2, are also single muscle fiber discharges and can be differentiated by their rhythm and rate of firing.

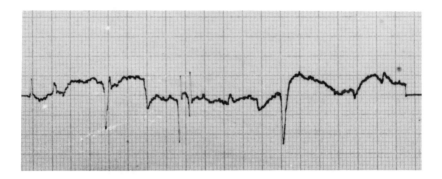

Figure 1.4. Fibrillation potentials and positive wave. Monopolar needle electrode in ext. dig. 1. (Caliber: Each square = 5 msec, 50 μV.)

These single muscle fiber discharges (fibrillations) are presumably the result of altered excitability of the muscle cell membrane. This instability results in a spontaneous activation of the muscle fiber from a variety of stimuli, including mechanical (moving the needle or tapping the muscle in the vicinity of the needle), chemical, and electrical. Fibrillation potentials are not characteristic of any single disease, but are seen in a variety of conditions in which the muscle cell membrane becomes hyperirritable. These include denervation (i.e., separation from its nerve supply), hypo- and hyperkalemia, local trauma, inflammatory states, certain stages of upper motor neuron diseases, and myopathies, among others. In some instances this intrinsic instability in the muscle cell membrane is present without any apparent disease. This may be a forme fruste of paramyotonia congenita (See Weichers and Johnson study (27) on the increased insertional activity or presence of positive waves in a family constellation.)

STEP 2: INSERTIONAL ACTIVITY

The gain setting should be 50 to 100 microvolts/cm and a sweep speed of 5 to 10 msec/cm. Note that the gain setting should always be adjusted so that the entire potential is seen. Filter setting should be from 20 Hz to 10 KHz so that needle electrode movement will not cause the trace to move off the screen.

This is a much-misinterpreted step in the needle examination. Insertional activity by definition results from moving the electromyographic needle briskly through the muscle and mechanically discharging some muscle fibers resulting in a burst of injury potentials. These potentials are single muscle fiber discharges resulting from disruption of the muscle cell membrane by the tip of the needle. The character of the insertional activity may be described as reduced, normal, or increased.

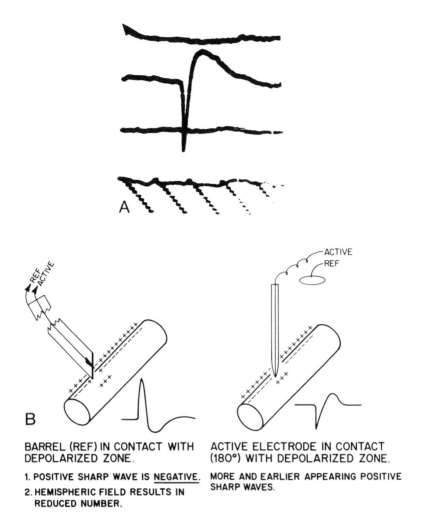

Figure 1.5. *A*, The positive sharp wave. (Caliber: Each slanted line = 10 msec. Height = 50 µV.) *B*, Diagrammatic representation of hypothesis explaining recording differences between monopolar and coaxial needle electrodes. (Not drawn to scale.) Note that monopolar needle electrode records positive waves earlier and in more profusion.

Reduction in insertional activity occurs when the muscle tissue has been replaced by fibrosis, necrosis, or even edema. In this instance the number of muscle cell membranes is not normal, so that there is a reduction of disrupted membranes when the needle is briskly moved through this area of the muscle.

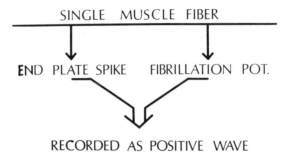

Figure 1.6. Origin of positive sharp wave.

In normal insertional activity, the duration of the insertional activity results from the movement of the electromyographer's hand. Some electromyographers whose hands move very quickly may produce a burst of injury potentials having a duration of 75 to 100 msec of insertional activity; other electromyographers who move the needle slowly and for a somewhat more prolonged time may produce a burst of 300 or 400 msec of insertional activity. Thus, the characterization of insertional activity by duration is entirely inappropriate and refers only to the technique of moving the needle through the muscle.

Increase in insertional activity results when the muscle cell membranes are extraordinarily hyperirritable in such diseases as acute polymyositis, myotonia, etc. This, however, should not be reported as increased insertional activity but better described as the positive waves and spike discharges that occur after the needle movement stops.

When the tip of the needle is in the endplate zone, some rather characteristic discharges occur (Fig. 1.7). First, the tip of the needle provokes discharge of the packets of acetylcholine that then migrate across the synaptic cleft and depolarize postsynaptic sites, resulting in an increase in the miniature endplate potentials. These are nonpropagated, monophasic, negative, high frequency (up to 1000 Hz) discharges that have been referred to as a seashell murmur. A more accurate description would be an increase in the noise level of the oscilloscope trace, perhaps increasing it from 5 μV at a gain setting of 50 μV/cm to 15 to 20 μV. As the endplate potential reaches threshold, the single muscle fiber discharges, resulting in an endplate spike. This has exactly the same characteristics as the fibrillation potential with the exception that, because it originates at the endplate, the initial deflection is negative instead of positive (Fig. 1.8). Also, although the fibrillation discharges in a regular rhythm at 2–20 Hz, the endplate spike discharges irregularly at 20–150 Hz (Fig. 1.9).

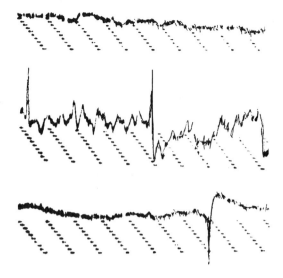

Figure 1.7. Caliber: Each slanted line = 10 msec., height = 50 µV. Upward deflection indicates negativity. Top trace: monopolar needle in relaxed muscle. Middle trace: in endplate zone. Note monophasic, low amplitude, negative waves (seashell murmur). Also two endplate spikes are present. Bottom trace: endplate spike is recorded as a positive wave.

Should the needle be in the presence of a cramp, there would be recorded a high frequency up to 150 Hz synchronous discharge of motor units or portions thereof (Fig. 1.10).

THE POSITIVE WAVE

= Single Muscle Fiber Disch.

W/ Electrode Tip At Injury Site

<u>ABNORMAL</u> If Rhythm Regular
Rate - 2-20Hz

NORMAL If Rhythm − Irregular
Rate − Rapid 20-150 Hz

Figure 1.8. Characteristics of abnormal and "normal" positive sharp waves.

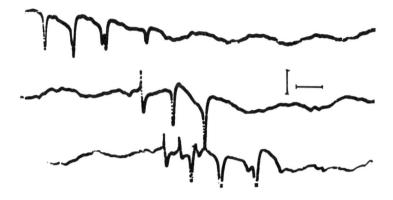

Figure 1.9. Endplate spikes being recorded as positive waves as needle electrode is advanced through endplate zone. (Caliber: 100 μV, 10 msec.)

Complex Repetitive Discharges

In areas involved by motor unit diseases of various types ranging from muscular dystrophy to amyotrophic lateral sclerosis, or even in chronic radiculopathy, the needle electrode occasionally records a discharge that has now been termed *complex repetitive discharge* (formerly "bizarre high frequency discharge") (Fig. 1.11).

Other names used in the past to describe these potentials include bizarre high frequency discharges and pseudomyotonic discharges; the latter term is inappropriate because these potentials lack the waxing and waning quality of myotonic discharges.

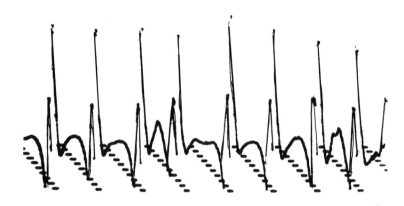

Figure 1.10. Cramp. Monopolar needle electrode in soleus. (Caliber: Each slanted line = 10 msec. Height = 500 μV.)

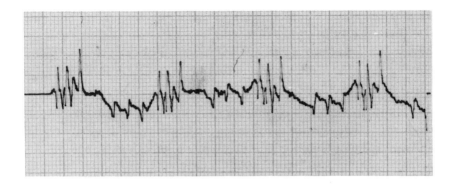

Figure 1.11. Complex repetitive discharge in Duchenne muscular dystrophy. Monopolar needle electrode in extensor digitorum longus. (Caliber: Each square = 5 msec, 50 μV.)

A complex repetitive discharge is spontaneous muscle fiber activity that appears as a continuous train of spikes at a regular frequency (5–150 Hz). The waveform is complex and is relatively uniform from one discharge to another. The discharge begins and ends abruptly, sounding like a motor boat.

The potentials can occur spontaneously, but appear to be provoked readily by movements of the needle electrode or percussion of the muscle. They are a nonspecific finding seen in conditions of chronic denervation (motor neuron disease, long-standing radiculopathy, chronic polyneuropathy) and in myopathies (muscular dystrophy, polymyositis) (Fig. 1.12).

When studied with single fiber electromyography, the discharges are

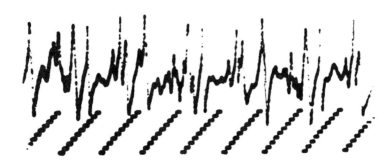

Figure 1.12. Complex repetitive discharges in chronic L5 radiculopathy. Monopolar needle electrode in anterior tibial muscle. (Caliber: Each slanted line = 10 msec. Height = 100 μV.)

seen as complex potentials containing up to ten or more distinct single fiber action potentials.

Repetitive discharges with low repetition rates (less than 20 Hz) occasionally had highly irregular interdischarge intervals but showed no other differences from higher frequency discharges.

Jitter between individual spikes is less than 5 microseconds and is never seen when impulse transmission occurs across a motor endplate. Therefore, the low jitter between individual spike components and consecutive discharges is felt to be evidence of ephaptic or direct electrical activation from muscle fiber to muscle fiber. The discharge is initiated by a fibrillating pacemaker muscle fiber, which activates one or several adjacent fibers. One of these fibers then reactivates the principal pacemaker, creating a closed loop. This cycle continues until the pacemaker fibers become subnormally excitable and blocks. The electromyographer must be careful to distinguish these discharges from similar findings of myotonia, neuromyotonia, and cramp syndrome.

Stalberg in 1982 with single fiber EMG studies has shown this to be the activation of a pacemaker denervated or very hyperirritable single muscle fiber that acts by ephaptic transmission to discharge neighboring hyperirritable fibers. This discharge begins abruptly and discontinues abruptly. It is referred to additionally as "high frequency" if it is discharging at a rate of 50 Hz or above.

STEP 3: MINIMAL CONTRACTION OF A MUSCLE

When the recording needle electrode is in an identified muscle, the patient is asked to think only about contracting that muscle. Doing so will activate a low threshold motor unit at about 5 Hz. These low threshold units are generally the smaller ones and are referred to as Type I motor units. As the individual continues to increase the strength of contraction, this first recruited unit begins to fire more rapidly, and then concomitantly an additional motor unit is recruited. The point at which this second motor unit is recruited is referred to as the *recruitment frequency* or *recruitment interval* (Fig. 1.13). That is, the recruitment interval is the time between succeeding activations of the first motor unit at the moment that the second one is recruited. The reciprocal of the recruitment interval is the recruitment frequency. Most of the commercially available electromyographs have digital memory with the capability of storing up to 400 or 500 msec of discharges so that the recruitment frequency or interval can be easily determined.

The recruitment interval actually could be a more sensitive diagnostic index of weakness. In neuropathic disease the recruitment interval would be shortened; that is, because there are fewer motor units available, the first unit will be firing more rapidly at the moment that the second is recruited. This would shorten the recruitment interval or in-

RECRUITMENT INTERVAL (RI)

Time between succeeding contractions of 1st MU at moment of 2nd MU recruited

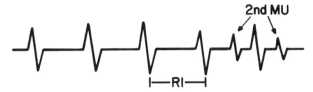

= Reciprocal of firing rate of 1st MU at moment of 2nd MU recruitment /

Figure 1.13. Recruitment interval (reciprocal of recruitment firing rate).

crease the recruitment frequency. Conversely, in early myopathic disease, the recruitment interval would be increased (Fig. 1.14). That is, the first unit would be firing more slowly at the moment that the second unit is recruited because each motor unit has fewer muscle fibers functioning and therefore is weaker.

The gain setting for Step 3 should be 50 to 100 μV/cm and a faster sweep at 2 to 5 msec/cm. These changes provide an opportunity to examine in detail the amplitude, duration, number of phases, and stability of the motor unit potential. The polyphasic MUP has more than five phases because it crosses the baseline more than four times (Figs. 1.15 and 1.16).

In reinnervation, the motor unit polyphasic (MUP) may be prolonged in duration, have low amplitude, and be highly polyphasic. As the axon sprouts mature, the muscle fibers discharge more synchronously, thus making the MUP larger and less polyphasic. Ultimately, a reinnervated motor unit will only be larger than normal particularly if it adopted more muscle fibers than in the original motor unit.

Type II motor units are generally recruited later and are larger in amplitude and of longer duration. The Type II motor units are activated in a vigorous contraction (see Step 4), which is referred to as *ballistic recruitment.* Note that the amplitude of the recorded motor unit potentials is measured from peak to peak. A trigger-and-signal delay line can help make accurate measurements of the motor unit potentials.

In some chronic reinnervation states, a satellite potential will occur 10–15 milliseconds later than the major potential but is time-locked. This is presumably due to incomplete myelination of an immature twig (Figs. 1.17 and 1.18).

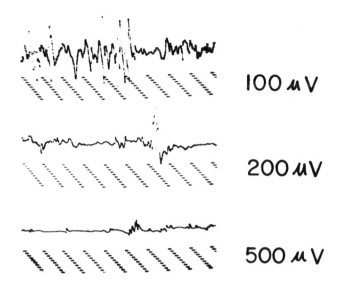

Figure 1.14. Recruitment pattern in vastus medialis in patient with Duchenne muscular dystrophy. (Caliber: Each slanted line = 10 msec. Height = as indicated.)

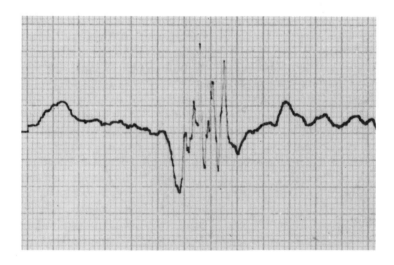

Figure 1.15. Polyphasic motor unit potential in Duchenne muscular dystrophy. Monopolar needle electrode in anterior tibial muscle. (Caliber: Each square = 5 msec, 50 μV.)

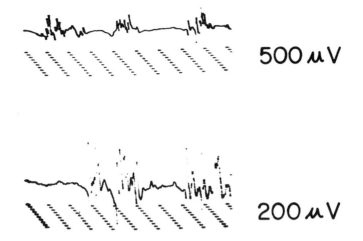

500 μV

200 μV

Figure 1.16. Polyphasic MUP recorded from anterior tibial muscle in 14-year-old Duchenne muscular dystrophy patient. (Caliber: Each slanted line = 10 msec. Height = as indicated.)

Satellite Potential
Time-locked to first component
May appear 5–50 msec later
Slow conduction in sprouting immature twig

Obviously in those conditions in which the Type II motor units are predominant, the first recruited potentials would be larger. In those where Type I motor units predominate (e.g., steroid myopathy), the Type II motor units may never appear even in a substantial contraction (see Step 4).

STEP 4: MAXIMAL EFFORT

In order that maximal effort may be exerted by the patient, the electrode should be placed superficially in the muscle so that making a maximal contraction will not be painful. The muscle should be a single joint muscle because it is extraordinarily difficult to generate a maximal effort with a two joint muscle when the patient is in a recumbent position. For example, the vastus medialis (a single joint muscle) should be used instead of the rectus femoris, which crosses both hip and knee.

The gain should be set at 200 to 500 μV/cm and the sweep speed at 10 msec/cm. It is essential that all of the potentials be visualized on the

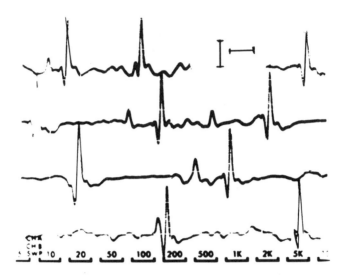

Figure 1.17. Reduced recruitment in patient with Charcot-Marie-Tooth disease. Monopolar needle electrode in abductor dig. V. (Caliber: 10 msec, 5 millivolts.)

screen; thus the gain setting should be adjusted during the contraction. In neuropathic conditions, during the maximal contraction, there is a reduced number of motor units as compared to strength of contraction (Fig. 1.19). The effort of the patient can be gauged by the rate of firing. One should not indicate that there is a reduced number of motor units or a reduced recruitment pattern unless there is a maximal rate of firing (Fig. 1.20). It is estimated that the tip of the electrode can record, at a maximum, portions of eight to ten motor units; therefore, if only two motor units are present on the screen, one could estimate that there is a substantial degree of weakness present. Because a grade of 4 out of 5 or G on the manual muscle test has been shown when only approximately 40% of the motor units remain, it will be extraordinarily difficult to detect degrees of weakness representing a loss of 30% or fewer motor units on the Step 4.

This difficulty in detecting weakness suggests that the recruitment interval or frequency is a more sensitive electromyographic technique than simply Step 4. When considerable notching at the peaks of the motor unit potentials is seen during maximal contraction, one should return to Step 3 for further estimation of the proportion of polyphasic potentials (Fig. 1.18). If increased more than 10%, they should be reported as "an increased proportion of polyphasics." The audio signal can suggest a reduction in duration of the motor unit potentials in Step 4.

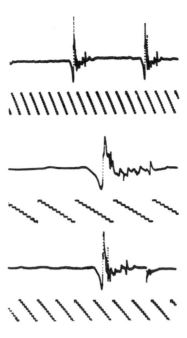

Figure 1.18. Complex motor unit potential recorded in reinnervating peripheral nerve injury (S/P 5 MO.) Monopolar needle electrode in deltoid. Note the satellite potential evident in bottom trace 10 msec after main complex. (Caliber: Each slanted line = 10 msec. Height = 200 μV.)

In so-called hysterical weakness Step 4 reveals the electrical correlate of the ratchety response that is so characteristic; that is, groups of MUPs discharge separated by a space, similar to a tremor.

STEP 5

When an abnormality has been detected, then one must explore other muscles to determine whether the disease or injury is limited to a branch of the peripheral nerve, a root level, or the abnormality is more generalized. This must be accomplished by a systematic needle exploration of the extremity muscles. A knowledge of surface and functional anatomy is necessary for completion of this step.

Usually, if a generalized disease is suspected, all four extremities should be explored, and certainly, in motor neuron disease (ALS), the tongue and soft palate should be studied as well.

Knowledge of the clinical patterns of disease is also essential in order to explore those areas of muscle that are most likely to be involved early in disease; for example, the upper trapezius in facioscapulohu-

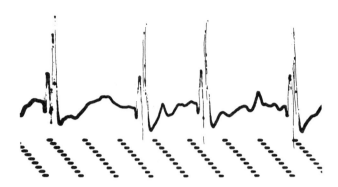

Figure 1.19. Reduced recruitment in severe axonal neuropathy. (Monopolar needle in ext. dig. 1.) Note firing rate is 36 Hz. (Caliber: Each slanted line = 10 msec. Height = 200 μV.)

meral muscular dystrophy. Varying muscles in different parts of the body have substantially different characteristics in terms of duration, amplitude, and firing rates (Table 1.1). For example, the extrinsic eye muscle has very tiny, short duration potentials, perhaps 100 to 200 μV and 1 msec duration and rates of firing up to 100 Hz. On the other hand, motor unit potentials in the vastus medialis may be 1500 to 2000 μV and 12 msec duration. As a rule, the more centrally located muscle have smaller amplitude and shorter duration potentials.

SPECIAL CONSIDERATIONS OF ANATOMY

Accessible muscles for needle exploration include most of the 434 skeletal muscles in the body. The trapezius and facial muscles are extraordinarily thin so that an exploring electrode may penetrate through the muscle unless meticulous care is taken. This is particularly true in certain diseases, for example, facioscapulohumeral muscular dystrophy, in the trapezius or trauma to the 11th cranial nerve with denervation of this muscle.

There have been reports of penetration of the pleural space by careless electromyographers who are unfamiliar with surface anatomy. This has occurred when exploring the proximal portion of the supraspinatus muscle or the lateral extent of the paraspinal muscles in the cervical area in a thin individual. The abdominal muscles should also be explored extraordinarily carefully so that the peritoneal cavity is not compromised. In the abdominal muscle it is well to insert the needle parallel to the skin into the muscle, rather than at a right angle.

The serratus anterior is easily explored in the midaxillary line. Because its attachments are on the rib, fingers can be placed in the in-

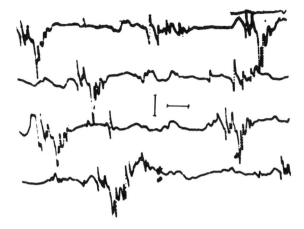

Figure 1.20. Complex motor unit potentials recorded in convalescent Guillain-Barré Syndrome (S/P 5 MO.) Monopolar needle electrode in V. med. (Caliber: 10 msec, 200 µV.)

tercostal space above and below a rib and the needle inserted in between. This is also the proper site to place a surface electrode for recording the compound muscle action potential of the serratus anterior.

The external anal sphincter is skeletal muscle and can be explored easily with a needle. It is difficult to get it to relax, however; in fact there is usually activity present, so more important diagnostically is the presence of a full recruitment pattern or whether fibrillation potentials and positive waves are easily seen, particularly if there is substantial compromise to the pudendal nerve or the roots (S3 and S4) that innervate that muscle.

Extrinsic Eye Muscles

The inferior oblique muscle is explored without going through the conjunctiva because it is accessible in the inferior medial aspect of the orbit through the skin. This would be a useful muscle in ocular paresis of various types.

GENERAL COMMENTS

The needle examination can be better accomplished with a monopolar electrode because it has been shown that the area of recording of a monopolar needle is about twice that of the coaxial needle. Furthermore, because of the dimensions and configuration of the monopolar needle electrode, it has been experimentally and clinically shown to record more profuse positive waves and at an earlier time than a

Table 1.1. Normal Amplitudes of MUP 1st Recruited/Monopolar Electrode

Muscle	Microvolts
Pect. maj.	429 ± 12
Biceps br.	490 ± 11
Glut. max.	533 ± 17
Abd. dig.	926 ± 63
Gastroc.	1133 ± 34
Triceps br.	1157 ± 45
Quads. fem.	1217 ± 43

coaxial needle (if disease or injury is present). Theoretically this difference could be explained by the beveled tip of a coaxial needle that records only a hemispheric field. Furthermore, the advancing tip of the coaxial needle is the barrel (i.e., reference), rather than the recording electrode, and thus the positive wave would be recorded as an initial negative deflection with a subsequent low amplitude, long duration positive deflection and may not be recognized as a positive wave. It is generally believed that the monopolar needle is less painful; however, it does have the disadvantage of insulation retraction at the tip with a reduction in the amplitude of the motor unit potential. This requires frequent needle electrode inspection.

The time and extent of the needle examination can be minimized with a careful and detailed planning of the electromyogram. This is particularly true in children and apprehensive patients. However, if the examination is explained carefully, the amount of discomfort associated with monopolar needle electromyography is sufficiently minimal to enable the electromyographer to complete the examination in most instances.

References

1. Bailey J, et al: A clinical evaluation of electromyography of the anal sphincter. *Arch Phys Med Rehabil* 51:403, 1970.
2. Buchtal F, et al: Motor unit territory in different human muscles. *Acta Physiol Scand* 45:72, 1959.
3. Buchtal F, Pinelli P: Action potentials in muscular atrophy of neurogenic origin. *Neurology* 3:591–603, 1953.
4. Denny-Brown D: Interpretation of the electromyogram. *Arch Neurol Psychiatr* 61:99, 1949.
5. Jensan S F: Spontaneous electrical activity in denervated extraocular muscles. *Acta Ophthalmol* 50:827, 1972.
6. Johnson E, et al: Use of electrodiagnostic examination in a university hospital. *Arch Phys Med Rehabil* 46:1965.
7. Johnson E, et al: EMG abnormalities after intramuscular injections. *Arch Phys Med Rehabil* 52:250, 1971.
8. Johnson E, et al: Sequence of electromyographic abnormalities in stroke syndrome. *Arch Phys Med Rehabil* 56:468, 1975.

9. Kimura J, et al: Reflex response of orbicularis oculi muscle to supraorbital nerve stimulation. *Arch Neurol* 21:193, 1969.
10. Kugelberg E: Electromyograms in muscular disorders. *J Neurol Neurosurg Psychiat* 10:122, 1947.
11. Kugelberg E, Cobb W: Repetitive discharges in human motor fibers during post schaemic state. *J Neurol Neurosurg Psychiat* 14:88, 1954.
12. Kugelberg E, Petersen I: "Insertional activity" in electromyography. *J Neurol Neurosurg Psychiat* 12:268–273, 1949.
13. Lambert E, McMorris R: Size of motor units potentials in neuromuscular disorders. *Fed Proc* 13:263, 1953.
14. Lambert E, et al: Studies on the origin of the positive wave in electromyography. *Newsletter Am Assoc EMG EDX* 3:3, 1957.
15. Landau W: The essential mechanism in myotonia: an electromyographic study. *Neurology* 2:369–388, 1952.
16. Lederman RJ, Wilbourn AJ: Brachial plexopathy: recurrent cancer or radiation? *Neurology* 34:1331–1335, 1984.
17. Mechler F: Changing electromyographic findings during the chronic course of polymyositis. *J Neurol Sci* 23:237–242, 1974.
18. McMorris R: Amplitudes and durations of 1st recruited motor unit potentials. Thesis, Mayo Foundation, Graduate Education, University of Minnesota, 1952.
19. Petajan J: Clinical electromyographic studies of diseases of the motor unit. *Electroencephalogr Clin Neurophysiol* 36:395, 1974.
20. Petajan J, Philip B: Frequency control of motor unit action potentials. *Electroencephalogr Clin Neurophysiol* 27:66, 1969.
21. Rosen J, et al: Electromyography in spinal cord injury. *Arch Phys Med Rehabil* 50:271, 1969.
22. Schwartz M, et al: The reinnervated motor unit in man. *J Neurolog Sci* 27:303, 1976.
23. Stohr M: Benign fibrillation potentials in normal muscle and their correlation with endplate and denervation potentials. *J Neurol Neurosurg* 40:765, 1977.
24. Taylor RG, Kewairamani LS, Fowler WM: Electromyographic findings in lower extremities of patients with high spinal cord injury. *Arch Phys Med Rehabil* 55:16–23, 1974.
25. Trontel J, Stalberg E: Bizarre repetitive discharges recorded with single fibre EMG. *J Neurol Neurosurg Psychiat* 46:310–316, 1983.
26. Wiechers D: Mechanically provoked insertional activity before and after nerve section in rats. *Arch Phys Med Rehabil* 58:402, 1977.
27. Wiechers DO, Johnson EW: Diffuse abnormal electromyographic insertional activity: a preliminary report. *Arch Phys Med Rehabil* 60:419–422, 1979.
28. Wiederholt W: "End-plate noise" in electromyography. *Neurology* 20:214, 1970.

2

Normal and Abnormal Motor Unit Potentials

DAVID O. WIECHERS

Normal Motor Unit

Skeletal muscles are divided into groups of fascicles that are separated by connective tissue. Each fascicle is comprised of individual muscle fibers that are 60–80 microns (μ) in diameter. Each of these muscle fibers is comprised of myofibrils that are the protein contractile elements—myosin and actin—over which physical movement occurs. Each muscle fiber has one endplate structure where the muscle fiber's membrane is chemically sensitive to acetylcholine. This endplate is the site of neural contact. Many muscle fibers are connected together by nerve twigs to a nerve trunk or axon that is 40–80 μ in diameter. These muscle fibers connected by one axon are rarely arranged side by side, but are usually greater than 300 μ apart. Each axon has a nerve cell body of approximately 20–80 μ in diameter located in the anterior horn of the spinal cord. These nerve cell bodies are called *motor neurons.* The motor neurons are divided into alpha and beta depending upon their size, with the alpha motor neuron being the larger in diameter.

The motor neuron with its axon and all of its connected muscle fibers is referred to as the *motor unit.* The exact number of muscle fibers per motor unit is currently unknown. Electrophysiologic recordings do demonstrate that the number varies from muscle to muscle, as well as within the same muscle. One way to determine the number of muscle fibers per motor unit is to count the number of motor neurons supplying a muscle and divide that number by an estimate of the total number of muscle fibers in the muscle. Studies using this technique reveal 110 muscle fibers per motor unit in the lumbricals and 1770 in the medial gastrocnemius (29).

Muscle fibers have been found to have different physiologic and biochemical characteristics. Most classification studies of muscle fibers

22

have been performed on animals and only to a limited extent on humans. The major physiologic classification has been based on the muscle fiber's contractile property or, more specifically, the time to peak tension in a twitch (7, 8, 9). Contraction studies done in humans demonstrate a bimodal distribution of time to peak tension of approximately 36 msec for fast twitch (FT) and 90 msec for slow twitch (ST).

The major determinant of the twitch properties of muscle is the rate at which myosin splits ATP. This ATPase activity of myosin is related to the presence of various forms of myosin or myosin isozymes (39, 40). These various isozymes are characterized by their loss of ATPase activity with changes in pH. Myosin from FT muscle is acid labile but alkaline stable. Myosin from ST muscles is acid stable but alkaline labile. Two classes of slow and three classes of fast ATP-splitting myosin have been identified. The muscle fiber usually contains either fast or slow myosin, but the proportion of different isozymes in the fast or slow class can vary.

Human biopsy materials are routinely preincubated at pH 9.4, 4.6, or 4.3 prior to ATPase staining (28). Preincubation at pH 9.4 results in a loss of stain to the ST whose myosin is alkaline labile. The FT muscle therefore stains darker. Preincubation in pH 4.3 results in loss of ATPase activity in the FT muscle fibers, and the ST fibers stain darker. Preincubation at pH 4.6 results in a subdivision of FT fibers into three groups based on their resistance to loss of ATPase activity with lower pH values (25). This histochemical ATPase staining technique separates ST and FT and reveals three subtypes of FT muscle.

The biochemical characteristics of FT and ST muscle fibers also differ. ST muscle is high in oxidative enzyme activity, whereas FT muscle is high in glycolytic enzyme activity. Quantification of mitochondrial enzyme activity can be used to differentiate three subtypes of FT fibers. Some FT muscle fibers are higher in oxidative enzyme activity and less glycolytic (FOG), whereas others are high in glycolytic (FG) activity. A third group is intermediate (FI). Whether these three subgroups of FT muscle fibers are related to differences in myosin isozymes and/or energy metabolism is not fully understood at this time. As would be expected from their metabolic enzyme concentration, ST muscle fibers are resistant to fatigue with repetitive firing as compared to FT. FOG muscle fibers are more fatigue resistant than FI. FG fibers, therefore, are the easiest to fatigue with repetitive discharge.

In routine medical practice the nonphysiologic classification of Type I for ST and Type II for FT is frequently utilized. Type IIA for FOG, Type IIB for FG, and Type IIC for FI are the designations used for the subgroups of FT muscle fibers.

All of the muscle fibers comprising one motor unit are of the same histochemical fiber type. Motor units can then be referred to as ST

(Type I) or FT (Type II). Fibers of a motor unit are distributed throughout a large area of the muscle and are rarely side by side. There is a central area of the motor unit where the density of fibers is greater (26, 63). Studies with a multielectrode by Buchthal demonstrate 15–30 motor units within a 5–10 mm^2 area of muscle (10, 12).

Under certain conditions, muscle fibers can change histochemical type. Reinnervation of deinnervated ST muscle fibers with axon sprouts from FT motor units results in a conversion of ST muscle fibers into FT (15, 43, 59). Exercise and electrical stimulation can also alter the metabolic properties of muscle. Electrical stimulation of a slow tonic nature to the axon or muscle fiber directly results in an increase in oxidative enzymes (50). In humans, it has not been possible to demonstrate a change from ST (Type I) to FT (Type II) with exercise or electric stimulation. However, change has been demonstrated within the subgroups of FT (Type II) fibers with exercise and electrical stimulation. Endurance exercise and low rates of stimulation result in a conversion of FG (Type IIB) to FOG (Type IIA).

The firing characteristics of FT and ST motor units are also different. Warmolts studied the firing characteristics of large reinnervated ST and FT motor units in neuropathic conditions (66). The ST motor units fired steadily and rhythmically at 6–10 Hz; the rate increased to a maximum of 18–20 Hz. They were also fatigue resistant. The FT motor units required a sudden or vigorous contraction for activation and discharged in brief bursts lasting 0.5–5.0 sec at 10–25 Hz with a maximum of 16–50 Hz.

Other studies demonstrated that ST motor units are capable of prolonged activity, producing ATP by the oxidative pathways of mitochondria. Slow twitch motor units develop approximately the same force per unit of cross-sectional area as do FT fibers (24). Therefore, FT motor units do not have to be recruited early to provide increased tension, and the oxidative capacity of FOG (Type IIA) is significantly lower than ST motor units.

The recruitment of motor units to perform a specific physiologic task is orderly, related to the level of tension demanded, and no doubt is controlled by the central nervous system. Motor unit recruitment is related to the size of the motor neuron (35, 36). Smaller motor neurons have a lower threshold of excitation and are activated first. They have smaller diameter axons, innervate fewer muscle fibers, and are resistant to fatigue. The recruitment of additional motor units proceeds in an orderly manner according to motor neuron size (20–23). The larger motor neurons have larger diameter axons and innervate a greater number of muscle fibers. They develop higher twitch tension and faster twitch contraction times. Larger motor units also fatigue more rapidly and are activated at higher strengths of contraction (30, 34, 52–55).

RECORDING THE MOTOR UNIT ACTION POTENTIALS

The recorded summated electrical depolarizations of the muscle fibers belonging to one motor neuron is the *motor unit action potential* (MUAP). The characteristics of the MUAP are dependent upon the number of action potentials generated by individual muscle fibers and their geometric arrangement, the volume-conduction properties of the muscle, and the type of electrode with its recording system. The MUAP is recorded routinely with monopolar or concentric electrodes. These intramuscular electrodes record the depolarization of only a few muscle fibers that comprise the whole motor unit. Because the monopolar and concentric electrodes record from less than 2 mm^2, they are recording the algebraic summation of mainly only 2 to 8 muscle fibers and, totally, fewer than 12 muscle fibers of the motor unit (64).

The depolarization of a single muscle fiber is a biphasic spike with an initial positive deflection having a duration of less than 1 msec. The amplitude of this extracellular single fiber action potential is increased by the square of the fiber diameter, and the amplitude is reduced exponentially by the distance of the recording electrode from the fiber (27, 31, 32). These single fiber recordings are made with special electrodes and recording equipment to be discussed later and in Chapter 10 on single fiber EMG. It is the summation, then, of these biphasic spikes and their geometric arrangement within the muscle volume conductor that determines the size and shape of the MUAP.

The type of electrode and the recording equipment has a direct effect on the recorded MUAP. In clinical electromyography there are basically two electrode types, monopolar and concentric. The monopolar electrode is a stainless steel wire coated with Teflon except for the tip, which has an exposed surface area of approximately 0.1 mm^2 (70). This electrode is used with a surface reference electrode of about 1 cm in diameter.

The concentric electrode was developed by Adrian and Bronk in 1929 (1). It is a platinum wire placed in the center of a needle. The wire is usually 0.1 mm in diameter, and the exposed tip is cut on a 15° angle that results in an elliptical surface area of 0.07 mm^2. The shaft of the needle or cannula becomes the reference electrode. The disadvantages of the concentric electrode, in addition to the pain of repetitive insertion, are that it has distinct directional properties and the cannula, which is also active, will affect the MUAP recording. The deeper the cannula is inserted, the less effect it will have on the recording. Because the concentric electrode is cut on a 15° angle it does not record from as many close fibers as the monopolar electrode, the pointed tip of which is the recording surface. As a result, the size of the MUAP recorded by the two electrodes is different.

The positive feature of the concentric electrode is that its recording

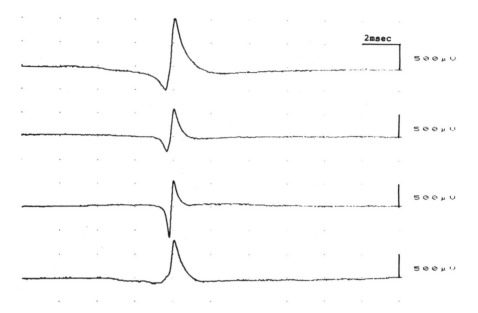

Figure 2.1. Normal low threshold MUAPs recorded from the biceps are usually of simple biphasic or triphasic shape. (Monopolar recording 20 Hz to 10 KHz.)

surface remains essentially unchanged, whereas the Teflon surface of the monopolar electrode does tend to peel back with repetitive use. Our studies reveal that the lead-off surface area is not as critical as once thought and that as many as 200 skin insertions can be made without any significant change in the electrode's lead-off surface. An increase in area from 0.10 mm^2 to 0.30 mm^2 was necessary to produce a significant change in the recorded MUAP duration (69). By the time such an increase occurs, the actual recording surface has become obviously visible to the naked eye, and skin insertion of the electrode becomes difficult.

The normal MUAP is the algebraic summation of the individual single muscle fiber action potentials and is usually triphasic when recorded with a monopolar or concentric needle electrode (Figs. 2.1 and 2.2). The initial positive deflection or the initial portion of the MUAP is a volume-conducted wave generated by the approach of the action potential to the recording electrode. This initial wave positivity is only seen when the recording electrode is away from the endplate zone (11, 48). The duration of this initial positive deflection is dependent upon the distance of the recording electrode from the endplate zone. The main spike is the algebraic summation of the muscle fiber action potentials as they pass the recording electrode. The terminal portion or

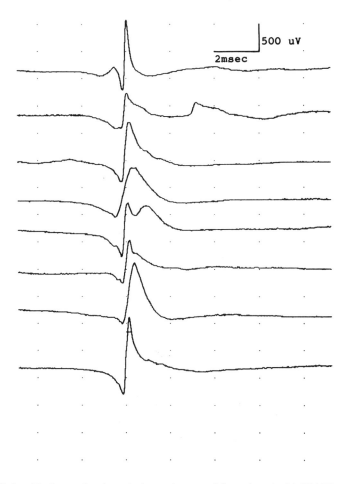

Figure 2.2. Various sized and shaped normal low threshold MUAPs recorded from biceps. Note the normally occurring late component in the second recording. (Monopolar recording 20 Hz to 10 KHz.)

the return to the baseline is the recording of the action potential moving away from the electrode and is analogous to the initial positive deflection. No terminal portion is seen with the recording electrode at the tendon (44).

In about 3–10% of normal MUAPs, potentials that have the characteristics of single fiber discharges are seen occurring several milliseconds later and are time-locked to the main MUAP. They are more commonly seen in reinnervation or other pathologic conditions and are referred to as parasites, satellites, or, more appropriately, late components (18, 47).

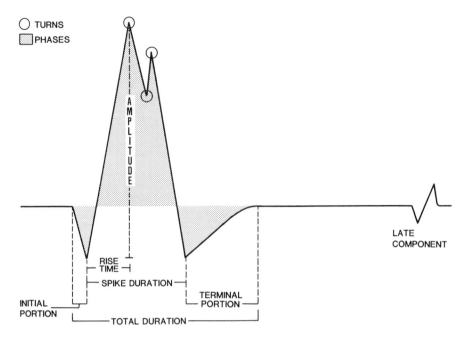

Figure 2.3. MUAP components and parameters.

MUAP PARAMETERS

The extensive work of Buchthal established the three basic MUAP parameters of total duration, amplitude, and number of phases. In the past decade, the parameters of spike duration and stability were added (6, 51, 68). MUAP parameters can be measured only after the electrode has been manipulated to the electrical center of the motor unit where the amplitude is maximized and the rise time minimized (Fig. 2.3). The *rise time* of the MUAP is the shortest interval from the nadir of the initial positive phase to the peak of the negative phase. It is used to determine if a MUAP is acceptable for inclusion in analysis. Rise time reflects the distance that the recording electrode is from the electrical center of the MUAP. The rise time should be 100–300 microsec, but definitely less than 500 microsec.

Total Duration

Total duration is defined as the initial deviation from the baseline to the return to the baseline. From multielectrode studies the duration seems to be dependent upon the distribution or spread of the endplate zone (4, 12). Computer-simulated studies seem to demonstrate that the number of muscle fibers in the motor unit may also be responsible for the total duration (2). Total duration is very dependent on the amplification, gain, filter, and whether or not the units are averaged. To date, no agreement has been reached among electromyographers as to whether to include late components within the total duration or simply to note their presence.

Spike Duration

Spike duration or the central spiky component is the time from the onset of the initial negative spike to the last most positive directed spike. Jasper and Ballem felt that spike duration was a measure of the degree of synchronization of the individual muscle fiber potentials (42). They felt this spike part should be of greater value than the total duration or the portions of the MUAP related to the conduction to and away from the electrode. A new interest in spike duration has surfaced in the past several years. This is due to the application of the computer to neurophysiology and the ease with which spike duration can be calculated. Unlike spike duration, the calculation of total duration varies considerably, depending on the electromyographer's determination of MUAP onset and return to baseline. No doubt computer analysis of MUAPs in the near future will help determine the value of spike duration in comparison to total duration.

Amplitude

The amplitude is the maximum voltage as measured peak to peak. Amplitude is determined by the density of muscle fibers, their diameters, and how synchronously they discharge or how close together are their endplates (13). Amplitude varies greatly in normal muscles. The main spike component of the MUAP is probably derived from 2–8 single muscle fibers and certainly fewer than 12 (64).

Phases

Motor units are usually biphasic (recorded at the endplate zone) or triphasic (recorded away from the endplate zone). The total number of phases is determined by adding one to the number of baseline crosses. A MUAP is considered polyphasic if it has greater than four phases. Normally there is a low percentage of polyphasic MUAPs in a muscle, but this is very dependent on physiologic and physical factors, to be discussed later. Frequently, the MUAPs have a sawtooth-like pattern where there are many changes of direction or "turns," but not actual baseline crosses. These potentials are referred to as *serrated MUAPs* and, as are polyphasics, are measurements of the synchronicity of the muscle fibers discharging. The percentage of motor units with polyphasic shapes should be reported for each muscle.

Stability

Motor unit stability is a parameter that has developed from the use of single fiber EMG (68). MUAP size and shape should be stable with repetitive discharge. Instability or variability of the motor unit size and shape (assuming the electrode is held perfectly still) is a result of impulse transmission problems in the terminal axon, across the neuromuscular junction, or with propagation down the muscle fiber membrane. As with polyphasic potentials, the percentage of MUAPs that are unstable is reported for each muscle.

PHYSIOLOGIC FACTORS AFFECTING MUAP

The physiologic factors that affect MUAP recordings include age, temperature, specific muscle, and strength of contraction (14).

Age

The total duration of MUAP increases rapidly from birth until the age of 15–20. The total duration then seems to remain essentially unchanged until the sixth to seventh decade and then increases to a milder degree. Amplitude, as does duration, increases rapidly through the growth period and then remains essentially unchanged until later years. The percentage of polyphasic MUAPs increases in older age groups (60).

Temperature

Intramuscular temperature greatly affects the MUAP parameters. Duration is increased as temperature decreases. At 30°C there is about a 10% per degree increase in duration when compared to duration at 37°C. The amplitude falls 2–5% per degree. The percentage of polyphasic potentials increases from 3% at 37°C to 10–15% at 30°C (14).

Muscle

MUAP parameters also vary greatly from muscle to muscle. Duration and amplitudes are reduced for facial and laryngeal muscles when compared to limb muscles (6, 42).

Strength of Contraction

First recruited MUAPs have lower amplitudes than second and third recruited potentials. Because it is difficult to isolate high threshold MUAPs from the interference pattern, it is difficult to state if their duration is increased. Theoretically, it would be expected to increase because higher threshold motor units have a greater number of muscle fibers (36).

Table 2.1. Biceps Brachii (Low Threshold MUAP)

	Amplitude	Duration	Polyphasics
Concentric (Buchthal) 2–10 KHz	μV 180 (120–390)	msec 10.3	% < 12%
Monopolar (Wiechers') 20–10 KHz	689 ± 133	4.3 ± 0.6	< 14 ± 7%

PHYSICAL FACTORS AFFECTING MUAP

With today's microprocessor-based digital equipment and the initial development of industry standards, the main physical factors affecting the MUAP are related to the selection of frequency response and electrode type by the electromyographers (11).

Frequency Response

The greatest amount of quantitative data for MUAP parameters has been produced by the Buchthal laboratory at Rigs Hospital in Copenhagen over a 25-year period. These data were obtained with concentric electrodes, recorded with a frequency response of 2 Hz to 10 kHz, with skin surface temperature maintained at 36–38°C and at weak voluntary contraction. The monopolar electrode has been more popular because of its painlessness with multiple insertions into muscles in a search for the presence of positive sharp waves and fibrillation potentials. If, however, a low frequency filter of 2 Hz is employed, the amplifier is blocked with electrode insertion. In routine clinical settings, the low frequency filter is set at 20 Hz and in some centers at 32 Hz. This raising of the low frequency in routine clinical practice greatly changes the motor unit parameters as established by the Buchthal laboratory. The slow return to the baseline of the terminal portion of the MUAP is frequently converted into another phase, and the percentage of normally occurring polyphasic potentials is increased. The total duration of the MUAP is reduced by raising the low frequency response.

Electrodes

The recording characteristics of the monopolar and concentric electrodes are different primarily due to the directional properties of the concentric electrode and the cancelling effect of the active cannula reference. The MUAP parameters are also different for monopolar and concentric electrodes. (See Table 2.1 data for 20–30 year olds.) Normal MUAP parameters must be developed for each laboratory based upon the electrodes and equipment used, the recording technique employed, and the patient population.

RECRUITMENT OF MUAPS

There is an orderly recruitment of MUAPs. First recruited motor units begin to fire at 4–6 per second. As the strength of contraction increases, the first recruited motor units increase in their rate of firing. When they reach a firing rate of 6–10 Hz a second motor unit is then recruited. The onset frequency of this second recruited MUAP is usually higher than that of the first recruited MUAP. The time between discharges of the first recruited MUAP when the second recruited MUAP is activated is referred to as the *recruitment interval* of the second recruited MUAP (56) (see Chapter 1). Likewise, as the strength of contraction increases, the rate of fire of the second recruited MUAP increases and then a third MUAP is activated. Usually four to five MUAPs can be followed and recruitment intervals calculated before the oscilloscope screen is saturated with MUAPs. The second recruited motor unit should be activated long before the first recruited motor unit reaches a rate of 15 Hz. The oscilloscope screen is normally filled when high threshold motor units are recruited. As a result, currently only the parameter of amplitude can be applied to high threshold MUAPs. Determining if the number of MUAPs recruited per strength of contraction is normal, increased, or reduced is, in many instances, the most difficult part of the EMG exam. This determination is based on visual and auditory impressions developed over years of experience.

QUANTITATIVE MUAP ANALYSIS

In routine clinical practice utilizing a trigger-and-delay device, the electromyographer can repetitively insert and manipulate the electrode to examine quickly 20–30 first recruited or low threshold MUAPs in each muscle. In most cases, abnormalities in MUAP parameters can be easily seen. This "impressionistic" technique is adequate for most clinical settings. On occasion questions arise as to the presence of subtle abnormalities that suggest neuropathy and myopathy. With such questions, quantitative analysis of MUAPs may be helpful. For statistically significant analysis, at least 20 MUAPs are recorded and the MUAP parameters are measured. Before a MUAP is accepted for analysis, the electrode is manipulated into the electrical center of the motor unit where the amplitude of the major spike is maximized and the rise time is minimized to less than 500 microsec. To avoid recording the MUAPs from different areas of the same anatomic motor unit usually less than five MUAPs are recorded from the same skin insertion.

Once the 20 MUAPs have been recorded, means for each parameter are calculated and compared to normative data. Each electromyographer or laboratory should have normal MUAP parameters established. The normative data of another laboratory can only be used if similar electrode, equipment, and recording techniques that are used by that laboratory are employed.

AUTOMATED ANALYSIS

Although quantitative analysis gives reproducible data, it is extremely time consuming to record MUAPs on paper and to make measurements of MUAP parameters by hand. This is especially true when several muscles per patient need evaluation. With advances in computer technology, automated analysis is the logical means to provide rapid quantitative analysis. Several EMG manufacturers are currently developing such analysis programs. The goal appears to be to provide an analysis of 20 motor units in less than 3 minutes per muscle or the time usually required to employ the "impressionistic" visual inspection method. Many automated methods have already been tried, but most are still too time consuming to aid the clinical electromyographer. One major difficulty is MUAP selection. Some methods use a simple averaging of three to eight discharges of the same MUAP before analysis. Other methods utilize a pattern recognition or template method that accepts MUAPs for analysis when their shape reappears repetitively. Another major difficulty in automated analysis is establishing standards that most electromyographers will accept to determine the onset and return of the motor units to the baseline. It seems only a matter of time until several good computer analysis programs are developed to provide the clinical electromyographer with a rapid, reliable, quantitative analysis of MUAPs.

Abnormal Motor Unit

Pathologic abnormalities that affect and alter the normal physiology of the motor unit will change the MUAP parameters. Which parameters and to what degree they are altered give clues to the site and extent of pathologic compromise within the motor unit. The five sites of motor unit compromises that can be determined by EMG are at the motor neuron, the axon, the terminal axon, the neuromuscular junction, and the muscle fiber.

MOTOR NEURON COMPROMISE

Compromise of the motor neuron can result in a loss or reduction of recruitment of MUAPs with increasing strength of contraction. Fasciculation potentials can be recorded when motor neurons are diseased or injured. Although fasciculation potentials are not pathognomonic of disorders affecting the motor neuron, they are so common in amyotrophic lateral sclerosis that, if they are not present, the diagnosis is suspect. A mild reduction in recruitment can be difficult to identify on EMG recordings during muscle contraction. The presence, however, of positive sharp waves and fibrillation potentials, when accompanied by fasciculation potentials, 3 weeks after the loss of a motor neuron may be the earliest findings in developing motor neuron disease.

Deinnervated and now fibrillating muscle fibers, in most instances, will result in the process of reinnervation by terminal axon sprouting or "collateral" reinnervation in the surviving motor units (71). Motor units, the terminal axons of which are in the vicinity of orphaned or fibrillating muscle fibers, will sprout a new axon twig. This axon sprout will grow toward the fibrillating muscle fiber. Wherever the axon sprout comes in contact with the fibillating fiber the new endplate will form. There seems to be a limit to the number of orphaned muscle fibers that a surviving motor unit can reinnervate, but the exact number is not known in humans. Under ideal condition it takes at least 3 weeks for an axon sprout to grow and make initial contact with a deinnervated muscle fiber (33).

Initially, the budding site of the new axon sprout will only be able to transmit intermittently the wave of depolarization out into the new sprout as the impulse passes by travelling down the rescuing motor unit. As a result, the reinnervated muscle fiber frequently does not receive a depolarization impulse every time the motor neuron fires. The axon sprout is initially unmyelinated, and the propagation of the impulse is slowed. The newly formed neuromuscular junction is immature, and failures and delays in transmission occur. After approximately 3-6 months, the impulse transmission to the rescued muscle fiber has matured (33). The end result of the process of reinnervation by terminal axon sprouting is that the motor unit now has an increased number of muscle fibers than it had originally. The geographical area of the motor unit may not necessarily be enlarged, but the number of fibers in one area belonging to the same motor unit, or the fiber density, is increased.

A change in MUAP parameters can be recorded during the process of reinnervation. With the early capture of orphaned muscle fibers, the MUAP will be a composite of the algebraic summation of the orig-

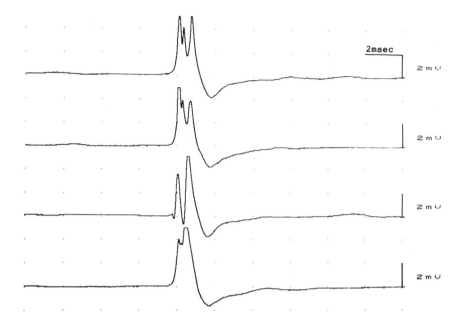

Figure 2.4. Marked variability of MUAP shape with repetitive discharge as seen early in the course of reinnervation. (Monopolar recording, 20 Hz to 10 KHz.)

inal biphasic spikes plus the biphasic spikes of the muscle fibers just rescued. The resultant MUAP's increased duration, amplitude, and number of phases are dependent on several factors. These include the number, geographic arrangement, and the physiologic functioning of the reinnervation structures of those fibers added to the original motor unit within the recording area of the electrode. Early during the rein- nervation process while the anatomic reinnervation structures are im- mature, the MUAP size and shape are variable or unstable with repetitive discharge (Fig. 2.4) (68). The main body of the MUAP, es- pecially its late components comprised of several or an individual mus- cle fiber on one axon sprout, demonstrates great variability in its appearance over time (*jitter,* see Chapter 10 on single fiber EMG) and frequently disappears with repetitive firing (*blocking*) of the motor unit (Fig. 2.5). With maturation of the reinnervation structures, the MUAP duration appears to decrease and the amplitude increases as the depolarization of the reinnervated fibers becomes more synchronous. The motor unit variability in size and shape generally resolves over a period of 3–6 months and is usually stable by 1 year in muscles that regain normal or near-normal strength. After this period, late components or those portions of the MUAP greater than 4 msec from the main MUAP components may have very mild variability or increased jitter but no blocking due to variations in muscle fiber propagation velocity. How long the MUAP remains unstable in a very weak muscle where there are more fibrillating fibers than can be reinnervated remains unknown. Muscle fiber propagation velocity can vary and is affected by the timing sequence of previous depolarizations when the motor unit is not firing at a steady rate. This changing muscle fiber propagation velocity is referred to as the velocity recovery function of muscle or the VRF (62).

With progressive motor neuron loss, the process of reinnervation by terminal axon sprouting continues until there are not enough remaining motor units to rescue all of the deinnervated muscle fibers. The loss of motor units results in an alteration of the normal systematic recruitment of motor units of increasing size with increasing strength of contraction. The loss of motor units and subsequent reinnervation is a focal process and does not necessarily affect the muscle in a homogeneous pattern. In some areas of muscle there can be only a few surviving motor units and the first recruited MUAPs can be extremely large, whereas in other areas the first recruited MUAP may be normal in amplitude. This increase in size of the first recruited MUAP may be the result of reinnervation by terminal axon sprouting or the loss of all the lower threshold motor units and the availability of only large, high threshold motor units for recruitment.

Motor nerve conduction studies are dependent upon the degree of involvement of the muscle used as the recording site. The motor nerve conduction velocity will remain normal until the faster conducting motor units are lost. Changes in the compound muscle action potential's amplitude, duration, shape, or area may be recorded long before the velocity is reduced to below normal levels. If only the motor neuron is affected by the disease process, the sensory conduction studies will remain normal.

MUSCLE FIBER COMPROMISE

Disorders affecting the muscle fiber directly are referred to as myopathies. Myopathies include not only the classical muscular dystrophies and inflammatory muscle diseases but also the congenital or structural abnormalities of muscle fibers, the mitochondrial myopathies, and the myopathies associated with systemic disease. Patients

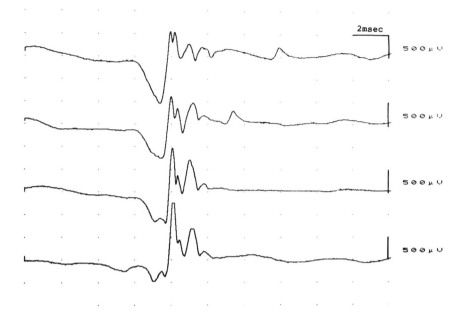

Figure 2.5. MUAP instability in an ALS patient demonstrating ongoing reinnervation. Note the last component, which "blocks" in the third and fourth discharge. (Monopolar recording, 20 Hz to 10 KHz.)

with Duchenne muscular dystrophy have been studied and were found to have MUAPs of low amplitude, short duration, and an increased percentage of polyphasic shapes (45, 46, 57). Subsequently, these electrical abnormalities were felt to be diagnostic of all myopathies in general. We now know that these same MUAP characteristics also occur in disorders of the terminal axon or the neuromuscular junction (58, 67).

Classically, muscular dystrophies result in a progressive loss of individual muscle fibers from a motor unit. As the disease progresses, some MUAPs are reduced to only one or two muscle fibers. Ultimately, an entire motor unit is lost. In end-stage muscle disease, there is a marked loss or dropout of MUAPs on maximal contraction, and large areas of muscle are not functional and are electrically silent (37).

The loss of individual muscle fibers from a motor unit alters the recorded MUAP. The normal triphasic MUAP is the algebraic summation of about two to eight single muscle fibers (64). The loss of an individual muscle fiber's depolarizations results in a summated MUAP of lower amplitude and shorter duration (Fig. 2.6). The algebraic summation of

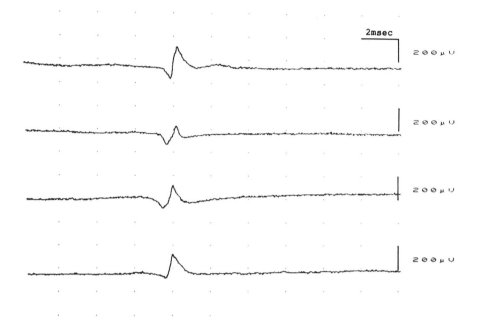

Figure 2.6. Four different low amplitude, short duration, simple shaped MUAPs from a 3-year-old boy with Duchenne dystrophy. (Monopolar recording, 20 Hz to 10 KHz.)

the depolarization of the remaining muscle fibers is no longer a smooth triphasic wave. Frequently, the potential is polyphasic and is composed of three or four biphasic spikes, each having characteristics of isolated single fiber discharges compressed together (Fig. 2.7). A loss of muscle fibers per motor unit implies that the motor unit is unable to produce normal tension with contraction. Additional motor units are now needed more rapidly to provide increasing strength of contraction. The rapid increase in number of motor units recruited per strength of contraction and an increased number of polyphasic MUAPs of low amplitude and short duration have been the characteristic EMG finding of myopathies.

The development of analog to digital conversion technology has made it possible to trigger electrically and delay in time a MUAP and to analyze its parameters. Many polyphasic MUAPs in muscular dystrophies have been found to be of normal or long duration, contrary to our previous understanding. Some MUAPs have late components that occur 10–40 msec after the main MUAP component and were, no doubt, previously felt to have been an entirely different MUAP (19). These

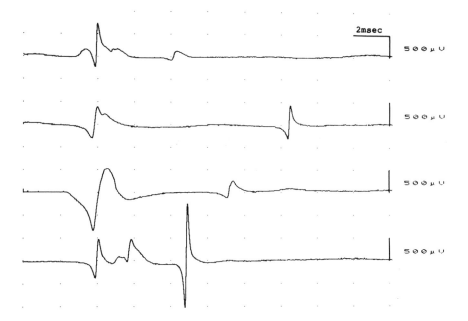

Figure 2.7. Four different MUAPs of various durations recorded from the biceps of a 42-year-old man with limb-girdle dystrophy. (Monopolar recording, 20 Hz to 10 KHz.)

long duration MUAPs are most commonly seen in Duchenne, Becker, and limb-girdle muscular dystrophies, but vary with the course of the disease (Fig. 2.8). Several of these MUAPs of long duration, which are composed of several individual components, can provide what seems to be full recruitment, despite an overall reduced number of MUAPs recruited. This may explain why in some weak muscles there seems to be an increased number of motor units recruited at low strengths of contraction, whereas at higher strengths of contraction there is an obvious loss of motor units. Similarly, single fiber EMG (SFEMG) demonstrates an increase in fiber density in Duchenne, Becker, and limb-girdle dystrophies (see Chapter 10). What possibilities exist to explain these long duration, polyphasic MUAPs in some myopathies? Certainly, the atrophy and loss of intermingling muscle fibers will result in a shrinkage of the remaining functional motor unit territory. However, this compacting of the motor unit territory alone is not enough to explain some of the 40–50 msec duration MUAPs recorded in some dystrophies.

Anatomically, myopathies are characterized by a variation in fiber

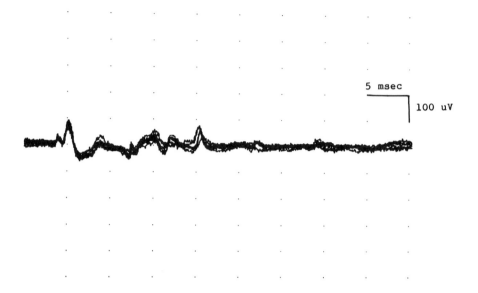

Figure 2.8. Six superimposed discharges of a MUAP from a teenaged boy with Becker dystrophy demonstrating long duration late components. (Monopolar recording, 20 Hz to 10 KHz.)

size (25). SFEMG demonstrates that one motor unit may contain fibers of various sizes in myopathies. In muscular dystrophy, the individual muscle fiber's ability to propagate the wave of depolarization down its membrane is slowed. This slowing is probably a result of the disease's effect on the muscle fiber membrane, but is amplified in some fibers of abnormally small diameter. Myopathic muscle fibers' propagation velocity is further compromised by the effect of time on the membrane since the previous depolarization or the VRF (62). These factors slowing individual muscle fiber propagation tend to increase the duration of the MUAP.

Fiber splitting is a common finding on biopsy in myopathies. This phenomenon explains an increase in fiber density and MUAP duration. Isolated areas of focal muscle cell necrosis result in a deinnervated segment of a muscle fiber. Terminal axon sprouting to these deinnervated segments, as well as to regenerating muscle fibers, causes focal areas of reinnervated muscle of a high fiber density and increased MUAP duration. Another factor explaining this seemingly surprising finding of increased MUAP duration may be the recruitment of adjacent muscle fibers by ephaptic transmission (38). The increase in fiber density and long duration MUAPs in some myopathies does not mean that the anatomic motor unit contains a greater number of muscle fibers than normal. However, it implies that focal architectural rearrangement has occurred in some areas of the motor unit while there is a loss of muscle fibers in other areas.

The MUAPs in myopathies vary with the type and state of the disease process. The MUAPs in a myopathy can be of short, normal, or long duration; low or normal amplitude; and demonstrate an increase in polyphasic shapes. These motor units tend to be relatively stable on repetitive firing when recorded with monopolar or concentric electrodes. SFEMG recordings demonstrate a mild increase in jitter in some recordings, which is probably related to these same factors surrounding the presence of long duration MUAPs (see Chapter 10).

COMPROMISE TO THE AXON

Motor unit axons are contained within large conduits known as peripheral nerves. There they travel with sensory fibers, sympathetic fibers, and the fibers controlling muscle spindle function. The axon of the motor unit is most commonly compromised by trauma, but also may be compromised by acquired or toxic or inherited disorders. In almost all of these conditions, the motor axon is not preferentially affected, and sensory as well as motor symptoms are present. Compromise to the axon has been classically divided into axonal (direct involvement of the nerve filament) or segmental demyelination (primary involvement of the Schwann cell and the axon's supportive structures). However, in later stages of demyelination, there is axon loss, and in some conditions the pathology is mixed. Nerve conduction techniques can usually be helpful in determining whether the disorder is axonal with normal or mild nerve conduction slowing of less than 70%, or demyelinating with slowing usually of 30–40% across the affected segments. Presence of conduction block and abnormalities of the evoked and compound muscle action potential can also be helpful and are discussed in the chapter on peripheral neuropathies.

The major difficulty in understanding the pathophysiology of these conditions affecting the axon is that they do not affect every axon simultaneously to the same degree. This is especially true in traumatic compromise where some axons may be destroyed with Wallerian degeneration following, some may be mildly damaged and ultimately recover, other axons remain intact anatomically but cease physiologic functioning, and still others simply escape compromise.

In axonal compromise and some cases of neurapraxia lasting longer than 14 days, positive sharp waves and fibrillations potentials are recorded (65). In conditions of segmental demyelination where the axon degeneration occurs, positive sharp waves and fibrillation potentials are also present. EMG reveals motor unit loss and MUAP parameter changes produced by reinnervation by terminal axon sprouting, as discussed previously under motor neuron disease.

Under certain conditions, the terminal axon may be the first to be affected. This is the so-called dying-back neuropathy that has been demonstrated for experimental acrylamide neuropathy (61), acute intermittent porphyria (17), triorthorocresyl phosphate neuropathy (16), and theorized for other neuropathies. If conduction block begins in the terminal axon, then early on most affected MUAPs will have parameter changes consistent with muscle fiber loss per motor unit. Under this condition, it may then be difficult early in the course of the neuropathy to differentiate these MUAP abnormalities from those seen in a myopathy (67).

What happens, months later, when the traumatically compromised axon finally grows back to its previously orphaned muscle? Does it reacquire its previously orphaned muscle fibers from the motor units that had reinnervated them? Studies in animals do seem to show that this does, indeed, happen (3, 41, 49). If this phenomenon does occur in humans, one could expect a second period of several months duration during which the MUAP of the returning motor unit would be unstable with repetitive discharge. Some of the previously large MUAPs would then theoretically revert to more normal size.

COMPROMISE TO THE NEUROMUSCULAR JUNCTION

Disorders affecting the production, release, or uptake of acetylcholine have an effect on the time delay to reach threshold at the muscle endplate. As a result, some muscle fibers of a motor unit fire asynchronously. This delayed discharge of an individual muscle can vary greatly with each depolarization of its nerve terminal. The position of this single muscle fiber's depolarization within the normal triphasic summated MUAP can vary with each consecutive discharge of the motor unit. If several muscle fibers of the same motor unit are also affected, great changes in the size and shape of each MUAP can occur with repetitive firing.

When this delay becomes too great (approximately 50 microsec), transmission to the muscle fiber will fail and the summated MUAP will be absent one fiber, further affecting its size and shape. This variability in neuromuscular transmission and blocking can vary with the rate of discharge. As in myasthenia gravis, at high firing rates abnormalities are exacerbated, whereas at very low rates of fire, the abnormalities may be minimal.

When the disease severely affects many muscle fibers of the same motor unit, only a few fibers may depolarize with each motor neuron discharge. The resulting MUAP parameters reveal a reduced number of muscle fibers per motor unit. The MUAP can now have the same characteristics as those seen in myopathies, although instability or variability of size and shape can be seen with repetitive discharge (58). It is possible that the motor endplate degenerates to such a degree that it is nonfunctional and the muscle fiber falls away. This may explain why fibrillation potentials are occasionally seen in myasthenia gravis.

SUMMARY

Abnormalities of the MUAP are dependent not only on the disease process but also on the location of the compromise. Many disorders that affect the motor unit are progressive. Likewise, changes in the MUAP parameters will also occur during the course of the disorder to reflect the underlying pathophysiology. Each clinical EMG study is only a snapshot during the course of the disease process. Repeated studies are most likely necessary for an accurate diagnosis and an appropriate course of management and rehabilitation.

References

1. Adrian E, Bronk D: The discharge of impulses in motor nerve fibers. II. The frequency of discharge in reflex and voluntary contraction. *J Physiol* 67:119, 1929.
2. Andreassen S, Jorgensen N: A model for the motor unit potential. *Electroenceph Clin Neurophysiol* 52:S116, 1981.
3. Brown H: Sprouting of motor nerves in adult muscles: a recapitulation of ontogeny. *Trends Neurosci* 7:10, 1984.
4. Buchthal F: The general concept of the motor unit. In Adams R, Eaton L, Shy G (eds): *Neuromuscular Disorders*. Baltimore, Williams & Williams, 1960.
5. Buchthal F: Diagnostic significance of the myopathic EMG. In Rowland (ed): *Pathogenesis of Human Muscular Dystrophies*. Amsterdam, Excerpta Medica 1977, p 404.
6. Buchthal F, Rosenfalck P: Action potential parameters in different human muscles. *Acta Psychiat Scand* 30:125, 1955.
7. Buchthal F, Schmalbruch H: Spectrum of contraction times of different fiber bundles in the brachial biceps and triceps muscles of man. *Nature* (London) 22:89, 1969.
8. Buchthal F, Schmalbruch H: Contraction times and fiber types in intact human muscles. *Acta Physiol Scand* 79:435, 1970.
9. Buchthal F, Dahl K, Rosenfalck P: Rise time of spike potential in fast and slowly contracting muscles of man. *Acta Physiol Scand* 87:261, 1973.
10. Buchthal F, Ermind F, Rosenfalck P: Motor unit territory in different human muscles. *Acta Physiol Scand* 45:72, 1959.
11. Buchthal F, Guld C, Rosenfalck P: Action potential parameters in normal human muscle and their dependence on physical variables. *Acta Physiol Scand* 32:200, 1954.
12. Buchthal F, Guld C, Rosenfalck P: Multielectrode study of the territory of a motor unit. *Acta Physiol Scand* 39:83, 1957.
13. Buchthal F, Guld C, Rosenfalck P: Volume conduction of the spike of the motor unit potential investigated with a new type of multielectrode. *Acta Physiol Scand* 38:331, 1957.
14. Buchthal F, Pinelli P, Rosenfalck P: Action potential parameters in normal human muscle and their physiological determinants. *Acta Physiol Scand* 32:219, 1954.
15. Buller A, Eccles J, Eccles R: Interactions between mononeurons and muscles in

respect of the characteristic speeds of their responses. *J Physiol* (London) 150:417, 1960.

16. Cavanagh J: Peripheral nerve changes in ortho-cresyl phosphate poisoning in the cat. *J Path Bacterial* 87:365, 1964.

17. Cavanagh J, Mellick R: On the nature of the peripheral nerve lesions associated with acute intermittent porphyria. *J Neurol Neurosurg Psychiat* 28:320, 1965.

18. Desmedt J, Borenstein S: Collateral reinnervation of muscle fibers by motor axons of dystrophic motor units. *Nature* 246:500, 1973.

19. Desmedt J, Borenstein S: Regenerative phenomena in muscular dystrophy and polymyositis: an electromyographic study. In Milhort A (ed). *Exploratory Concepts in Muscular Dystrophy II* Excerpta Medica 333:555, 1974.

20. Desmedt J, Godaux E: Ballistic contractions in man: characteristic recruitment pattern of single motor units of the tibialis anterior muscle. *J Physiol* (London) 264:673, 1977.

21. Desmedt J, Godaux E: Fast motor units are not preferentially activated in rapid voluntary contractions in man. *Nature* (London) 267:717, 1977.

22. Desmedt J, Godaux E: Recruitment patterns of single motor units in the human masseter muscle during brisk jaw clenching. *Arch Oral Biol* 24:171, 1979.

23. Desmedt J, Godaux E: Voluntary motor commands in human ballistic movements. *Ann Neurol* 5:415, 1979.

24. Donaldson S, Bolitho S, Hermansen L: Differential, direct effects of H^+ and Ca^{2+} activated force of skinned fibers from soleus, cardiac and adductor magnus muscles of rabbits. *Pfleugers Arch* 376:55, 1978.

25. Dubowitz V, Brooke M: *Muscle Biopsy: A Modern Approach.* London, WB Saunders, 1973.

26. Edstrom L, Kugelberg E: Histochemical composition, distribution of fibers and fatigability of single motor units. *J Neurol Neurosurg Psychiat* 31:424, 1968.

27. Ekstedt J: Human single muscle fiber action potentials. *Acta Physiol Scand* 61 (suppl 226):1, 1964.

28. Engel WK: The essentiality of histo- and cytochemical studies of skeletal muscle in the investigation of neuromuscular disease. *Neurology* 12:778, 1962.

29. Feinstein B, Lindegard B, Nyman E, Wohlfart G: Morphologic studies of the motor units in normal human muscles. *Acta Anat* 23:127, 1955.

30. Freund H, Budingen H, Dietz V: Activity of single motor units from human forearm muscles during voluntary isometric contractions. *J Neurophysiol* 38:933, 1975.

31. Gath I, Stalberg E: The calculated radial decline of the extracellular action potential compared with in situ measurements in the human brachial biceps. *Electroenceph Clin Neurophysiol* 44:547, 1978.

32. Hakansson C: Action potentials recorded intra and extracellularly from isolated frog muscle fiber in Ringers solution and in air. *Acta Physiol Scand* 39:291, 1957.

33. Hakelius I, Stalberg E: Electromyographical studies of free autogenous muscle transplant in man. *Scand J Plast Reconstr Surg* 8:211, 1974.

34. Hannerz J: Discharge properties of motor units in relation to recruitment order in voluntary contraction. *Acta Physiol Scand* 91:374, 1974.

35. Henneman E, Clamann H, Gillies J, Skinner R: Rank order of motoneurons within a pool: law of combination. *J Neurophysiol* 37:1338, 1974.

36. Henneman E, Sumjen G, Carpenter D: Functional significance of cell size in spinal motoneurons. *J Neurophysiol* 28:560, 1965.

37. Hilton-Brown P, Stalberg E: Motor unit size in muscular dystrophy, a macro EMG and scanning EMG study. *J Neurol Neurosurg Psychiat* 46:996, 1983.

38. Hilton-Brown P, Stalberg E: The motor unit in muscular dystrophy, a single fiber EMG and scanning EMG study. *J Neurol Neurosurg Psychiat* 46:981, 1983.

39. Hoh J: Neural regulation of mammalian fast and slow muscle myosins: an electrophoretic analysis. *Biochemistry* 14:747, 1975.

40. Hoh J, McGrath P, White R: Electrophoretic analysis of multiple forms of myosin in fast-twitch and slow-twitch muscles of the chick. *Biochem J* 157:87, 1976.
41. Jansen J, Lomo J: Development of neuromuscular connections. *Trends Neurosci* 4:178, 1981.
42. Jasper H, Ballem G: Unipolar electromyograms of normal and deinnervated human muscle. *J Neurophysiol* 12:231, 1949.
43. Karpati G, Engel W: "Type grouping" in skeletal muscles after experimental reinnervation. *Neurology* 18:447, 1968.
44. Katz B, Miledi R: Propagation of electric activity in motor nerve terminals. *Proc Roy Soc* (Great Britain) 161:453, 1965.
45. Kugelberg E: Electromyography in muscular disorders. *J Neurol Neurosurg Psychiat* 10:122, 1947.
46. Kugelberg E: Electromyography in muscular dystrophies. *J Neurol Neurosurg Psychiat* 12:129, 1949.
47. Lang A, Partanen V: "Satellite potentials" and the duration of motor unit potentials in normal, neuropathic and myopathic muscles. *J Neurol Sci* 27:513, 1976.
48. Lang A, Tuomola H: The time parameters of motor unit potentials recorded with multi-electrodes and the summation technique. *Electromyogr Clin Neurophysiol* 14:513, 1974.
49. Lomo T: What controls the development of neuromuscular junctions? *Trends Neurosci* 3:126, 1980.
50. Lomo T, Westgaard R, Engebresten L: Different stimulation patterns affect contractive properties of deinnervated rat soleus muscle. In Pette D (ed): *Plasticity of Muscle.* New York, de Gruyter, 1980, p 297.
51. Melvin J, Wiechers D: Measurement of motor unit action potentials. *Arch PM&R* 57:325, 1976.
52. Milner-Brown H, Stein R, Lee R: Contractive and electrical properties of human motor units in neuropathies and motor neuron disease. *J Neurol Neurosurg Psychiat* 37:670, 1974.
53. Milner-Brown H, Stein R, Yemm R: Changes in firing rate of human motor units during linearly changing voluntary contractions. *J Physiol* (London) 230:317, 1973.
54. Milner-Brown H, Stein R, Yemm R: The contractive properties of human motor units during voluntary isometric contractions. *J Physiol* (London) 228:285, 1973.
55. Milner-Brown H, Stein R, Yemm R: The orderly recruitment of human motor units during voluntary isometric contractions. *J Physiol* (London) 230:359, 1977.
56. Petatan J: Clinical electromyographic studies of diseases of the motor unit. *Electroenceph Clin Neurophysiol* 36:395, 1974.
57. Pinelli P, Buchthal F: Muscle action potentials in myopathies with special regard to progressive muscular dystrophy. *Neurology* 3:347, 1952.
58. Pinelli P, Arrigo A, Moglia A: Myasthenic decrement and myasthenic myopathy. A study on the effects of thymectomy. *J Neurol Neurosurg Psychiat* 38:525, 1975.
59. Romanul F, Van DerMeulen J: Slow and fast muscles after cross innervation enzymatic and physiological changes. *Acta Neurol* 17:387, 1967.
60. Sacco G, Buchthal F, Rosenfalck P: Motor unit potentials and different ages. *Arch Neurol* 6:44, 1962.
61. Schaumburg H, Wisniewski H, Spencer P: Ultrastructural studies of the dying-back process. I. Peripheral nerve terminal and axon degeneration in systemic acrylamide intoxication. *J Neuropathol Exp Neurol* 33:260, 1974.
62. Stalberg E: Propagation velocity in human muscle fibers in situ. *Acta Physiol Scand* 70(suppl 287):1, 1966.
63. Stalberg E, Antoni L: Electrophysiological cross section of the motor unit. *J Neurol Neurosurg Psychiat* 43:469, 1980.
64. Thiele B, Boehle A: Anzhal der spike-komoponenten in motor-unit potential. *EEG and EMG* 9:125, 1978.

65. Trojaborg W: Early electrophysiologic changes in conduction block. *Muscle Nerve* 1:400, 1978.

66. Warmolts J, Engel W: Open biopsy electromyography. I. Correlation of motor unit behavior with histochemical muscle fiber type in human limb muscle. *Arch Neurol* 27:572, 1972.

67. Warmolts J, Mendell J: Open-biopsy electromyography. Direct correlation of a pattern of excessively recruited, pathologically small motor unit potentials with histologic evidence of neuropathy. *Arch Neurol* 36:406, 1979.

68. Wiechers D: Single fiber EMG with a standard monopolar electrode. *Arch Phys Med Rehabil* 66:47, 1985.

69. Wiechers D, Blood J: Monopolar electrodes: lead off surface versus motor unit characteristics. *Muscle Nerve* 3:185, 1980.

70. Wiechers D, Blood J, Stow R: EMG needle electrodes: electrical impedance. *Arch Phys Med Rehabil* 60:364, 1979.

71. Wohlfart G: Collateral regeneration from residual motor nerve fibers in amyotrophic lateral sclerosis. *Neurology* 7:124, 1957.

3

Motor Unit Potentials in Disease

DAVID O. WIECHERS

DISORDERS OF THE MOTOR NEURON

Motor neuropathies are a group of disorders that result primarily in degeneration of the anterior horn cells of the spinal cord. Such disorders can either be inherited or acquired. Motor neurons can also be compromised as the result of a vascular insult, infection, mechanical compression, or direct trauma. The EMG findings in all of these disorders affecting the motor neuron are essentially identical. There are no specific EMG findings or pathognomonic potentials that are diagnostic of any disorder affecting the motor neuron or anterior horn cell. The function of the EMG is to localize the site of pathology within the motor unit to the motor neuron; it is used in conjunction with other laboratory data to confirm the clinical diagnosis.

Those disorders of the motor neuron that are progressive have dynamic, ongoing EMG abnormalities. In these cases, EMG can be used to help determine the state and rate of progression of the disorder within a specific muscle. The extent of major motor unit loss in a muscle can be judged clinically by manual muscle testing. More subtle abnormalities of motor unit loss in a muscle can be determined by EMG changes in recruitment, nerve conduction, and the parameters of the compound muscle action potential. The rate of progression of the disorder in a muscle can be determined by the density of free fibrillating muscle fibers and the extent of ongoing reinnervation as analyzed by MUAP stability or single fiber EMG. Repeating EMG studies in a progressive disorder can give additional clues to the anticipated need for rehabilitative intervention with braces, hand splints, and respiratory assistive devices.

Disorders that clinically and physiologically affect motor neurons can be divided into two broad categories: those with motor neuron involvement only and those in which motor neuron involvement is part of a more generalized neurologic disturbance. Only those disorders affecting primarily the motor neuron are addressed here.

Motor Neuron Disease

Disorders primarily affecting motor neurons can be of a hereditary or sporadic nature. The most common disorder affecting primarily the motor neuron is amyotrophic lateral sclerosis (ALS), with its clinical variants of progressive bulbar palsy, progressive muscular atrophy, and primary lateral sclerosis (47, 87). The term "motor neuron disease" is gaining wide acceptance in place of ALS for describing only the clinical syndrome of asymmetrical, painless muscle atrophy and hyperreflexia, with adult onset and relentless progression.

The etiology of motor neuron disease remains unknown. A possible genetic transmission or common toxic origin has been postulated in an ALS-like syndrome that occurs with high frequency among Chamorro Indians on Guam (75, 88). A hereditary pattern of autosomal dominance is seen in 5–10% of all motor neuron disease patients. In this hereditary form there appears to be good penetrance, but the expression can vary greatly within the same family (46, 76). The presence of this inherited form of the disease raises the possibility of an enzyme defect as the etiology of this disorder. Intoxication by heavy metals and other organic compounds has been implicated, but never proven as the cause of the disease. A slow or latent virus, immunologic abnormalities directly affecting motor neurons, or acceleration of the aging process have all been suggested as possible etiologies (11). To date, however, attempts to find a virus have been unsuccessful (132). Others have suggested that the disease syndrome may be the result of multiple different causes that are entirely unrelated.

Motor neuron disease, which is not rare, occurs worldwide. The incidence of the disease is felt to be approximately 1/100,000 per year. The male-to-female ratio is approximately 2:1 (88). The disease is relatively rare before the age of 30, and the median age of onset is at 66 years (67).

Motor neuron disease, or ALS, is progressive and usually begins as a painless asymmetric weakness and atrophy occurring in either proximal or distal limb muscles or in the bulbar muscles. In some rare instances, the disease process may begin first with upper motor neuron symptoms. The disease progresses at a variable rate in various muscles. Symptomatic lower motor neuron involvement of the opposite extremity at the same spinal levels is common before the disease becomes generalized. In light of its painless nature, weeks to months often pass before the patient seeks medical attention. Fasciculations are frequent in affected muscles, but may range from being completely unnoticed by the patient to being of greater concern than the weakness itself.

Muscle cramps are also a frequent and often painful symptom and may be the reason the patient seeks medical assistance. The bulbar musculature may be involved early, resulting in dysarthric speech characterized by imprecise articulation and reduced ability to sustain phonation. Weakness of tongue and palate can result in problems of swallowing and eating. At this point, a feeding gastrostomy may be necessary and should be performed early before the patient is too weak to tolerate the surgery. At some point during the course of the disease, the pyramidal system becomes affected. The patient develops hyperflexia or spasticity. The Babinski reflex is frequently present, but may not be obtainable due to weakness that has progressed in the extensor hallucis longus and other foot musculature.

As atrophy progresses there is loss of weight. Fatigue increases steadily, and cold temperatures may reduce the patient's endurance. The patient does maintain bowel and bladder control. Eventually the muscles of respiration become involved, and associated respiratory problems are usually the cause of death.

Laboratory examinations, including a search for disorders known to produce such mimicking syndromes as heavy metal intoxication, CNS syphilis, diabetic amyotrophy, late effects of polio, postradiation myelitis, paraneoplastic and paraproteinemic syndromes, and spinal cord compression, are normal. Muscle enzyme levels, however, may be elevated in about half of the patients with motor neuron disease (126). Patients usually do not complain of sensory abnormalities. However, quantitative measurements of cutaneous touch-pressure sensation and peripheral nerve biopsy demonstrate mild involvement of peripheral sensory neurons (30).

Because laboratory and x-ray findings are normal, the diagnosis of motor neuron disease is a clinical diagnosis that is confirmed by the EMG examination. In light of the grave prognosis, care and concern should be given before reaching such a diagnosis. Repeated follow-up and EMG examinations are necessary to confirm the diagnosis.

In many cases, the patient fails to notice early weakness and does not go to the physician until several months after the onset of the disease process. By this time, essentially one-half of the motor units of an affected muscle may have been lost, and the EMG is grossly abnormal. A plethora of positive sharp waves and fibrillating potentials are seen with electrode insertion into these affected muscles. Normal-strength muscles examined in the same spinal segments as the atrophic muscles usually also demonstrate profuse positive sharp waves and fibrillation potentials. Some of the fibrillation potentials are of small amplitude, implying fiber atrophy. Fasciculation potentials are also present to varying degrees. The fasciculation potentials tend to occur at low discharge frequencies, usually not faster than one every 3–5 seconds (120). The fasciculation potential can be of any size or shape. However,

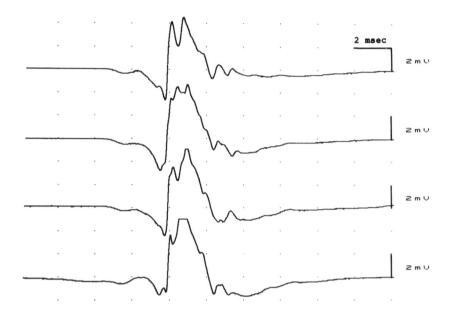

Figure 3.1. A first recruited MUAP in an ALS patient of increased amplitude and duration, polyphasic and unstable with repetitive discharge. (Monopolar recording 20 Hz to 10 KHz)

if the same fasciculation potential is electronically stored and its size and shape are analyzed with repetitive discharge, it is almost always found to be unstable (129). The origin of this instability in fasciculation potentials is, no doubt, due to impulse transmission abnormalities within the MUAP with the ongoing deinnervation and reinnervation.

In motor neuron disease, MUAPs are of increased amplitude, duration, and phases, frequently with many late components (Fig. 3.1). The percentage of unstable MUAPs reflects the extent of active ongoing reinnervation. This extent of MUAP instability, at least in the earlier stages of the disease, is an indirect reflection of motor neuron loss or the rate of progression of the disease (Fig. 3.2) (115).

Recruitment of MUAPs in motor neuron disease is usually grossly abnormal in affected muscles (Fig. 3.3). Low threshold MUAPs are larger in amplitude and duration as a result of reinnervation or a loss or dropout of previously lower threshold MUAPs. The early recruitment of abnormally very large MUAPs is not uncommon, reflecting a moderate to marked loss of MUAPs. High threshold MUAPs can be extremely abnormal with amplitudes of 20–30 μV and firing rates of 30–40 Hz (Fig. 3.4). The disease spreads to muscles of the same spinal segment on the opposite extremity while at the same time proximal and distal muscles in the initially affected limb are becoming involved.

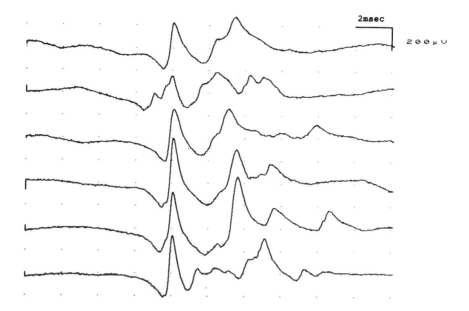

2msec

200μV

Figure 3.2. Extreme instability of this low threshold MUAP with repetitive discharge 7 months after the onset of weakness. (Monopolar recording 20 Hz to 10 KHz)

Electrical abnormalities in clinically unaffected limbs involving multiple spinal segments help confirm the diagnosis. A four-extremity EMG examination in this disease is almost routine, but certainly does not have to be performed at the time of the initial visit.

Examination of the tongue, sternocleidomastoid, digastric, or other cranial nerve innervated muscles is probably of greatest diagnostic significance. EMG demonstration of involvement of the cranial innervated muscles precludes the need for a myelogram in most cases. The examination of the tongue can be approached by two different methods. In one method, the protruded tongue is grasped with a gauze sponge, and the electrode is inserted in the long axis, either along the lateral surface or underneath. The patient relaxes the tongue, carrying the inserted electrode back into the mouth. The tongue musculature is examined for fasciculations, positive sharp waves, and fibrillation potentials, taking care to ensure that the muscle is relaxed. Insertional activity can be examined by grasping the electrode, with the tongue relaxed in the floor of the mouth or held with a gauze sponge by the examiner's hand. One should be sure to hold the electrode throughout the study of insertional activity so that tongue movements will not be confused with provokable positive sharp waves or fibrillations due to pathologic abnormalities.

A second approach to the examination of the tongue is to enter from under the chin, staying in the midline and passing through the digastric

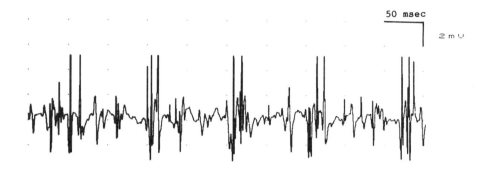

Figure 3.3. Recruitment of MUAPs at maximal contraction in motor neuron disease demonstrates a loss or dropout of units.

muscle. This technique is most helpful when looking for spontaneous activity in a person who has difficulty relaxing.

Nerve conduction studies are also helpful in the diagnosis of motor neuron disease. Sensory nerve conduction studies are normal. Motor nerve conduction studies are also normal early in the course of the disease. With loss of some of the fastest conducting motor units, mild slowing can occur. Nerve conduction velocity in this disorder does not fall lower than 75% of normal for age value (77). As the disease progresses, the compound motor nerve action potential recorded from an affected muscle will change in size and shape to reflect the muscle fiber loss. Repetitive stimulation studies may be abnormal and are a reflection of motor unit instability. The finding of EMG abnormalities in muscles of multiple spinal segments in multiple extremities and/or cranial innervated muscles with normal nerve conduction studies confirms the clinical impression of motor neuron disease.

Single fiber EMG (SFEMG) can be an adjunct to routine EMG studies in revealing information about the continuous process of deinnervation and reinnervation (114). Fiber density or the mean of the number of single fiber potentials recorded within the SFEMG electrode's 300 μm recording area with 20 different recording sites is increased in affected muscles. The presence of normal or mildly increased fiber density and a large percentage of motor unit instability (increased jitter or blocking) imply that the disease process is moving rapidly in that muscle. Likewise, a very high fiber density and only a few motor units with instability or increased jitter and blocking imply that the disease process is moving at a slow rate in that specific muscle.

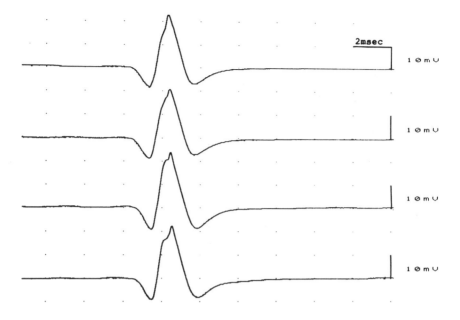

Figure 3.4. An extremely large MUAP recorded in motor neuron disease of normal triphasic shape. (Monopolar recording 20 Hz to 10 KHz)

Repeat EMG examinations throughout the course of the disease may be helpful in following the activity of the disease process. The number and location of affected muscles, their number of active motor units, the presence or absence of reinnervation, the percentage of unstable MUAPs, the density and extent of fibrillation potentials are all helpful prognostic indicators. These abnormalities can be correlated with the clinical picture in determining the time to institute bracing, inpatient rehabilitation programs, and/or ventilatory assistance.

As the disease process continues and specific muscles become very weak, the remaining motor units become extremely unstable. The greatly enlarged reinnervated motor unit territory appears at the end stage actually to be decreasing toward normal size as the few remaining motor neurons become affected and are unable to maintain all the rescued reinnervated muscle fibers (106).

Histologically, there are no pathognomonic changes. The muscle biopsy demonstrates a fairly typical neuropathic picture (12). The presence of small angulated fibers with atrophy of both Type I and Type II muscle fibers is seen in most patients. Some Type II muscle fiber hypertrophy may be seen early in the disease process. Groups of fibers of the same histochemical type suggest collateral reinnervation. Nonspecific nuclear changes with an occasional targetoid fiber are common.

Teased fiber preparations from peripheral motor nerves reveal primary axonal degeneration with secondary segmental demyelination and remyelination. This explains why nerve conduction velocities remain essentially within normal limits, even in later stages of the disease process (57). Histologic studies of sensory nerves demonstrate axon degeneration, despite the clinical absence of sensory complaints, implying subclinical sensory nerve involvement (7). Recent somatosensory evoked potentials reveal abnormalities in 60% of ALS patients (6).

Treatment of the patient, as is treatment of most medical problems, is one of strict management. Although there is no specific treatment for the disease, a total and comprehensive rehabilitation program needs to be maintained continuously to allow the patient to function independently for as long as possible. A decision regarding feeding gastrostomy needs to be discussed early in the disease's course with the patient and family. Likewise, the decision to use mechanical ventilation needs to be made early to avoid last-minute efforts.

The clinical variants of ALS are progressive bulbar palsy, primary lateral sclerosis, and progressive muscular atrophy; they differ electrically only in the site and extent of EMG abnormalities. Progressive bulbar palsy is the clinical diagnosis when the muscles innervated by the medulla are principally involved. This disorder usually begins in the fifth and sixth decade. Several inherited forms of the disease have also been described in childhood and adolescence. Primary lateral sclerosis, as the name implies, begins with corticospinal and corticobulbar involvement and little or no involvement of the motor neurons. Progressive muscular atrophy is a rare, usually sporadic disorder that can be diagnostically very confusing. It is a focal, asymmetrical, and very slowly progressing motor neuron disorder. It frequently begins in the hand and must be differentiated from a distal pure motor ulnar nerve lesion or the early symptoms of motor neuron disease. The disease progresses slowly, and hyperflexia and upper motor neuron involvement do not occur.

The hereditary form of motor neuron disease or ALS is autosomal dominant and is felt to comprise 5-10% of all cases (76). Clinically, the mean age of onset is earlier, and the male:female ratio is about equal. Although the disorder has not been thought to skip generations, some affected parents can be only mildly inconvenienced while their children die with a rapidly progressive course of the disease in their early thirties. It is therefore of importance to examine family members of patients with suspected acquired motor neuron disease, especially when it occurs in early life. At the current time there is no way to differentiate the acquired from the inherited form of the disease electrically or histologically.

Hereditary Motor Neuron Disorders

The remaining primary motor neuron disorders are of a hereditary nature. They are either of autosomal recessive or dominant inheritance and vary in age of onset, severity, and rate of progression. They involve primarily the motor neurons of the spinal cord, often the bulbar motor nuclei, but rarely the pyramidal tracts. Weakness is proximal at onset, and clinical differentiation must be made from myopathies and spinal cord tumors or injury. Until the actual genetic abnormalities are localized, these disorders are classified according to their age of onset and clinical findings. There are, however, many overlapping characteristics. For the purpose of this text and because they are currently electromyographically nondescript, these disorders are considered as varying degrees of spinal muscular atrophy. The rare occurrence of distal hereditary motor neuropathy, facioscapulohumeral, and the scapuloperoneal variety are mentioned separately.

The most common of these disorders is the autosomal recessive Werdnig-Hoffmann disease or acute infantile progressive spinal muscular atrophy. The disease may occur in utero and has been associated with a decrease in fetal movements. Approximately one-third of the cases are diagnosable at birth. Most cases begin early in the first year of life. In general, the earlier the presentation of weakness, the more rapid the course and the poorer the prognosis. The more severely affected infant is hypotonic, inactive, and areflexic. Paradoxical respiratory movements due to severe intercostal weakness are frequent. Fasciculations may be visible only in the tongue because of the thick layer of subcutaneous fat. The cry is weak. The infant, however, is alert and appears to have normal intellectual functions. If the infant does not succumb to early respiratory complications, some motor skills, such as hand control and sitting in a forward, leaning position, may be possible. The patient's survival time, however, can be as short as 2–4 years.

If the disease has its onset later in the first year, generally a less acute form of the disease is observed (45). The patient may even develop the capacity to scoot about in the sitting position using the upper extremities, but will almost never walk. Paralysis of the trunk muscles leads to chest wall deformity and scoliosis and may even lead to cardiac decompensation through mechanical deformation of the heart. With the passage of time, the motor skills are lost, and the patient's demise is usually secondary to respiratory infection and failure. The serum muscle enzyme levels, although normal in most cases, may be elevated. The EMG examination of the infant usually confirms the clinical impression, and a biopsy is not usually needed.

The most prominent finding on EMG is the presence of profuse positive sharp waves and fibrillations. These are frequently not appreciated because they may be extremely small in amplitude due to small atrophic fiber size. They are best recorded with monopolar electrodes and with the instrument amplitude gain at 20 μV per division. The infant cannot provide a requested, graded, voluntary contraction so waiting for voluntary movements or evoking movements by cutaneous stimulation, such as recording from tibialis anterior while stroking the sole of the foot, may be necessary. Motor unit dropout or loss is usually apparent, and MUAPs demonstrating early reinnervation can be seen. Fasciculation potentials, although present, are not usually prominent. Buchthal and Olsen were the first to describe a finding of spontaneous rhythmic motor unit activity in relaxed muscles of these infants occurring at 5–15 Hz (14). This activity was found to persist for hours and even during sleep. Motor and sensory nerve conduction studies are normal for age. On muscle biopsy, the histologic pattern shows large seas of round atrophic fibers of both histochemical fiber types in proximity to groups of normal-sized or hypotrophic fibers. Fibrosis is seen in bands surrounding the fascicles. Interspersed with groups of atrophic fibers are groups of hypertrophic fibers that are almost all Type I.

The other forms of spinal musculature atrophy are extremely variable in their age of onset, severity, and rate of progression. Their clinical picture as a whole represents a more benign disease with a slower course.

A more chronic form of Werdnig-Hoffmann disease has an onset before the age of 2 and survival for usually more than 10 years (45, 56). This group of children seems to have a more chronic form of the disease with less severe bulbar involvement. These children have prominent muscle atrophy, scoliosis, and other bone deformities. Some learn to sit independently. A few of these individuals learn to stand with assistance, but are generally unable to walk.

Kugelberg and Welander in 1956 described 12 cases of a more chronic, but progressive proximal spinal muscular atrophy occurring between the ages of 2 and 17 years (73). The majority of these cases had an autosomal recessive inheritance. Wohlfart in 1942 (134) and 1949 (135) described two similar cases. Weakness characteristically occurs in the proximal musculature of the lower extremities. Because the weakness is ongoing during the skeletal growth period, problems with scoliosis often occur. A pseudohypertrophy of the calf and gluteal muscles is common. These individuals can have a long life-span. The presence of fasciculations and the typical EMG picture of a motor neuron disorder help differentiate this process from a myopathy.

Many other chronic forms of spinal muscular atrophy are described with onset in later life. Their differentiation from ALS or motor neuron disease is based on their inheritance pattern, symmetry, more proximal involvement, absence of hyperflexia, and a more benign and less rapid progression.

There are many reports of families in which the severity of the disease is greatly variable in the affected siblings. One child may be severely affected, whereas the other may have only mild symptoms. Or, one child in the family may have a more classical form of Werdnig-Hoffmann disease, whereas another child may have a Kugelberg-Welander type picture.

The EMG findings in the various forms of spinal muscular atrophy are at present felt to be nonspecific, but are being analyzed to determine if quantitative analysis of MUAPs will aid in their differentiation at the time of the initial examination (55). The extent of motor unit loss tends to follow the course of the disease, and following the rate of loss may be helpful. The slower the disease process in a muscle, the greater the percentage of stable MUAPs and the fewer fibrillating muscle fibers. In the slower progressive forms of spinal muscular atrophy, SFEMG demonstrates a higher fiber density, with a lower percentage of motor units demonstrating increased jitter and blocking. It is not uncommon to see extremely long duration potentials composed of many components with firing rates of 30–40 Hz on SFEMG and routine recordings. The slower loss of motor neurons results in fewer deinnervated muscle fibers and more stable impulse transmission in the now mature reinnervated motor units.

There is a rare occurrence of distal hereditary motor neuropathy. The disease is found in both autosomal dominant and recessive forms (52, 98). Onset is before the age of 20 years and usually begins distally in the legs. Pes cavus foot deformity is common. Differentiating the disorder from Charcot-Marie-Tooth or hereditary motor sensory neuropathy is based on the finding of normal motor and sensory nerve conduction studies. EMG findings confirm the motor unit loss with ongoing reinnervation.

Facioscapulohumeral hereditary motor neuropathy is a rare disorder and only a few cases have been reported (39, 42). Clinically, the disorder is extremely similar to facioscapulohumeral muscular dystrophy, and differentiation is made by EMG and/or muscle biopsy. Facioscapulohumeral hereditary motor neuropathy is an autosomal dominant disorder. Facial weakness is prominent with involvement of shoulder and pelvic girdle muscles. The muscle weakness may be asymmetrical, and the ankle dorsiflexors can be affected. Creatine kinase blood levels are elevated. The disorder usually has its onset in the second or third decade of life. The weakness can be quite variable within the same family as demonstrated by a family being followed by the author. In this family, the affected father only has mild facial and ankle dorsiflexor weakness, whereas one of the affected sons has severe facial, pelvic girdle, and ankle dorsiflexor weakness. Fasciculations are not uncommon and may be unnoticed by the patient. EMG demonstrates positive sharp waves and fibrillation potentials to varying degrees. There is motor unit loss with overall MUAPs of normal to increased amplitude, long duration, and polyphasic shape.

Scapuloperoneal hereditary motor neuropathy is usually autosomal dominant with onset in early adult life. As the name implies, the distal lower limbs and shoulder girdle muscles are involved. Differentiation from the myopathic form of the disorder may be difficult, and the EMG abnormalities may demonstrate a mixed picture (68, 84, 103). Facial muscles may be mildly affected in some patients, which adds further confusion to diagnosing these rare conditions based on clinical presentation when we do not understand their exact etiology.

Myelitis and Myelopathies

Disorders affecting the spinal cord as a whole may have their primary effect on the ventral horn. Infections, lesions from direct trauma, and pressure or infiltration from tumors, radiations, and vascular insults may have a more selective effect on the anterior horn or motor neurons, producing an EMG picture that can be identical with motor neuron disease. Recently, the association of pure motor neuropathies with monoclonal gammopathy and various cancers has been recognized and must be added to the differential diagnosis of the patient presenting with a motor neuron disorder.

Poliomyelitis and its Late Effects

Poliomyelitis in developed countries is now only seen in occasional outbreaks in nonimmunized groups, mainly those who object to immunization for religious reasons. Vaccine-related disease is more common and was reported in 21 individuals in this country in 1982 and 1983 (95). Eight of these cases occurred in infants following their first oral vaccine dose. Six cases occurred among household contacts, mainly parents who were not properly immunized. Three cases were in immune-deficient individuals.

The disease is caused by an enterovirus, and only a very small percentage of patients who develop symptomatic illness of fever and/or diarrhea proceed to nervous system involvement (63). The virus has a predilection for the motor neurons in the spine and brainstem. In a brainstem nucleus at least one-third of the motor neurons can be lost without clinical weakness, and in the spine approximately 50% of the motor neurons can be lost with normal strength still being maintained. The virus attacks motor neurons throughout the spine, although the lumbar area is most frequently involved. The resulting weakness is a function of where and how many motor neurons are lost. It is common to find EMG abnormalities in upper extremity muscles of patients who clinically only have leg paralysis. The EMG findings in acute polio are the result of deinnervation followed by reinnervation by terminal axon sprouting. Fasciculation potentials are common. Frequently there are only a few surviving motor units in a muscle, and there are more fibrillating fibers available than can be reinnervated. The resultant MUAPs of these reinnervated motor units are some of the largest recorded. Surprisingly, fewer than 20 of these reinnervated motor units can give a muscle a Grade F or 3/5 MRC.

Over the past several years there has been an increased interest regarding the late effects of polio or what has been referred to as the *postpolio syndrome*. Many patients who have recovered from polio 30–40 years ago are now complaining of slowly progressing fatigue, weakness, and muscle pain (51). About 25% of older polio patients experience significant problems (50). The progressive weakness occurs not only in weak muscles but also in those muscles that were initially weakened but had regained normal strength. Because these reinnervated motor units activate a larger portion of the affected muscle, the natural loss with aging of a few motor neurons can result in significant changes in strength. The MUAPs of these old, reinnervated muscles are unstable (Fig. 3.5) (128). This instability may be due to a peripheral disintegration of the motor unit as the overworked motor neuron is unable to supply all of its muscle fibers with increasing age since reinnervation. The EMG findings in late polio are then centered around reinnervated MUAP instability, the continuing presence of fasciculations, and the variable presence of positive sharp waves and fibrillations (127). Because these EMG abnormalities are seen in almost all older polio patients, the EMG alone cannot be used to make the diagnosis of postpolio syndrome.

The clinical progression of these late effects of polio is relatively slow. The serum creatine kinase level has been elevated in a few cases. Upper motor neuron signs, however, are not seen. If the postpolio patient does present with hyperflexia and upper motor neuron signs, other conditions need to be considered, including the possibility of motor neuron disease occurring in an older polio patient.

Herpes Zoster

There are many other pathogenic organisms that can and do intermittently attack the spinal cord. They usually present, however, with a clinical picture of transverse myelitis, evidence of upper motor neuron disease, and sensory abnormalities. Rarely are they selective in affecting only the motor neurons, and differentiation from motor neuron disease is based on the presence of sensory and/or bowel and bladder abnormalities.

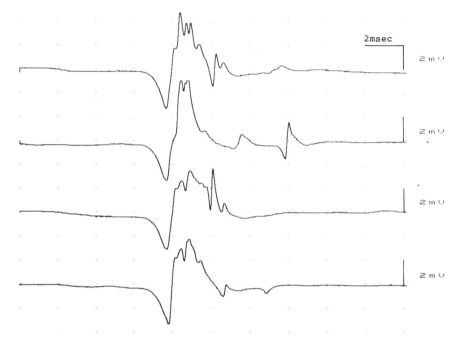

Figure 3.5. MUAP instability in a patient now 31 years postpolio. (Monopolar recording 20 Hz to 10 KHz).

One virus, however, is being recognized more commonly in its selective attack on the motor neurons (10, 48, 118, 124). Herpes zoster primarily affects the dorsal root ganglion, but it does spread into the anterior horn, not infrequently in older patients, cancer patients, and patients on immunologic-compromising pharmacologic agents. The motor involvement in most cases is at the same spinal segment as the sensory involvement and usually follows the rash. The paralysis can spread to involve multiple motor segments or produce a transverse myelitis. If the rash is missed or forgotten by the patient, diagnostic differentiation from motor neuron disease may require waiting to note the lack of progression.

Cervical Spondylosis and Direct Spinal Cord Compromise

Because few spinal cord injuries produce only localized or segmental neurologic defects, they are therefore usually easily diagnosed. However, cervical spondylosis can frequently result in a myelopathy that can be confused with motor neuron disease. With the development of degenerative joint disease and osteophyte formation, the cervical canal can become markedly narrowed. Flexion or extension of the neck can result in the anterior compression of the spinal cord over anteriorly developed osteophytic bars. Extension, on the other hand, can result in a buckling of the ligament flava and trauma to the ventral spinal cord. Clinically, the patient demonstrates evidence of an associated cervical radiculopathy and spastic paraparesis. The EMG, then, presents abnormalities consistent with a motor neuropathy, and a myelogram may be necessary to make an accurate diagnosis.

Compression of the spinal cord and/or infiltration by both primary and secondary tumors can produce a myelopathy. Direct metastases to the spinal cord are rare. However, the cord can frequently be compressed by tumor invasion of surrounding areas. Primary tumors of the spinal cord are also relatively rare, but are most commonly of glial tissue origin. Associated neurologic abnormalities, sensory loss, spastic paraparesis, and bowel and bladder incontinence rarely make the differentiation from motor neuropathy difficult, except early in cases where tumor growth may be centrally located or limited solely to the anterior horn. More commonly, treatment of tumors by radiation may result in a delayed (as long as several years) myelopathy. The onset may be slow and progressive, but the whole cord is most frequently involved with sensory abnormalities, spastic paraparesis, and bowel and bladder incontinence. Occasionally a patient has a clinical picture of a pure motor neuropathy that is progressive (80, 107).

Vascular insults to the spinal cord are being recognized with increasing frequency. Arterial insufficiency secondary to generalized arterial sclerosis is the most common vascular insult and can result in acute onset of a rapidly progressive loss of motor function. The thoracic area of the cord is most susceptible due to its poor arterial supply. The patient usually rapidly develops paraplegia. Associated pain and dysesthesias at a segmental level due to involvement of the spinothalamic and corticospinal tracts are common and aid in the diagnosis. Venous thrombosis, though infrequent, rarely produces selective involvement of the motor neurons.

Developmental Abnormalities

Developmental abnormalities of the spinal cord can produce a myelopathy. Syringomyelia and hydromyelia, because of their central location, can produce a significant motor neuropathy. The associated findings of segmental pain and temperature loss due to compromise of crossing fibers are major clues to the diagnosis. Many patients present, however, with pure motor symptoms. Dysrhaphism of the cord and more specifically diastematomyelia may remain asymptomatic until rapid growth causes increased pressure on the spinal cord. Usually sensory and bladder symptoms are associated, but the condition may present with motor neuron involvement of the foot or leg, making the diagnosis then dependent upon myelography (65).

Paraneoplastic and Paraproteinemic Syndromes

A pure motor neuropathy mimicking motor neuron disease is being recognized in patients who have undiagnosed cancers and in patients with serum protein abnormalities. In some cases, the motor neuropathy improves with treatment of the cancer or protein abnormality. The association between cancer and ALS has been recognized to be greater than would be expected by coincidence (8, 92). This raises the question as to whether some motor neuron abnormalities are due to a nonmetastatic or "remote" effect of cancer. Carcinoma of the lung is the most common, although breast and ovarian cancer, lymphomas, and others have been described to produce these paraneoplastic syndromes. Treatment of the cancer in most cases does not alter the neurologic abnormalities. Isolated cases are reported, however, where removal of the tumor has resulted in a dramatic improvement in neurologic symptoms, implying that the cancer has a "remote" effect on the motor neuron (86).

The association between a pure motor neuropathy or ALS-like syndrome and plasma cell dyscrasia or monoclonal gammopathy has received recent widespread interest because many of these patients diagnosed as having ALS improve with treatment of the serum protein abnormalities (37, 97, 100, 105). Abnormalities of IgG and IgM are most common (96, 112). These rare associations of gammopathy and ALS syndromes may be coincidental, but the fact that they respond to immune therapy implies a direct relationship. The possibility of a paraproteinemic syndrome must be included in the differential diagnosis of motor neuron disorders.

The EMG in the paraneoplastic and paraproteinemic syndromes does not differ from those seen in other motor neuron disorders. Occasionally, the patient with these syndromes is not capable of reinnervation by terminal axon sprouting. Motor unit dropout without a change in MUAP size or shape may be a helpful clue in evaluating these patients. Because the best-known neurologic disorder of cancer and plasma cell disorders is a sensorimotor peripheral neuropathy, nerve conduction studies are most helpful in the evaluation of these patients.

MYOPATHIES

Disorders producing weakness where the muscle fiber appears to be the primary site of abnormality are referred to as myopathies. Myopathies can be subdivided into dystrophic, inflammatory, congenital forms and those associated with electrical evidence of myotonia, intermittent paralysis, or metabolic enzyme deficiencies. Histologically, myopathies are characterized by the presence of a variation in fiber size. The EMG recordings of these disorders vary greatly from one to another and with the stage or course of the individual disease. The motor unit action potentials (MUAPs) overall tend to be stable, polyphasic, of low to normal amplitude, and of varying durations. The duration of the MUAP, though usually short at the time of initial diagnosis, later in the course of the disease may become quite long with late components. The EMG variations recorded in myopathies are, no doubt, due to the great variation in the pathophysiology of the diseases themselves. Although these disorders primarily affecting the muscle fibers are referred to as myopathies, the exact etiology in most incidences is unknown. In these known or unknown disorders, not all muscle fibers are equally affected, and the degree of involvement varies from muscle to muscle. Due to a loss of produced tension with contraction of the affected motor units, the rapid recruitment of additional motor units is needed to produce a specific strength of contraction. As the disorder progresses, electrical excitability of some muscle fibers is lost, and over time, areas of muscles become nonfunctional and electrically silent. Electromyographers are attracted to those areas where electrical activity continues, and the EMG in end-stage disease reflects the architectural changes of the surviving motor units.

Muscular Dystrophies

Muscular dystrophies are the most common form of myopathies and are characterized by a progressive loss of muscle strength. They are inherited disorders, but to date, the specific genetic defects and resultant pathologic effect on muscles are not known. Histologically these patients demonstrate a variation in muscle fiber size and degeneration and regeneration of muscle fibers. Electrically, there are no pathognomonic potentials, and the EMG varies with the course of the disease. Consequently, diagnosis is based primarily on the history and physical examination, with confirmation by EMG, laboratory work, and, when necessary, biopsy and biochemical data.

Duchenne Muscular Dystrophy

Duchenne muscular dystrophy is the most common and rapidly progressive dystrophy. It is inherited as a X-linked recessive disorder. The recent use of DNA markers has localized the genetic abnormality to the X_p 21 region of the X chromosome. The female, as the carrier of the disease, rarely demonstrates any signs or symptoms of the disorder, but will pass it to 50% of her male offspring. Fifty percent of her female offspring will also then be carriers. The mutation rate may be as high as one-third of new cases. The affected male usually demonstrates clinical abnormalities by the age of 3 years. The serum creatine kinase

(CK) is elevated from birth and is usually ten times the normal value. Walking may be delayed. Weakness is usually first clinically detected in the hip extensor muscles (66). The child, by this time, may be clumsy, be falling frequently, and have difficulty running and climbing stairs. The calf muscles appear to be hypertrophied with a hard rubbery consistency but, in reality, are a proliferation of connective tissue and fat-replacing necrotic muscle, indicating that the disease process has been long-standing. A reduced mental capacity is commonly associated with the disease, and IQ scores are about 20 points lower than those of their siblings (102).

As the weakness progresses, the child assumes a hyperlordic waddling gait. With the onset of proximal lower extremity weakness, the weakness in the shoulder musculature becomes apparent. Hip extensor muscle weakness makes rising from the floor difficult, and children display the characteristic Gower's maneuver as they climb their own legs to right their trunk. The disease continues with relentless progression, and daily stretching exercises are required to slow the development of calf, hamstring, tensor fascia latae, and pronator contractures. By the age of 9 to 12, the child has stopped walking. A scoliosis develops, further compromising lung function. Death is usually the result of pulmonary complication in the third decade.

The muscle biopsy is rather characteristic, with degenerating fibers and small groups of regenerating fibers intermixed in fields of normal fibers. There is a marked increase in the variability of muscle fiber size. Endomysial and perimysial connective tissue proliferation and muscle fiber fibrosis become increasingly prominent with progression of the disease. Type I fiber predominance is common, with an overall deficiency of Type IIB fibers. A recent serial section study demonstrates signs of regeneration after segmental necrosis. Most prominent are the multiple branchings and small fiber diameters. Many short noninnervated fibers are seen (108).

Performing an EMG on a 2- or 3-year-old boy can be challenging. The use of a tape recorder for the later review of MUAPs is invaluable. The muscle at rest often demonstrates complex repetitive discharges. Positive sharp waves and fibrillation potentials are not prominent, but can usually be detected with searching.

With monopolar recordings at 20 Hz to 10 KHz, the low threshold motor units are low in amplitude in the 50–200 μV range in proximal muscles. High threshold motor units are approximately 1000–1500 μV and rarely over 2500 μV. The duration at this early stage of the disease is short, and motor units of 1–3 msec duration are common. The shape of these potentials is frequently polyphasic and commonly has the characteristics of two or three single fiber discharges (Fig. 3.6). In some areas of muscle and especially later in the disease, long duration MUAPs

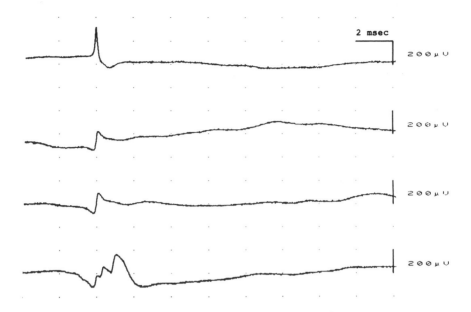

Figure 3.6. Short duration MUAPs recorded from a 3-year-old boy with Duchenne dystrophy. (Monopolar recordings 20 Hz to 10 KHz)

are seen comprised of complexes of late components that, without electronic delay and triggering, would have been perceived as several different MUAPs (Fig. 3.7). Early in the disease the recruitment is rich with what seems like the entire muscle being activated to produce a low strength of contraction. With progression of the disease, a marked loss of high threshold MUAPs is noted. As a muscle becomes very weak at end stage, some areas actually become electrically silent during contraction and are no doubt nonfunctional (Fig. 3.8). Single fiber EMG (SFEMG) in Duchenne muscular dystrophy has been rarely performed before the age of 6 years (see Chapter 10). As a result, most SFEMG recordings are of normal or long duration. Using SFEMG stimulation techniques instead of voluntary contraction to record reveals many single fiber pairs with extremely low jitter values, indicating that there are many more split fibers than originally thought from routine voluntarily activated recordings (61). This finding correlates with the extensive branching of fibers observed on serial biopsy section studies (108).

Becker Muscular Dystrophy

The Becker variety of muscular dystrophy is an x-linked recessive disease with later onset and slower progression of symptoms than

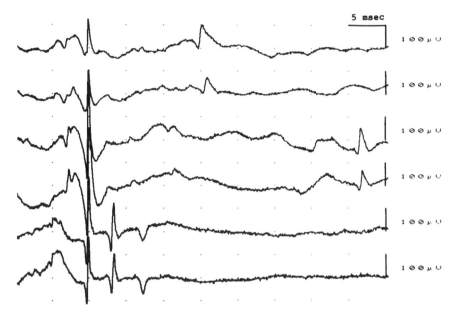

Figure 3.7. Long duration MUAPs from an 8-year-old boy with Duchenne dystrophy. Three different MUAPs, two recordings of each to emphasize late components. Note second MUAP in recordings 3 and 4 has a 45 msec total duration when including late components. (Monopolar recordings 20 Hz to 10 KHz)

Duchenne dystrophy (3). As with Duchenne dystrophy, the genetic abnormality is also located in the X_p 21 region. Although the clinical signs of the disease may be present as early as in Duchenne dystrophy, some cases do not present until the late teens and early twenties. In contrast to those with Duchenne, these boys generally continue walking through their early teenage years and many continue to walk until the fifth or sixth decade. As in Duchenne dystrophy, the serum muscle enzymes are elevated. Histologically, except for a more normal distribution of Type IIB fibers, the biopsy has essentially the same characteristics as that for Duchenne (28). Electrically, EMG abnormalities are also similar (Fig. 3.9). Some of the longest duration (40–50 msec) late components have been recorded in this disorder using SFEMG.

Facioscapulohumeral Muscular Dystrophy

Facioscapulohumeral muscular dystrophy (FSH) is inherited as an autosomal dominant trait with marked variations in expression from generation to generation. Because of this variability of expression, it is not

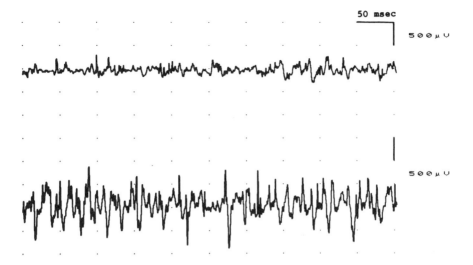

Figure 3.8. *Top,* Low threshold contraction reveals an increased number of MUAPs recruited per strength. *Bottom,* High threshold contraction reveals a reduced number of MUAPs or muscle fibers recruited.

uncommon for the disorder to remain undiagnosed in a family until a child in the first or second decade of life develops significant face or shoulder weakness. As the name implies, the muscles of the face and shoulder girdle are selectively involved. The ankle dorsiflexor muscles are also affected. Unlike the other muscular dystrophies, the weakness is frequently asymmetrical. Weakness in the trapezii muscles is usually the first to be noticed by the patient. This weakness results in a winging of the scapula. Clinically, the patient appears to have deltoid weakness, but when tested with the scapula stabilized it is usually of normal strength.

The typical facial weakness produces a flat facial expression with an unlined forehead. A transverse smile with only minimal elevations of the corners of the mouth is evidence of the predominant involvement of the orbicularis oris muscle. This facial weakness, however, in some patients is not prominent, and examination of other family members is necessary to make an accurate diagnosis. The disease generally progresses very slowly and does not usually affect a normal life-span. Weakness of truncal and pelvic muscles occurs in more severely affected individuals later in life.

Biopsy findings are variable and depend on the muscle examined. The biceps muscle is commonly selected for study and demonstrates

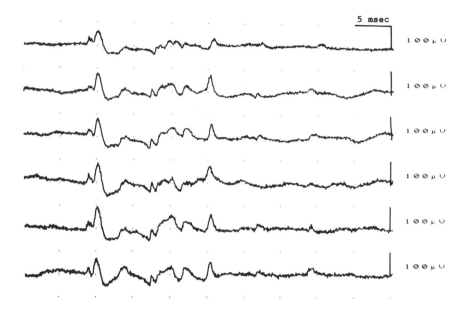

Figure 3.9. Long duration MUAP recorded from a teenage boy with Becker dystrophy. (Monopolar recording 20 Hz to 10 KHz)

fiber size variability with overall fiber hypertrophy. Moth-eaten and whorled fibers are frequently found. An inflammatory response is also occasionally present.

The EMG abnormalities may be minimal, and it is most important to examine the clinically weak muscles. Recordings from deltoid and biceps may be normal, whereas recordings from pectoralis major, infraspinatus, and orbicularis oris are abnormal. The upper trapezius is very thin but careful EMG exploration will reveal abnormalities. Fibrillation potentials and positive sharp waves, although present, are difficult to locate. MUAPs are of low amplitude, short duration, and polyphasic in shape. The MUAPs are stable on repetitive firing, with monopolar and concentric recording. Recruitment abnormalities reflect the stage of the disease process. It may be normal or demonstrate an increased number recruited per strength. In more end-stage disease and with significant weakness, there is a loss of motor units.

Limb-Girdle Muscular Dystrophy

Limb-girdle muscular dystrophy represents, most likely, several different nonspecific disorders characterized by a distribution of weakness in proximal pelvic and shoulder girdle musculature. It is usually of autosomal recessive inheritance, but many cases appear to be sporadic. Most commonly, there are two major ages of onset: in the second or third decade, or later in life. The rate of progression is usually slow, although there are exceptions. Muscle enzymes may be mildly elevated. Surprisingly, when the disease begins in the fifth and sixth decade, the patient may present with a complaint of low back pain. This is most likely due to the hyperlordotic posture caused by weak hip extensor and abductor muscles and underlying degenerative joint disease in the lumbosacral spine. Weakness in this disorder is proximal and symmetrical. Quadriceps weakness is common, and atrophy can be severe.

Muscle biopsy is nonspecific. There is a pronounced variation in fiber size with many hypertrophied fibers. Moth-eaten and whorled fibers, as a whole, are more commonly found in limb-girdle dystrophy than in FSH. Fiber splitting is common, as are internal nuclei.

EMG abnormalities are variable and correlate with the extent of clinical involvement. Examination of the clinically weak muscles is most revealing. Positive sharp waves and fibrillation potentials can be difficult to find even with searching. In mildly affected muscles, MUAP abnormalities of low amplitude, short duration, and an increased percentage of polyphasics are minimal and require quantitative analysis. Early recruitment of additional MUAPs may also be minimal. In severely weak patients or patients who have an early onset and rapid course, the EMG abnormalities may be profound and similar to those recorded in Duchenne or Becker muscular dystrophy (Fig. 3.10).

Myotonic Muscular Dystrophy

Myotonic muscular dystrophy is a multisystem disorder of autosomal dominant inheritance. The disease is characterized by stiffness and delayed relaxation of a contraction, facial weakness, and initially distal limb weakness and atrophy. Myotonia or the painless, delayed relaxation of muscle following contraction or percussion may initially worsen with voluntary activity, but may then improve as the activity continues. The patient usually complains of stiffness and the inability to release a tightly gripped object. The myotonia is worsened by cold temperatures. As the disease progresses, ptosis, weakness of the sternocleidomastoids and neck flexors, atrophy of the masseter and temporalis, and frontal balding result in a characteristic facial appearance. Clinically, weakness and myotonia are most prominent in hand and forearm and foot and lower leg musculature. In addition to frontal balding, associated abnormalities include cataracts, cardiac conduction abnormalities, mental slowness or deficiency, esophageal motility problems, testicular or ovarian atrophy, structural abnormalities of the skull, low basal metabolic rate, abnormal glucose tolerance test, and abnormalities of IgG

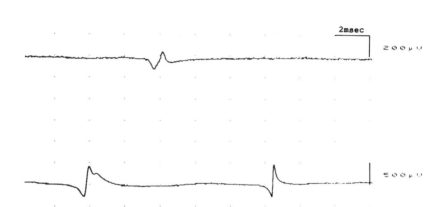

Figure 3.10. Marked variability in duration of these two different MUAPs recorded from the biceps of a 42-year-old man with limb-girdle dystrophy 5 years after onset of weakness. (Monopolar recording 20 Hz to 10 KHz)

(53). As with autosomal dominant neuromuscular disorders, the expression of the genetic abnormalities varies greatly from patient to patient within the same family. Affected infants of myotonic mothers may be floppy at birth with frequent respiratory and feeding difficulties (54).

The muscle biopsy shows typically Type I fiber atrophy with Type II fiber hypertrophy. As the disease progresses, Type II fibers become equally affected. Internal nuclei are common.

Electromyographically, the myotonic phenomenon is recorded in most muscles but is marked in distal musculature. The myotonic discharge is a repetitive discharge of 20–80 Hz (Fig. 3.11). The discharge is composed of either biphasic spikes of less than 5 msec duration or positive waves of 5–20 msec. The amplitude and frequency of the biphasic spikes or positive waves wax and wane. The potential is generated from a single muscle fiber recorded with needle insertion, percussion, or following voluntary contraction. The myotonic discharge is not characteristic of myotonic dystrophy and can be recorded in myotonia congenita, paramyotonia congenita, myotubular myopathy, hyperkalemic periodic paralysis, and other metabolic muscle disorders (4, 44, 122). The myotonic discharge in myotonic muscular dystrophy is most frequently found in distal muscles. However, it can be difficult or impossible to find in some clinically affected relatives.

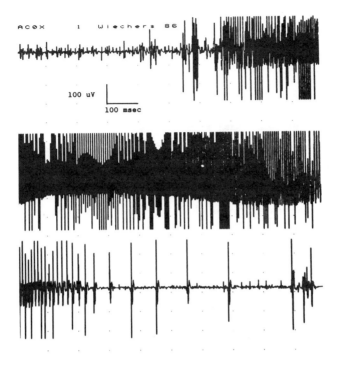

Figure 3.11. Myotonic discharge recorded from a patient with myotonic dystrophy.

MUAP abnormalities may only be seen in distal muscles, and analysis can be challenging, with frequent ongoing myotonic discharges. In affected muscles, low amplitude, short duration, polyphasic MUAPs indicate a loss or dropout of muscle fibers per motor unit and confirm the dystrophic disorder. Rapid recruitment of additional motor units per strength of contraction is very difficult to determine in some muscles where myotonic discharges are prominent. Repetitive stimulation may demonstrate a decrement due to depolarization block.

Distal Muscular Dystrophy

This disorder, although very rare in this country, is quite frequent in its appearance in other parts of the world. The largest number of reported cases are from Sweden (81, 125). The disorder is autosomal dominant with symptoms usually appearing between 40–60 years, and it affects males more frequently than females. Hand and foot intrinsic muscles and finger extensor muscles are most commonly affected first. The disorder is slowly progressive, and significant proximal weakness is rare except in cases that have their onset in youth (26).

Muscle biopsy demonstrates variation in fiber size and vascular changes (32, 81). Muscle enzymes are mildly elevated. EMG confirms the diagnosis with normal nerve conduction studies, the absence of myotonic discharges, and the presence of motor units of low amplitude, short duration, and an increased number recruited per strength of contraction.

Ophthalmoplegic Muscular Dystrophies

This term does not describe a specific disorder but rather a group of several different neuromuscular diseases that are all extremely rare and primarily involve the ocular muscles. Differentiating these disorders from the treatable myasthenia gravis is most important. There are several other neurogenic disorders that also affect the ocular muscles that must be differentiated.

Pure ocular dystrophy (9, 72) begins at any age, but most commonly within the first 25 years of life. The disorder begins with ptosis and progresses to weakness of eye muscles. The disorder is slowly progressive and will eventually involve facial muscles. Neck and limb muscles are occasionally involved. The disease can be inherited as an autosomal dominant or recessive. Sporadic cases have been described.

The EMG of extraocular eye muscles is technically difficult. Normal MUAPs in the orbicularis oculi are of low amplitude, short duration, and polyphasic as compared to normal limb muscles, and care must be taken in EMG interpretation of abnormalities in this muscle. In contrast, changes of MUAPs recorded from affected orbicularis oculi demonstrate reduced amplitude, duration, and increased proportion of polyphasics when compared to normals.

Oculopharyngeal dystrophy (9, 123) is usually an autosomal dominant disorder occurring most commonly in French Canadians and in focal areas among Spanish-American families in southwest America. Onset is usually in the third and fourth decade with bilateral or unilateral ptosis. Extraocular muscle weakness with normal pupillary reactions and facial weakness then develops slowly. Dysphagia occurs early in the course of the disease and becomes progressively worse with age. Proximal limb muscle weakness develops with age in some patients. Serum muscle enzymes may be elevated. EMG demonstrates MUAPs of low amplitude, short duration, and increased polyphasics in affected muscles. Biopsy reveals variability of fiber size and small angulated fibers. The presence of vacuoles in many of the fibers is seen in most biopsies and appears to be somewhat characteristic.

Oculocraniosomatic Neuromuscular Disease with Ragged Red Fibers

Ophthalmoplegia plus, Kearns-Sayres syndrome, or oculocraniosomatic neuromuscular disease with ragged red fibers are terms used to describe a mitochondrial disorder with associated progressive weakness of extraocular muscles and ptosis (27, 69, 71, 94). Although this disorder is not a dystrophy, it is included here for completeness in understanding the myopathic disorders primarily affecting ocular muscles. The disorder can be sporadic or autosomal dominant. The symptoms usually begin as ptosis in childhood or young adult life. There is usually a progression of weakness with time to involve the extraocular and proximal musculature. The patient may develop some or all of the associated abnormalities of sensorineural deafness, cardiac conduction abnormalities, pigmentary degeneration of the retina, cerebellar or pyramidal tract abnormalities, endocrine abnormalities, or mental retardation.

The muscle biopsy reveals variation in fiber size and an increase in the number of mitochondria that stain red with modified trichrome and have been called "ragged red" fibers. Ragged red fibers are not specific to this disorder and occur in other disorders (28).

The EMG abnormalities, as expected, follow the course of the disorder. In a symptomatic family the affected mother, who is severely weak with nonfunctional extraocular motion and proximal muscles of just antigravity strength, demonstrates severe abnormalities on EMG. There were positive sharp waves and fibrillation potentials with searching. MUAPs were of low amplitude with polyphasic shape and of short and long duration. Recruitment demonstrates an increased number per strength of contraction at low threshold and a loss or dropout at high threshold. Areas of some muscles were electrically silent. Her son, who was first examined in his early twenties, clinically demonstrates ptosis but without the extraocular or systemic weakness and demonstrated EMG abnormalities only in the orbicularis oculi. A 28-year-old daughter with ptosis and mild proximal weakness demonstrated mild MUAP changes only in the deltoid, biceps, and orbicularis oculi. This family typifies the clinical and EMG variability that can be seen in this disorder.

Inflammatory Myopathies

An inflammatory response in muscle may be the result of many different conditions. The term *inflammatory myopathies* is used here to refer to the conditions of polymyositis and dermatomyositis (31, 83, 99). The exact etiology of these acquired disorders is unknown. They are frequently seen in association with collagen vascular diseases and some cancers. They can occur at any age, although it is more common to see dermatomyositis in childhood and after the fifth decade. Both disorders may begin with systemic manifestations of fever, malaise, weight loss, or gastrointestinal upset. The onset of weakness may be sudden over several days, but more commonly is progressive over several weeks to months. Muscle aching and pain to palpation and repetitive motion, although prominent complaints in some patients, are totally absent in others.

Both conditions are serious disorders, and one-third of patients may die, one-third recover, and one-third linger on to wheelchair ambulation and loss of independence. Steroids and immunosuppressive therapy, although not completely proven to alter the course of the disease, are not withheld from sick patients, and the true natural history of the disease may never be fully known (133).

Dermatomyositis is found equally as commonly in males and females. The characteristic rash that distinguishes this disorder from polymyositis is erythematous and edematous with telangiectasia. The eyelids are most frequently affected, and the characteristic "heliotropic" or deep violaceous discoloration is prominent. Extensor surfaces of the joints, especially knees and fingers and periungual areas, are also affected by the rash. The rash may precede the weakness by several weeks. The weakness is mainly proximal, and with the exception of problems with dysphagia, cranial muscles and respiratory muscles are not usually involved. In the patient population over 40 years of age, the association of dermatomyositis and the presence of malignancy varies from 10–50% (1, 2). Myalgia and muscle soreness to palpation are present in about 50% of patients. Subcutaneous calcinosis is common in later stages of the disease and is usually seen when the disease is inactive.

Polymyositis, as does dermatomyositis, begins frequently with systemic manifestations and associated elevated sedimentation rate, CK, or serum gammaglobulin. As with dermatomyositis, scleroderma and Raynaud's phenomenon also occur; however, in polymyositis, other collagen vascular disorders may also be present. In inflammatory myopathy there is usually a sudden onset of proximal weakness in pelvic muscles followed by shoulder muscle weakness. The presentation of weakness without a rash can be a diagnostic problem in differentiating polymyositis from limb-girdle dystrophy. The occurrence of a myopathy with collagen vascular diseases, cancer, alcoholism, endocrine abnormalities, and other disorders makes the term "polymyositis" somewhat of a "wastebasket" classification. Better understanding of the etiology of this disorder will lead to more distinct classifications in the future.

Because the inflammatory myopathies are so spotty in involvement of the muscle, the first biopsy can frequently be normal while a second biopsy taken from the same muscle can be severely affected. The biopsy demonstrates variability of fiber size with evidence of degeneration and regeneration (28). Inflammatory changes are seen in about 75% of biopsies. Perifascicular atrophy of fibers is seen and suggests that the myopathy may be vascular in origin.

The EMG recordings in dermatomyositis and polymyositis change dramatically with the course of the disease. The pathophysiology of these disorders is felt to be segmental muscle cell necrosis (21). The muscle fiber with its one motor endplate is now divided into several segments by segmental necrosis, only one of which contains neural connection. The now deinnervated segments fibrillate. Early in the course of the disease, areas of muscle have a large number of positive sharp waves and fibrillation potentials. Once treatment of the disease with steroids is instituted, the abnormal muscle membrane irritability is reduced, and although positive sharp waves and fibrillations can usually still be found, they are no longer exuberant. With many segments of muscle fibers deinnervated, the process of reinnervation by terminal axon sprouting begins. Single fiber recordings demonstrate an increase in fiber density with histochemical evidence of reinnervation (59). Early on, motor units are losing muscle fibers, and short duration polyphasic potentials are recorded (15, 22).

As the reinnervation process continues, the motor units become of longer duration and remain polyphasic. Long duration potentials composed of many late components are not uncommon. If the disease process continues, the whole process of muscle fiber segmental necrosis and reinnervation continues until areas of muscle become nonfunctional and electrically silent. Recruitment abnormalities of MUAPs also follow the pathophysiology of the disease. Early on, there is an increased number of units recruited per strength of contraction. Later, as more and more of the muscle is destroyed, a loss of motor units is recorded.

Congenital Myopathies

The congenital myopathies comprise a group of fairly benign muscle disorders that are characterized and classified by the biopsy finding of a structural abnormality of the muscle cell or an abnormal distribution of muscle fiber types. Whether these neuromuscular disorders are the result of faulty or arrested muscle cell development or the lack of proper trophic influences of their nerve supply remains to be determined. In most cases, the affected child is floppy at birth, but unlike other muscle disorders, the weakness is nonprogressive and muscle strength usually improves. Muscle strength usually plateaus by the early to late teens. Frequently associated with the muscle weakness is a series of other congenital abnormalities, ranging from a long narrow face with a high arched palate to chest wall deformities. It is most important to identify these children early to begin an aggressive program of physical therapy. It may be many years before the child gains enough strength to walk or perform other functional activities. By this time the seemingly rapid development of contractures and scoliosis may limit the child's ability to function despite adequate strength.

Central Core Disease

In 1956 Shy and Magee described a nonprogressive myopathy characterized by the histochemical presence of central areas within muscle fibers that were composed of compact myofibrils, but devoid of enzymatic activity (111). This disorder is usually of autosomal dominant inheritance, although sporadic cases have been identified.

Clinically, the patient is floppy at birth or noted to be weak shortly thereafter. Motor milestones are delayed. Weakness is usually mild and nonprogressive. The patient is usually weaker proximally, although generalized weakness, including the facial musculature, has been described. Reflexes may be normal. Congenital dislocation of the hips is frequent, and kyphoscoliosis may be a problem later in life. The CK level is normal.

Histologically there is a central area or core of the muscle fiber that is devoid of oxidative enzyme activity. These cores are usually more prominent in Type I muscle fibers. Some patients are Type I predominant. The cores can be structured or unstructured, demonstrating a loss of myofibular pattern (90).

Electromyographically, the EMG may be normal in the areas examined. An increase in the frequency of polyphasic potentials or an increased discharge frequency per effort exerted may be the only abnormality. Motor units have been described in individual cases to be of low or high amplitude and short and long duration (29, 64). Spontaneous and insertional activity are normal.

Nemaline Myopathy

Using Gomori trichrome staining techniques in 1963, Shy and others observed a rod or thread-like structure in the muscle fibers of patients with a clinical diagnosis of congenital myopathy (110). These rods, or threads—thus, nemaline—structures could not be seen or were easily overlooked with the routine H & E staining.

Clinically, there are two somewhat distinct presentations (74). The most common presentation is a floppy infant or a child with diffuse weakness beginning early in life. More typically, the children are dysmorphic and have a long narrow face with a high arched palate. These patients have a reduced muscle bulk or very slender musculature. The disorder in most cases is nonprogressive, and weakness is mild. Facial muscles may be affected. Reported cases have demonstrated pigeon breast or high arched feet and kyphoscoliosis. The disorder may also present in adolescence or adult life. These patients have mild weakness in a scapuloperoneal distribution. Autosomal dominant inheritance and sporadic cases have been reported. CK may be slightly elevated.

Histologically, the rod-like structures in the muscle fibers have been shown to be in continuity with the Z band, and it has been postulated that they represent an abnormal deposition of Z band material. Rods involve predominantly either Type I or Type II muscles. Both muscle fiber types may, however, be affected (109). Rod structures themselves are nonspecific and have been seen in association with other structural abnormalities of muscle.

Electromyographically, spontaneous and insertional activity have been reported in the literature to be normal (110). The author has recorded fibrillation and positive sharp waves of a mild degree in one of his patients and complex repetitive discharges of high frequency in another patient. Amplitudes of both low threshold and high threshold MUAPs are reduced with an overall reduction in the duration. There is an increased percentage of polyphasic potentials, many of short duration. Recruitment demonstrates an increased number of voluntary units per strength of contraction.

Myotubular Myopathy (Centronuclear Myopathy)

In 1966 Spiro, Shy, and Gonatos saw what they felt resembled the fetal myotubes in the muscle biopsy of a patient with a clinical presentation of a congenital myopathy (113). Classically, the patient is floppy at birth or noted to be weak in childhood by delays in reaching motor milestones. Varying degrees of facial weakness, ptosis, and ophthalmoplegia are frequently present. CNS abnormalities with seizure disorder and apneic episodes are reported. Weakness may be severe and can be primarily of proximal or distal distribution. Like those with nemaline myopathy, these children may appear somewhat dysmorphic with long narrow faces and pectus excavatum. Autosomal dominant, recessive, and x-linked patterns of inheritance have been described (122). The CK may be mildly elevated.

Histologically, the fibers are of normal diameter, but contain central nuclei, as does fetal muscle. Central nuclei vary in number, but are seen in the majority of fibers examined. There is an area devoid of myofibrils and thus of myofibular ATPase activity around the central nuclei. Oxidative enzyme activity has been shown to be absent or increased in these central areas of muscle fiber.

Electromyographically, these patients are abnormal. Positive sharp waves and fibrillation potentials are frequent. Myotonic discharges are seen and may lead to confusion in the diagnosis (58). Because the patient clinically may present with distal weakness and ptosis, the findings of myotonic discharges may lead to an erroneous diagnosis of myotonic dystrophy. Clinical myotonia has not been present in the patients with this disorder who have been examined by the author. MUAPs are abnormal. Amplitudes of high and low threshold potentials are reduced as are durations. An increased percentage of polyphasic potentials of short to normal duration is recorded. An increased recruitment of voluntary motor units per strength of contraction is observed. Single fiber EMG in one case demonstrated a mild increase in fiber density with an increase in jitter and occasional blocking.

Abnormal Distribution of Fiber Types

A group of the clinically diagnosed congenital myopathies are characterized by abnormalities in muscle fiber type distribution. Human muscles that are most often studied by biopsy are generally composed of one-third Type I muscle fibers and two-thirds Type II muscle fibers. Type I muscle fibers in humans are an average 50 μ in diameter. Type II muscle fibers are slightly larger, approximately 60 μ in diameter. In this group of disorders the biopsy demonstrates variation in size and distribution of fiber types.

Congenital Fiber Type Disproportion

Brooke in 1973 recognized a group of patients with a fairly consistent clinical picture whose biopsy demonstrated Type I smallness and predominance and Type II hypertrophy (12). Inheritance is autosomal dominant in some families and in others is unknown. Clinically, these children are almost all floppy at birth or noted not to be progressing normally according to the motor milestones. About one-half of the patients have congenital dislocations of the hip. Contractures are a major source of functional limitation and are present at birth in some patients. Weakness in respiratory musculature in the first year of life can lead to recurrent respiratory infections. As the children grow older, their strength improves. In the usual case, the strength plateaus, but on occasion, normal strength musculature is obtained. Weakness tends to be more proximal. Kyphoscoliosis is common. CK is normal or only slightly elevated. Hip and knee flexion contractures may inhibit brace wearing and walking. In one of the author's patients, walking was not achieved until age 12, following an intensive rehabilitation program with extreme stretching of contractures.

The EMG is abnormal. Spontaneous and insertional activity are usually normal. One of the author's cases has demonstrated positive sharp waves and fibrillation potentials upon diligent search. In another case the rare occurrence of complex repetitive potentials was recorded. MUAPs are of reduced amplitude in both low and high threshold potentials. Overall, durations of MUAPs are reduced. There is an increase in polyphasic potentials. Recruitment in some muscles may be normal, whereas others demonstrate increased number recorded per strength of contraction. SFEMG in one case demonstrated a normal fiber density with a mild increase in jitter and a rare occurrence of blocking.

Type I Smallness and Predominance and Normal Type II. Although this condition is not recognized as a specific syndrome, the author has been following four patients with this biopsy picture who have a similar clinical manifestation. They were floppy at birth or had early delays in motor milestones. Walking was delayed, but achieved by all four. Two have subsequently lost the ability to walk: one due to a necessary spinal fusion and the other due to the development of contractures. Weakness is mild, and strength appears to have plateaued by mid-to-late childhood. Contractures are common, and hypermobility of finger and wrist joints is seen. Scoliosis is present in two of the cases. CK is normal.

On EMG, spontaneous and insertional activity are normal. MUAPs are abnormal in three cases personally studied. Amplitudes are normal or slightly reduced in both low and high threshold units. Overall duration is reduced. An increase in the percentage of polyphasic potentials is prominent. An increased number of motor units are recruited per strength of contraction on mild to moderate force. At maximal contraction in two patients, there appeared a reduction in high threshold units available for recruitment. SFEMG in two cases demonstrated a mild increase in fiber density. Jitter is increased in approximately 50% of motor units examined, and less than half of these motor units with abnormal jitter show evidence of blocking.

MYOTONIAS

Myotonia is a painless delay in muscle relaxation that is recorded electrically as the repetitive discharge of a single muscle fiber following its initial activation. This initial activation can be by voluntary contraction following a period of rest, percussion, or needle electrode insertion. The myotonia or resultant muscle stiffness increases initially with movement and then improves. Cold tends to increase the myotonia. The underlying defect of the muscle fiber responsible for the myotonic phenomenon is unknown. Electrically, the myotonia is recorded as a biphasic spike or positive sharp wave that waxes and wanes in frequency and amplitude. Myotonic discharges are found in various muscles and to varying degrees in a number of disorders in addition to the classical myotonic dystrophy, myotonia congenita, and paramyotonia that are characterized by its presence. Myotonic discharges are frequently recorded in muscles of patients who may have little or no clinical evidence of myotonia, as in hyperkalemic periodic paralysis (44), myotubular myopathy (58), acid maltase deficiency (34), and hyperthyroidism (93).

Myotonia Congenita

There are basically two different forms of this disorder that are characterized clinically by myotonia, occasionally muscle hypertrophy, but no dystrophy. The autosomal dominant form was originally described by Dr. Thomsen as occurring in his own family (119). This variety affects males and females equally, and the clinical myotonia becomes noticeable in infancy or early childhood. The autosomal recessive form of the disease described by Becker (4) seems to affect males most commonly and has much more profound myotonia. Clinically, stiffness that occurs after resting is the major complaint. The stiffness is most prominent when arising from a chair or starting to walk. It seems to resolve with a warmup period of activity. Once the clinical myotonia is resolved with activity, manual muscle testing reveals normal strength. The major differential in this clinical diagnosis is myotonic dystrophy. The absence of true distal weakness and the other systemic abnormalities associated with myotonic dystrophy usually makes this differentiation relatively easy. Overall, the myotonia or complaints of stiffness by the patients are worse in the legs. With severe myotonia, muscle hypertrophy can occur in certain muscles.

The diagnosis, as in most neuromuscular disorders, is clinical and is confirmed by the biopsy, laboratory work, and EMG. Muscle biopsy demonstrates an absence of Type IIB fibers in some patients and various degrees of nonspecific changes, such as internal nuclei (20). The EMG is most helpful in confirmation of this diagnosis. Myotonic discharges are usually abundant and easy to elicit from needle electrode insertion. MUAPs are normal, but are difficult to evaluate with the concurrent myotonia and until after muscle warmup. Repetitive stimulation may demonstrate a decrement of the evoked compound muscle action potential as a result of the refractory nature of the individual muscle fibers to repetitive discharge. The decrement increases with the rate of stimulation and does not tend to diminish toward the end of the train of stimulation.

Paramyotonia Congenita

Originally described by Eulenburg, this is a rare disorder of autosomal dominant inheritance (38). Clinically, the myotonia is dramatically increased by the cold, and some individuals only have myotonia after cold exposure. The myotonia is usually most prominent in the face and upper extremities. Unlike other disorders characterized by myotonia, repetitive activity may make the myotonia worse and can provoke weakness in some individuals. These episodes of weakness can resemble those seen in hyperkalemic periodic paralysis.

Electrical recordings reveal myotonic discharges. Unlike in the other disorders characterized by myotonia, with cooling, the discharges disappear despite increased stiffness (49). A simple test to distinguish paramyotonia congenita from myotonia congenita is to immerse the patient's hand in ice water for 10 minutes (91). In paramyotonia, the myotonic discharges disappear, and the muscle goes into a stiff electrically silent contracture. In myotonia congenita, the myotonic activity increases and recruitment is unchanged. Repetitive stimulation and intense exercise result in a decrement of the evoked compound muscle action potential most easily seen at high rates of stimulation of 25 to 50 Hz (17, 116).

Hyperkalemic Periodic Paralysis

Hyperkalemic periodic paralysis or adynamia episodica hereditaria is characterized by episodes of weakness or paralysis associated with an elevation of the serum potassium (43, 78). The disorder is autosomal dominant, affects both sexes equally, and can appear in early infancy. It presents as attacks of paralysis or weakness usually lasting less than 1 hour. Although the exact mechanism of weakness is unknown, it is most likely induced by a release of intramuscular potassium. The episodes of weakness are frequently associated with myotonia and seem to occur with exposure to cold, rest following vigorous exercise, or after potassium loading. During the attack, spontaneous discharges, positive sharp waves, and fibrillation potentials are recorded. MUAPs reveal a loss of muscle fibers per motor unit with low amplitude, short duration, and increased polyphasia (16). Recruitment demonstrates a marked decrease in functioning MUAPs. Nerve stimulation will result in a reduced or absent muscle response depending on the extent of the paralysis. Between attacks, MUAPs are usually normal or slightly reduced in duration. Nerve stimulation studies between attacks are normal.

Several families have been described who have hyperkalemic periodic paralysis with clinically prominent myotonia (44, 121). The author has been following a family in whom several affected members have significant neck hypertrophy as a result of the myotonia. The presence of myotonia in many affected individuals with this disorder has raised the question of a relationship between this disorder and paramyotonia congenita (41). Indeed, some families' specific hereditary defect may cause some overlapping between the myotonias and the periodic paralysis. Acetazolamide, which is effective in the prophylaxis of periodic paralysis, however, has been shown to produce severe weakness in a patient with paramyotonia congenita, implying that the disorders are indeed distinct (104). Normokalemic periodic paralysis has been described in a few cases and appears to resemble hyperkalemic periodic paralysis closely, except for the lack of a rise of the serum potassium during attacks (101).

Hypokalemic Periodic Paralysis

Hypokalemic periodic paralysis, also an autosomal dominant disorder, affects males more than females and has an onset usually in the teens (33, 36). In this condition, the paralysis tends to occur with rest following exercise, early morning walking, or a heavy sodium or carbohydrate meal. Weakness starts in the legs and progresses to involve the trunk and arms. During attacks, which usually last less than 1 day, the serum potassium is low, and there is a dropout of MUAPs with contraction. Insertional abnormalities on EMG are not recorded. During a severe attack, nerve stimulation reveals no muscle response. Abnormalities of repetitive stimulation are dependent on the degree of weakness of the recording muscle (18).

Syndrome of Diffuse Abnormal Insertional Activity

The author has observed a total of 20 patients to date who demonstrate the diffuse presence of provoked positive sharp waves in almost all muscles (130, 131). The positive sharp waves vary in frequency but not in amplitude and tend to be descrescendo in nature. Their number varies from time to time, from muscle to muscle, and in different locations of the same muscle. Fasciculation potentials are not found, and MUAPs are normal. Nerve conduction studies and repetitive stimulation studies are also normal. Three of the patients said that on occasion they had difficulty releasing their grip after holding on for long periods of time with full tension. This phenomenon could not be reproduced clinically, nor was there any clinical or electrical evidence of myotonia in other muscles. In families in whom we were able to examine completely at least two generations, an autosomal dominant inheritance was demonstrated. There are no abnormalities on clinical exam, and the EMG abnormality of provoked positive sharp waves was detected when the patient was referred to rule out an unrelated problem, such as a possible radiculopathy following trauma. Extensive laboratory studies have been normal. Muscle biopsy in four patients has been normal with the normal presence of Type IIB fibers. This seemingly insignificant muscle membrane abnormality is of importance only to the patient who unfortunately goes through endless testing until the syndrome is recognized.

METABOLIC MYOPATHIES

Disorders of the metabolism of glycogen and lipids can result in a myopathy. These rare disorders are usually the result of a genetic defect in the enzyme system that makes glycogen available for intense initial rapid exercise, blood glucose available for continued intense activity, and free fatty acids available for low intensity endurance activity. Although the clinical, laboratory, and EMG data are helpful, the disorders can only be confirmed by demonstrating the specific biochemical defect in the muscle or other tissue. The disorders of glycogen and lipid metabolism have no specific clinical presentation, but in general present with either progressive weakness or recurrent muscle aching or cramps frequently associated with myoglobinuria. Although the number of abnormalities of glycogen and lipid metabolism continue to increase as isolated cases of new enzyme deficiencies appear, only those disorders that are substantiated by multiple cases in several different families that have significant EMG abnormalities are discussed here.

Acid Maltase Deficiency

Referred to as Pompe's disease when occurring in infancy, this autosomal recessive disorder is characterized by an accumulation of glycogen in tissue lysosomes (34, 60). This is a devastating disease involving many organ systems. The infant appears normal for several weeks and then develops weakness, cardiomegaly, and hepatomegaly. The respiratory muscles become affected as the weakness progresses. These children usually die in the first year of life. A more benign form of disease occurs in childhood and later life clinically with proximal muscle weakness (24, 34). A vacuolar myopathy is seen with muscle biopsy.

EMG demonstrates a tremendous amount of spontaneous and abnormal insertional activity including not only positive sharp waves and fibrillation potentials, but also myotonic discharges and complex repetitive potentials (34, 62). MUAPs are of low amplitude, short duration, and polyphasic shape. Recruitment early of additional MUAPs is seen with increasing strength of voluntary contractions.

Debrancher Deficiency

This autosomal recessive enzyme deficiency of glycogenosis results in the accumulation of glycogen in the liver, the limb, and cardiac muscles. Typically, the child is hypotonic with proximal weakness, hypoglycemic, and has failure to thrive (40). Although the child may improve clinically, distal weakness may also develop as time passes. An adult form of the disorder is seen with distal weakness and atrophy (13, 23). Muscle biopsy demonstrates vacuoles in the subsarcolemma. EMG demonstrates abundant positive sharp waves and fibrillation potentials with complex repetitive potentials. Short duration and reduced amplitude MUAPs have been reported.

Myophosphorylase Deficiency

This disorder, originally described by McArdle and called McArdle's disease for many years, is usually inherited as an autosomal recessive condition, although autosomal dominant inheritance has been described (19, 82).

In this disorder, there is a defect in myophosphorylase that results in the inability to convert muscle glycogen to glucose. This is of clinical significance during vigorous exercise or heavy work, especially under ischemic conditions. The disorder typically presents as progressive fatigue and muscle cramping in early childhood. A wide variability of symptoms exists, and some patients do not experience cramps until young adulthood. With a severe cramp there can be resultant muscle cell injury expressed as myoglobinuria. The cramps are painful, and if exercises are slowed and the muscles are slowly stretched, the pain will decrease and activity can be continued. If the muscles are not stretched, the cramps can last for several hours. Some patients may develop a proximal muscle weakness with age, whereas others continue to have normal strength. Ischemic exercise testing demonstrates a loss of the normal rise in blood lactate (89). The diagnosis is confirmed by a biochemical analysis of phosphorylase activity in muscle. The cramped muscle is in a true contracture and is electrically silent on EMG. Positive sharp waves and fibrillation potentials may be recorded, as well as MUAPs of short duration, implying a loss of muscle fibers per motor units. These EMG abnormalities are not seen in all patients and, no doubt, reflect the degree of muscle cell damage.

Phosphofructokinase Deficiency

This very rare autosomal recessive disorder results in the inability to convert fructose-6-phosphate to fructose-1-6-diphosphate. This disorder was first described by Tarui and has been called Tarui disease (79, 117). This enzyme defect is a more distal step in the entry of glucose into the glycolytic pathway than myophosphorylase, but clinically and electromyographically they are essentially the same condition. Pretreatment of patients with McArdle's myophosphorylase deficiency with glucagon improves their muscle symptoms with exercise, whereas in Tarui's phosphofructokinase deficiency, no improvement occurs (85). This difference is most likely due to the fact that blood glucose enters the glycolytic pathway below the myophosphorylase defect, but above the phosphofructokinase abnormality.

Carnitine Deficiency

Carnitine is the transporter of medium and long chain fatty acids across the inner mitochondrial membrane. It is synthesized predominantly in the liver, but is also available in certain foods. With prolonged fasting or prolonged exercise of greater than 40 minutes, the muscle relies on free fatty acids as a fuel source. Carnitine is therefore necessary for continued normal muscle function. Carnitine deficiency appears to result in two main syndromes.

Myopathic carnitine deficiency is characterized by a reduced concentration of carnitine in muscle but normal or slightly decreased concentration in serum (25). Clinically, a proximal limb-girdle type weakness begins in childhood and is slowly progressive. Creatine kinase is elevated in most patients. Biopsy reveals a marked accumulation of lipid droplets that are most prominent in Type I muscle. EMG demonstrates MUAPs of low amplitude, short duration, increased polyphasic shape, and an increased recruitment per strength of contraction. Positive sharp waves, fibrillation potentials, and complex repetitive potentials are recorded in most patients.

Systemic carnitine deficiency is characterized by a low carnitine concentration in serum and muscle, implying a defect in liver biosynthesis (25, 70). These patients have a systemic form of liver dysfunction with hepatic encephalopathy. Associated with the proximal limb-girdle type weakness may also be cardiac and respiratory muscle involvement. The disorder appears to be of autosomal recessive inheritance. Mixed forms of systemic and myopathic types exist. EMG abnormalities are the same as in the myopathic form.

Carnitine Palmityltransferase Deficiency

Carnitine palmityltransferase is an enzyme necessary to allow carnitine to transfer fatty acids across the inner mitochondrial membranes. It exists in several different forms. Clinically, this disorder is characterized by muscle pains and recurrent myoglobinuria beginning in childhood that are usually precipitated by prolonged fasting and/or exercise (25). Unlike myophosphorylase deficiency, there is no difficulty with sudden vigorous, short duration activity and cramps are unusual. It appears to be of autosomal recessive inheritance. EMG in the majority of cases studied has been normal, although an increase in polyphasic MUAPs and high frequency repetitive discharges have been reported (5).

References

1. Arundell F, Wilkinson R, Haserick J: Dermatomyositis and malignant neoplasms in adults. *Arch Derm* 82:772, 1960.
2. Barnes B: Dermatomyositis and malignancy. *Ann Intern Med* 84:68, 1976.
3. Becker P: Eine neve x-chromosomale muskeldystrophie. *Arch Psychiat Nervenkr* 193:427, 1955.
4. Becker P: Generalized non-dystrophic myotonia. In Desmedt J (ed): *New Developments in Electromyography and Clinical Neurophysiology*, vol 1. Basel, S Karger, 1973, p 407.
5. Bertorini T, et al: Carnitine palmityl transferase deficiency: myoglobinuria and respiratory failure. *Neurology* 30:263, 1980.
6. Bosch E, Yamada T, Kimura J: Somatosensory evoked potentials in motor neuron disease. *Muscle Nerve* 8:556, 1985.
7. Bradley W, Good P, Rasool C, Adelman L: Morphometric and biochemical studies of peripheral nerve in amyotrophic lateral sclerosis. *Ann Neurol* 14:267, 1983.

8. Brain W, Croft P, Wilkinson M: Motor neuron disease as a manifestation of neoplasm. *Brain* 88:479, 1965.
9. Bray G, Kaarsoo N, Ross T: Ocular myopathy with dysphagia. *Neurology* 15:678, 1965.
10. Leading article: paralysis in herpes zoster. *Br Med* 2:ii, 1970.
11. Brody J, Hirano A, Scutt R: Recent neuropathologic observations in amyotrophic lateral sclerosis and parkinsonism-dementia of Guam. *Neurology* 21:528, 1971.
12. Brooke M: A neuromuscular disease characterized by fiber type disproportion. In Kakulas B (ed): *Clinical Studies in Myology.* Amsterdam, Excerpta Medica, 1973, p 295.
13. Brunberg J, McCormick W, Schochet S: Type III glycogenosis: an adult with diffuse weakness and muscle wasting. *Arch Neurol* 25:171, 1971.
14. Buchthal F, Olsen P: Electromyography and muscle biopsy in infantile spinal muscular atrophy. *Brain* 93:15, 1970.
15. Buchthal F, Pinelli P: Muscle action potentials in polymyositis. *Neurology* 3:424, 1953.
16. Buchthal F, Engaek L, Gamstorp I: Paresis and hyperexcitability in adynamia episodica hereditaria. *Neurology* 8:347, 1958.
17. Burke D, Skuse N, Lethvean A: Contractile properties of the abductor digiti minimi muscle in paramyotonia congenita. *J Neurol Neurosurg Psychiat* 37:894, 1974.
18. Campa J, Sanders D: Familial hypokalemic periodic paralysis, local recovery after nerve stimulation. *Arch Neurol* 31:110, 1974.
19. Chui L, Munsat T: Dominant inheritance of McArdle syndrome. *Arch Neurol* 33:636, 1976.
20. Crews J, Kaiser K, Brooke M: Muscle pathology of myotonia congenita. *J Neurol Sci* 28:449, 1976.
21. Desmedt J, Borenstein S: Relationship of spontaneous fibrillation potentials to muscle fiber segmentation in human muscular dystrophy. *Nature* 258:531, 1975.
22. Devere R, Bradley W: Polymyositis: its presentation, morbidity and mortality. *Brain* 98:637, 1975.
23. Dimuro S: DeBrancher deficiency: neuromuscular disorder in five adults. *Ann Neurol* 5:422, 1978.
24. Dimuro S, et al: Adult onset acid maltese deficiency: a postmortem study. *Muscle Nerve* 1:27, 1978.
25. Dimuro S, Trevisan C, Hays A: Disorders of lipid metabolism in muscle. *Muscle Nerve* 3:369, 1980.
26. Does De Willebois A, Bethlem J, Meyer A, Simons A: Distal myopathy with onset in early infancy. *Neurology* 18:383, 1968.
27. Drachman D: Ophthalmoplegia plus. *Arch Neurol* 18:654, 1968.
28. Dubowitz V, Brooke M: *Muscle Biopsy: A Modern Approach.* London, W.B. Saunders, 1973.
29. Dubowitz V, Roy S: Central core disease of muscle: clinical, histochemical and electron microscope studies of an affected motor and child. *Brain* 93:133, 1970.
30. Dyck P, Stevens J, Mulder D, Espinosa R: Frequency of nerve fiber degeneration of peripheral motor and sensory neurons in amyotrophic lateral sclerosis. *Neurology* 25:781, 1975.
31. Eaton L: Perspective of neurology in regard to polymyositis: study of 41 cases. *Neurology* 4:245, 1954.
32. Edstrom L: Histochemical and histopathological changes in skeletal muscle in late-onset hereditary distal myopathy. *J Neurol Sci* 26:147, 1975.
33. Engel A, Lambert E: Calcium activation of electrically inexcitable muscle fibers in primary hypokalemic periodic paralysis. *Neurology* 19:851, 1969.

34. Engel A, et al: The spectrum and diagnosis of acid maltase deficiency. *Neurology* 23:95, 1973.
35. Engel A, Gomez M, Seybold M, Lambert E: The spectrum and diagnosis of acid maltase deficiency. *Neurology* 23:95, 1973.
36. Engel A, Lambert E, Rosevear T, Tauxe M: Clinical and electromyographic studies in a patient with primary hypokalemic periodic paralysis. *Am J Med* 38:626, 1965.
37. Engel W, Linton L, Bradley J: Fasciculating progressive muscular atrophy (F-PMA) remarkably responsive to antidysimmune treatment (Adit)—a possible clue to more ordinary ALS. *Neurology* 35(suppl 1):72, 1985.
38. Eulenburg A: Ueber eine familiare durch 6 generationen verfolgbare form congenitaler paramyotonie. *Neurologisches Centralblatt* 5:265, 1886.
39. Fenichel G, Emery E, Hunt P: Neurogenic atrophy simulating facioscapulohumeral dystrophy. *Arch Neurol* 17:257, 1967.
40. Forbes G: Glycogen storage disease: report of a case with abnormal glycogen structure in liver and skeletal muscle. *J Pediatr* 42:645, 1953.
41. French E, Kilpatrick R: A variety of paramyotonia congenita. *J Neurol Neurosurg Psychiat* 20:40, 1957.
42. Furukawa T, Tsukagosht H, Sugita H, Toyokura Y: Neurogenic muscular atrophy simulating facioscapulohumeral muscular dystrophy. *J Neurol Sci* 9:389, 1969.
43. Gamstorp I: Adynamia episodica hereditaria. *Acta Scand Paed* 45(suppl 108):1, 1956.
44. Gamstorp I: Adynamia episodica hereditaria and myotonia. *Acta Neurol Scand* 39:41, 1963.
45. Gamstorp I: Progressive spinal muscular atrophy with onset in infancy or early childhood. *Acta Paed Scand* 56:408, 1967.
46. Gardner J, Feldmahn A: Hereditary adult motor neuron disease: report of 154 year genealogy with eighteen cases. *Trans Am Neurol Assoc* 91:239, 1966.
47. Goldblatt D: Motor neuron disease: historic introduction. In Norris F, Kurkland L (eds): *Motor Neuron Diseases: Research on Amyotrophic Lateral Sclerosis and Related Disorders.* New York, Grune & Stratton, 1969, pp 3–11.
48. Gordon I, Tucker J: Lesions of the central nervous system in herpes zoster. *J Neurol Neurosurg Psychiat* 8:40, 1945.
49. Haass A, et al: Clinical study of paramyotonia congenita with and without myotonia in a warm environment. *Muscle Nerve* 4:388, 1981.
50. Halstead L, Wiechers D: *Late Effects of Poliomyelitis.* Miami, FL, Miami Symposia Foundation, 1984.
51. Halstead L, Wiechers D, Rossi C: Late effects of poliomyelitis. Part II: results of a survey of 201 polio survivors. *South Med J* 78:1281, 1985.
52. Harding A, Thomas P: Hereditary distal spinal muscular atrophy. A report on 34 cases and a review of the literature. *J Neurol Sci* 45:337, 1980.
53. Harper P: *Myotonic Dystrophy.* Philadelphia, W B Saunders, 1979.
54. Harper P: Presymptomatic detection and genetic counseling in myotonic dystrophy. *Clin Genet* 4:134, 1973.
55. Hausmanowa-Petrusewicz I, Karwanska A: Electromyographic findings in different forms of infantile and juvenile proximal spinal muscular atrophy. *Muscle Nerve* 9:37, 1986.
56. Hausmanowa-Petrusewicz I, Fidzianska-Polot A: Clinical features of infantile and juvenile spinal muscular atrophy. In Gamstorp I, Sarnat H, (eds): *Progressive Spinal Muscular Atrophies.* New York, Raven Press, 1984, p 31.
57. Hausmanowa-Petrusewicz I, Drac E, Sawick E, Kopec J: The possible mechanism of the motor conduction velocity changes in the anterior horn cells involvement. (electrophysiological and histological studies). In Hausmanowa-Petrusewicz I, Je-

drzejowska H (eds): *Structure and Function of Normal and Diseased Muscle and Peripheral Nerve, Proceedings of the Symposium in Kazimerz Upon Vistula.* Poland, Polish Medical Publishers, 357, 1972.

58. Hawkes C, Absolon M: Myotubular myopathy associated with cataract and electrical myotonia. *J Neurol Neurosurg Psychiat* 38:761, 1975.
59. Henriksson K, Stalberg E: The terminal innervation pattern in polymyositis: a histochemical and SFEMG study. *Muscle Nerve* 1:3, 1978.
60. Hers H: a-Glacosidase deficiency in generalized glycogen storage disease (Pompe's disease). *Biochem J* 86:11, 1963.
61. Hilton-Brown P, Stalberg E, Tronteli J, Mihelin M: Cause of the increased fiber density in muscular dystrophies studied with single fiber EMG during electrical stimulation. *Muscle Nerve* 8:383, 1985.
62. Hogan G, Gutmann L, Schmidt R, Gilbert E: Pompe's disease. *Neurology* 19:894, 1969.
63. Horstman D: Epidemiology of poliomyelitis and allied diseases. *Yale J Biol Med* 36:5, 1963.
64. Isaacs H, Heffron J, Badenhorst M: Central core disease. *J Neurol Neurosurg Psychiat* 38:1177, 1975.
65. James C, Lassman L: Diastematomyelia. *Arch Dis Child* 39:125, 1964.
66. Johnson E: Pathokinesiology of Duchenne muscular dystrophy: implications for management. *Arch Phys Med* 58:4, 1977.
67. Juergens S, Kurkland L, Okazaki H, Mulder D: Amyotrophic lateral sclerosis in Rochester, Minnesota, 1925–1977. *Neurology* 30:463, 1980.
68. Kaeser H: Scapuloperoneal muscular atrophy. *Brain* 88:407, 1965.
69. Karpati G, et al: The Kearns-Shy syndrome. A multisystem disease with mitochondrial abnormality demonstrated in skeletal muscle and skin. *J Neurol Sci* 19:133, 1973.
70. Karpati G, et al: The syndrome of systemic carnitine deficiency. *Neurology* 25:16, 1975.
71. Kearns T: External opthalmoplegia, pigmentary degeneration of the retina and cardiomyopathy: a newly recognized syndrome. *Trans Am Opthalmol Soc* 63:559, 1965.
72. Kiloh L, Nevin S: Progressive dystrophy of the external ocular muscles (ocular myopathy). *Brain* 74:115, 1951.
73. Kugelberg E, Welander L: Heredofamilial juvenile muscular atrophy simulating muscular dystrophy. *Arch Neurol Psychiat* 75:500, 1956.
74. Kuitunen P, Rapola J, Noponen A, Donner M: Nemaline myopathy. *Acta Paed Scand* 61:353, 1972.
75. Kurkland L, Mulder D: Epidemologic investigations of amyotrophic lateral sclerosis. 1. Preliminary report on geographic distribution, with special reference to the Mariana Islands, including clinical and pathologic observations. *Neurology* 4:355, 438, 1954.
76. Kurkland L, Mulder D: Epidemiologic investigations of amyotrophic lateral sclerosis. 2. Familial aggregations indicative of dominant inheritance. *Neurology* 5:182, 249, 1955.
77. Lambert E, Mulder D: Electromyographic studies in amyotrophic lateral sclerosis. *Proc Staff Meet Mayo Clinic* 32:441, 1957.
78. Layzer R, Lovelace R, Rowland L: Hyperkalemic periodic paralysis. *Arch Neurol* 16:455, 1967.
79. Layzer R, Rowland L, Ranney H: Muscle phosphofructokinase deficiency. *Arch Neurol* 17:512, 1967.
80. Maier J, et al: Radiation myelitis of the dorsolumbar spinal cord. *Radiology* 93:153, 1969.

81. Markesberry W, Griggs R, Leach P, Lapham L: Late onset hereditary distal myopathy. *Neurology* 24:127, 1974.
82. McArdle B: Myopathy due to a defect in muscle glycogen breakdown. *Clin Sci* 10:13, 1951.
83. Medsger T, Dawson W, Masi A: The epidemiology of polymyositis. *Am J Med* 48:715, 1970.
84. Medsger R, Demester J, Martin J: Neurogenic scapuloperoneal syndrome in childhood. *J Neurol Neurosurg Psychiat* 43:888, 1980.
85. Mineo I, et al: A comparative study on glucagon effect between McArdle disease and Tarui disease. *Muscle Nerve* 7:552, 1984.
86. Mitchell D, Olczak S: Remission of a syndrome indistinguishable from motor neuron disease after resection of bronchial carcinoma. *Br Med J* 2:176, 1979.
87. Mulder DW: *The Diagnosis and Treatment of Amyotrophic Lateral Sclerosis.* Boston, Houghton-Mifflin Professional Publishers, 1980.
88. Mulder D, Espinosa R: Amyotrophic lateral sclerosis: comparison of the clinical syndrome in Guam and the United States. In Norris F, Kurkland L (eds): *Motor Neuron Diseases: Research on Amyotrophic Lateral Sclerosis and Related Disorders.* New York, Grune & Stratton, 1969, pp 12–19.
89. Munsat T: A standardized forearm ischemic exercise test. *Neurology* 20:1171, 1970.
90. Neville H, Brooke M: Central core fibers; structured and unstructured. In Kakolas B (ed): *Basic Research in Myology.* Amsterdam, Excerpta Media, 1973.
91. Nielsen V, Friis M, Johnsen T: Electromyographic distinction between paramyotonia congenita and myotonia congenita: effect of cold. *Neurology* 32:827, 1982.
92. Norris F, Engel W: Carcinomatous amyotrophic lateral sclerosis. In Brain W, Norris F (eds): *The Remote Effects of Cancer on the Nervous System.* New York, Grune & Stratton, 1965, p 81.
93. Okuno T, et al: Myotonic dystrophy and hyperthroidism. *Neurology* 31:91, 1981.
94. Olson W, et al: Oculocraniosomatic neuromuscular disease with "ragged-red" fibers. *Arch Neurol* 26:193, 1972.
95. Paralytic poliomyelitis—United States, 1982 and 1983. *Mort Morb Weekly Rep* 33:635, 1984.
96. Parry G, Hultz S, Ben-Zeev D, Drori J: Gammopathy with proximal motor axonopathy simulating motor neuron disease. *Neurology* 36:273, 1986.
97. Patten B: Neuropathy and motor neuron syndromes associated with plasma cell disease. *Acta Neurol Scand* 69:47, 1984.
98. Pearn J, Hudgson P: Distal spinal muscular atrophy—a clinical and genetic study of 8 kindreds. *J Neurol Sci* 43:183, 1979.
99. Pearson C: Polymyositis. *Ann Rev Med* 17:63, 1966.
100. Peters H, Clatanoff D: Spinal muscular atrophy secondary to macroglobulinemia: reversal of symptoms with chlorambucil therapy. *Neurology* 18:101, 1968.
101. Poskanzer D, Kerr D: A third type of periodic paralysis with normokalemia and a favourable response to sodium chloride. *Am J Med* 31:328, 1961.
102. Prosser E, Murphy E, Thompson M: Intelligence and the gene for Duchenne muscular dystrophy. *Arch Dis Child* 44:221, 1969.
103. Ricker K, Mertens H, Schimrigk K: The neurogenic scapulo-peroneal syndrome. *Eur Neurol* 1:257, 1968.
104. Riggs J, Griggs R, Moxley R: Acetazolamide-induced weakness in paramyotonia congenita. *Ann Intern Med* 86:169, 1977.
105. Rowland L, et al: Macroglobulinemia with peripheral neuropathy simulating motor neuron disease. *Ann Neurol* 11:532, 1982.
106. Rydin E, Stalberg E, Sanders D: Dynamic changes of the motor unit in amyotrophic lateral sclerosis. *EEG Clin Neurophysiol* 56:S164, 1983.

107. Sadowsky C, Sachs E, Ochoa J: Post-radiation motor neuron syndrome. *Arch Neurol* 33:786, 1976.
108. Schmalbruch H: Regeneration muscle fibers in Duchenne muscular dystrophy: a serial section study. *Neurology* 34:60, 1984.
109. Shafiq S, Dubowitz V, Peterson H, Milhorat A: Nemaline myopathy: report of a fatal case, with histochemical and electron microscope studies. *Brain* 90:817, 1967.
110. Shy G, Engle W, Somers J, Wanko T: Nemaline Myopathy; a new congenital myopathy. *Brain* 86:293, 1963.
111. Shy M, Magee K: A new congenital non-progressive myopathy. *Brain* 79:610, 1956.
112. Shy M, Trojaborg W, et al: Motor neuron disease and plasma cell dyscrasia. *Neurology* 35 (suppl 1):107, 1985.
113. Spiro A, Shy G, Gonatas N: Myotubular myopathy. *Arch Neurol* 14:1, 1966.
114. Stalberg E, Trontelj J: *Single Fiber Electromyography*, Old Working United Kingdom, Mirvalle Press, 1979, p 112.
115. Stalberg E, Schwartz M, Trontelj J: Single fiber electromyography in various processes affecting the anterior horn cell. *J Neurol Sci* 24:403, 1975.
116. Subramony S, Malhotra C, Mischra S: Distinguishing paramyotonia congenita and myotonia congenita by electromyography. *Muscle Nerve* 6:374, 1983.
117. Tarui S, Okuno G, Ikura Y: Phosphofructokinase deficiency in skeletal muscle: a new type of glycogenosis. *Biochem Biophys Res Commun* 19:517, 1965.
118. Thomas J, Howard F: Segmental zoster paresis—a disease profile. *Neurology* 22:459, 1972.
119. Thomsen J: Tonische Krampfe in Willkurlich Beweglichen Muskeln in Folge von Ererbter Psychischer Disposition. *Arch Psych Nervenka* 6:702, 1876.
120. Trojabrg W, Buchthal F: Malignant and benign fasciculations. *Acta Neurol Scand* 41(suppl 13):251, 1965.
121. Van Der Meulen J, Gilbert G, Kane C: Familial hyperkalemic paralysis with myotonia. *N Engl J Med* 264:1, 1961.
122. Van Wijngaarden G, Fluery T, Bethlem J, Meijer A: Familial myotubular myopathy. *Neurology* 10:901, 1969.
123. Victor M, Hayes R, Adams R: Oculopharyngeal muscular dystrophy: a familial disease of late life characterized by dysphagia and progressive ptosis of the eyelids. *N Engl J Med* 267:1267, 1962.
124. Weiss S, Streifer M, Weiser H: Motor lesions in herpes zoster. *Eur Neurol* 13:332, 1975.
125. Welander L: Myopathia distalis tarda hereditaria. *Acta Med Scand* 141(suppl 256):1, 1951.
126. Welch K, Goldberg D: Serum creatine phosphokinase in motor neuron disease. *Neurology* 22:697, 1972.
127. Wiechers D: Acute and latent effects of poliomyelitis on the motor unit as revealed by electromyography. *Orthopedics* 8:870, 1985.
128. Wiechers D, Hubbell S: Late changes in the motor unit after acute poliomyelitis. *Muscle Nerve* 4:524, 1981.
129. Wiechers D, Johnson E: Characteristics of malignant fasciculations. *EEG Clin Neurophysiol* 49:17, 1980.
130. Wiechers D, Johnson E: Diffuse abnormal electromyographic insertional activity: a preliminary report. *Arch PM&R* 60:420, 1979.
131. Wiechers D, Johnson E: Syndrome of diffuse abnormal insertional activity. *Arch PM&R* 63:538, 1982.
132. Wiener L, Stohlman S, Davis R: Attempts to demonstrate virus in amyotrophic lateral sclerosis. *Neurology* 30:1319, 1980.
133. Winkelmann R, Mulder D, Lambert E, Howard F, Diessner G: Dermatomyositis-

polymyositis: comparison of untreated and cortisone-treated patients. *Mayo Clin Proc* 34:545, 1968.

134. Wohlfart G: Muscular atrophy in diseases of the lower motor neuron. *Arch Neurol Psychiat* 61:599, 1949.

135. Wohlfart G: Zwe Falle Von Dystrophia Musculorum Progressiva Mit Fibrillaren Zuchungen und Atypischen. *Muskelbefund Dentsch Z Nervenheilk* 153:189, 1942.

4

Motor and Sensory Conduction and Entrapment Syndromes

ROBERT J. WEBER

The first part of this chapter describes the physiology of nerve conduction, techniques for nerve stimulation, factors in recording evoked responses, and the interpretation of conduction results. The final portion covers conduction studies for specific nerves and entrapments, beginning with the upper extremity. Because the "basic science" sections are very helpful in interpreting clinical results, a complete review of the chapter is recommended before employing the techniques described.

Discoveries related to the functional anatomy and physiology of peripheral nerves are one of the major accomplishments of 20th-century medical science. Progress in this field has been closely linked with the development of new instrumentation, and the rapid development of computer technology will yield further advances, including information on the central control of peripheral nerve function. The reader is referred to Dr. Licht's excellent review of early developments in nerve conduction studies for an account of the history of our specialty (36). Many nerve conduction techniques rely on computer-based control or processing of data. Only a few of these techniques are now widely employed in practice, but others may be expected to enter general use. Further information on developments in computer-assisted conduction studies is available in Desmedt (15).

PHYSIOLOGY OF NERVE CONDUCTION

Past explanations for the acquisition of sensation and the control of movement in complex organisms were varied and imaginative. Both the need for an internal communication system and the fact that such a system would involve some form of electrical conduction seem natural to us today. It is well established that both sensory signals and motor and various other control signals are carried through a "hard wired" system of extensions from the cell bodies of the nervous system, the axon. *Axons* are fine tubes containing cytoplasm and organelles surrounded by a lipoprotein cell membrane. Mechanical transport of cell constituents is necessary to maintain the axon, but actual signal transmission is accomplished by means of an electrical depolarization wave moving along the cell membrane.

Transmission of a signal is possible because the neuron and axon maintain an ionic charge differential between the exterior and the interior of the cell of approximately -60 to -90 millivolts. The cell membrane separates the intra- and extracellular environments, preventing the charged proteinaceous molecules from leaving the cell and limiting the diffusion of electrolytic ions—principally potassium, sodium, chloride, and calcium—through it. This charge gradient (i.e., high extracellular $Na+$, $CL-$, high intracellular $K+$, $Ca++$) is maintained by an active transport system that is mediated by protein structures injected into the cell membrane. The electrical potential developed by this process is described by the Nernst equation.

These membrane "pores" regulate ionic flow and thus control membrane depolarization in order to produce a sustainable depolarization wave. Approximately 200 of these pores per square micron are found in unmyelinated axon membranes. The shape (i.e., opening or closing) of the pore is controlled by the electrical field surrounding the pore. Thus, ion flow through the pore is regulated by the membrane charge. The electrical field controlling pore activation and deactivation is affected by various physiologic or toxic molecules, permitting chemical mediation of initiation or blocking of the membrane depolarization wave. Once depolarization begins along the axon, the electrical field generated by ion flow at one point is sufficient to cause activation of the adjacent pore, resulting in the "rolling" movement of depolarization along the membrane.

In unmyelinated axons, the rate of propagation of the depolarization signal along the axon increases in proportion to the square root of the axon diameter. This increase results from two opposing factors—the larger an increase proportional to the increase in diameter because of reduced resistance to flow, counteracted by a decrease in the propagation rate because of increasing capacitance proportional to the increasing axon diameter. Bare axons must be of enormous diameter in order to conduct rapidly enough to permit control of complex body movements. Because this is not consistent with effective function in large organisms, their nerve fibers have fortunately been modified by the addition of an insulating myelin sheath that increases their conduction velocity.

Myelination is produced by supporting Schwann cells, which wrap a thin, membranous cellular process up to 100 times around the axon. Each of these insulated segments may be up to 2 mm in length and is separated from its neighbor by a micron-sized gap of bare axon, the *node of Ranvier*. Myelination tremendously increases the conduction rate along the nerve fiber by permitting the excitation-depolarization signal to jump from node of Ranvier to node of Ranvier (saltatory conduction), rather than conducting along each part of the membrane. This results in a conduction velocity of up to 100 meter/sec, compared to that of fractions of a meter/sec in unmyelinated axons.

In order to sustain saltatory conduction along the nerve, the depolarization flux at each node of Ranvier must produce a sufficient electrical field to cause depolarization (pore opening) at the adjacent node. This field intensity (degree of ion flux) is obtained by concentrating the ion-controlling pores at the nodes of Ranvier. Studies show essentially no pores in the internodal region, whereas densities of from 2–12,000 pores per square micron at the nodal gap have been estimated (9). These facts explain the sensitivity of nerve conduction to demyelination, because interference with the saltatory conduction severely slows conduction and the discontinuity of pores along the axon immediately after demyelination results in conduction block.

Peripheral nerves are composed of mixtures of large-diameter myelinated fibers, small-diameter myelinated fibers, and unmyelinated fibers. Nerve conduction studies examine only the very large-diameter, myelinated fibers. These are classified as A-type fibers, with afferents in the subgroups I and II and efferents in the subgroup alpha.

Each peripheral nerve is composed of thousands of individual nerve fibers (axon plus Schwann cell-myelin sheath). Within the nerve itself, the fibers are grouped into bundles (i.e., fascicles), each of which is surrounded by its own connective tissue sheath (perineurium). The median nerve at the wrist contains approximately 6000 individual fibers grouped into 150 fascicles, whereas the sciatic nerve contains as many as 175,000 individual fibers. Features of this anatomic arrangement are important in clinical decision making related to conduction studies.

Temporal Dispersion

Nerve conduction studies begin with a stimulus (usually electrical) that is sufficient to initiate simultaneous depolarization in all tested axons. Although only the large Type A nerve fibers are tested, even this "homogenous" collection of fibers contains significant variation in individual fiber conduction velocities. Therefore, the resultant depolarization wave conducted down the nerve does not arrive in perfect

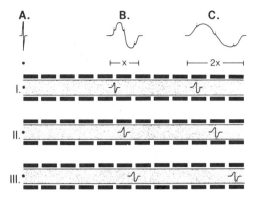

Figure 4.1. Temporal dispersion. Three axons of various conduction speeds, I (fastest) to III (slowest), are illustrated. The summated response of the signals from each of these axons is shown *(A* through *C)* at distances along the nerve. Conduction begins at the left and proceeds to the right. At point *A,* the signals in each axon arrive almost simultaneously, producing a very compact recorded response. At point *B,* the signals are less well synchronized, producing a smaller amplitude and longer duration response, and this spreading is increased by the time the signals arrive at point *C.* The greater the number of axons contributing to the signal, the smoother is the curve of the recorded evoked response.

synchronization at the recording electrode. Instead, arrival is "spread out" over a short period of time. This is referred to as *temporal dispersion* and is the reason that the evoked potential is not recorded as a single spike, but is seen as a bi- or multiphasic curve. The recorded signal is the algebraic summation of the biphasic spikes from each axon volume-conducted through body tissue to the recording electrode. The temporal dispersion of the recorded signal is proportional both to the range in conduction velocities of the nerve fibers that make up the peripheral nerve and to the distance over which the signal is conducted, i.e., the longer the nerve segment tested, the greater the temporal dispersion (Fig. 4.1). The amplitude of the recorded signal is also dependent upon the synchronization of the signal's arrival—the more synchronized the signal, the greater (more spike-like) the amplitude. Thus, amplitude varies inversely with the dispersion of the evoked response.

This normal dispersion of the signal is exaggerated by pathophysiologic processes, such as demyelination, remyelination, and axon regeneration, which increase desynchronization of the depolarization wave by slowing conduction in individual axons (increasing range of values). The increased temporal dispersion in the signal is often as clinically important as changes in the absolute nerve conduction velocity (fastest axon) in detecting abnormalities of nerve function.

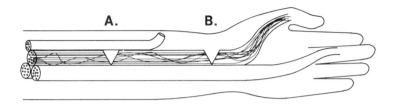

Figure 4.2. Hypothetical nerve in which all axons stay in a single fascicle until they exit the nerve. Note that a lesion at *A* or *B* would appear identical on EMG examination both on distal examination and on examination of the mid-forearm branch.

Fascicular Arrangement

One of the more important features of the fascicular arrangement of axons in nerves is that axons frequently shift from one fascicle to another, rather than following the same fascicle throughout the course of the nerve. This shifting disperses fibers throughout the nerve that supply a specific muscle or function, rather than permitting them to run as an isolated group throughout the course of the nerve. Such functionally related fibers only join into a discrete bundle a few centimeters proximal to the point at which they will exit from the nerve. Because of this dispersion of fibers, proximally located partial injuries of the nerve do not produce complete denervation in a narrowly isolated portion of the distal distribution of the nerve. Instead, abnormalities are seen throughout the distribution of the nerve below the level of the lesion, and this dispersion of findings below the point of injury is used clinically to localize the point of injury. Without it, localization would be impossible (Figs. 4.2 and 4.3).

Of lesser clinical importance is the fact that nerve fascicles located in the center of the nerve are less susceptible to compression from chronic entrapments than are those located around its periphery. This may result in the relative sparing of some functions of the nerve in entrapment syndromes when fibers serving these functions are centrally located at the level of the entrapment. This occurs occasionally in carpal tunnel syndrome, where the fibers serving the lumbricals may be centrally located at the point of entrapment as compared to the exiting fascicles to the thenar muscles.

Nerve Fiber Pathology

Individual nerve fibers undergo only a limited number of electrophysiologically demonstrable changes, which are detailed below. The proportion of fibers within the nerve exhibiting each of these changes will determine the findings in conduction studies, and the electromyogra-

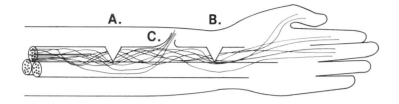

Figure 4.3. Typical nerve illustrating the movement of axons from one fascicle to another during their course. Here lesions at *A* and *B* may be easily distinguished electromyographically by the fact that lesion *A* produces changes in the distribution C, whereas the lesion at *B* does not.

pher must interpret these findings in a clinically useful form. The characteristics for each possible fiber status are listed below.

A *normal* nerve fiber is a metabolically intact, fully myelinated axon of normal diameter. The distance between nodes of Ranvier is normal, and the fiber conducts the depolarization wave through saltatory conduction.

A *neurapraxic* fiber (conduction block) is one in which transmission of the depolarization impulse is blocked over a short segment, but the viability of the axon is maintained. Normal signal propagation is possible in a neurapraxic axon above the area of the block and also below the area of the block, but not across the block (Fig. 4.4). Neurapraxia may persist for some time and then resolve or progress to axonotmesis. Causes include mechanical deformity of the fiber with "telescoping," as demonstrated in experimental tourniquet palsies (1) (Fig. 4.4) and demyelinated nerve segments in which no ion pores are present.

Axonotmesis (axon death) causes failure of axon conduction and therefore loss of the motor or sensory evoked response. Normal conduction of the nerve with stimulation below the point of nerve injury continues for at least 4 days following an axonotmetic injury. After this, the distal axon segment loses its ability to conduct (Wallerian degeneration) (Fig. 4.5). The response to electrical stimulation both above and below the lesion of neurapraxic and axonotmetic fibers is the same until after Wallerian degeneration occurs (Figs. 4.4A and 4.5A). Therefore, it is not possible to distinguish between a neurapraxic and axonotmetic fiber in a peripheral nerve for at least 4 days following injury.

Nerve fiber *demyelination* results in loss of saltatory depolarization with slowing or blocking of nerve conduction. The axon remains viable (Fig. 4.6). Studies in rat sciatic nerve have shown that conduction completely fails across fiber segments undergoing demyelination and remains blocked until several days after the complete removal of all myelin debris (Figs. 4.6A) (59). Waxman's computer simulations indi-

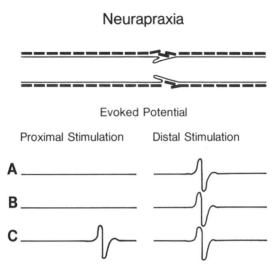

Figure 4.4 *A, B*, and *C* show the evoked responses from stimulation proximally and distally to the lesion: *A*, immediately postinjury; *B*, 7 days postinjury; *C*, some weeks following injury after neurapraxia has resolved.

cate that this failure of conduction may be secondary to impedance mismatch between the nonmyelinated fiber segment and the adjacent myelinated segments (60). Smith showed that conduction would resume when debris-free Schwann cells, but not necessarily myelin, were present (50). Computer simulations suggested that shortening the two internodes immediately preceding the demyelinated segment to one-third their normal length might eliminate the impedance mismatch and permit conduction. Recent studies suggest that insertion of membrane pores in the denuded segments is required to restore conduction.

Remyelination is a repair process in which Schwann cells restore the myelin coating of the axon (Fig. 4.7). Remyelinated fibers have a thinner myelin sheath and shorter-than-normal distances between the nodes of Ranvier. Although remyelination restores saltatory conduction, the thinner myelin and shorter internode distance result in a less-than-normal conduction velocity.

Axon regeneration can successfully occur in nerve fibers that have undergone Wallerian degeneration, provided that the support architecture of the nerve is preserved to channel regrowth. Regeneration produces smaller diameter, more thinly myelinated axons with shorter internodal distances. Therefore, conduction in these fibers remains below normal values (Fig. 4.8).

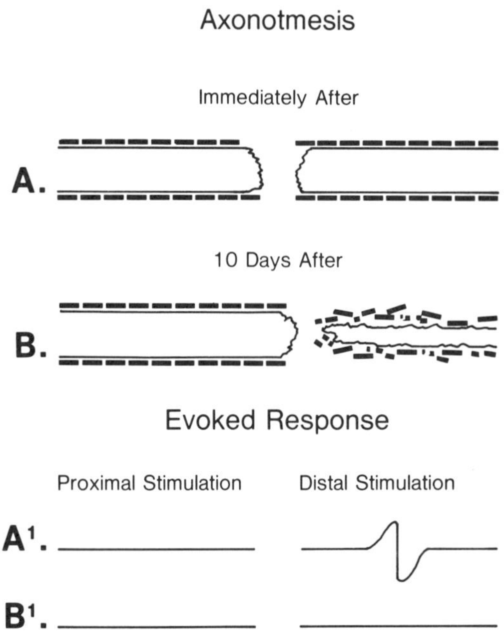

Axonotmesis

Immediately After

10 Days After

Evoked Response

Proximal Stimulation   Distal Stimulation

Figure 4.5. Axonotmetic lesion with axon changes demonstrated *A,* immediately after injury and *B,* 10 days after injury. The evoked response obtained by stimulation proximally and distally to the lesion at the corresponding times *(A¹ and B¹)* are demonstrated below.

Composite Action Potential

Clinical conduction studies are performed on nerves containing thousands of individual axons, not on individual nerve fibers. The recorded potential is a composite of the contributions from each of the large Type A fibers stimulated (Fig. 4.1). Although conduction along a single axon is an all-or-nothing phenomenon, conduction along a nerve can show gradations of abnormality, with conduction in some axons blocked, some slowed, and some normal. The amplitude, duration, and number of phases of the composite action potential are determined by the proportion of the type of fibers present.

Nerve function is tested by stimulating the nerve at points above and below the injury or entrapment site and observing the evoked responses. In general, conduction slowing occurs when axons are demyelinated, have remyelinated, or have regenerated. If all of the axons in the nerve are affected, the conduction velocity across the segment will be slowed; however, if even a few normal axons are present, normal velocity will be maintained. However, an increase in temporal dis-

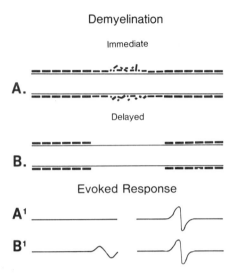

Figure 4.6. Demyelination pictured immediately following the onset of injury *(A, A¹)* and some weeks later *(B, B¹)* after myelin debris has been removed. The evoked responses with stimulation proximal to and distal to the lesion are demonstrated at *A¹* and *B¹* below.

persion of the compound action potential across the lesion will be observed whenever a significant number of damaged fibers are present. In those cases, the amplitude of the proximally generated evoked response will be smaller and its duration longer than that obtained with distal stimulation.

Because axonotmesis and neurapraxia produce conduction block, the evoked potential produced by stimulation proximal to the lesion is smaller (or absent) than that produced by stimulation distal to the lesion immediately after injury. They differ in that, after 4 days have passed, the axonotmetic axons will no longer produce a response when stimulated distal to the lesion because they will have undergone conduction failure (Wallerian degeneration) by that time. In contrast, neurapraxic fibers will continue to conduct when stimulated distal to the level of the lesion and will remain excitable until they recover (or are further injured and die) (Figs. 4.5B and 4.4C).

General Factors Affecting Nerve Conduction

Temperature

There is a direct relationship between intraneural temperature and conduction *velocity* of myelinated nerves throughout the physiologic

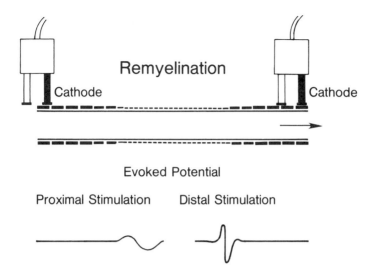

Figure 4.7. Remyelinated axon: note the decreased internodal distance and decreased thickness of myelin. The evoked potential with stimulation above and below the lesion that would be obtained from a nerve with all axons remyelinated is seen at bottom. Conduction is slowed, and the response is temporally dispersed across the lesion.

temperature range. Henriksen reported a drop in conduction velocity of approximately 2.4 m/sec for every degree centigrade of temperature decrease in the forearm (measured by needle thermistor at a depth of 2 cm) (24). Johnson, using intramuscular temperature, found a decrease of 5% per degree centigrade (29). Haller found a linear correlation in normals among skin, subcutaneous, and intramuscular temperatures of the calf with various induced temperatures (23). He suggested that the skin temperature be measured 15 cm proximal to the medial malleolus and that an arithmetic correction for conduction velocity then be made to an equivalent of 32° C.

Arithmetic correction for temperature is effective for small variations from normal, but may have drawbacks in circumstances where the temperature is significantly lower. The correlation in normals be-

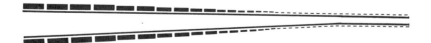

Figure 4.8. Axon regeneration: Diameter is decreased, myelin has shorter internodal distances and is thinner.

tween surface, subcutaneous, and deep temperature and their relation to conduction velocity has been shown to exist, but it is uncertain whether these relationships hold in all pathologic circumstances. For this reason and for those cited in the next section, it is perhaps better to warm an extremity to an acceptable value before performing nerve conduction studies when the temperature decrease exceeds several degrees.

Reported studies in normal subjects show a very wide range of normal *amplitudes* for both sensory and motor conduction studies. These variations are not only due to biologic causes but also are greatly affected by such technical factors as skin/electrode impedance, depth of the nerve from the skin surface, location of the recording electrodes in relation to the nerve and other anatomic structures, variation in nerve size among individuals, stimulation technique, and nerve temperature. It is because of the wide variation in the normal values that comparison of amplitudes side to side and along the course of the nerve (above and below entrapment points), combined with following changes occurring over time after injury, is more clinically useful than is the absolute value of the amplitude of the evoked response.

It is been demonstrated that the amplitude and duration of evoked potentials (and therefore the area under the negative spike) decrease with increasing nerve temperature throughout the physiologic range. Because in the same circumstances nerve conduction velocity increases, we might expect this velocity increase to result in better summation of the evoked response and thus a larger amplitude. This paradoxical change observed may be due to disproportionate changes in the rate of conduction of the various diameters of axons during temperature change or the summated effects of the reduction of individual axon depolarization durations (4).

The preceding discussion demonstrates the importance of both recording and attempting to control temperature in the usual clinical situation. Recording the temperature from a standard location for each examination provides an excellent reference point for serial studies in individual patients. This extra step may not be necessary to demonstrate that such an entrapment as carpal tunnel is not present if the latencies recorded are normal. However, the information may prove invaluable for comparison years later, when one re-examines the patient for signs of an early peripheral neuropathy.

Age

The relationship of conduction velocity to age is most dramatically seen in individuals younger than age 4 and older than 60. At birth, motor conduction velocities are approximately one-half those of the normal adult. They reach the low end of the normal range for adults

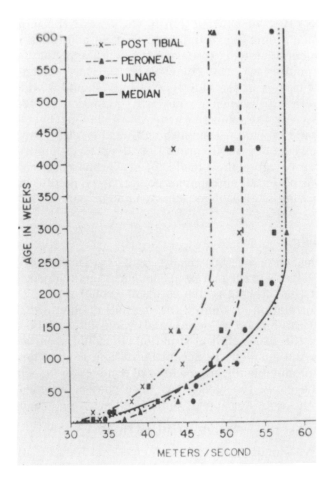

Figure 4.9. Conduction velocity as a function of age in children.

by the age of 2 and are in the midnormal range by the age of 4 (Fig. 4.9) (3). Nerve conduction velocity studies have been used to determine the degree of prematurity in infants and to distinguish between prematurity and low weight for gestational age infants (47).

A distinct correlation has also been established between advancing age, decreased conduction velocity, and decrease in the amplitude of the evoked response. The slowing is due to the loss of large myelinated fibers, which is a normal part of aging. Reports vary as to the age at which this slowing can be detected with clinical studies, ranging from the early forties to the sixties (17). Norris found a decrease in conduction velocity of 1.5% per decade after the age of 60 (43).

Aging produces a proportionate (i.e., affecting all segments of the nerve equally) type of slowing due to the loss of the largest axons. However, some studies have indicated that an additional, disproportionate (segmental) slowing can also occur with aging at the standard entrapment points (43). This complicates the electrodiagnosis of entrapment syndromes in the elderly. Not only should a wider latitude be used in defining "normal" values for conduction in older patients to compensate for the expected generalized slowing but also greater attention should be paid to establishing that the full spectrum of clinical and electrodiagnostic abnormalities are present before the diagnosis of nerve entrapment is made. In borderline cases, comparisons among various potential entrapment points can be helpful in determining if the slowing is an isolated entrapment or part of a generalized process.

Sex and Height

Campbell has shown a statistically significant slowing of peripheral conduction velocity with increasing height of individuals tested. He believes that this slowing is due to distal axonal tapering (8). In his study, this correlation accounted for one-half of the normal variation in peripheral conduction velocities and would have to be considered significant in the usual clinical situation. It would seem wise, therefore, in very tall subjects, to accept borderline conduction values as normal. A reproducible difference in both conduction velocity and amplitude of the evoked response has been shown between men and women, but this does not appear to be of clinical importance (26).

NERVE STIMULATION

Proper nerve stimulation creates an electrical field of sufficient intensity to depolarize simultaneously all large diameter, myelinated axons. By convention, this supramaximal stimulation intensity is obtained by increasing the voltage of the stimulus 25% above that necessary to produce the maximum recorded amplitude of the evoked response. A bipolar surface stimulator is used. The cathode is placed closest to the direction along which conduction is to be measured, because hyperpolarization of the nerve can occur under the anode and block depolarization wave propagation. Depolarization proceeds in both directions along the nerve after supramaximal stimulation.

Theoretical evaluations of the nature of the electrical field produced by bipolar surface stimulators indicate that it is a downward-directed cone with an angle of approximately 70° (Fig. 4.10) (13). Depolarization of the nerve or nerves can begin anywhere within the volume of this cone. Irregularities in the shape of the cone are created in the patient by connective tissue planes, bones, etc. It follows that the deeper the nerve is located, the more uncertain we are of the exact point on the

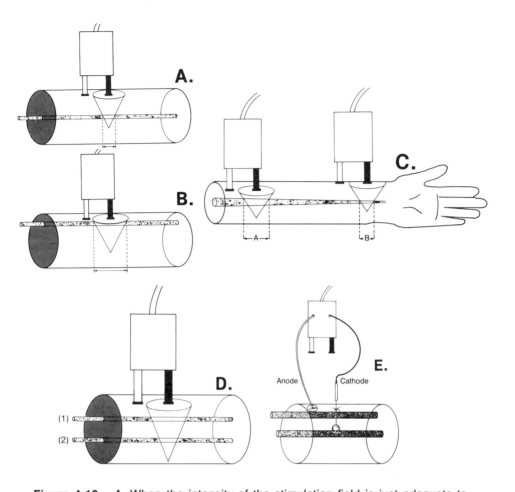

Figure 4.10. *A,* When the intensity of the stimulation field is just adequate to produce nerve depolarization, the initial depolarization point in more likely to be directly below the cathode. B, Very large stimulation intensities increase the uncertainty of this location and increase the changes of stimulation of nearby nerves. *C,* The cone approximates the volume of tissue in which the electrical field produced by the cathode is sufficient to initiate nerve depolarization. Initial depolarization may begin anywhere along the nerve within this volume. *D,* The high intensity stimulation required to produce depolarization of nerve *(2)* causes depolarization of the adjacent nerve *(1).* This often occurs when attempting to stimulate a deep-lying nerve from the surface. *E,* A needle electrode can be used to produce a small, localized stimulation field *(sphere).* Needle stimulation can ensure stimulation of a specific nerve (while excluding others) or permit stimulation of deep-lying nerves. The lower intensity of the stimulation is better tolerated by the patients.

nerve at which depolarization begins—due both to the increased volume of the stimulating field and to the increased chance that the field shape may be distorted.

This small uncertainty about the exact point of initial depolarization of the nerve creates a measurement error for the length of the nerve segment used in the conduction study (increased by the use of two stimulation points) and contributes to the normal fluctuation in conduction velocity values (Fig. 4.10C). Using higher-than-necessary stimulus intensities increases the uncertainty about the exact point of nerve depolarization, because doing so further increases the size of the stimulation electrical field (Fig. 4.10A and B).

Increases in the stimulation intensity, whether accidental or necessary for stimulation of deeply situated nerves, also increases the chances that the depolarization stimulus will spread to adjacent nerves (Fig. 4.10D). Unintended stimulation of multiple nerves is a major source of error in conduction studies. It should be suspected when there is a change in the configuration of the evoked potential between two points of stimulation along the nerve (nerve injury and anatomic variation are two other frequent causes).

It is often helpful to use needle electrodes to stimulate deeply situated nerves or when trying to isolate the stimulation to a specific nerve (Fig. 4.10E). These electrodes are usually Teflon-coated monopolar EMG needles from which a small additional amount of the Teflon has been removed at the tip. They are inserted at a point near the nerve; thus stimulation can then be produced using a very small electrical field and will bypass the very large skin resistance (3-400K Ohms). Duration of stimulus may be shortened to 50 microseconds. Properly inserted needle electrodes do not cause excessive bleeding or infection. Theoretical analysis indicates that there is no risk of electrical injury to the nerve as a result of this technique (41).

Nerve conduction studies can be performed either by stimulating the nerve at a single point and recording the evoked potential from the appropriate location or by stimulating the nerve at two separate points and observing the changes in the evoked potential recorded at the single appropriate point. The second technique provides not only a latency value but also a conduction velocity and the possibility of comparing the two evoked potentials. When entrapments are suspected, stimulation both proximal and distal to the entrapment point is most helpful. Distal latencies should be used only when the suspected entrapment point is too distal to permit effective stimulation beyond it.

The Evoked Potential

The electrical signal recorded from nerve or muscle following stimulation is termed an *evoked potential*. That signal recorded from the muscle endplate area following full stimulation of the motor nerve is termed the *compound motor action potential.* Sensory nerve action potentials are obtained by recording over purely sensory nerves, such as the sural, whereas compound nerve action potentials can be obtained by recording from mixed nerves, such as the median, in which both the sensory and motor axons have been stimulated. Conduction can be measured in either the normal conducting direction of the axon, which is termed *orthodromic,* or in the opposite direction, which is termed *antidromic.* Obviously, the antidromic and orthodromic direction in a mixed nerve are opposite for motor and sensory fibers.

The evoked potentials recorded during nerve conduction studies are the summated electrical fields generated by the depolarization wave moving along the nerve or muscle membranes. This field is located within the volume-conducting medium of the body, and the medium considerably modifies the shape of the potential from that seen with intercellular recording techniques. The evoked potential can be recorded at considerable distances from the generating membrane, but in clinical conduction studies, recording is usually done from a point as close to the generator as possible. In motor conduction studies, the generator is the muscle fiber, whereas in sensory conduction studies, the generator is the nerve axon.

When the nerve is stimulated at two locations and the evoked potentials are recorded from a single location, there are slight differences in the evoked potential generated from the two stimulation points. In normal individuals, the evoked potential obtained from the stimulation point closest to the recording electrode is of greater amplitude and shorter duration than that obtained from the stimulation point further from the recording electrode. In the usual clinical situation, these two points would correspond to the distal and the proximal stimulation points of a motor (or sensory) conduction study. This normal change in the evoked potential is referred to as *temporal dispersion* (Fig. 4.1). As previously discussed, it occurs because of the difference in the conduction velocities of the various axons within the nerve; with longer conduction distances, there is a greater difference in the arrival time between the fastest and the slowest conducting fibers of the nerve. In typical clinical studies, one is recording only from the large myelinated A-alpha fibers, and the temporal dispersion results from the range of values in their conduction velocities. Although physiologic temporal dispersion produces a decrease in the amplitude of the evoked potential, there is also a corresponding increase in the duration of the potential, so that in normals, the area under the negative spike of the evoked potential remains about the same when recorded from stimulation at different points along the nerve (Fig. 4.11). This physiologic dispersion is amplified in peripheral neuropathy and must be distinguished from that resulting from entrapment (see Fig. 4.76).

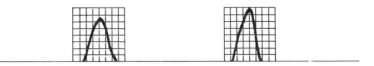

Figure 4.11. The negative spike of the evoked potential recorded when stimulating a motor nerve proximally *(left)* and distally *(right).* Normal temporal dispersion results in decreased amplitude at the proximal stimulation point, but the area under the curve of the two evoked potentials is essentially the same.

In clinical conduction studies, it is important to determine not only the conduction velocity between two points but also the changes that occur in the evoked potential. In chronic entrapments (or acute compression syndromes in which some nerve function is preserved) a decrease in the amplitude of the evoked potential is obtained when stimulating proximally as compared to distally to the site of compromise. Analysis of the evoked potential changes provides crucial information as to the nature of the lesion. In general, there are three possible results of the comparison:

1. Evoked potentials show only slight changes consistent with normal temporal dispersion. This may be seen where no nerve injury is present or when a few large axons have been lost, but conduction remains normal in the surviving axons. Figure 4.66 illustrates this in an individual with loss of some large diameter axons due to aging.
2. The evoked potential obtained from the proximal stimulation point shows a decrease in amplitude and an increase in duration compared to that obtained at the distal stimulation point, but the area under the evoked potential curves are similar. This results from slowing of conduction from demyelination and/or remyelination across the damaged segment. Conduction is preserved in all or most axons. As in No. 1, there may have been some loss of axons (i.e., not contributing to either the proximal or distal stimulation evoked potential) but this loss can only be judged by comparison with the evoked potential in the opposite limb and by needle electromyography.
3. There is a drop in amplitude of the evoked potential obtained at the proximal as compared to the distal stimulation, and there is a decrease in the area under the negative spike of the evoked potential obtained from the proximal stimulation site. In this instance, in addition to the changes seen in Nos. 1 and 2, there is a block in conduction of some axons between the two points of stimulation. The change in the area of the compound evoked potential curve is proportional to the number of axons that are unable to conduct across

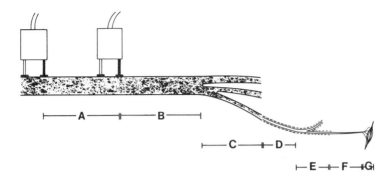

Figure 4.12. Conduction "environments" of a typical motor axon.

the point of injury (20). When the injury is acute, the conduction block may be due to either neurapraxia or axonotmesis. If testing is done at least 4 days or longer after an injury, axonotmetic fiber will have undergone Wallerian degeneration and will no longer contribute to the evoked potentials from either the proximal or the distal stimulation. Therefore, this type of change seen in patients more than 4 days after the injury indicates that the axons that do not conduct across the lesion but can still be stimulated at the distal point are neurapraxic. They should recover function, provided no additional injury occurs. This information can help determine the appropriateness of surgical treatment and is crucial in determining the prognosis for recovery or residual weakness. Review Figures 4.21 and 4.67 for illustrations of these postinjury changes.

Latency

Motor latencies are obtained by stimulation near the terminal end of a nerve and recording the compound motor action potential. The time required for this distal conduction represents a number of different physiologic events, as described below:

1. Latency of activation—the time between the initiation of the electrical discharge in the stimulator and the actual beginning of saltatory conduction along the axon;
2. Fast, saltatory conduction along the large, myelinated axon (Fig. 4.12B);
3. Slower conduction along the smaller diameter of the myelinated axon as it tapers distally (Fig. 4.12C);
4. Slower conduction along the still smaller diameter of the axon as it branches distally (Fig. 4.12D);

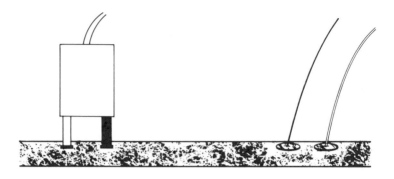

Figure 4.13. Conduction along a sensory axon showing stimulation and recording electrodes. Note the contrast between this rather uniform conducting medium and that illustrated for the motor axon in Fig 4.12.

5. Very slow conduction along the nonmyelinated, terminal twigs of the axon (Fig. 4.12E);
6. Chemical transmission of the signal across the myoneural junction—approximately 0.2 to 0.5 msec (Fig. 4.12F).

Residual latency is a term applied to the difference between the observed terminal (distal) latency and the calculated time for the depolarization signal to travel along the terminal segment of the nerve using the conduction velocity obtained with standard nerve conduction studies. For example, if the median nerve forearm conduction velocity is 50 m/sec and the distal segment is 8 cm, then the calculated time for conduction along this segment would be 0.08m/50m/s = 0.0016 sec = 1.6 msec. If the actual measured latency is 3.5 msec, then 3.5 msec − 1.6 msec = 1.9 msec, which is the residual latency.

In sensory latencies, the evoked potential recorded is directly generated by the nerve, and the latency (conduction time) required consists only of these factors: (a) the latency of activation, (b) saltatory conduction along the myelinated axon, and (c) slower saltatory conduction along the smaller diameter distal portion of the myelinated axon (Fig. 4.13).

Because the sensory latency principally consists of "nerve factors," it can be arithmetically converted into a conduction velocity. Authors may or may not correct for the latency of activation in this process by subtracting 0.1 msec from the latency, and comparisons of normal values among authors must be adjusted for this factor. Because motor latencies include residual latency factors, they cannot be arithmetically converted into conduction velocities.

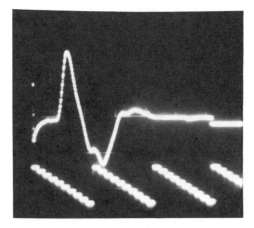

Figure 4.14. Motor nerve evoked potential with recording electrode over motor point of a single muscle. Note initial negative deflection.

Evoked Potential Recording

Evoked potentials are recorded using a recording and a reference electrode attached to the separate grids of the differential amplifier. The signal that appears simultaneously at the two electrodes is cancelled by the differential amplifier. This makes the placement of the two electrodes in relation to the generator source (nerve or muscle) and to each other important. Surface (silver cup) electrodes are usually used because they record a signal that permits quantitative analysis of the evoked potential.

In motor conduction studies, the recording electrode is placed over the motor point of the muscle, and the reference electrode is placed distally over the tendon or another electrically silent area. Placement of the recording electrode off the motor point produces distortion of the recorded potential. The initial deflection of motor responses should be sharply negative, and the signal should be a smooth, biphasic curve (Fig. 4.14). Signals that show initial positive deflection are volume conducted and should not be used. They may originate from the muscle under investigation, but may also be from a distant muscle that was accidentally cross-stimulated. Polyphasic signals may be produced by recording simultaneously from two muscles by placing the recording electrode between them (Figs. 4.15 and 4.16).

In sensory conduction studies, both the recording electrode and the reference electrode are placed directly along the course of the nerve, with the recording electrode closest to the stimulator. The ground electrode should always be placed between the stimulating and the record-

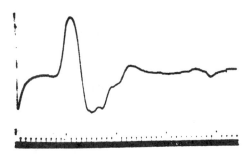

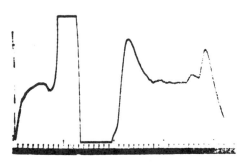

Figure 4.15. Median evoked response in a patient with carpal tunnel syndrome recorded at amplifier settings of 1 millivolt *(above)* and 100 microvolts *(below)* per division (division equals height of time base). Estimate of latency can be affected by the amplification.

ing electrode to reduce the shock artifact. The impedance of dry skin is high and may result in excessive shock artifact. The use of a standard electrode paste or gel is usually sufficient to overcome this difficulty, but occasionally light abrasion of the skin may be necessary to obtain satisfactory recording. This step is required most often for short segment sensory conduction studies.

The distance between the recording and reference electrodes alters the measured latency and the amplitude of the recorded evoked potential (Fig. 4.17) (57). In sensory studies, the distance chosen is usually 3 to 4 cm. This separation can be controlled by embedding the two electrodes in a plastic bar. An alternate technique of recording is to place the recording electrode directly over the nerve as above, but to place the reference electrode approximately 3 cm away from the recording electrode directly perpendicular to the course of the nerve. This "monopolar" recording results in a lower-amplitude, but more reproducible, evoked potential (Fig. 4.18) (35).

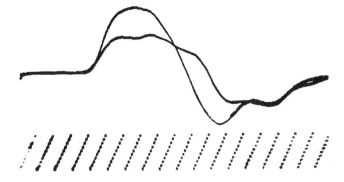

Figure 4.16. Superimposed are evoked potentials recorded at the median thenar motor point and a more medial site over motor point of three muscles. The larger amplitude response is from the single muscle. The separate components of the smaller response result from recording responses from three separate median-innervated muscles.

Needle electrodes offer advantages in certain circumstances because they enable the investigator to isolate the stimulation to a specific nerve or the response to a specific muscle. When placed intermuscularly, the needle electrode records the muscle fiber spike potentials from a few motor units located very close to the needle tip. The negative rise time of the potential for a fiber located near the needle tip is fast (Fig. 4.19).

Needle electrodes are most useful for confirming that the evoked potential that is recorded originates in the muscle under investigation and is not a volume-conducted potential from nearby nerves or muscles. Because the spike response recorded by a needle electrode originates in only a few nearby motor units, conduction velocities from this technique represent those of only a few (not necessarily the fastest

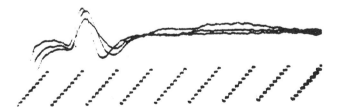

Figure 4.17. Three sensory evoked responses recorded with increasing separation of the reference from the recording electrode along the nerve axis. Separation is 3 cm (largest amplitude, shortest duration), 6 cm, and 8 cm (smallest amplitude, longest duration), respectively.

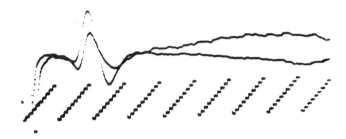

Figure 4.18. Sensory evoked response obtained using standard recording electrode placement of the reference electrode (large amplitude response) and off-nerve placement (monopolar technique) of the reference electrode (small amplitude response).

conducting) axons and may not be representative for that of the whole nerve. Therefore, these values cannot readily be compared with those of control groups. Small movements of the needle electrode may drastically change the latency of the response and its amplitude, and no useful information regarding amplitude is contained in the signal.

INTERPRETATION OF FINDINGS

Entrapment or compression neuropathies interfere with nerve conduction over a short segment of the nerve. An *entrapment neuropathy* is defined as a chronic process in which nerve injury occurs through continuous or repeated compression by another anatomic structure. A compression neuropathy is usually a more acute process, often due to nerve compression from external causes. Direct trauma to the nerve can also produce conduction changes similar to those from entrapments.

As previously discussed, the peripheral nerve is a compound structure, much like a large telephone cable, containing numerous, separate fascicles of individual nerve fibers. The amount and type of injury can vary among fascicles and, indeed, among fibers. Injuries can occur at several locations along the course of the nerve, affecting different combinations of axons at each point.

Nerve conduction studies show the cumulative effect of injuries on the entire nerve, not just individual fibers. Thus, in nerve compressions, the measured conduction velocity may be normal if just a small number of the fastest conducting fibers remain functional, despite severe nerve injury. In that instance, the amplitude and size of the evoked response would be reduced. In contrast, in a chronic entrapment syndrome, there may be significant slowing due to demyelination of the fastest conducting fibers, whereas evoked response amplitude

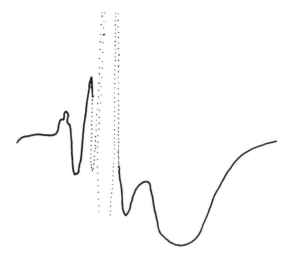

Figure 4.19. Evoked motor response recorded using a needle electrode in the muscle. Note that the initial deflection is of low amplitude (full screen deflection represents 6 millivolts), indicating that the needle tip is not directly against fibers depolarized by the fastest conducting axons.

changes may not be as striking, because the number of fibers conducting and their synchrony remain good.

In most injuries and entrapments, combinations of axonotmesis, neurapraxia, and demyelination coexist. An estimate of the number of axons that remain viable can be obtained by comparing (a) the area under the negative spike of the evoked response obtained with stimulation distal to the injury to (b) the response obtained from stimulation performed in a analogous way on the opposite limb. The loss of area under the curve on the injured side is proportional to the number of axons that have undergone axonotmesis and that no longer contribute to the evoked response (Fig. 4.11). Comparison of the areas under the curves of evoked potentials obtained from stimulation proximal to and distal to the lesion (after Wallerian degeneration has occurred) indicates the proportion of remaining axons that are neurapraxic, because neurapraxic axons contribute to the evoked potential from stimulation distal to but not proximal to the lesion. The severity of the demyelinating process can be estimated from the conduction slowing (i.e., slowing of the fastest conducting fibers) and from the degree of temporal dispersion of the evoked response. This latter value is often a good indication of the proportion of axons that have been demyelinated/remyelinated.

In acute injuries, by far the most valuable piece of information is the size of the evoked potential that can be recorded 4 to 7 days postinjury,

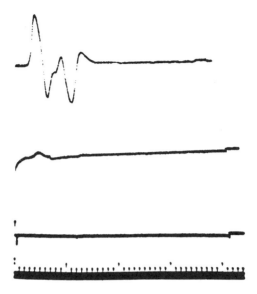

Figure 4.20. Evoked potential recorded from the thenar eminence with median nerve stimulation at the wrist in an individual with surgically demonstrated complete section of the median nerve following a stab wound in the upper arm. *Upper* response was recorded 4 days postinjury, the *middle,* 7 days postinjury, and the *bottom* response, 10 days postinjury. The time base is in msec divisions, and the amplitude of the time base is 1 millivolt.

i.e., post-Wallerian degeneration (Figs. 4.20 and 4.21). The maintenance of a significant response, even if only a tenth the area of that obtainable on the opposite side, demonstrates the survival of a functionally significant proportion of the nerve axons (and indicates continuity of the nerve). In these instances, the prognosis for useful motor recovery is good, even though some residual weakness might be expected.

In interpreting studies, it is important to be certain that each result is consistent with the overall clinical interpretation. The clinician may vary the importance given each part of the study in light of experience, but inconsistency in the findings should lead to a careful reevaluation of the diagnosis. Emphasis on internal consistency in examination results is the major safeguard against error in electrodiagnosis.

Special Conduction Techniques

H and F Wave Use in Proximal Conduction Studies

Peripheral nerves are routinely evaluated by stimulating the nerve at two separate locations and recording the evoked potential from a

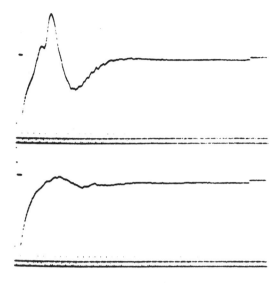

Figure 4.21. Evoked potential of the facial nerve 3 days *(upper tracing)* and 10 days *(lower tracing)* following the onset of clinically complete Bell palsy. The amplitude and area changes seen are roughly proportional to the number of axons undergoing Wallerian degeneration. (Caliber: 1 msec, 200 µV.)

more distal point. In this way, the conduction velocity of the segment can be calculated, and changes in the various parameters of the evoked response caused by pathology in the segment can be studied. This technique is not easily applicable to proximally located nerve lesions, e.g., those seen in the Guillain-Barré syndrome, injuries at the root or plexus level, in thoracic outlet syndrome, or intragluteal sciatic nerve injuries. These lesions are more easily studied using F and H waves. These waves are generated from peripheral stimulation of the nerve, but their conduction pathway includes the proximal portion of the nerve.

The F wave is believed to be a recurrent discharge of a small percentage (approximately 1-5%) of the alpha motor neurons that are antidromically activated during peripheral nerve stimulation. Thus, both the afferent and the efferent arcs of this late wave must follow the same alpha motor neuron axons (Fig. 4.22). Which anterior horn cell redischarges varies from stimulation to stimulation; thus, the latency, shape, and amplitude of the F response vary slightly from stimulation to stimulation (14,39). If a number of stimulations are recorded and the shortest latency selected, a consistent value, representing the fastest conducting motor fibers, is obtained. Other techniques for evaluating F waves are listed in Chapter 6.

F - Wave

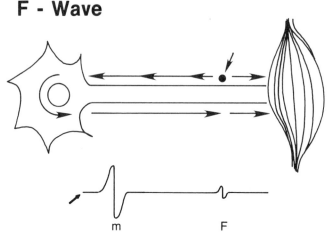

Figure 4.22. F response. The course of the depolarization following stimulation *(dot)* is shown by the arrows. Initially, depolarization travels both directly to the muscle fiber, producing the M response, and retrograde up the axon to the neuron, where it is repropagated in a small percentage of neurons back down the axon to produce the delayed F response.

The F wave is not suppressed by a high intensity or frequency of stimulation. Its amplitude is smaller than that of the H wave and is usually less than 500 μV. Care must be taken to ensure that the shortest latency (earliest takeoff) of the wave is used; thus, recording multiple responses is essential for accurate use of this technique. This is accomplished by using a direct paper recorder, digital storage, memory scope, or Polaroid film to record ten successive stimulations. It is best to displace slightly the vertical axis of the sweep after each three or four superimpositions to facilitate reading the results (Fig. 4.23).

The F wave occurs in all motor nerves and often remains present even in the face of severe disease. Weber has developed the following formula for predicting the F wave in the ulnar nerve (62):

$$\left\{ \begin{array}{l} 0.31 \times \text{(the distance in centimeters from the spine of C7} \\ \text{to the tip of the ulnar styloid)} + \text{(the constant 11.05)} - \\ \text{(0.123 times the forearm velocity of the ulnar nerve)} \end{array} \right.$$

The predicted value may also be obtained from a nomogram (Fig. 4.24). The normal latency should not exceed the predicted value by more than 2.5 msec (mean + 2 SD). Side-to-side variation on the ulnar nerve should not exceed 1 msec (mean + 2 SD), and side-to-side com-

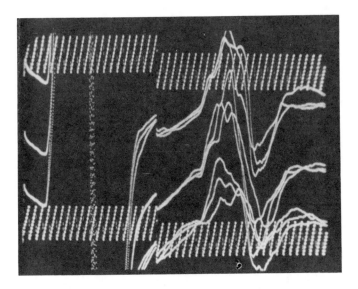

Figure 4.23. Recording of ulnar F responses obtained in nine sequential stimulations of the nerve. (Caliber: Each slanted line = 1 msec. Height = 200 µV.)

parisons in other nerves remain within this general range. For this technique, the ulnar nerve is stimulated at the wrist just as for the usual ulnar motor latency, except that the anode and the cathode positions are reversed (Fig. 4.25). Stimulation at the wrist avoids the necessity of recording an F wave on the upslope of the M wave, which results from proximal stimulation unless special (collision) techniques are used. For testing and for distance measurement, the arm is positioned with the elbow extended and the shoulder abducted approximately 20° (Fig. 4.26).

The inclusion of ulnar forearm velocity in the formula to predict latency compensates for the normal variation in peripheral nerve conduction velocity among individuals. It also negates the effect of distal slowing from proximal entrapment. Therefore, these predicted values should be used only for entrapments, not for investigation of generalized neuropathy.

The H wave results from a monosynaptic spinal reflex with an afferent arc comprised of I-a afferent fibers of the muscle spindle and an efferent arc that is the axon of the alpha motor neuron (Fig. 4.27). In infants, the H wave is found in many nerves but in normal adults, it is seen only in a few.

The tibial H wave latency for an individual can be predicted from the following formula, which was developed by Braddom (5):

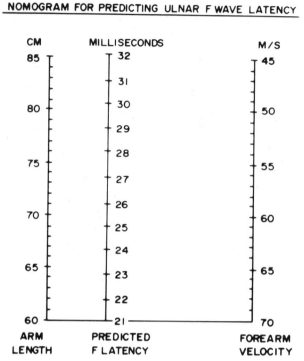

NOMOGRAM FOR PREDICTING ULNAR F WAVE LATENCY

Figure 4.24. Multiple regression technique derived F-wave formula.

(0.46 × the length in centimeters from the midpopliteal crease to the tip of the medial malleolus) + (one-tenth the patient's age) + (the constant, 9.14).

This value may also be obtained from a nomogram. The normal variation from the predicted value is rather large (4.8 msec), but it can be reduced in unilateral problems by comparison of the symptomatic to the nonsymptomatic side. In this instance, the sides should vary by no more than 1.2 msec.

The H wave is elicited by stimulating at an intensity below that which is necessary to evoke muscle contraction (M response) because the larger-diameter I-a afferent axons are more easily stimulated. It is suppressed by supramaximal stimulation intensities and by stimulation frequencies greater than 1/sec. Therefore, it can be distinguished from the F wave by use of a slowly increasing stimulation intensity (40). When this technique is used, the H wave will appear before or near the threshold stimulation intensity for eliciting the M response, in-

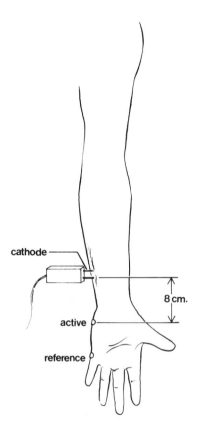

Figure 4.25. Stimulation and recording technique for obtaining the F wave in the ulnar nerve. Note that the cathode is placed proximally to the anode.

crease in amplitude to several millivolts, and finally disappear as the intensity of the stimulation increases (the F wave will then be seen).

Although these techniques offer a method of confirming distal conduction abnormalities (particularly useful in ulnar lesions at the elbow), they should not be routinely relied upon to replace direct stimulation studies for segments of the nerve that are easily accessible.

Spinal Nerve Stimulation

Direct stimulation of spinal nerves as they exit the neural canal provides an excellent means of testing conduction of the proximal segments of the plexus or peripheral nerves. Stimulation requires the use of a needle electrode, which is most frequently a monopolar needle electrode from which several millimeters of the distal Teflon coating have been removed. The needle is employed as the stimulating cath-

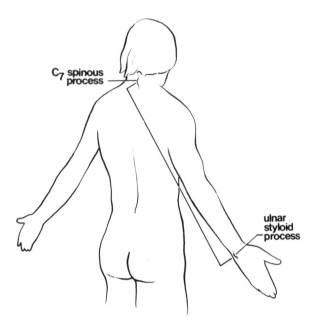

Figure 4.26. Distance measurement for ulnar F wave.

ode, and a large surface electrode serves as the anode. A stimulation intensity of 50–100 volts and a duration of 0.05 to 0.10 msec are used.

H - Wave

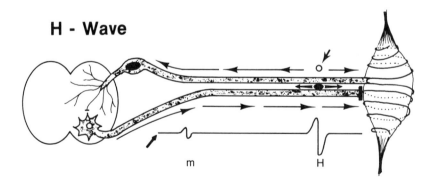

Figure 4.27. The H response is obtained by stimulation of the afferent sensory fiber *(top),* resulting in orthodromic conduction to the spinal cord. There, synaptic stimulation of the alpha motor neuron occurs, resulting in the evoked H response in the muscles. A few motor axons are often directly stimulated, producing the rudimentary M response illustrated.

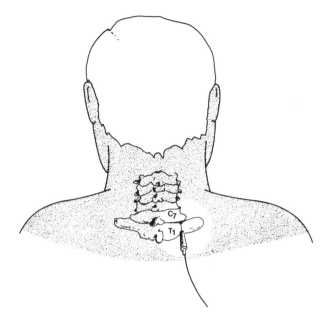

Figure 4.28. Needle stimulation of the C8 root.

The procedure is safe and relatively painless, particularly if limited to several stimuli.

The most clinically useful technique is that of a C8 spinal nerve stimulation. The stimulating needle is inserted into the paraspinal muscles 1 inch lateral to the caudal border of the dorsal spine of C7. The needle is oriented perpendicular to the skin and then angled toward the midline 30 to 45 degrees. It is inserted through the paraspinal muscles until it makes contact with the transverse process (Fig. 4.28).

Recording may be from any C8 muscle, but the abductor digiti V is usually chosen. It is important to have some means of recording the evoked potential to ensure accurate assessment of the response and to avoid multiple stimulations. When recording from the ulnar nerve, the conduction distance is measured from the point of stimulation at the neck to a distal stimulation point 8 cm proximal to the recording electrode (standard ulnar motor conduction study distal stimulation point). The arm is positioned for measurement in the plane of the body and abducted approximately 10 degrees from the side of the body; the elbow is fully extended as for the ulnar F wave study (Fig. 4.26). The normal value for this conduction study is 68 m/sec ± 3.0 m/sec (lower limit of normal, 62 m/sec, Weber) (61). See also Chapter 6 for an alternate method.

A similar standardized technique is available for the median nerve. Stimulation is as above. Recording and distal stimulation are the same as for the standard median motor latency study. Distance is measured from the C8 stimulation point to the distal stimulation point, as previously described. The normal conduction velocity is 70 m/sec ± 2.7 m/sec (lower limit of normal, 65 m/sec, Weber). The mean latency difference between C8 root stimulation to the median versus the ulnar hand intrinsics, as described above, is zero (0.0 ± 0.86 m/sec, upper limit, 3 SD = 1.8 m/sec, Weber).

If the C8 conduction study result is abnormal, conduction must be tested along the more distal segments of the nerve in order to localize the point of nerve injury or entrapment.

Techniques have also been described for stimulation of the lower lumbar and first sacral nerve roots in a similar manner and for stimulation of sacral roots 3 and 4 with recording of the response from the anal sphincter (37,55).

Errors in Nerve Conduction

Whenever an error is made in electrodiagnosis, whether an error in diagnosis or the failure to detect pathology when present, the cause can usually be traced to the use of improper technique or to error in interpretation of the study results. Some of the common, clinically important errors are listed below, and further details concerning them can be found earlier in the chapter. The importance of consistency and care in the application of techniques and the advantage of a good pretesting clinical examination for helping interpret test results and guide testing are obvious.

1. Inadequate examination—insufficient number of nerves studied may result in the failure to detect a generalized conduction abnormality with resultant false diagnosis of a localized entrapment, etc. It is always wise to test several nerves for both a general screening and for testing the hypothesis of multiple entrapment syndromes before reaching diagnostic conclusions.
2. Measurement error—perhaps the simplest mistake, but one that can produce substantial errors.
3. Failure to recognize that one has measured an extraneous evoked potential either because of improper stimulation technique with spread to a different nerve or recording from the wrong location, or failure to recognize that the desired response is absent due to pathology and that an alternate generator source is being recorded. The last cause is best avoided by an adequate clinical examination, because it tends to occur in patients with the most obvious clinical deficits.

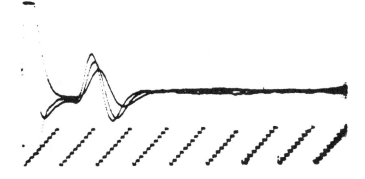

Figure 4.29. Sensory evoked response recorded from identical stimulation and recording electrode placements with shifts in the high frequency filter settings. The largest amplitude response with shortest latency was obtained with the high frequency cut at 3.2 kHz. Settings at 1.6 and 0.8 kHz produced the intermediate and low amplitude response, respectively. Note the clinically significant shift in the recorded peak latency. (Caliber: Each slanted line = 1 msec. Height = 20 µV.)

4. Failure to correct conduction values for limb temperature.
5. Systematic modification of the testing parameters used to establish normal values. Attention is often given to the importance of careful patient positioning and choice of stimulation and recording locations used in the control series, because changing these variables can alter the results obtained. Less often appreciated is the fact that variation in such mundane equipment settings as frequency filters, amplification, and sweep speed also will significantly affect the values recorded or the reading of the conduction parameters by the electromyographer (Figs. 4.15, 4.29, and 4.30). When comparing clinical values to a control series, the techniques, equipment, etc., should be copied in every detail.
6. Failure to appreciate the presence of anatomic variation.
7. Failure to obtain internally consistent results in all components of the electrodiagnostic study. Although there are exceptions, every effort should be made to explain all electrodiagnostic values by a single pathologic problem; when multiple diagnoses are invoked, strong supporting evidence should be present.

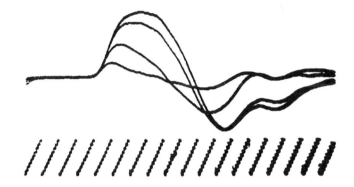

Figure 4.30. Motor evoked responses obtained with low frequency filter cutoffs of 16, 32, 160, and 500 Hz (largest to smallest amplitude response). Note that there is no shift in the latency of the initial deflection but that the accuracy of identification of the deflection becomes more difficult as amplitude decreases. (Caliber: Each slanted line = 1 msec. Height = 2 µV.)

SPECIFIC NERVE EXAMINATIONS

Phrenic Nerve

Anatomy

The phrenic nerve is supplied principally by the fourth cervical root, with contributions from C3 and C5, and is the sole motor supply for the diaphragm. The right and left phrenic nerves follow different courses to the diaphragm, the right nerve being shorter and more vertical.

Loss of diaphragmatic function is a catastrophic event, occurring most frequently with spinal cord injury, peripheral nervous system disease, and trauma. Electrodiagnostic studies are often crucial in determining both the prognosis and the appropriate treatment.

Standard Motor Conduction Technique

The phrenic nerve is easily stimulated using a standard bipolar surface stimulator pressed deeply along the lateral edge of the sternocleidomastoid in the supraclavicular space (Fig. 4.31). MacLean has noted the benefits of stimulation in this location using a needle electrode, which he believes is both safe and more effective in isolating the stimulus to the phrenic nerve (38). The recording electrode is placed over the xiphoid, and the reference electrode is placed in the eighth intercostal space at the costochondral junction (Fig. 4.32). This location helps isolate the diaphragmatic response from those that occur through inadvertent brachial plexus stimulation. The normal latency on the right

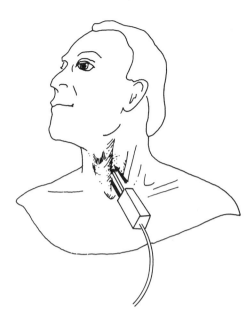

Figure 4.31. Stimulation technique for the phrenic nerve.

is 7.4 ± 0.73 msec, and on the left, it is 7.5 ± 0.97 msec (38). The highest normal latency seen was 8.6 msec, although some authors have reported slightly higher values, up to 9.4 msec (2).

Suprascapular Nerve

The suprascapular nerve (C5,C6) enters the suprascapular fossa through the suprascapular foramen (Fig. 4.33), a U-shaped bony notch bridged by the superior transverse scapular ligament.

The nerve forms two branches, one to the supraspinatus muscle, branching to the glenohumeral and acromioclavicular joints. The second passes around the lateral margin of the scapular spine, supplying the infraspinatus muscle, the scapula, and the glenohumeral joint.

Compromise may be due to isolated "neuritis"; compression by the transverse scapular ligament; relatively minor, repeated trauma to a metabolically compromised nerve; or stretching of the nerve during an extreme motion of the scapula (forced scapular protraction). The infrascapular branch can be stretched or compressed as it passes around the scapular spine.

Supraspinatus weakness disrupts normal glenohumeral motion by decreasing stabilization of the humeral head, and paralysis may prevent initiation of shoulder abduction. Patients may substitute for this weak-

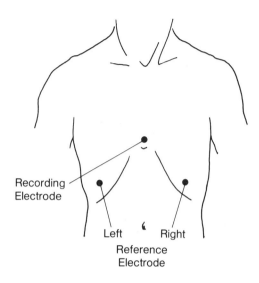

Figure 4.32. Evoked potential recording technique from the diaphragm for phrenic nerve stimulation.

ness by dipping the shoulder and flexing the trunk toward the side of the injury, because the resultant pendular motion of the arm will initiate abduction. Infraspinatus weakness decreases external rotator strength, but is not functionally limiting.

There are no cutaneous sensory symptoms from suprascapular nerve injury, because it provides no cutaneous innervation.

Suprascapular nerve injury may result in a prolongation of motor latency to or loss of the evoked response in the supraspinatus and/or infraspinatus muscles. Needle EMG examination must always be performed in order to confirm the diagnosis. Positive waves, fibrillation potentials, motor unit loss, etc., should be confined to the appropriate muscles. Careful exploration of the C5, C6 paraspinals must always be included because C5 radiculopathy can mimic suprascapular nerve entrapment. Investigation of the infraspinatus muscles is essential when the supraspinatus is normal and shoulder pain is the major complaint.

Standard Motor Conduction Techniques.

Because of its short length and the inaccessibility of the distal portion of the nerve for stimulation, standard studies utilize only a motor latency determination. Stimulation is in the supraclavicular fossa using a standard bipolar surface stimulator that is pressed deeply into the space behind the clavicular head of the sternocleidomastoid just above the clavicle (Fig. 4.34). The cathode is situated lateral to the anode.

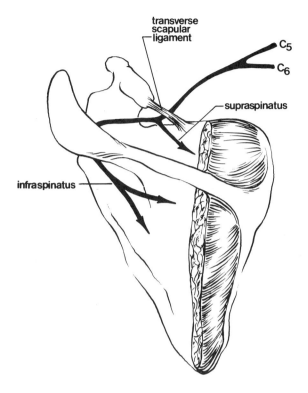

Figure 4.33. Suprascapular nerve anatomy.

Due to patient discomfort, efforts should be made to organize the examination so that the study can be limited to two stimulations per recording point: therefore, electronic storage of the responses facilitates this study.

Surface electrodes are adequate for recording in normal individuals, but in abnormals, a needle electrode may be required to ensure that the recorded signal originates from the appropriate muscle (see the section on recording technique) and not from other adventitiously activated muscles (Fig. 4.35).

Kraft reported normal latencies to the supraspinatus of 2.7 ± 0.5 msec (upper limit of normal, 3.7 msec) and to the infraspinatus of 3.3 ± 0.5 msec (upper limit of normal, 4.3 msec.) (33). (Fig. 4.36)

There are no standard sensory conduction techniques.

Axillary Nerve

The axillary nerve (C5, C6) forms an anterior branch that supplies branches to the deltoid and overlying skin and a posterior branch that

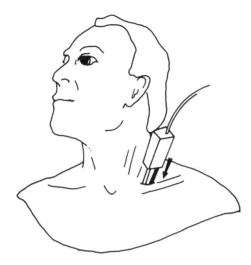

Figure 4.34. Technique of supraclavicular stimulation of the upper brachial plexus utilized in various upper extremity nerve conduction studies.

supplies the teres minor and the posterior portion of the deltoid. Its sensory continuation pierces the deep fascia along the lower part of the posterior deltoid border and continues as the upper lateral cuta-

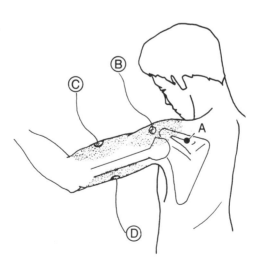

Figure 4.35. Motor recording points illustrated for various upper extremity nerve conduction studies. *A*, Supraspinatus; *B*, axillary; *C*, musculocutaneous; *D*, radial.

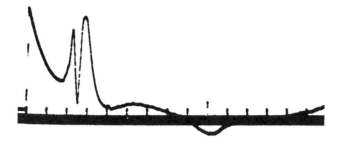

Figure 4.36. Motor response recorded with needle electrode in the supraspinatus muscle with suprascapular nerve stimulation. (Caliber: Each slanted line = 2 msec. Height = 200 µV.)

neous nerve of the arm, supplying an oval-shaped area over the lateral aspect of the upper arm.

The axillary nerve is infrequently injured, with gunshot wounds, shoulder dislocations, and errant intermuscular injections accounting for most injuries. Loss of the teres minor is not functionally significant; however, denervation of the deltoid limits shoulder abduction. Although some authors disagree, abduction can occur in the absence of a functioning deltoid, particularly in muscular individuals (33). Sensory loss can occur independent of motor loss.

Standard Motor Conduction Technique

Stimulation is the same as for the suprascapular and musculocutaneous nerves (Fig. 4.34). Recording is done with surface electrodes: active electrode over the most prominent portion of the middle deltoid, and reference over the junction of the deltoid tendon and the humerus (Fig. 4.35, point B). The mean latency is 3.9 ± 0.5 msec, with a normal range of 2.8 to 5.0 msec (33).

Standard Sensory Conduction Technique

Direct recording of a sensory response from the axillary nerve is not practical; however, somatosensory evoked potential recording from this nerve is possible.

Musculocutaneous Nerve—Lateral Cutaneous Nerve of the Forearm

The musculocutaneous nerve (C5, C6) supplies the biceps, coracobrachialis, and brachialis minor muscles and provides sensation to the lateral aspect of the forearm through its terminal branch, the lateral cutaneous nerve of the forearm. The latter proceeds obliquely across the arm and emerges through the deep fascia several centimeters above

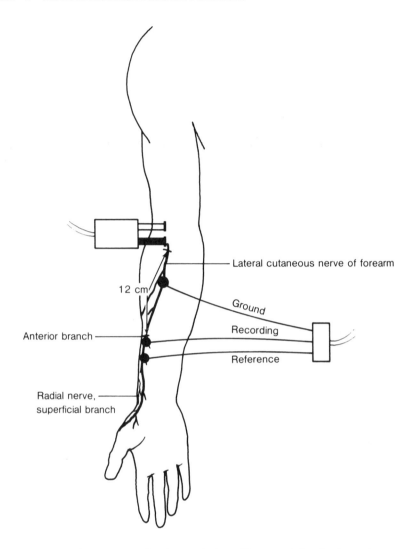

Figure 4.37. Sensory conduction technique illustrated for the lateral cutaneous nerve of the forearm (musculocutaneous nerve).

the elbow crease. There, it lies in close relationship to the antecubital veins—usually medial and deep to their confluence. There the nerve divides into posterior and anterior branches, which proceed along the forearm, providing cutaneous sensation to the volar and dorsal aspects of the radial side of the forearm (Fig. 4.30). In some individuals, it also supplies sensation to the radial side of the hand.

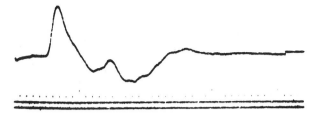

Figure 4.38. Motor evoked response recorded from the biceps with musculocutaneous nerve stimulation. Height of the time base equals 1 m.; 1-msec division.

Clinical Pathology

The proximal portion of the musculocutaneous nerve is infrequently entrapped or injured. Gunshot wounds are the most frequent cause of proximal injury and usually damage both the nerve and the lateral cord of the plexus. Injury occasionally occurs in shoulder dislocation, violent compressive injuries to the anterior portion of the shoulder, or stretch injuries of the arm. Compression during surgery has been reported, as has spontaneous palsy occurring in weightlifters. In weightlifters, compression probably takes place during the nerve's passage through the coracobrachialis or the biceps muscle (6).

Injury to the terminal sensory portion, the lateral cutaneous nerve of the forearm, is more frequent. That nerve may be tethered as it passes through deep fascia and where it forms its two terminal branches. It is occasionally injured during phlebotomy in the antecubital space. Most frequently, injury occurs during cardiac catheterization in association with canalization of the vein.

Because there is much overlap among sensory nerves supplying the forearm and hand, injury to this nerve may produce only a small area of numbness or dysesthesia. Paralysis of the motor portion leads to loss of strength for elbow flexion, but the pronator teres and other forearm muscles are still able to carry out effective elbow flexion, albeit with more pronation than supination.

Standard Motor Conduction Technique

The musculocutaneous nerve is stimulated in the supraclavicular fossa at the lateral attachment of the sternocleidomastoid to the clavicle (Fig. 4.34). Recording is by means of surface electrodes recording electrode just distal to the midpoint of the biceps over the area of its greatest mass, and reference at the elbow (Fig. 4.35, point C). The mean normal latency is 4.5 ± 0.6 msec, with a normal range of 3.3 to 5.7 msec (33) (Fig. 4.38).

Standard Sensory Conduction Technique

Sensory studies can be performed using surface stimulation and recording. The antidromic technique reported by Spindler involves stimulation in the antecubital space just lateral to the biceps tendon, with recording 12 cm distal along the course of the nerve (Fig. 4.37) (52). Latency is measured to the negative peak, and the normal latency is 2.3 ± 0.1 msec, the upper limit of normal is 2.5 msec, and the mean amplitude, 24 ± 7.2 μV. In the reported study, the comparison side to side of latencies gave a mean plus 2 SD of 0.30 msec, whereas the mean plus 2 SD comparison side to side of the ratio of the smaller over the larger amplitude was 0.73 (52).

Long Thoracic Nerve (of Bell)

Anatomy

The long thoracic nerve (C5,C6,C7) supplies only the serratus anterior muscle, innervating each muscle slip as it passes vertically down the chest wall. It is anchored proximally at the scalenus medius and on each slip of the serratus. This increases its susceptibility to stretch injury from either contralateral bending of the neck or depression of the ipsilateral shoulder. Palsies may result from use of a heavy knapsack depressing the shoulders or from inappropriate positioning during surgery. The nerve is frequently damaged during competitive wrestling.

The serratus assists the trapezius in elevation of the shoulder and pulls the medial border of the scapula against the chest wall during elevation of the arm. Paralysis results in winging of the scapula, i.e., separation from the thoracic wall. This is demonstrated by having the patient place the extended arms directly in front of him or her and press forward against a wall with the hands.

Standard Motor Conduction Technique

The long thoracic nerve can be stimulated in the supraclavicular space using a surface stimulator. The technique is similar to that used for the other proximal portions of the plexus (Fig. 4.34). Recording is done from the serratus muscle slips at the midaxillary line using needle or surface electrodes. Kaplan reported a mean latency of 3.9 ± 0.6 msec (upper limit of normal, 5.1 msec) using surface recording electrodes (32). Side-to-side comparison of the evoked potential and latency and needle EMG examination should be included in the evaluation. Needle exploration of the muscle may be more useful than conduction studies in following the progress of recovery.

There are no standard sensory conduction techniques.

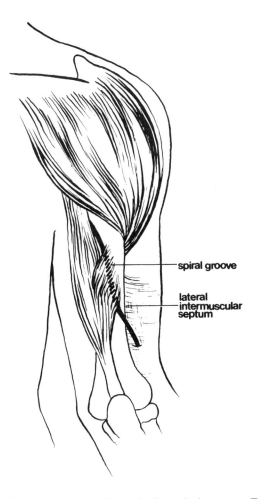

Figure 4.39. Radial nerve course through the spiral groove. The immobility of the nerve in this location makes it vulnerable to injury during upper arm trauma and fractures.

Radial Nerve

The radial nerve (C5 though D1) is more likely to be damaged by trauma or acute compression and is less frequently involved in chronic entrapment syndromes than are other upper extremity nerves. Crutch palsy occurs from compression in the axilla. It is the nerve most frequently damaged with arm fractures, occurring in perhaps 10% of mid-humeral shaft fractures (spinal groove) and, less frequently, with fractures of the proximal third of the radius (posterior interosseus branch) (Fig. 4.39). With fractures and open trauma, proper treatment

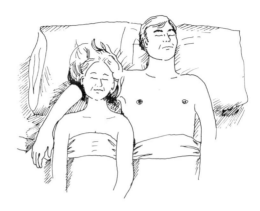

Figure 4.40. Compression of the radial nerve in sleep palsy—an alternative method involves compression from the sharp edge of the back of a bench or chair.

is dependent upon knowing if the nerve remains in continuity (no surgery required), and this question commonly occurs with regard to the radial nerve in humeral fractures. Evoked potential analysis and needle EMG are most useful in answering that question.

In the "sleep" palsies, the radial nerve is compressed near its penetration of the intermuscular septum (lower humerus) by the hard edge of furniture or by pressure from a companion's head while the individual sleeps (Fig. 4.40).

The nerve is vulnerable to compression in its course from the lateral epicondyle to the supinator muscle (radial tunnel). In this area, it passes the radiohumeral joint, where it may be tethered by connective tissue and thus more easily injured, and it may be compressed by the tendon of the overlying extensor carpi radialis brevis (Fig. 4.37).

Because the radial nerve divides into its two major branches (superficial and posterior interosseus) in the tunnel, either the entire nerve or either separate branch can be entrapped there. The purely sensory superficial branch can be damaged near the wrist by handcuffs or watchbands (18,45).

Posterior Interosseus Nerve Syndrome

This purely motor nerve arises in the radial tunnel from the division of the radial nerve. Injury has been reported from direct trauma, compression by ganglia or vascular anomaly, and rheumatoid synovitis. The nerve seems to be most vulnerable to repeated trauma from firm wrist extension where it passes through the supinator muscle at the tendinous arcade of Frohse. Additionally, full pronation of the forearm may exert pressure on the nerve at the sharp, tendinous edge of the extensor carpi radialis brevis muscle. Paresis following Frisbee throwing has been reported (19).

The patient has difficulty extending the fingers and thumb and frequently complains of a dull, aching pain, i.e., lateral epicondylitis. The radial wrist extensors are normal, and there is no superficial sensory loss.

Needle EMG may be positive in several of the supplied muscles: extensor digitorum, extensor digiti minimi, extensor carpi ulnaris, abductor pollicis longus, extensor pollicis longus, extensor pollicis brevis, and extensor indicus proprius.

The Sleep Palsies

These palsies have two forms: the "Saturday night palsy," in which the individual sleeps with the arm draped over or pressed against the hard edge of a piece of furniture, and the "honeymoon palsy," in which the weight of another individual's head compresses the nerve against the patient's arm as both parties sleep together (Fig. 4.40). In both instances, the individual suffering the radial nerve injury is often in a deeper-than-normal sleep from the use of alcohol or sedatives.

Wrist and finger extension is compromised, but the triceps is spared; therefore, triceps involvement indicates a more proximal lesion. Occasionally the brachioradialis and, less often, the extensor carpi radialis longus muscles may be spared.

Sensory loss (hypesthesia and hypalgesia) is seldom prominent in radial nerve palsy, because the area of exclusive radial nerve sensory innervation is often confined to the dorsum of the thumb.

Nerve conduction across the lesion may be slowed or partially or completely blocked, whereas the forearm conduction usually remains normal. Special care is necessary to avoid confusion caused by volume-conduction spread of the stimulus to adjoining nerves; one should watch to see which muscles are responding or use needle recording electrodes to confirm the signal source.

Needle EMG following sleep palsy may be markedly abnormal, but despite, that, prognosis for recovery (generally within 2 months) is excellent if a radial evoked response can be obtained with stimulation at the elbow 7 days after the injury or if there continue to be some voluntary motor units present in the extensor muscles on needle EMG (22).

Recovery from intra-axillary compression, humeral fractures, intermuscular injections, etc., is less satisfactory than those associated with the sleep palsies, and residual weakness is frequent.

Standard Motor Conduction Technique

The radial nerve has less well-defined landmarks for stimulation points, and the muscles used for recording are less isolated than for

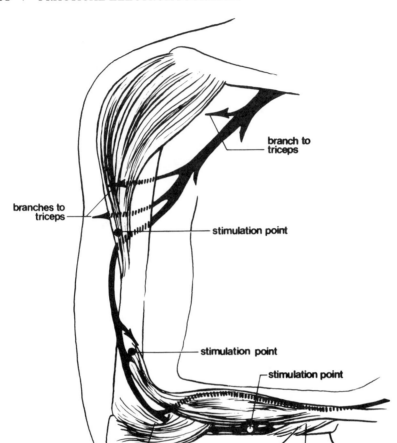

Figure 4.41. Radial nerve with major motor distributions, stimulation points, and recording points marked.

many other nerves. Radial motor conduction studies are therefore less reproducible or precise than those of the median and ulnar nerves. Potential stimulation points include the supraclavicular space, axilla, posterior to the deltoid insertion at the beginning of the spiral groove, between the brachioradialis and biceps, and in the midforearm (Figs. 4.40 and 4.41). The last site requires needle electrode stimulation. Recording has been reported from the triceps, anconeus, brachioradialis, extensor communis, and extensor index muscles. The latter is the most practical for general use, although certain problems may dictate the use of another recording site.

When investigating the proximal portion of the nerve, surface recording from the extensor index is usually satisfactory; however, needle recording may be necessary when studying the segment from just above the elbow to the midforearm. The three stimulation points for the standard study are the supraclavicular space, the groove between the brachioradialis and the biceps just above the elbow crease, and approximately 3–4 cm proximal to the recording electrode in the midforearm. The first two points can be stimulated using a hand-held surface stimulator pressed deeply between muscles, whereas the distal point requires needle electrode stimulation (Fig. 4.41). The arm is positioned in 10° abduction, the elbow flexed 10–15°, and the forearm pronated.

Normal conduction velocity for the proximal segment is 72 m/sec ± 6.3 m/sec (lower limit of normal, 50 m/sec). For the distal segment, the normal value is 61.6 ± 5.9 m/sec (lower limit of normal, 50 m/sec) 27.

Conduction to the triceps has been reported by Gassel using Erb point stimulation and surface recording (Fig. 4.35, point D) (21). Normal motor latency is dependent on the distance to the recording electrode, because the motor endplates are spread out along the muscle. Distance was measured with the arm at the side using obstetric calipers, which better approximates the nerve length (22). At 21.5 cm, the latency is 4.5, SD = 0.42 msec (upper limit of normal, 5.3 msec), and at 31.5 cm, 5.3 msec, SD = 0.5 (upper limit of normal, 6.3 msec).

To investigate the midarm segment in cases of trauma or the sleep palsies, it is helpful to stimulate proximally just posterior to the insertion of the deltoid, rather than at Erb point, thus confining the stimulus to the radial nerve. Normal velocities are essentially the same as described above, with the proximal segment conduction velocity approximately 10% faster than that of the distal segment. Loss of this velocity relationship is suggestive of nerve entrapment.

To investigate entrapments in the radial or supinator tunnels, the distal radial segment is tested using needle recording and often using stimulating electrodes. In sleep palsies and fractures, voluntary motor function is often absent, and evoked potential analysis is used to determine prognosis.

Standard Sensory Conduction Technique

The superficial radial nerve, formed by radial nerve bifurcation in the radial tunnel, is most frequently used for radial sensory conduction studies. The orthodromic technique utilizes stimulation of the digital branches on the dorsum of the thumb. Recording is done 14 cm proxi-

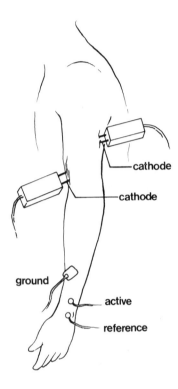

cathode

cathode

ground

active

reference

Figure 4.42. Standard stimulation and recording locations for radial nerve motor conduction studies. G-1 over ext. ind. prop., G-2 over tendon.

mally along the nerve using surface electrodes (Fig. 4.42). The forearm is positioned in neutral, and the recording electrodes are placed over the crest of the radius. A hand-held surface stimulator should be used, rather than ring electrodes, to reduce the overflow of stimulation to the median nerve branches that supply the palmar surface of the thumb. Because of this potential for median nerve stimulation, Trojaberg preferred to stimulate the nerve at the wrist for conduction studies of the more proximal segments of the nerve (54). Antidromic techniques have been described for the distal segment using stimulation at the wrist and recording with ring electrodes at the thumb. Normal values are essentially the same as those for the orthodromic technique.

Computer averaging is usually necessary to obtain conduction values for segments proximal to the wrist. Using a surface stimulator at the wrist, recording can be done by means of surface electrodes placed in the groove between the biceps and brachioradialis, posterior to the insertion of the deltoid, or in the axilla.

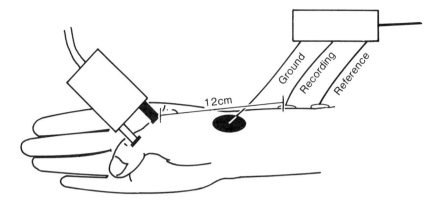

Figure 4.43. Standard stimulation and recording locations for orthodromic sensory conduction studies of the radial nerve. Note that individual digital nerve branches may be stimulated.

The orthodromic distal latency is 3.3 ± 0.5 msec (upper limits of normal, 4.1 msec (Fig. 4.43). Using needle stimulation, measuring from the initial deflection, proximal conduction values (Trojaberg) are wrist to elbow, 66 ± 3.5 m/sec (lower limits of normal, 50 m/sec); to the axilla, 67 ± 6.5 m/sec (lower limits of normal, 54 m/sec) (54).

Ulnar Nerve

Testing ulnar nerve (C7,C8,D1) problems is perhaps the most challenging task that the electromyographer faces. The nerve's length and mobility, coupled with the number of potential points of entrapment, make testing difficult while similarity of symptoms from other causes further complicates the diagnosis.

Proximal entrapment occurs in thoracic outlet syndrome (which is discussed elsewhere in the chapter), in Pancoast tumor, by axillary lymph nodes, vascular aneurysms, and from deformed clavicles, cervical ribs, and other anatomic structures. These can be studied by means of F waves, C8 root stimulation, somatosensory evoked potentials (Fig. 4.44), and in many instances by direct conduction studies using stimulation in the supraclavicular space. As is the median nerve, it is seldom injured in the upper arm, but may occasionally be entrapped as it passes through the intermuscular septum or the arcade of Struthers.

Compromise at the elbow is most frequent and occurs from two basic problems—constriction by fibrous bands or by pressure or trauma to the nerve in the ulnar groove. The importance of nerve subluxation in the latter process is unknown. True entrapment by fibrous bands oc-

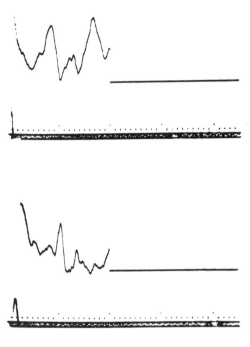

Figure 4.44. Evoked nerve potential in the ulnar nerve recorded at supraclavicular point using a signal averager: technique for somatosensory evoked potentials. Upper response latency is 8.5 msec, whereas that obtained from the opposite side is pictured below and is delayed to 10.5 msec. (Caliber: 1 msec, 10 µV.)

curs up to 6 cm above the groove and produces nerve injury by both constriction and repeated trauma as the nerve is pulled to and fro. Entrapment can often be localized by moving the stimulator sequentially at 1- to 2-cm intervals along the nerve and looking for changes in the evoked potential.

Direct compression at the elbow is often associated with weight loss or prolonged bedrest. It may occur from position during anesthesia or during unconsciousness. Injury from acute compression is more easily demonstrated than that from chronic compression. In the latter, some fast conducting fibers may be preserved, leaving conduction velocity normal. Evoked potential analysis, sensory conduction, and needle electromyography may be needed to identify chronic injury changes (Figs. 4.45–4.47).

Limited help in localization of abnormalities is obtained from the status of various branches: The flexor carpi ulnaris may be supplied above, in, or below the ulnar groove. Thus, when it is involved, it indicates ulnar injury at or above the elbow, but normal findings in this muscle

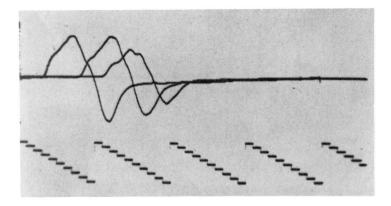

Figure 4.45. Hypothenar motor evoked responses from ulnar nerve stimulation at the wrist, below the elbow, and above the elbow. Note the loss of amplitude and area of the evoked response with conduction across the elbow. (Caliber: each slanted line = 10 msec. Height = 5 millivolts.)

do not preclude injury at the elbow. Forearm ulnar lesions are difficult to localize because of the absence of nerve branches in the forearm and because of the occurrence in 15–20% of people of an anastamosis (Martin-Gruber) from the median to the ulnar nerve in the upper forearm (Fig. 4.48). When this anastamosis is present, the evoked response obtained by stimulating the ulnar nerve below the level of the anastamosis is larger than that obtained from stimulating the nerve above the anastamosis—in direct proportion to the number of axons that join the ulnar from the median nerve (Figs. 4.49 and 4.50). Thus, sequential

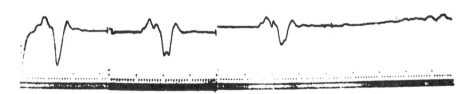

Figure 4.46. Ulnar nerve conduction series in severe, chronic ulnar nerve entrapment at the elbow. Evoked potentials obtained from left to right with stimulation at the wrist, below elbow, and above elbow. Note that all responses are small and velocities slowed due to loss of many of the large-diameter axons. In this instance, it is difficult to determine if the entrapment at the elbow is ongoing or resolved, in view of the lack of dramatic change in conduction in this segment. This picture often confronts the electromyographer in patients with long-standing ulnar injuries both before and after surgical decompression. The height of the time base equals 1 millivolt, and the intervals are 1 msec. Forearm conduction velocity equals 34 m/sec, and across the elbow was 30 m/sec.

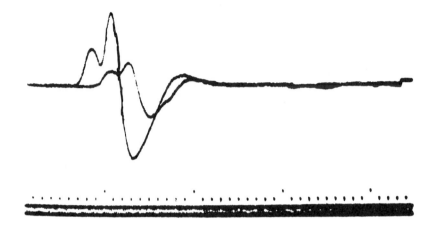

Figure 4.47. Evoked response with ulnar nerve stimulation below and above elbow. Note loss of response and slowing across elbow. (Caliber: same as Figure 4.46.)

stimulation along the course of the ulnar nerve from distal to proximal would produce a point of sudden drop in the amplitude and area of the evoked response similar to that which would be seen in the presence of a partial ulnar palsy. The ulnar nerve enters the forearm between the two heads of the flexor carpi ulnaris (cubital tunnel) and may be entrapped here.

The ulnar nerve gives off its dorsal cutaneous branch (hand) approximately 6 cm above the ulnar styloid, and preservation of sensation (and normal conduction) in this branch indicates a more proximal problem.

The next more distal branch is the palmar sensory branch. This arises several centimeters proximal to the wrist crease and supplies sensory innervation to the ulnar aspect of the palm. It serves as another marker of the point of nerve injury.

Already present in Guyon's canal is the terminal separation into the superficial branch (sensation to little and ring fingers and palm, motor to palmaris brevis muscle) and the deep branch (motor innervation to the remaining ulnar-innervated muscles). The deep branch lies on the bony roof of the canal and is more susceptible to compression. Handlebar palsy from bicycling compresses the nerve in the canal and may produce painless weakness of the interossei and/or numbness, demonstrating that unequal compromise of the two branches can occur at any point from the beginning of the canal distalward.

The deep branch gives off motor twigs to the hypothenar muscles and then exits the canal. It must pass over the pisohamate ligament

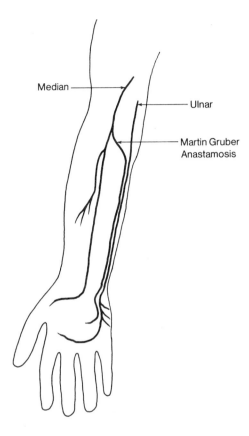

Figure 4.48. Communication in the forearm between the median and ulnar nerve: the Martin-Gruber anastomosis.

and under the fibrous arch from which the abductor and opponens digiti V originate. It turns sharply around the hook of the hamate and proceeds as the deep palmar branch, supplying the ulnar interossei, the two ulnar lumbricals, and the adductor pollicis brevis. These points are potential sites of entrapment (Fig. 4.51).

Unfortunately, from the standpoint of localizing lesions along the course of the deep branch, it divides into its terminal motor fascicles quite proximally in Guyon's canal. Thus, proximal partial injuries of the deep branch may involve all or only some of the distal fascicles and can produce falsely localizing distributions of abnormalities. Thus, it is not possible to localize the injury based on the distribution of abnormalities in the deep palmar branch.

Conduction studies to the abductor V and to the adductor pollicis

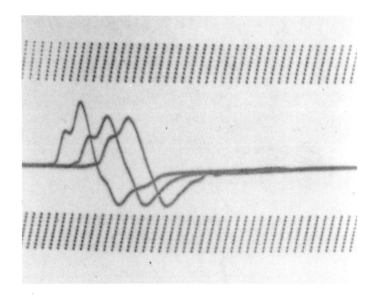

Figure 4.49. Evoked response recorded with stimulation of the ulnar nerve at the wrist, below the elbow, and above the elbow in an individual with the Martin-Gruber anastomosis. This must be distinguished from the changes seen in ulnar entrapment.

brevis are helpful, but needle exploration of both these muscles and several of the dorsal interossei should also be routinely done in suspected ulnar lesions. Sampling of many muscles is necessary, both because of the possibility of specific branch injury or entrapment and because of the prevalence of anatomic variation in the nerve supply of the hand.

Standard Motor Conduction Technique

Numerous cadaver studies have shown that arm position greatly affects the actual versus the surface measured length of ulnar nerve segments. Because of this, clinical studies show great variations in calculated conduction velocities depending on the arm position used. A technique in which the shoulder is abducted approximately 45°, the elbow is acutely flexed so that the angle between the arm and forearm is less than 70° and the forearm is supinated gives surface measured distances closest to actual nerve segment lengths. The recording electrode is placed at the midpoint between the proximal wrist crease and the metacarpal phalangeal joint over the abductor digiti V, and the reference is placed on the little finger. Distal stimulation is 8 cm proximal to the recording electrode—lateral to and under the flexor carpi

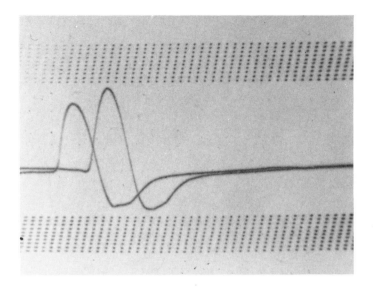

Figure 4.50. Paradoxical response to median nerve stimulation in same patient (as in Fig. 4.49). Proximal stimulation here produces larger evoked potential. Note also the initial positive deflection with elbow stimulation. (Caliber = each slanted line = 1 msec. Height = 5 millivolts.)

ulnaris tendon. Proximal stimulation points are just distal to the ulnar groove at the elbow, a point approximately 12 cm proximal to this at the junction of the mid and distal third of the arm, and in the supraclavicular space (Fig. 4.52). The mean value for the distal latency is 3.2 ± 0.5 msec (upper limits of normal, 4.2 m/sec). The mean value for the forearm segment (below elbow to wrist) is 61.8 ± 5m/sec (lower limits of normal, 52 m/sec) and, for the across-elbow segment, 61.7 ± 5.5 m/sec (lower limits of normal, 51 m/sec) (12).

Checkles noted that variation was still considerable when comparing the across-elbow to below-elbow segment conduction velocities. The 95% confidence interval for normal was a slowing of up to 7% in the across-elbow segment as compared to the forearm segment of the nerve. Thus, a small amount of slowing is acceptable in the across-elbow segment when using this technique. This compares to the finding of up to 45% slowing in normal individuals when this conduction comparison is made by testing with the elbow fully extended. (28,51) This reinforces the importance of using evoked response analysis in addition to velocity changes in electrodiagnosis.

Jebsen reported a mean value of 62.8 ± 6 M/sec for conduction between the supraclavicular and above-elbow stimulation points (28).

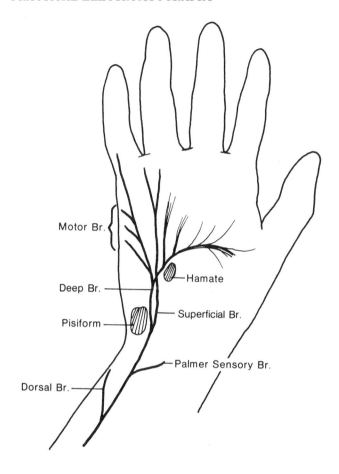

Figure 4.51. Distal branching pattern of the ulnar nerve.

Calipers were used to measure this distance, and the lower limit of normal obtained by this technique was 51 m/sec.

Investigation of entrapment of the deep palmar branch of the ulnar nerve can be accomplished by recording over the adductor pollicis brevis in the dorsal web space. The mean latency for this response, stimulating as above, was found by Johnson and Melvin (unpublished data) to be 3.34 ± 0.6 msec (Fig. 4.53) (upper limit of normal, 4.6 msec).

Standard Sensory Conduction Technique

Both orthodromic and antidromic techniques have been reported for the ulnar nerve. Checkles used an antidromic technique with arm po-

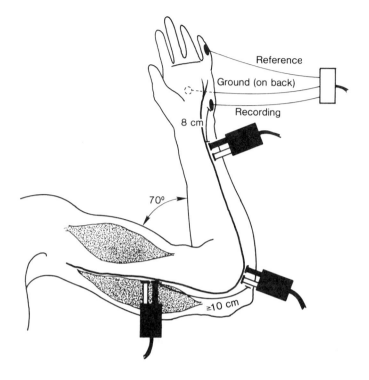

Figure 4.52. Standard motor conduction technique for the ulnar nerve.

sitioning similar to that described for the motor conduction studies above. The mean conduction velocity of the forearm segment was 61.9 m/sec, and, for the across-elbow segment, 64.0 m/sec (10). All of the problems of positioning mentioned for the motor studies hold true for the sensory study. After analyzing their data, Checkles et al. felt the most reliable means of determining abnormal conduction at the elbow (95% confidence) was the use of an absolute conduction velocity in the across-elbow segments of not less than 50 m/sec.

With the ready availability of electronic averaging equipment and better amplifiers, orthodromic techniques have become more popular. Stimulating the digital nerves on the little and ring fingers (ring electrodes, cathode proximal, 4 cm separation of anode and cathode) and recording 14 cm proximally, Johnson and Melvin (unpublished data) found a mean latency value to the peak of 3.2 ± 0.25 msec (Fig. 4.54) (upper limit of normal, 3.7 msec) (Fig. 4.47). They also recorded proximally at the elbow and found a mean conduction velocity of 57.0 ± 5.0 m/sec (lower limit of normal, 47 m/sec).

The use of shorter segments may improve sensitivity in entrapments.

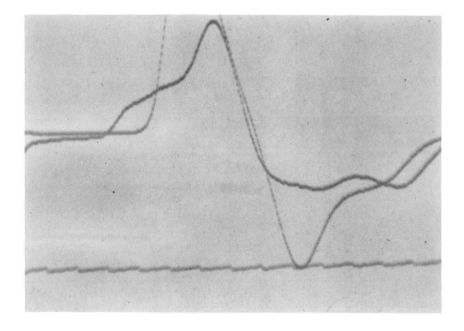

Figure 4.53. Motor evoked response from ulnar nerve stimulation at the wrist recorded with surface electrodes in the first dorsal interosseous (longer latency) and the abductor digiti quinti. (Caliber: 1 msec.)

Weber used a technique in which the common digital nerve between the fourth and fifth metacarpals was stimulated with a bipolar surface stimulator at the palmar crease (cathode proximal) (Fig. 4.55). Recording was at a point 8 cm proximal along the course of the nerve, and the mean latency was 1.86 ± 0.16 msec (upper limit of normal, 2.2 msec, greater than 30° C).(54) The difference between this and the analogous median conduction study was 0.02 ± 0.18 msec, with a maximum acceptable difference of 0.38 msec (mean plus 3 SD) (Figs. 4.55 and 4.56).

The superficial ulnar branch and the dorsal cutaneous branch can be tested and compared. Palmar stimulation was as above, but the recording point was 12 cm proximal along the course of the nerve (Fig. 4.57). This same recording point was then used for the dorsal cutaneous branch. A flexible tape was used to measure distally 12 cm along the course of the nerve onto the dorsal area of the hand between the ring and little fingers. There, stimulation was performed in a method analogous to that described in the palm (Fig. 4.58). In both cases, low intensity stimulation is used in order to avoid volume-conduction spread of the stimulus. With this technique, the mean latency from stimula-

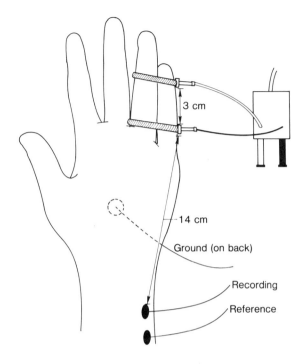

Figure 4.54. Standard orthodromic ulnar stimulation technique using ring electrodes over the fingers (cathode proximal).

tion of the palm was 2.4 ± 0.2 msec (upper limit of normal, 2.7 msec), whereas that from the dorsal cutaneous branch was 2.2 ± 0.2 msec. (upper limit of normal, 2.6 msec). The difference between the two in the same hand is 0.2 ± 0.3 msec, i.e., acceptable variation between the superficial and dorsal sensory branches was 0.5 msec (mean plus 3 SD) (Weber, unpublished data).

Median Nerve

The median nerve (C6, C7, C8, D1) is formed by the union of the medial and lateral cords of the brachial plexus. It descends into the arm, lying lateral to the brachial artery, and crosses in front of the artery at about the insertion of the coracobrachialis muscle.

The nerve continues into the forearm between the two heads of the pronator teres and under the fibrous, arching origin of the flexor digitorum sublimis. In this area, it gives rise to the anterior interosseus branch that supplies the flexor pollicis longus, pronator quadratus, and the index and long finger slips of the flexor digitorum profundus. Entrapment here can involve either the anterior interosseus branch alone

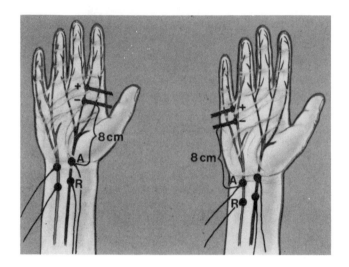

Figure 4.55. Palmar stimulation technique of the ulnar nerve *(right)*. This technique has the advantage of producing a large amplitude evoked response that is easy to detect without the use of a signal averager. Occasionally a shock artifact will obscure very short latency responses. This cause can be confirmed by increasing the separation between the cathode and recording electrodes. Low-intensity stimulation will decrease the shock artifact. The analogous technique for the median nerve is also illustrated.

or both it and the median nerve supply to the hand. The remaining portion of the median nerve, destined to innervate the hand, then passes between the flexor digitorum superficialis and the profundus, being adherent to the former. About 5 cm proximal to the flexor retinaculum, the nerve becomes superficial, lying just medial to the tendon of the flexor carpi radialis at the wrist.

Median nerve entrapment at the wrist—carpal tunnel syndrome—is discussed elsewhere. There are, however, a number of other causes of median neuropathy. In the upper arm, injury can occur by the same mechanisms affecting the radial nerve, i.e., sleep palsies, rifle slings, crutch compression, or trauma.

It may be entrapped by a supracondylar ligament (foramen) as it passes from the dorsal to the volar surface of the arm before entering the pronator canal. This ligament occurs in approximately 1% of individuals and may be associated with a supracondylar process that projects medially about 5 cm above the condyle. Injury can be from nerve constriction or by repeated trauma from back-and-forth motion. All median-innervated muscles are affected.

The median nerve may be entrapped or traumatized as it enters the

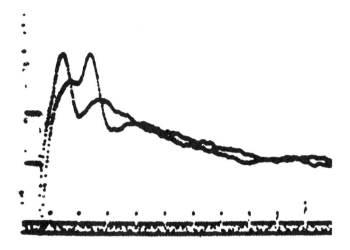

Figure 4.56. Sensory evoked potentials recorded from the ulnar nerve and from the median nerve using the palmar stimulation technique. Note the short latencies and large amplitudes of the evoked responses. Median response is delayed due to carpal tunnel syndrome. (Caliber: 1 msec, 10 µV.)

forearm between the heads of the pronator teres and passes under the edge of the retinaculum of the flexor sublimis (pronator syndrome). Entrapment here may include or spare the anterior interosseus branch. Innervation to the pronator teres occurs above this point, and that muscle is spared in the pronator syndrome.

The anterior interosseus branch may be entrapped in the pronator canal or more distally in the forearm (see anterior interosseus syndrome). This results in weakness of the long thumb flexor, flexor profundus slips to the index and long fingers, and the pronator quadratus.

The median nerve supply to the hand may be entrapped before entering the carpal canal by compression as it emerges from under the edge of the flexor digitorum sublimis (Figure 4.59). This so-called pseudo-carpal tunnel syndrome is clinically indistinguishable from the true carpal tunnel syndrome, because injury involves the same axons that pass through the carpal canal.

These proximal median entrapment syndromes produce symptoms similar to those of the carpal tunnel syndrome (CTS). Even entrapment of the anterior interosseus nerve, which lacks the cutaneous sensory supply to the hand, produces a vague aching and discomfort in the area similar to CTS. Thus full investigation of the median nerve is essential when CTS symptoms are present.

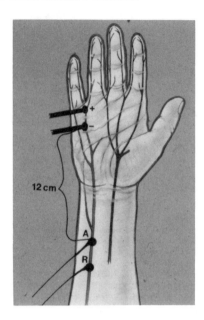

Figure 4.57. Technique for recording the sensory response from the volar branches of the ulnar nerve for comparison with that of the dorsal branch. Note that the same recording point is used for both studies. *A,* Active electrode; *R,* cathode.

Standard Motor Conduction Technique

Due to the strong interest in median entrapment syndromes, median nerve conduction values are perhaps the most documented in existence. The nerve is easily accessible, and the thenar eminence offers an excellent evoked response recording point. The recording electrode is placed over the motor point of the abductor pollicis brevis, and the reference is placed on the distal thumb. The distal stimulation point is 8 cm proximal to the recording electrode (W) measured along the approximate course of the nerve (Fig. 4.60). The normal distal latency is 3.7 ± 3 msec (upper limits of normal, 4.3 msec) (42). Conduction velocity is determined using surface stimulation at the supraclavicular point (N), 10 cm proximal to be elbow (AE), at the elbow (E), and 5 cm distal to the elbow (BE). Normal values are (28):

	Mean	Lower Limit
N-AE	62.9 m/sec	50.9 m/sec
N-E	61.8 m/sec	50.8 m/sec
E-W	58.6 m/sec	51.0 m/sec
BE-W	55.1 m/sec	44.7 m/sec

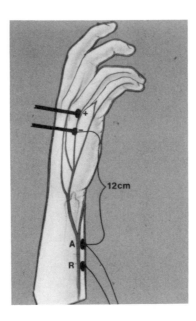

Figure 4.58. Technique for recording the sensory response from the dorsal branch of the ulnar nerve. *A* = active electrode; *R* = cathode.

The test is performed with the arm abducted approximately 10° at the shoulder and the elbow fully extended. All distance measurements are made with a steel tape, with the exception of the supraclavicular fossa, which is best measured with calipers. For routine clinical purposes, the above-elbow-to-wrist segment is the most crucial, because it includes the supracondylar ligament and the pronator canal and, depending on the size of the hand, the pseudocarpal tunnel syndrome entrapment points. When this segment is abnormal, shorter segments must be studied in order to isolate the point of entrapment.

The Martin-Gruber anastamosis is described more fully in the sections of the ulnar nerve and the carpal tunnel syndrome (Figure 4.48). It should be remembered that this diversion of median nerve fibers to the ulnar nerve in the forearm can cause confusion when investigating suspected forearm median nerve entrapment or trauma, because it produces a difference in the evoked motor response recorded in the hand when the median nerve is stimulated at the elbow and at the wrist. A larger response is generated from stimulation at the elbow in these patients, because all median nerve axons are activated there whether they travel to the median or to the ulnar nerve. They summate into a larger response regardless of which muscle fibers are activated, and the wave shape of the responses has an initial small positive deflection.

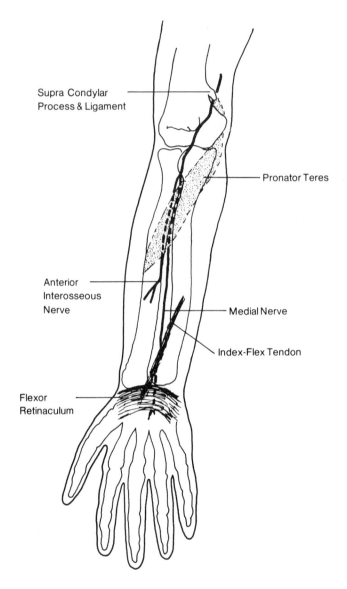

Figure 4.59. Course of the median nerve in the arm. Note the potential entrapment points at the supracondylar process and in the forearm.

A technique is available for determining conduction along the anterior interosseus branch of the median nerve and is described under anterior interosseus syndrome.

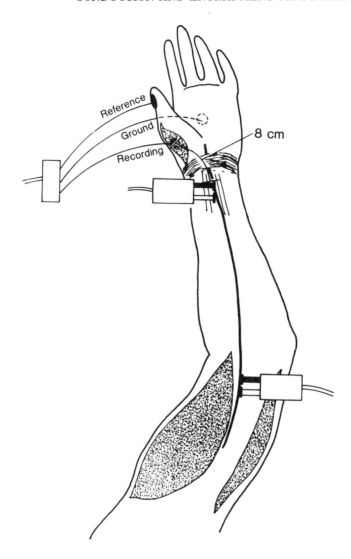

Figure 4.60. Standard technique for obtaining median conduction velocity in the forearm.

Standard Sensory Conduction Technique

The distal techniques of median sensory conduction are described in the section on carpal tunnel syndrome. Forearm conduction velocity can be obtained using either orthodromic or antidromic techniques. The standard antidromic technique consists of recording with ring electrodes from the index and long finger digital branches and stimulating at a point over the wrist 14 cm proximal to the recording electrode and then proximally at the elbow. Using this technique, the mean conduction velocity in the forearm, measuring to the peak, is 56.9 ± 4 msec (lower limits of normal, 49 M/sec) (42). Using computer averaging techniques, proximal orthodromic segment conduction velocities can be measured, stimulating at the hand or wrist and recording along the nerve as proximal to the Erb point or the spinal cord. More recently, the somatosensory evoked potentials using median nerve stimulation have been well defined and may be the best technique for determining median conduction proximal to the midarm segment.

Anterior Interosseus Syndrome

The anterior interosseus nerve arises from the posterior aspect of the median nerve as it passes between the two heads of the pronator teres. It runs with the interosseus artery along the anterior aspect of the interosseus membrane deep to and supplying the flexor pollicis longus, the flexor digitorum profundus (two lateral leads), and pronator quadratus (Fig. 4.59).

The most frequent cause of anterior interosseus nerve syndrome is repeated forceful use of the forearm muscles. It is occasionally seen bilaterally following floor-scrubbing with a hand brush. Some cases may represent a true entrapment neuropathy, because fibrous constricting bands have been reported. It can also occur from compression during unconsciousness.

The major complaint is that of vague aching in the forearm, developing either gradually or suddenly. Weakness, if present, is usually noticed during pinch grip. Physical examination reveals weakness of the flexor pollicis longus and other muscles supplied. In some cases, only a portion of the nerve distribution is compromised. Sensory examination is normal.

Needle electromyography is usually most helpful in defining the syndrome, because all terminal branches can be tested. It should be used in conjunction with the standard testing of the median and ulnar nerves to rule out other pathology. The flexor pollicis longus is most likely to be abnormal.

For conduction studies, the median nerve is stimulated at the elbow, and recording is from the pronator quadratus using a needle electrode. (Editor's note: Colachis has recently described surface recording of pron. quad. m. from the dorsal aspect of the distal forearm.) The electrode is inserted proximal and just volar to the ulnar styloid, parallel to the plane of the radius and ulnar with the forearm supinated (Fig. 4.61). The latency is 5.3 ± 0.5 msec (upper limit of normal, 6.3 msec).

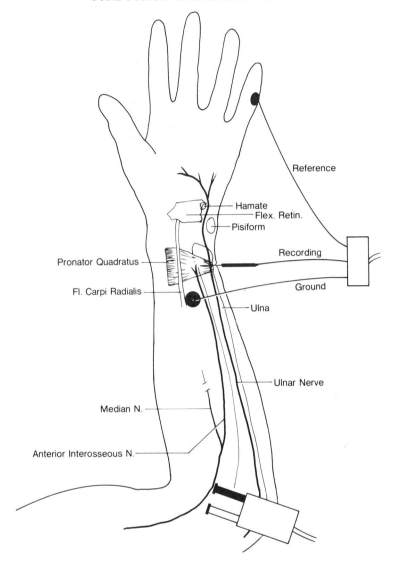

Figure 4.61. A technique for obtaining motor conduction in the anterior interosseous nerve.

Lateral Cutaneous Nerve of the Thigh

This purely sensory nerve (lumbar roots 2 and 3) supplies sensation to the lateral one-third of the thigh. It passes around the pelvis and emerges into the thigh beneath or through the inguinal ligament approximately 1 cm medial to the anterior superior iliac spine. Distally it

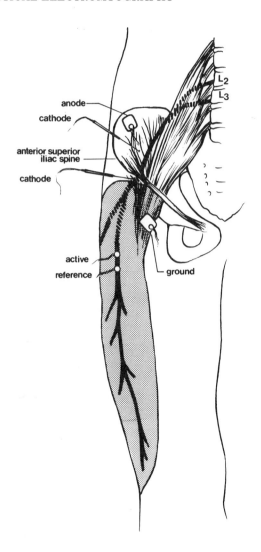

Figure 4.62. Anatomy and stimulation technique for the lateral cutaneous nerve of the thigh.

forms branches that travel some distance distally (Fig. 4.62) before penetrating the fascia lata and becoming subcutaneous.

Entrapment is usually at the inguinal ligament. Obesity, underlying metabolic or toxic neuropathies, direct trauma, and indirect trauma by corsets, belts, or braces have been implicated as causes of nerve injury at the ligament, but often no clear etiology is found. Another potential site of entrapment is the point of penetration of the distal branches

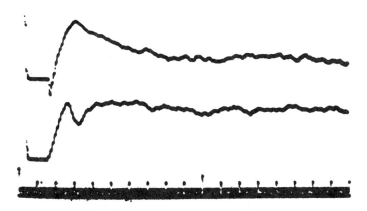

Figure 4.63. Evoked sensory response recorded antidromically from each side in the lateral cutaneous nerve of the thigh. Time base divisions are 1 msec, and the height is equivalent to 10 μV. The lower response is from the asymptomatic side. Note the slight prolongation of the latency on the symptomatic side *(top)*.

through the fascia lata. The nerve is sometimes compromised by intrapelvic masses or inflammatory processes.

Entrapment, regardless of its location, produces burning pain and numbness over the lateral thigh known as *meralgia paresthetica*. Sitting may exacerbate the symptoms, but anesthesia is rare. The presence of true thigh weakness is inconsistent with this diagnosis, because it is a purely sensory nerve.

Standard Sensory Conduction Technique

The nerve is evaluated antidromically using the anterior branch. A needle electrode is most effective for stimulation. It is inserted approximately 1 cm medially and distally to the anterior iliac spine. Depth depends on patient size. Surface recording is obtained 12 cm distal to the ligament (Fig. 4.62). Normal latency is 2.6 ± 0.2 msec, giving an upper limit of less than 3.1 msec. There should be little change in the latency across the ligament (Fig. 4.63). Amplitude ranges from 10 to 25 μV. Strip electrodes placed perpendicular to the course of the nerve are helpful for recording. Placing recording electrodes more distally on the lateral thigh may avoid the interfering motor artifact of the tensor fascia lata.

Mild chronic entrapments may produce a prolongation of the latency, but in most instances of true meralgia no evoked potential is recordable. Because there is anatomic variation in nerve location, the asymp-

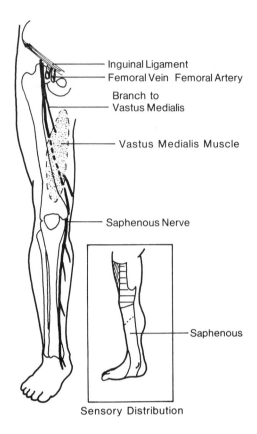

Figure 4.64. Anatomy of the femoral nerve and its distal sensory continuation of the saphenous nerve.

tomatic extremity should always be examined when the potential is absent on the symptomatic side to ensure that the recording technique is not the cause of the "abnormality."

Femoral Nerve

The femoral nerve (L2,L3,L4) passes through the psoas major and supplies the iliacus and pectineus muscles before passing beneath the inguinal ligament. In the thigh the anterior branch supplies the sartorius and gives off the intermediate and medial cutaneous branches to the thigh. The posterior branch forms the saphenous (sensory) nerve and also supplies the quadriceps and knee joint (Fig. 4.46).

Femoral neuropathy has many causes: alcoholism, diabetes, polyarteritis nodosa, trauma from hip fracture, pressure during the birth process, hemorrhage into the psoas muscle secondary to anticoagulation therapy, self-retaining surgical retractor blades, or during prolonged dorsal lithotomy position. Surgical tourniquets can produce injury, and as many as 40% of total hip procedures may result in some femoral injury.

Symptoms include medial leg and thigh sensory changes, knee instability, or frank quadriceps weakness. Hip flexor weakness is rare, because these muscles also receive direct root branches. The patellar reflex may be decreased or absent.

Standard Motor Conduction Technique

Conduction is studied using stimulation at three points: just above the inguinal ligament, just below the ligament, and distally along Hunter's canal. Recording is from the medialis, because it receives the most direct branch of the femoral nerve. Above the inguinal ligament, the nerve lies lateral to the pulsation of the femoral artery and can be easily stimulated with a needle electrode if surface stimulation proves inadequate (Fig. 4.65). Needle stimulation may be necessary in Hunter's canal, and this stimulation point is often omitted.

Johnson found a mean latency from the above-inguinal ligament stimulation point of 7.1 ± 0.7 msec (upper limit of normal, 8.5 msec) and a mean latency of 6.0 ± .07 msec (upper limit of normal, 7.4 msec) from the below-inguinal ligament stimulation point. The conduction velocity over the femoral nerve was found to be 66.7 ± 7.4 m/sec; however, in 25% of their controls, the evoked response was not well enough defined at all points of stimulation to enable the determination of a conduction velocity. It is often more practical to rely on latency values, rather than attempt to determine a femoral conduction velocity.

Johnson reported a mean latency difference of 1.1 ± 0.4 msec (upper limit of normal, 1.9 msec) for the clinically important transinguinal segment. There should be no significant loss of evoked potential amplitude or distortion of the evoked response between these two stimulation points. The mean distance across the inguinal ligament in their study was 5.5 ± 1.6 cm, and the mean distance from above the inguinal ligament site to the recording electrode was 35.4 ± 1.9 cm.

Needle EMG studies, late waves (H and F waves), or somatosensory evoked potentials are useful for injuries proximal to the ligament. Individual motor branches may be tested using needle recording electrodes to isolate the evoked response. Diabetic lumbar radiculopathy may simulate femoral neuropathy; therefore, needle examination of the paraspinals should always be performed when femoral neuropathy is suspected.

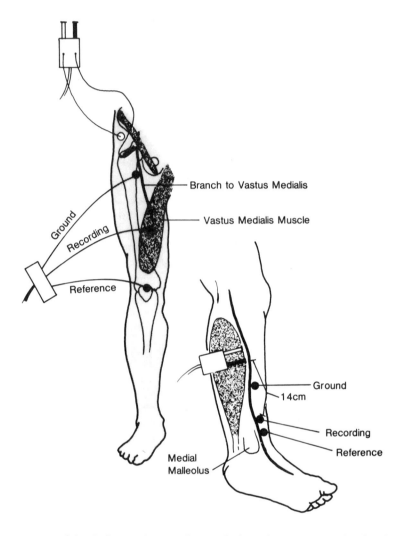

Figure 4.65. Stimulation and recording technique for motor conduction in the femoral nerve (note needle stimulation at the inguinal ligament). Lower insert shows technique for recording sensory evoked response antidromically in the saphenous nerve.

Standard Sensory Conduction Technique

See the section on the saphenous nerve for a discussion of this technique.

Saphenous Nerve

The saphenous nerve (L3,L4) provides sensation for the medial aspect of the knee, leg, and foot. Entrapment may occur as it penetrates the roof of the adductor canal. It can be injured by compression or improper support of the leg during surgery. Most frequently, injury occurs during vein stripping due to its position near the saphenous vein. Injury produces aching or burning pain on the medial aspect of the leg.

Standard Sensory Conduction Technique

The reference electrode (most distal) is placed just anterior to the medial malleolus in the space between the malleolus and the tibialis anterior tendon. The active recording electrode is placed 3 cm proximal to this, also just below the anterior tibialis tendon. The nerve is stimulated 14 cm proximal to the recording electrode using a standard bipolar surface stimulator (Fig. 4.65). It is usually necessary to press the stimulating electrodes firmly under the medial edge of the tibia, separating the gastroc soleus from the bone. The response is measured to the peak of the evoked potential. Wainapel reported a normal latency of 3.6 ± 0.4 msec, with an amplitude of 9.0 ± 3.4 μV, giving an upper limit of normal of 4.4 msec (58).

Sciatic Nerve

The sciatic nerve is actually two closely bound separate cords throughout its full course. The lateral division supplies the short head of the biceps and eventually becomes the peroneal nerve. The medial division becomes the tibial nerve after providing some twigs to the other hamstrings (Fig. 4.66).

Compression can occur during coma or narcosis from prolonged lying or sitting on the buttocks. Transient sciatic numbness or symptoms may occur from sitting on a hard seat or wallet. Compression from tightness of the piriformis muscle has been reported, but remains controversial. Injury is seen in femoral shaft fractures and other thigh trauma, but is most frequently seen in injection palsy (lateral division).

Standard Motor Conduction Technique

When sciatic nerve compromise occurs in the thigh, as with injury from femoral fracture, it can be evaluated using conventional conduction studies. A needle electrode is used for proximal stimulation. The nerve lies deeply, approximately one-third of the way from the ischial tuberosity to the femoral trochanter. The distal stimulation point is in the popliteal fossa (needle or surface stimulation), and recording is from the abductor digiti minimi (lateral division) (Fig. 4.67) Yap reported a

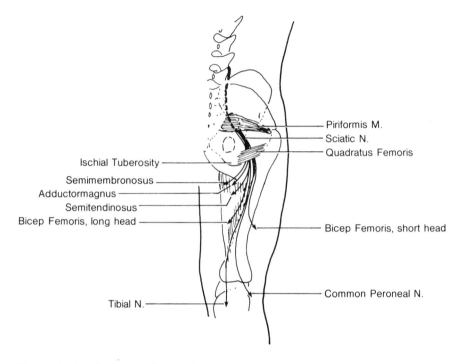

Figure 4.66. Anatomy of the sciatic nerve in the gluteal region.

normal conduction velocity for the thigh segment of 51.3 ± 4.4 m/sec, with a lower limit of normal of 42 m/sec (63). Responses can be recorded from any sciatic-innervated muscle; however, the normal conduction velocity varies to each muscle, e.g., medial gastrocnemius, 53.8 ± 3.3 m/sec; lower limit, 49.1 m/sec. Injury proximal to the ischium (wallet or narcosis-associated compression, injection palsy) shows only indirect changes, such as mild, generalized conduction slowing from large axon loss, by this direct conduction technique.

The most effective means of evaluating the function proximal to the ischium is the use of late waves. In this regard, H and F wave changes can be present in injection palsy or other proximal injuries. Both the tibial (H or F wave) and the peroneal (F wave) branches should be tested, because compromise of a single division of the nerve is possible (see H and F wave section). It is important to remember that direct conduction studies must be performed, if the late wave studies are abnormal, in order to localize the level of injury. Proximal stimulation using needle or magnetic electrodes for root stimulation may also prove helpful.

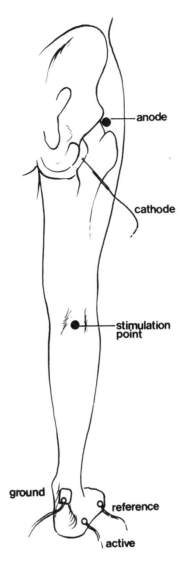

Figure 4.67. Stimulation technique for motor conduction studies in the sciatic nerve.

Standard Sensory Conduction Technique

Somatosensory studies recorded from the cortex or spinal cord provide another method of assessing sciatic sensory function.

Peroneal Nerve

The nerve originates at the "division" of the sciatic nerve at the apex of the popliteal fossa. It is vulnerable to compression as it spirals around the caudolateral margin of the fibular head before dividing into its two branches, the deep and the superficial peroneal nerves (Figs. 4.61, 4.68, and 4.69). There, "crossed leg palsy" results from compression of the nerve between the ipsilateral fibular head and the contralateral patella and femoral condyle when the legs are casually crossed while sitting. Recent weight loss, diabetic status, and neurotropic drug use increase susceptibility to compression. Trauma, cast pressure, or prolonged, unaccustomed squatting or kneeling can also cause compromise. Clinical localization is aided by the absence of involvement of the popliteal sensory branches in these entrapments (Figs. 4.68 and 4.70). Inversion ankle sprains may produce stretch injuries to the peroneal nerve, which should be suspected in individuals with repeated ankle sprains. Popliteal space masses and accessory ossicles can also produce nerve injury. Symptoms are painless foot drop, dorsiflexion or eversion weakness, and decreased sensation on the dorsum of the foot.

Standard Motor Conduction Technique

The common peroneal nerve is stimulated in the popliteal fossa and at the lower limit of the fibular head (Fig. 4.71). Distal stimulation of the deep branch is at the border of the anterior tibialis tendon and at the posterior border of the lateral malleolus when an accessory peroneal nerve (APN) is present. Calculation provides conduction velocities for the fibular head segment and for the leg segment distal to the fibular head.

The extensor digitorum brevis is composed of separate muscle slips, which in some individuals may be supplied by both the deep peroneal nerve branch and by a separate accessory peroneal nerve (22%) that originates from the superficial peroneal nerve. The APN passes behind the lateral malleolus, and its presence can be recognized by the unusual finding of a smaller evoked response when stimulating at the ankle than proximally (Fig. 4.72). These additional axons can be tested by stimulating behind the lateral malleolus.

Peroneal palsy from compression or entrapment at the fibular head results in slowing of conduction in the segment of the nerve across the fibular head. The normal peroneal conduction velocity is 49.9 ± 5.9 m/sec, lower limit of normal, 38 m/sec. The velocity of the proximal segment should be equal to or greater than that of the leg segment. In addition to conduction slowing, there should be changes in the evoked motor action potential with entrapment, as described earlier in the chapter.

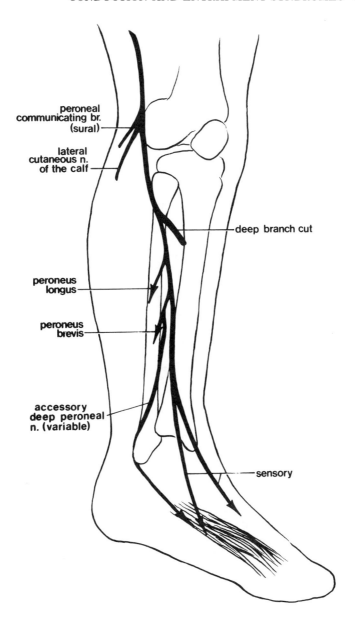

peroneal
communicating br.
(sural)

lateral
cutaneous n.
of the calf

deep branch cut

peroneus
longus

peroneus
brevis

accessory
deep peroneal
n. (variable)

sensory

Figure 4.68. Superficial branch of the peroneal nerve.

The peroneal nerve is particularly susceptible to compromise in neuropathies of various types. Figures 4.72–4.76 demonstrate frequent nonentrapment sources of evoked potential amplitude decrease.

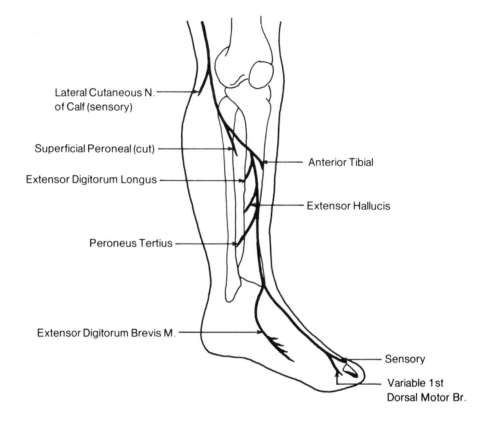

Figure 4.69. Deep branch of the peroneal nerve.

Before reporting complete axonotmesis of the nerve in cases of trauma, it is important to test both the deep and the superficial branches. When no clear response is detected using surface recording electrodes, needle recording electrodes should be used, and needle EMG exploration should be undertaken to achieve better sensitivity of the examination.

In peroneal compromise, needle EMG abnormalities are expected only in the peroneal nerve territory; however, the concomitant occurrence of a chronic peripheral neuropathy is possible. Thus, the presence of abnormalities in the distal tibially innervated muscles does not necessarily exclude peroneal nerve injury. Stretch injuries associated with ankle sprains may produce only mild distal segment conduction slowing. There, needle EMG is helpful, along with recording conduction from several distal muscles. Trauma can be confined to a single nerve branch; thus, conduction and needle electrode EMG should routinely

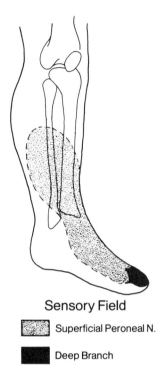

Sensory Field

▨ Superficial Peroneal N.

■ Deep Branch

Figure 4.70. Peroneal nerve sensory distribution.

be performed to several muscles supplied by the nerve. Conduction to the extensor hallucis longus can be studied when the more distal muscles are unavailable due to chronic neuropathy.

Standard Sensory Conduction Technique

DiBenedetto has described an antidromic technique for the superficial branch involving stimulation with a bipolar surface stimulating electrode at a point 2 cm medial and 5 cm proximal to the lateral malleolus (16). Recording is over the dorsum of the foot using two 1 cm by 3 cm silver straps. Light abrasion of the skin may be required, and in 2–3% of normal individuals no response was seen. Measurement was performed to the first negative deflection, rather than to the peak. Mean conduction velocity for individuals below the age of 15 is 53.1 ± 5.2 m/sec, lower limit of normal, 43 m/sec, and for those over the age of 15, 47.3 ± 3.4 m/sec, lower limit of normal, 40 m/sec. The mean amplitude was 13 μV.

In a group of patients with neuropathy, response was absent more

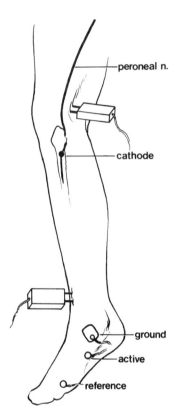

Figure 4.71. Standard motor conduction study technique for the peroneal nerve.

often in the superficial peroneal than in the sural nerve (68% versus 32%). The absence of response is, of course, more difficult to interpret than is the finding of a delayed response, as technical error must be considered. Thus, the better established sural or tibial nerve conduction studies would appear to be more reliable for screening uses.

Tibial Nerve

The tibial nerve (L4,L5,S1,S21) originates by the "division" of the sciatic nerve at the apex of the popliteal fossa. It lies quite superficially through the middle of the popliteal fossa (lateral to the popliteal vessels) and in the distal third of the calf. Distally, it forms the medial and lateral plantar nerves as it passes through the tarsal tunnel at the medial malleolus (see tarsal tunnel syndrome).

The tibial nerve above the tarsal canal is relatively free from entrapments. It can be compromised in the popliteal space by cysts, masses,

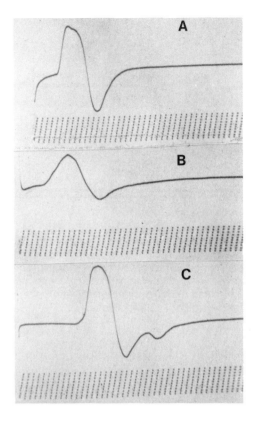

Figure 4.72. Accessory peroneal nerve: motor evoked response recorded from the extensor digitorum brevis with peroneal nerve stimulation at *C,* knee; *B,* behind lateral malleolus, and *A,* standard distal location anterior ankle. The drop in the evoked potential size with distal stimulation is the clue to presence of anomalous innervation.

or physical compression. In the leg, it is vulnerable to direct trauma and to ischemia during vascular compartment syndromes.

Standard Motor Conduction Technique

Johnson and Ortiz described stimulation of the nerve in the midpopliteal space using a standard bipolar surface stimulator (30). The distal stimulation point is just above the tarsal tunnel along the lower tibial border, at the upper edge of the medial malleolus. Recording is by means of a surface electrode placed over the motor point of the abductor hallucis (Fig. 4.77). This is located approximately 1 cm posterior and below the navicular tubercle. The normal conduction velocity is 49.8 ± 6.0 m/sec (lower limit of normal, 38 m/sec), and the motor la-

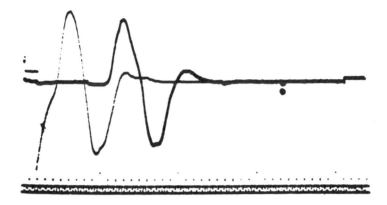

Figure 4.73. Evoked responses obtained by stimulation of the peroneal nerve at the ankle and above the fibular head in an 82-year-old man in good health. The slight amplitude loss is the result of increased temporal dispersion associated with aging. The proximal response *(right)* changes little above and below the fibular head. Minor changes between stimulation points are common in older people, and care should be exercised to avoid overinterpretation of such minor changes. (Caliber: 1 msec. Negative spike = 2.5 millivolts.)

tency to the abductor hallucis is 4.8 ± 0.8 msec (upper limit of normal, 6.4 msec). Motor conduction using the same stimulation points can also be performed for the lateral plantar branch. Recording is over the abductor digiti quinti motor point, which is directly below the lateral malleolus at the sole-regular skin junction (Fig. 4.77). The latency for this study is 5.8 ± 0.84 msec, with an upper limit of normal of 7.5 msec.

Standard Sensory Conduction Technique

See tarsal tunnel syndrome for a discussion of distal studies. Sensory conduction can be obtained along the leg segment using computer averaging techniques. Somatosensory studies provide an alternative means of assessing sensory conduction.

Tarsal Tunnel Syndrome (TTS)

The tarsal tunnel contains the tibial nerve and vessels and tendons of the posterior tibialis, flexor digitorum longus, and flexor hallucis longus covered by the flexor retinaculum (lancinate ligament). Unlike the transverse carpal ligament, it is composed of multiple deep fibrous septa to which the nerve may be attached and which blend with the periosteum (Fig. 4.78). The anchoring of the nerve makes it susceptible to traction or compression. Causes include posttraumatic fibrosis after ankle fracture, compression by a ganglion or varix of the posterior ti-

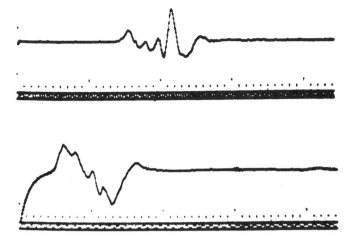

Figure 4.74. Motor evoked responses from the peroneal nerve in an 83-year-old adult-onset diabetic. The time base is 1 msec, and height is 500 µV. Such dispersion and changes in the form of the evoked potential between stimulation points are more related to the underlying disease than to any superimposed entrapment. Conservative interpretation of results regarding entrapment may be best when a long-standing peripheral neuropathy coexists. The peroneal evoked response using the extensor digitorum brevis as the recording point may be polyphasic and dispersed because of the presence of multiple muscle slips.

bial vein, tendon sheath cysts, valgus deformity of the ankle, and compression by an accessory or hypertrophied abductor hallucis muscle. TTS has also been described as associated with sudden weight gain or fluid retention. In the majority of surgically explored cases, however, no underlying cause has been identified.

The tibial nerve divides into medial and lateral plantar branches just after entering the tunnel. Either of these branches can be entrapped as it runs in its separate compartment. The nerve also gives off the calcaneal branch, providing cutaneous and deep sensation (another entrapment site). The medial plantar nerve supplies the abductor hallucis, the flexor digitorum brevis, flexor hallucis brevis, and the first lumbrical. The lateral plantar nerve has both a superficial (third plantar, fourth dorsal interosseous) and a deep (two or three lateral lumbricals, remaining interossei, adductor hallucis) branch.

In contrast to the carpal tunnel syndrome, females are affected only sightly more often than males. The patient typically complains of intermittent burning pain and tingling in the foot that usually worsens with prolonged standing. Symptoms may be most prominent at night and seem to be proportional to the amount of standing or walking done during the day. The distribution of sensory impairment depends on the

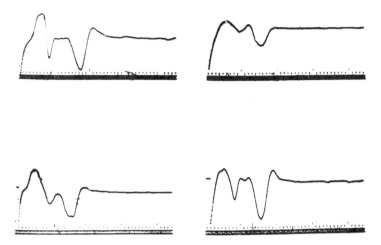

Figure 4.75. Evoked potentials recorded from the peroneal nerve with distal stimulation from the involved side *(upper two tracings)* and the uninvolved side *(lower two tracings)* 3 days *(left tracings)* and 7 days *(right tracings)* following the onset of an acute peroneal palsy. Recording was from the midpoint of the anterior tibialis muscle, and the time base is 1 msec, height is 2 millivolts. Note the excellent reproduction of the waveform in the uninvolved side 4 days apart, indicating the reliability of evoked response comparisons. The significant loss of amplitude in the upper right tracing and the evoked potential area decrease, when compared to the upper left tracing, are proportional to the percentage of motor axons that have undergone Wallerian degeneration. Had the patient not been seen at 3 days after the injury, late comparison between the two sides would have given essentially identical information concerning the proportion of axons lost.

site of compromise and may involve either the medial or the lateral plantar nerve or both. Sensation on the dorsum of the foot should be normal, with the exception of the distal phalanges of the toes. Tapping

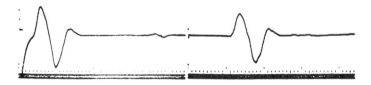

Figure 4.76. Evoked response change in a 73-year-old adult-onset diabetic man. Note the temporal dispersion and decreased amplitude of the motor evoked potential from proximal stimulation. The peroneal nerve, because of its length, is affected early in neuropathies, and the possibility of an underlying neuropathy should always be considered when small changes in the evoked potential are present between two stimulation points in this nerve. (Caliber: same as Figure 4.75.)

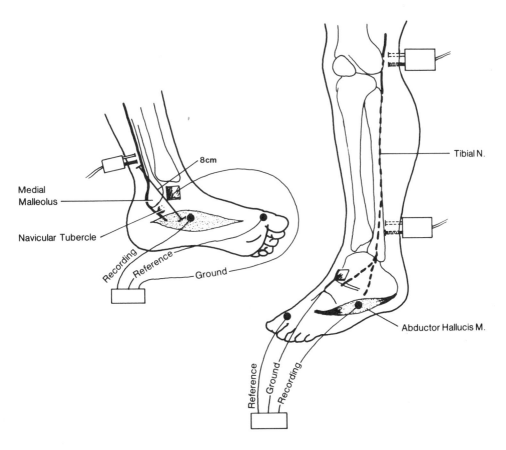

Figure 4.77. Motor conduction technique for the tibial nerve.

over the nerve may produce tingling in the foot (Tinel's sign), and tenderness, proximal and distal to the site of compression (the Valleix phenomenon), may be present. In addition, holding the ankle in forced inversion or application of a venous tourniquet on the calf may reproduce symptoms.

Standard Motor Conduction Technique

The tibial nerve is stimulated at the superior border of the medial malleolus, above the flexor retinaculum. Motor latencies to the abductor hallucis (medial plantar) and abductor digiti quinti pedis (lateral plantar) muscles can be recorded with surface electrodes (Fig. 4.77) Because both motor branches are stimulated, it is sometimes difficult to obtain a well-defined initial deflection for latency measurement for

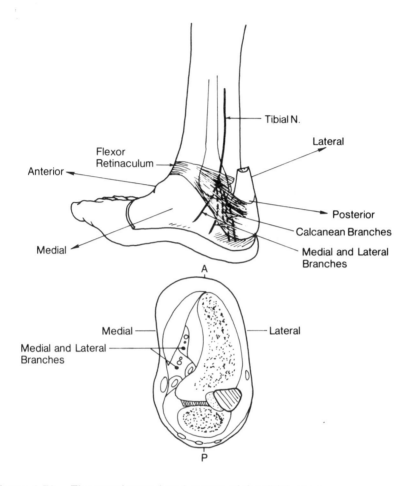

Figure 4.78. The tarsal tunnel and course of the tibial nerve.

each branch. Needle electrodes may be helpful in isolating the responses, but care must be taken to ensure that the shortest latency is obtained (see needle recording). Assuming that a normal conduction velocity is present in the proximal segment of the tibial nerve, the latency should not exceed 6.1 msec for the medial plantar and 6.7 msec for the lateral plantar branch. More than a 1.0 msec difference between the branch latencies suggests branch compromise.

Standard Sensory Conduction Technique

Sensory conduction studies are more sensitive to pathologic changes in conduction and can be recorded more precisely than motor studies. Although computer averaging is required to observe the response, the

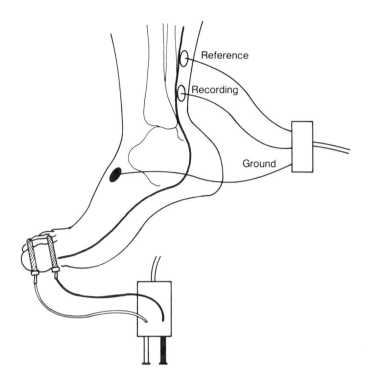

Figure 4.79. Orthodromic sensory conduction study in the distal tibial nerve. The illustrated technique employs the medial branch, whereas the analogous study may be performed on the lateral branch by placing the ring electrodes around the small toe.

technique is simple and is the one of choice in evaluating tarsal tunnel syndrome. Care must be exercised in distinguishing between tarsal tunnel syndrome and early peripheral neuropathy. The tibial sensory nerve is more sensitive than the sural nerve to the effects of peripheral neuropathy. Bilateral absence of the response (or symmetrical changes of any kind) is more likely due to peripheral neuropathy than to nerve entrapment.

Tibial sensory studies are performed orthodromically, recording the response from behind and just proximal to the medial malleolus from surface electrodes (Fig. 4.79). Studies of the medial and lateral branches are done using ring electrodes on the great and little toes respectively. A signal averager is required, because normal amplitudes range from 0.5 μV upward (Fig. 4.80). Normal values are medial branch—35.2 ± 3.6 m/sec, lower limit, 28 m/sec—and lateral branch—31.7 ± 4.4 m/sec, lower limit, 23 m/sec. A similar technique in recording over the tibial

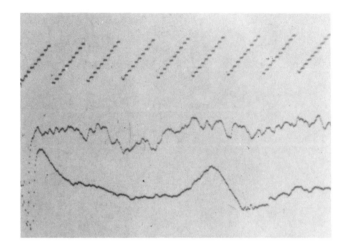

Figure 4.80. Averaged tibial orthodromic sensory response *(lower)* and real time response using technique illustrated (Fig. 4.26).

nerve can be used with stimulation of medial and lateral plantar nerves (compound nerve AP). No averaging is needed (48).

The minimal acceptable temperature recorded on the sole of the foot is 29.5° C (44). Other techniques, including stimulation at intervals along the nerve branches, have been reported. Because of the sensitivity of this study to foot temperature and to neuropathy, each electromyographer should establish standard values for the equipment and technique while simultaneously gaining practical experience in use of the technique.

Sural Nerve

The purely sensory sural (L5,S1,S2) nerve forms at midcalf with the junction of tibial and peroneal components. It is easily stimulated once it pierces the deep fascia to become subcutaneous. It runs posteriorly behind the lateral malleolus and along the lateral foot until it terminates at the lateral aspect of the small toe. The nerve supplies sensation to the posteriolateral aspect of the lower third of the leg and the dorsolateral aspect of the foot (Fig. 4.81).

Clinical Pathology

It is relatively free of entrapments, and therefore it is frequently used to assess the general physiologic status of the peripheral nervous system. Entrapment can occur as it passes through the deep fascia near its origin or by fibrous adhesions from ankle fractures at the medial

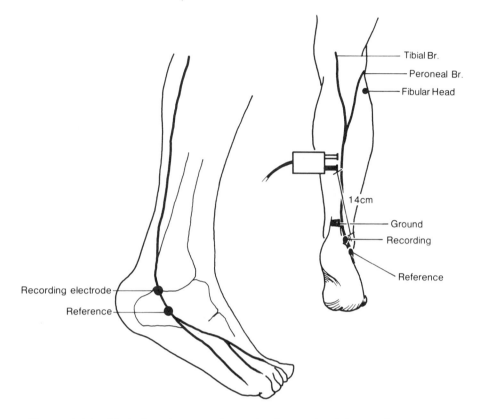

Figure 4.81. Technique for sensory conduction study of the sural nerve.

malleolus. Boot top compression also has been reported. Symptoms consist of numbness, burning, or dysesthesia in the appropriate distribution.

Standard Sensory Conduction Technique

Antidromic conduction studies are performed using surface stimulation and recording (Fig. 4.82). The recording electrodes are placed 3–4 cm apart along the course of the nerve as it passes around the lateral malleolus. It is best to maintain the ankle at approximately 90° (neutral position) during the study. The nerve can be stimulated along its course using a standard bipolar surface stimulator. A sweep speed of 2 msec/cm and amplification of 20 μV/cm for recording are used. Best results are obtained at 14 or 17 cm. At shorter distances, separating the evoked response from the shock artifact may be a problem, and at longer distances, the nerve may be too deeply located to stimulate.

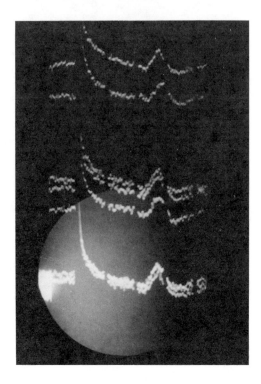

Figure 4.82. Sural sensory response. 20 μV = time base height *(lower left)*. Trace is interrupted at 1 msec intervals. Stimulus (14 cm) applied after 1 msec delay.

The mean latency value at 14 cm is 3.5 ± .25 msec (Fig. 4.83). giving an upper limit of normal of 4.0 msec. Particular care is required in ensuring that the foot temperature is above 29°C measured at the recording point. The mean amplitude of the evoked response is 23.7 ± 3.8 μV. Although technical problems may affect amplitude values, an amplitude below 10 μV peak to peak does suggest the presence of peripheral neuropathy. This impression should be confirmed through the use of multiple conduction studies, e.g., other sural, tibial sensory, peroneal sensory studies.

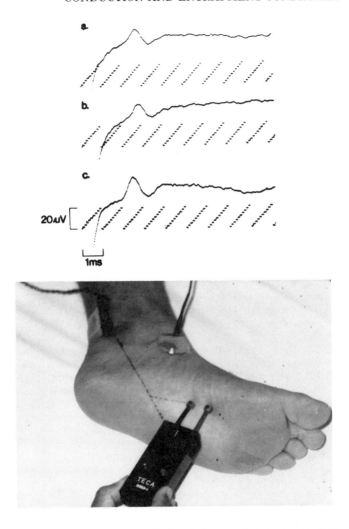

Figure 4.83. *A,* Compound nerve AP stimulating medial plantar N. *B,* Compound nerve AP stimulating lateral plantar N. *C,* Antidromic sural N. sensory AP (14 cm). *Bottom:* Medial plantar N. stimulation. (Courtesy of P. Gatens, M.D.)

References

1. Aguayo A: Neuropathy due to compression and entrapment. In Dyck P, Thomas P, Lambert E (eds): *Peripheral Neuropathy.* Philadelphia, WB Saunders, 1975.
2. Awad EA: Electrodiagnostic evaluation of phrenic nerve and diaphragm in high quadriplegia. Abstract, AAPM&R 40th Annual Assembly, 1978.
3. Baer RD, Johnson EW: Motor nerve conduction velocities in normal children. *Arch Phys Med Rehabil* 46:698–704, 1965.
4. Bolton CF: Factors affecting the amplitude of the human sensory compound action potentials. *AAEE Minimonograph (#17, October 1981.)*
5. Braddom RL, Johnson EW: Standardization of H reflex and diagnostic use in S-1 radiculopathy. *Arch Phys Med Rehabil* 55:161, 1974.
6. Braddom RL, Wolfe CV: Musculocutaneous nerve entrapment syndrome. Abstract, AAPM&R 37th Annual Assembly, 1975.
7. Butler ET, Johnson EW, Kaye Z: Normal conduction velocity in the lateral femoral cutaneous nerve. *Arch Phys Med Rehabil* 55:31–32, 1974.
8. Campbell WW, Ward LC, Swift TR: Nerve conduction velocity varies inversely with height. Abstract, AAEE 27th Annual Meeting, 1980.
9. Catterall WA: The molecular basis of neuronal excitability. *Science* 223:653–661, 1984.
10. Checkles NS, Balmaseda M: Standardization of ulnar sensory fiber conduction velocity. Abstract, AAPM&R 38th Annual Assembly, 1976.
11. Checkles NS, Bailey JA, Johnson EW: Tape and caliper surface measurements in determination of peroneal nerve conduction velocity. *Arch Phys Med Rehabil* 50-214–218, 1969.
12. Checkles NS, Russakov AD, Piero DL: Ulnar nerve conduction velocity—effect of elbow position on measurement. *Arch Phys Med Rehabil* 52:362–365, 1971.
13. Cockrell JL, Levine SP, Miller HF: Prediction of the excitation site resulting from surface electrical stimulation of a myelinated nerve. Abstract, AAPM&R 41st Annual Assembly, 1979.
14. Dawson G, Merton P: "Recurrent" discharges from motoneurones. Abstract, XX International Congress on Physiology, Bruges, Belgium, 1956.
15. Desmedt JE (ed): *Computer-Aided Electromyography,* Vol. 10 in *Progress in Clinical Neurophysiology.* Basel, S. Karger, Switzerland, 1983.
16. DiBendetto M: Sensory nerve conduction in lower extremities. *Arch Phys Med Rehabil* 51:253–258, 1970.
17. Dorfman LJ, Bosley TM: Age-related changes in peripheral and central nerve conduction in man. *Neurology* 29:38–44, 1979.
18. Dorfman L, Jayaramar: Handcuff neuropathy. *JAMA* 239:957, 1978.
19. Fraim CJ: Unusual cause of nerve entrapment. Letters to the Editor. *JAMA* 242:2557, 1979.
20. Gans BM, Kraft GH: Techniques of quantifying the stimulated M response and their clinical significance. Abstract, AAEE 23rd Annual Meeting, 1976.
21. Gassel MM: A test of nerve conduction to muscle of the shoulder girdle as an aid in the diagnosis of proximal neurogenic and muscular disease. *J Neurol Neurosurg Psychiat* 27:200–205, 1964.
22. Gassel MM, Diamantopoulous E: Pattern of conduction times in the distribution of the radial nerve. *Neurology* 14:222–231, 1964.
23. Haller EM, DeLisa JA, Brozovich FV: Nerve conduction velocity: relationship to skin, subcutaneous and intermuscular temperatures. *Arch Phys Med Rehabil* 61:199–203, 1980.
24. Henriksen JD: Conduction velocity of motor nerves in normal subjects and patients with neuromuscular disorders. M.S. Thesis, University of Minnesota, Minneapolis, 1956.

25. Hulley WC, Wilbourn AJ, McGinty K: Sensory nerve action potential amplitudes: alterations with temperature. Abstract, AAEE 24th Annual Meeting, 1977.
26. Izzo KL, Sridhara CR, Sharma R: Side, age, and sex influences on lower extremity sensory nerve conduction studies. Abstract, AAEE 27th Annual Meeting, 1980.
27. Jebsen RH: Motor conduction velocity in the proximal and distal segments of the radial nerve. *Arch Phys Med Rehabil* 47:597–601, 1966.
28. Jebsen RH: Motor conduction velocities in the median and ulnar nerves. *Arch Phys Med Rehabil* 48:185–194, 1967.
29. Johnson EW, Olsen KJ: Clinical value of motor nerve conduction velocity determination. *JAMA* 172:1–6, 1960.
30. Johnson EW, Ortiz PR: Electrodiagnosis of tarsal tunnel syndrome. *Arch Phys Med Rehabil* 47:776, 1966.
31. Johnson EW, Wood PK, Powers JJ: Femoral nerve conduction studies. *Arch Phys Med Rehabil* 49:528–532, 1968.
32. Kaplan RE: Electrodiagnostic confirmation of long thoracic nerve palsy. *J Neurol Neurosurg Psychiat* 43:50–52, 1980.
33. Kraft GH: Axillary, musculocutaneous and suprascapular nerve latency studies. *Arch Phys Med Rehabil* 53:383–387, 1972.
34. Lambert EH: The accessory peroneal nerve. *Neurology* 19:1169–1176, 1969.
35. Lambert EH: Principles of recording electrophysiological data: nerve action potential. Abstract, AAEE 24th Annual Session, 1977.
36. Licht, S: History. In Johnson EW (ed): *Practical Electromyography.* Baltimore, Williams & Wilkins, 1980.
37. MacLean IC: Nerve root stimulation to evaluate conduction across the lumbosacral plexus. Abstract, AAPM&R 41st Annual Assembly, 1979.
38. MacLean IC, Mattioni TA: Phrenic nerve conduction studies: a new technique MacLean IC, Mattioni TA: Phrenic nerve conduction studies: a new technique and its application in quadriplegic patients with high spinal cord injury. Abstract, AAPM&R 41st Annual Assembly, 1979.
39. Magladery JW, McDougal DB: Electrophysiological studies of nerve and reflex activity in normal man. *Bull Johns Hopkins Hosp* 86:265, 1950.
40. Magladery J, Porter W, Parka A, Teasdall R: Electrophysiological studies of nerve and reflex activity in normal man. IV. Two-neurone reflex and identification of certain action potentials from spinal roots and cord. *Bull Johns Hopkins Hosp* 88:499, 1951.
41. Martinez AC, Barrio M, Perez-Conde MS, Gutierrez AM: Electrophysiological aspects of sensory conduction velocity in healthy adults: *J Neurol Neurosurg Psychiat* 41:1092–1096, 1978.
42. Melvin JL, Schuchmann JA, Lanese RR: Diagnostic specificity of motor and sensory nerve conduction variables in carpal tunnel syndrome. *Arch Phys Med Rehabil* 54:69–74, 1973.
43. Norris AH, Shock NW, Wagman IH: Age changes in the maximal conduction velocity of motor fibers in human ulnar nerves. *J Appl Physiol* 5:589, 1953.
44. Oh SJ, Sarala PK, Cuba T, Elmore RS: Tarsal tunnel syndrome: electrophysiologic study. *Ann Neurol* 5:327–330, 1979.
45. Rask MR: Watchband superficial radial neurapraxia. *JAMA* 421:2702, 1979.
46. Roles NC, Maudsley RH: Radial tunnel syndrome. Resistant tennis elbow as a nerve entrapment. *JBJS Br* 54B:499–508, 1972.
47. Ruppert ES, Johnson EW: Motor nerve conduction velocities in low birth weight infants. *Pediatrics* 42:255, 1968.
48. Saeed MA, Gatens PF: Compound nerve action potentials of the medial and lateral plantar nerves through the tarsal tunnel. *Arch Phys Med Rehabil* 63:304–307, 1982.

49. Schuchmann JA: Sural nerve conduction and a standardized technique. *Arch Phys Med Rehabil* 58:166, 1977.
50. Smith KG, Hall SM: Nerve conduction during peripheral demyelination and remyelination. *J Neurol Sci* 48:201–219, 1980.
51. Spiegel MH, Johnson EW: Conduction velocity in the proximal and distal segments of motor fibers in the ulnar nerve of human beings. *Arch Phys Med Rehabil* 43:57–61, 1962.
52. Spindler HA, Felsentahl G: Sensory conduction in the musculocutaneous nerve. *Arch Phys Med Rehabil* 59:20–21, 1978.
53. Sunderlin: *Nerve and Nerve Injuries* Churchill Livingstone, 1978.
54. Trojaberg W, Sindrup EH: Motor and sensory conduction to different segments of the radial nerve in normal subjects. *J Neurol Neurosurg Psychiat* 32:354–359, 1969.
55. Turk MA, Weber RJ: EMG assessment of bladder function and rehabilitation potential. Abstract, 8th International Congress of PM&R, Stockholm, Sweden, 1980.
56. Turk MA, Burkhart JA, Traetow D, Waylonis GW: An alternate method of estimating peroneal motor nerve conduction velocity. Abstract, AAEE 23rd Annual Session, 1976.
57. Varghese G, Dulalas R, Rogof JB: Influence of inter-electrode distance on antidromic sensory potentials. Abstract, AAPM&R 39th Annual Assembly, 1977.
58. Wainapel SF, Kim DJ, Ebel A: Conduction studies of the saphenous nerve in healthy subjects. *Arch Phys Med Rehabil* 59:316–319, 1978.
59. Waxman SG: Conduction in myelinated, unmyelinated, and demyelinated fibers. *Arch Neurol* 34:585–589, 1977.
60. Waxman SG, Brill MH: Conduction through demyelinated plaques in multiple sclerosis: computer simulation of facilitation by shortening the nodes. *J Neurol Neurosurg Psychiat* 41:408–416, 1978.
61. Weber RJ, Bowers D: Determination of the anatomical distribution of the C-8 nerve root by percutaneous root stimulation. Abstract, AAEE 27th Annual Meeting, 1980.
62. Weber RJ, Piero DL: F wave evaluation of thoracic outlet syndrome: a multiple regression derived F wave latency predicting technique. *Arch Phys Med Rehabil* 59:464, 1978.
63. Yap CB, Hirota T: Sciatic nerve motor conduction velocity study. *J Neurol Neurosurg Psychiat* 30:233–239, 1967.

5

Carpal Tunnel Syndrome

ERNEST W. JOHNSON

Along with radiculopathy, carpal tunnel syndrome (CTS) cases comprise a majority of the clinical conditions seen by the electromyographer (Fig. 5.1).

Since the early 1970s, the use of many precise techniques has made the diagnosis of CTS more sensitive. Historically, the first detection of abnormality in CTS was the uncovering by needle examination of fibrillation potentials and a reduced recruitment pattern. The next advance in electrodiagnostic testing was the determination of the distal motor latency of the median nerve recording from the abductor pollicis brevis. Initially, the limit of 5 msec was determined to be the top normal latency. In CTS the distal median nerve motor latency was delayed under the carpal ligament.

This technique of determining distal motor latency was further refined. With more accurate measurements, the mean latency at 8 cm was found to be 3.7 $\pm$ .3 msec. Two SDs established the upper limit as 4.3 msec. In vivo recording of sensory nerve action potentials orthodromically was developed by Dawson and Scott and adapted clinically for CTS diagnosis (7). Age does not appreciably affect the sensory or motor latency.

Many electromyographers still compare the distal median motor latency with that of the ulnar nerve. Unfortunately, if one does not measure carefully (8 cm) from the motor point, one will obtain a shorter distance for the ulnar nerve and thus a shorter latency. If a precise measurement is made, the stimulation for the ulnar nerve will be more proximal than that for the median nerve, and there will be no difference between median and ulnar nerve latencies, i.e., normal value for both latencies is 3.7 $\pm$ .3 msec.

Although a difference of 1 msec from contralateral median latency has been used as a diagnostic indicator for CTS, this marker has been shown to be inappropriate because there is often bilateral involvement, with the dominant hand more severely affected.

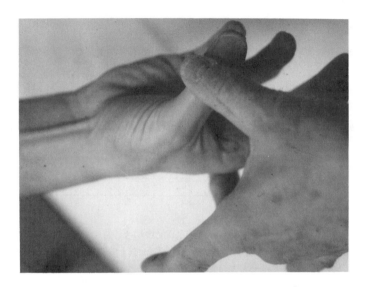

Figure 5.1. Testing the abductor pollicis brevis. Although it is impossible to isolate this muscle completely, this maneuver is the most reliable and valid one. (Courtesy of E.W. Johnson)

A frequent observation in chronic CTS is that the proximal median motor conduction velocity is low, even abnormally low. This had been considered to be a consequence of retrograde demyelination from the site of compromise; however, the low velocity is now felt to be simply a result of measuring the velocity of only those smaller diameter median motor axons (and slower conducting axons) that escape the compression under the carpal ligament that befalls the larger, more vulnerable, and thus faster conducting motor axons (Fig. 5.2).

If one measures the conduction velocity by evoking the compound nerve action potential recording over the median nerve at the wrist and elbow, the values are in the normal range.

MARTIN-GRUBER ANASTOMOSIS

A frequent anatomic anomaly (17–30% of cases) can make CTS motor determinations confusing unless the electromyographer appreciates its consequences.

In patients with the Martin-Gruber anastomosis, some ulnar motor fibers travel down the median nerve until the forearm where they rejoin the ulnar nerve. Therefore, stimulation of the median nerve at the elbow also stimulates those ulnar motor fibers traveling in the median nerve, whereas stimulating the median nerve at the wrist does not (Fig. 5.3).

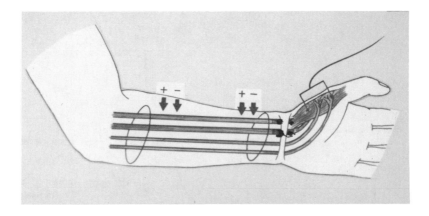

Figure 5.2. Diagrammatic representation of the reason for slowing of the median nerve motor conduction velocity in the forearm. Note that the only fibers conducting to the abductor pollicis brevis are the smaller diameter axons that escaped the compression in the carpal tunnel. The large diameter and thus faster conducting axons were blocked under the carpal ligament. However, conduction velocity of the nerve trunk between the wrist and elbow is normal.

The clues on electrodiagnostic testing to the presence of this anastomosis when CTS is present include the following:

1. An initial positive deflection of the compound motor action potential (CMAP) is obtained when stimulating at the elbow, but is not present when the median nerve is stimulated at the wrist. This is because the recording electrode is not over the motor point of the ulnar (muscle) portion of the nerve, whereas at the wrist only the median nerve is activated and the recording electrode is over the abductor pollicis brevis.
2. There is a larger CMAP when stimulating the median nerve of the elbow because the recording electrode is responding to ulnar-innervated muscles (presumably the deep head of the flexor pollicis brevis), whereas at the wrist the stimulus is restricted to median-innervated muscles. This is the only finding present in normal nerve conduction.
3. If motor conduction velocity is calculated it will be artifactually fast (100–150 m/sec) because the elbow stimulation activates the ulnar axons that escape the carpal tunnel.

More recent techniques that are more sensitive in diagnosis and also can assist in evaluation of the anastomosis severity, as well as provide prognostic information, have been described.

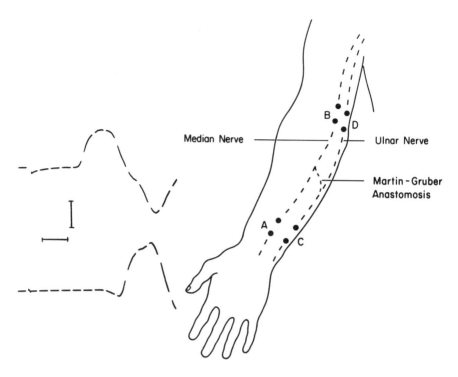

5.3. Martin-Gruber Anastomosis. *Top trace,* Median nerve stimulated at wrist. *Bottom trace,* Median nerve stimulated at elbow. Note larger CMAP and initial positive deflection (not present at wrist stimulation). (Caliber: 5 millivolt. Sweep is interrupted at 1-msec interval.)

MIDPALMAR STIMULATION

Stimulation of the median nerve at the wrist (14 cm) and then at the midpalmar site (7 cm) with recording antidromically of the sensory nerve action potential (SNAP) at Digit III or Digit II has been shown to be extraordinarily sensitive and reliable (Fig. 5.4). It can also provide objective evidence of neurapraxic block within the carpal tunnel and thus give prognostic information. Finally, this technique can assist in assessing the degree of underlying peripheral neuropathy (vulnerable nerve syndrome) when there is additional entrapment under the carpal ligament.

Orthodromic stimulation gives the same values at 14 cm, but midpalmar stimulation with orthodromic recording at the wrist involves both motor and sensory nerve fibers. This is not comparable to digital stimulation of only sensory fibers as is the case in antidromic (14 cm; 7 cm) stimulation.

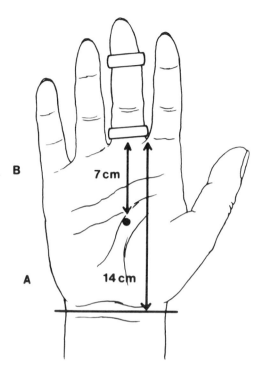

Figure 5.4. Technique for antidromic median sensory stimulation at 7 and 14 cm.

One should always measure the temperature of the hand because a cold hand may mask the diagnosis of mild CTS if the latencies and amplitudes are examined uncritically (Fig. 5.5). The reduced temperature usually increases the reduced amplitudes of SNAP in CTS, despite the prolonged latency across the carpal tunnel. The temperature should be measured at the surface of the palm at the distal palm crease and also over the palmar aspect at the distal middle phalanx. The relatively prolonged delay within the carpal tunnel can be masked by a disproportionate slowing in the distal 7-cm segment because the more distal fingers will be cooler than the proximal wrist and palm segment (Figs. 5.6–5.9).

COMPARISON OF ULNAR AND MEDIAN SENSORY LATENCIES

In the clinically confusing situation of a CTS with an underlying peripheral neuropathy, the comparison of antidromic sensory latency between ulnar and median nerve can be helpful with recording over Digit

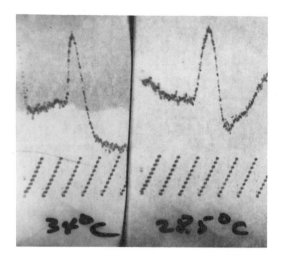

Figure 5.5. Effect of temperature on antidromic median snap. (Caliber: Each slanted line = 1 msec. Height = 20 μV.

IV (Fig. 5.10). Unfortunately there is almost always an interfering motor artifact when the ulnar nerve is stimulated antidromically.

Orthodromic recording at the wrist over the ulnar and median nerves with stimulation of Digit IV provides similar latencies and avoids the motor artifact. The amplitudes of orthodromically determined SNAP are smaller by 30–50%.

COMPARISON OF RADIAL AND MEDIAN SENSORY LATENCIES

The sensory territory of the thumb (Digit I) is supplied by both median and radial nerves (Fig. 5.11), thereby providing an opportunity to compare the antidromic or orthodromic sensory latency of the radial nerve with that of the median nerve. Note that the radial sensory action potential is quite a bit smaller than the median SNAP (approximately 50–70% smaller) (Fig. 5.12). A distance of 10 cm is used because the sensory branch of the radial nerve courses volarly until the distal forearm when it travels to the dorsal wrist and then to the thumb. A 10-cm distance approximates this change in the nerve's course and positions the electrode where it is possible to stimulate both median and radial nerves simultaneously. Should the median nerve be blocked in the carpal tunnel and thus delayed, it will appear later on the trace, making a double hump in the SNAP recording. The first SNAP is then the normal latency radial and the second (delayed) one is the median SNAP (Fig. 5.13). We have named this the Bactrian sign to call atten-

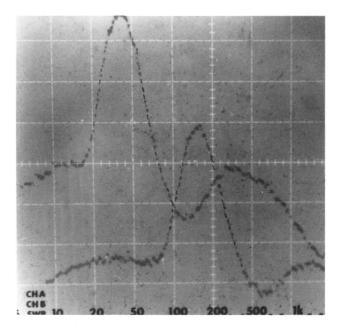

Figure 5.6. Median sensory nerve stimulation at 7 and 14 cm with recording over Digit III. This is a cold hand (25° C). Note that the duration and amplitude of snap are increased, and proportionately more on distal stimulation. (Caliber: Each horizontal division = 1 msec. Vertical division = 20 μV.)

tion to the double-humped camel (Asian or Bactrian camel), an endangered species. The values are as follows:

	Latency	Amplitude
Median	2.6 ± .2 msec	30 ± 12 μV
Radial	2.5 ± .15 msec	12 ± 5 μV

A difference of 1 msec is usually present even in mild CTS. Our recent studies suggest that this technique may be the most sensitive of the various distal latencies in the diagnosis of CTS.

This technique may also be done orthodromically although surface recording over the radial nerve is more difficult. Near-nerve needle electrode recording facilitates orthodromic recording.

Technique of Kimura

Antidromic sensory median latency can be determined with stimulation at 1-cm intervals. Ring electrodes are placed on Digit II or III, and surface bipolar stimulation is started at the wrist (14 cm) and then proceeding distally at 1-cm intervals (17). A block within the carpal

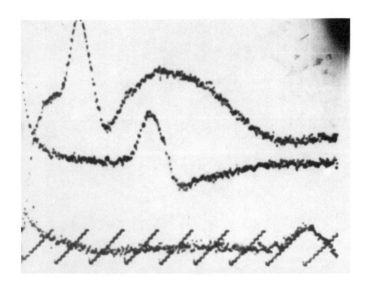

Figure 5.7. Normal median SNAP antidromically evoked with ring electrodes over Digit III. *Top trace,* stimulation at midpalmar site (7 cm). *Middle trace,* Stimulation at wrist (14 cm). *Bottom trace,* Stimulation at antecubital site (27 cm). Note that this is a normal tracing, yet the SNAP on proximal stimulation is smaller than expected as reported by Kimura. (Caliber: Each slanted line = 1 msec. Height = 20 µV.)

tunnel results in reduction in the SNAP in those stimulations proximal to the block and a prolonged latency with some restoration of both toward normal values as stimulation passes the site of the compromise (18).

However, this technique is best done with needle cathode stimulation because the depth of the median nerve varies as it courses from a superficial position at the base of the wrist, deeper through carpal tunnel, and then superficially again at the midpalm.

ANALYSIS OF COMPOUND MUSCLE ACTION POTENTIAL OF ABDUCTOR POLLICIS BREVIS WITH WRIST AND MIDPALMAR STIMULATION

The determination of the distal motor or sensory latency of the median nerve can confirm the diagnosis of CTS; however, only stimulation of the median nerve both proximally and distally to the carpal ligament can provide objective information about the prognosis. If the CMAP (>.5 millivolt) or SNAP (>30%) is larger when the median nerve is stimulated distally to the carpal ligament, then neurapraxic axons are present.

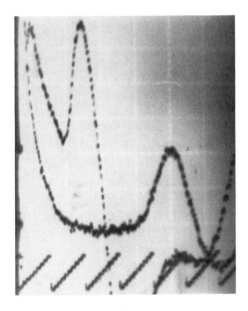

Figure 5.8. Seven and 14 cm. antidromic median SNAP ring electrode over Digit III in mild CTS. Note the temporal dispersion and reduced amplitude of the SNAP of wrist stimulation as compared to midpalmar stimulation. *Top trace,* 7 cm (midpalmar) stimulation. *Bottom trace,* 14 cm (wrist) stimulation. (Caliber: Each slanted line = 1 msec. Height = 20 μV.)

In contrast, the presence and number of fibrillation potentials in thenar muscles have little prognostic significance. Similarly, the reduced recruitment pattern on needle electrode examination does not

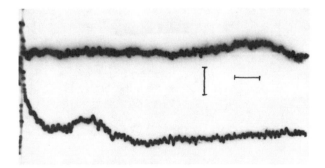

Figure 5.9. Median nerve antidromic SNAP in severe chronic CTS. *Top trace,* wrist stimulation 14 cm. *Bottom trace,* Midpalmar stimulation 7 cm. (Caliber: 20 μV; 1 msec.)

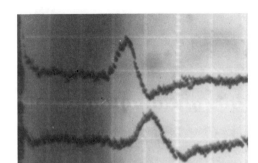

Figure 5.10. Antidromic median and ulnar SNAP in mild CTS (difference = .9 msec). *Top trace,* Ulnar. *Bottom trace,* Median. (Caliber: Each slanted line = 1 msec. Height = 20 µV.)

reflect the prognosis, but only the degree of block. The neurapraxic nerve fibers will still be excitable distal to the carpal ligament, a cir-

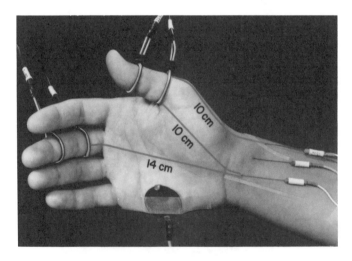

Figure 5.11. Needle antidromic stimulation of radial and median sensory nerves. Note the electrode placement. This permits comparison of the usual determination of the distal sensory latency to Digit III (14 cm), and the 10 cm antidromic latency of radial and median middle electrode stimulates the median and radial nerves simultaneously.

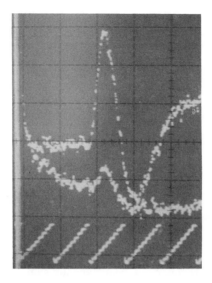

Figure 5.12. Normal antidromic radial (*bottom*) and median (*top*) SNAP to Digit I. (Caliber: Each slanted line = 1 msec. Height = 20 µV.)

cumstance easily assessed by midpalmar stimulation of motor nerve fibers. The point of stimulation distal to the carpal ligament is indicated by the tip of the ring finger flexed and touching the base of the palm (Fig. 5.14). Note that with needle stimulation the anode must be placed near to the needle cathode, e.g., ring electrode around Digit V (Fig. 5.15). Normal values are as follows:

	Mean Latency	Mean CMAP
	(msec)	(millivolt)
Wrist stimulation	3.7 ± .3 msec	9 ± .5 mV
Midpalmar stimulation	1.8 ± .2 msec	9.6 ± .5 mV
Increase distal to carpal ligament–.5 mV		

The degree of neurapraxia is proportional to the increase in the area under the negative spike of CMAP when stimulating distal to the carpal ligament (Figs. 5.16–5.18).

STEPS IN EVALUATING SUSPECTED CARPAL TUNNEL SYNDROME

The following steps should be taken when evaluating a suspected case of CTS.

1. Evaluate the sensation of the median nerve sensory territory, i.e. two-point discrimination, light touch.
2. Evaluate the weakness of the thenar muscles (see Fig. 5.1). Touch

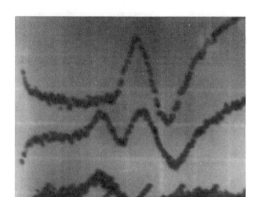

Figure 5.13. Median and radial antidromic SNAP (Digit I) *Top trace,* Median nerve at wrist (10 cm). *Middle trace,* Simultaneous stimulation of median and radial nerve (Bactrian sign). *Bottom trace,* radial nerve at wrist (10 cm). (Caliber: Each slanted line = 1 msec. Height = 20 μV.)

little finger to thumb (pad to pad). Examiner attempts to move proximal phalanx of thumb to second MP joint. Compare simultaneously with contralateral thumb.

3. Compare antidromic median and radial sensory latencies to Digit I.
4. Compare median latency at 14 cm antidromically to Digit III with midpalmar stimulation (7 cm).
5. Compare amplitude of the CMAP (area under negative spike of

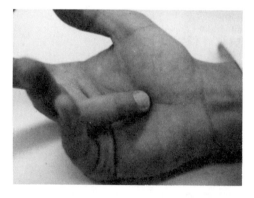

Figure 5.14. Point of stimulation of median motor branch to abductor pollicis brevis. Tip of flexed ring finger indicates site.

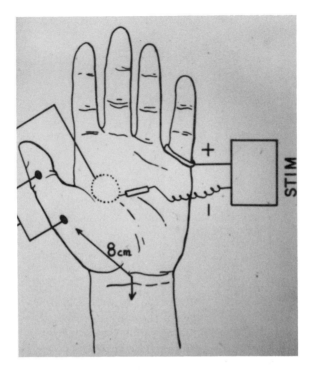

Figure 5.15. Electrode placement for median motor stimulation proximal and distal to carpal ligament. Note that the pin cathode is at midpalm and the ring anode is over Digit V. This placement keeps the stimulation current field away from the recording electrodes.

CMAP) of abductor pollicis brevis at both wrist and midpalmar stimulations (Fig. 5.19).

6. If there is any question about the diagnosis, compare Digit III with Digit II, at 7 and 14 cm.
7. If you suspect underlying peripheral neuropathy (Fig. 5.20) in addition to CTS, compare ulnar and median sensory latencies to Digit IV.
8. Screen the contralateral hand by median and radial sensory latencies to Digit I.

F waves and H waves (flexor carpi radialis) should only be used in CTS if one suspects proximal entrapment or peripheral neuropathy.

WRIST DIMENSIONS

The size of the wrist as a risk factor in the development of CTS has been investigated over the years. The original x-ray view (Gaynor-Hart)

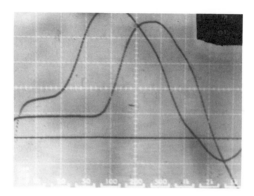

Figure 5.16. Wrist and midpalmar stimulation of median motor fibers (CMAP)—normal. *Top trace,* Midpalmar stimulation (2 cm). *Middle trace,* Wrist stimulation (8 cm). (Caliber: Each square = 1 msec, 2 millivolts.)

was designed to show the bony carpal tunnel. Recently, computed tomography has been used to assess the carpal tunnel and its contents.

We have compared the shape of the wrist with the distal antidromic median sensory latency and reported a statistically significant relationship between the "squareness" of the wrist and a prolonged distal sensory latency (Fig. 5.21). The anterior-posterior distance of the wrist (thickness) measured at the distal wrist crease was divided by the side-to-side measurement (width), again at the distal wrist crease. This cal-

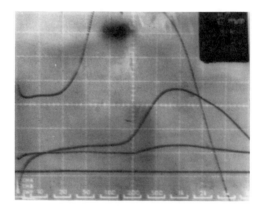

Figure 5.17. Median motor stimulation midpalmar (*top*) and wrist (*bottom*) in carpal tunnel syndrome. Note the larger CMAP on midpalmar stimulation (*top trace*) (substantial neurapraxia). (Caliber: Each square = 1 msec, 2 millivolts.)

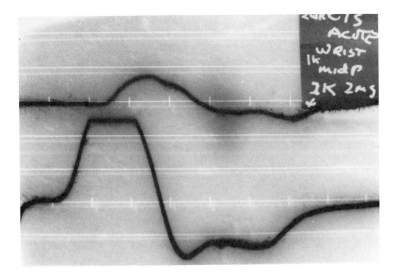

Figure 5.18. Wrist and midpalmar stimulation of median motor nerve in acute CTS. Substantial neurapraxia is present. Note that the top trace gain was 1 millivolt, whereas the lower trace (distal to carpal ligament) gain was 2 millivolts. Horizontal separation at 2-msec intervals.

culation results in an index. All wrists with an index greater than 0.7 had distal median sensory latencies of 4 msec or more.

This index has been used to place industrial workers at risk of developing CTS at workstations where activity was unlikely to cause CTS. A retrospective study at an automobile plant showed that 99 of 100

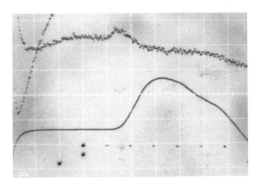

Figure 5.19. Comparison of CMAP and SNAP in moderate CTS. *Top trace,* Sensory antidromic (14 cm) to Digit III. (Caliber: 20 µV/square.) *Bottom trace,* Motor latency and CMAP (8 cm). (Caliber: 2 millivolts/square, 1 msec/square)

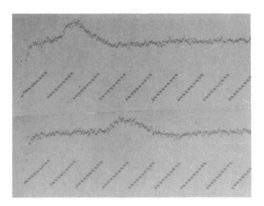

Figure 5.20. Seven and 14 cm median nerve antidromic SNAP in moderate diabetic neuropathy (record Digit III). Note that wrist latency (*bottom*) is low amplitude and dispersed yet is only 4 msec. Also the midpalmar stimulation (7 cm *top trace*) is one-half the latency and slightly larger. This is characteristic of moderate peripheral neuropathy (axonal). (Caliber: Each slanted line = 1 msec. Height = 20 µV.)

workers whose wrist index was 0.7 or greater (i.e., a more square wrist) developed classic CTS as diagnosed by electrodiagnostic testing.

ACUTE CARPAL TUNNEL SYNDROME

In industry, repetitive motions of the wrist can result in the development of CTS in a relatively short time, e.g. 1–2 weeks. The acute carpal tunnel syndrome is characterized by these features:

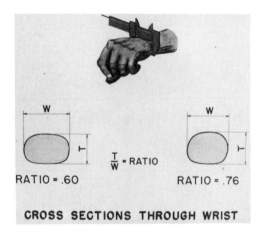

Figure 5.21. Determination of the wrist ratio index. Note that the larger (.76) wrist index indicates a "squarer" wrist. This correlates with a prolonged median sensory latency (CTS).

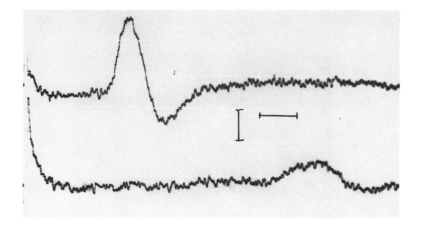

Figure 5.22. Median SNAP antidromic at 7 and 14 cm. This is an acute carpal tunnel syndrome (symptoms—2 weeks duration) ring electrodes over Digit III. Note the relatively normal SNAP when stimulated at the midpalmar site (7 cm). (Caliber: 1 msec, 20 µV.)

1. There is a disproportion between the latency and amplitude of either the CMAP or SNAP. The latency may be quite short, yet the amplitude is very small.
2. There can be a large component of neurapraxia when stimulating proximally and distally to the carpal ligament on both motor or sensory nerves, or either (Fig. 5.22).
3. Selective involvement of only motor nerve fibers with relatively normal sensory can be a frequent finding (Fig. 5.23).
4. Occasionally the latency may be greatly prolonged on wrist stimulation, yet distal to the carpal ligament it may be relatively normal.

MANAGEMENT

Treatment of acute CTS and mild to moderate degrees of CTS can be either by a splint to hold the wrist in a neutral position (we use a bowling glove) or an injection of 2 mg (.5 ml) of Decadron in the carpal tunnel. Follow-up electrodiagnostic study can provide objective evidence of improvement or lack thereof. Decisions regarding surgical correction are made primarily with clinical data supported by electrodiagnostic studies and not on the basis of electrodiagnostic studies alone. Electrodiagnostic abnormalities can still be present, although to a lesser degree, at 1 year postsurgery (20).

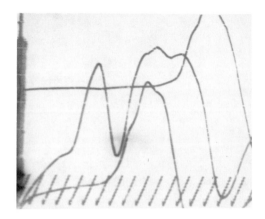

Figure 5.23. Effect of increasing stimulating current intensity in severe carpal tunnel syndrome. *Top trace,* Median nerve stimulation at elbow. *Bottom trace,* Median nerve stimulation at wrist. Motor latency is 6.7 msec. *Middle trace,* Current intensity stimulation is increased with field of stimulation exciting the ulnar nerve with surface electrode now recording ulnar-innervated muscle (flexor pollicis brevis, deep head).

References

1. Bailey D, Carter FFB: Median nerve palsy associated with acute infections of the hand. *Lancet* 1:530, 1955.

2. Bleecker M, Bohlman M, Moreland R, Tipton A: Carpal tunnel syndrome: role of carpal canal size. *Neurology* 35:1599–1604, 1985.

3. Brain WR, Wright AD, Wilkinson M: Spontaneous compression of both median nerves in the carpal tunnel. *Lancet* 252-277, 1947.

4. Buchthal F, Rosenfalck A: Sensory conduction from digit to palm and from palm to wrist in the carpal tunnel syndrome. *J Neurol Neurosurg Psychiat* 34:243–252, 1971.

5. Cannon BW, Love JG: Tardy median palsy; median neuritis; median thenar neuritis amendable to surgery. *Surgery* 20:210, 1946.

6. Casey EB, LeQuesne PM: Digital nerve action potentials in healthy subjects, and in carpal tunnel and diabetic patients. *J Neurol Neurosurg Psychiat* 35:612–623, 1972.

7. Dawson G, Scott J: The recording of nerve action potentials through skin in man. *J Neurol Neurosurg Psychiat* 12:259–262, 1949.

8. Gilliatt RW, Sears TA: Sensory nerve action potentials in patients with peripheral nerve lesions. *J Neurol Neurosurg Psychiat* 21:109, 1958.

9. Gutmann L: Mediam-ulnar nerve communications and carpal tunnel syndrome. *J Neurol Neurosurg Psychiat* 40:982–986, 1977.

10. Gutmann L, Gutierrez A, Riggs J: The contribution of median-ulnar communications in diagnosis of carpal tunnel syndrome. *Muscle Nerve* 9:319–321, 1986.

11. Hunt JR: The thenar and hypothenar types of neural atrophy of the hand. *Am J Med Sci* 141:224, 1911.

12. Johnson EW, Wells RM, Duran RJ: Diagnosis of carpal tunnel syndrome. *Arch Phys Med* 6:137, 1961.

13. Johnson EW, Kukla RD, Wongsam PE, Piedmont A: Sensory latencies to the ring finger: normal values and relation to carpal tunnel syndrome. *Arch Phys Med Rehabil* 62:206–209, 1982.

14. Johnson EW, Gatens T, Poindexter D, Bowers D: Wrist dimensions: correlation with median sensory latencies. *Arch Phys Med Rehabil* 64:556–557, 1983.

15. Johnson EW, Sipski M, Lammertse T: Radial and median latencies to dig. I: value in carpal tunnel syndrome. *Arch Phys Med Rehabil* 68:140, 1987.

16. Kimura J: The carpal tunnel syndrome—localization of conduction abnormalities within the distal segment of the median nerve. *Brain* 102:619–635, 1979.

17. Kimura J: A method for determining median nerve conduction velocity across the carpal tunnel. *J Neurol Sci* 38:1–10, 1978.

18. Kimura J, et al: Relationship between size of compound sensory or muscle action potentials and length of nerve segment. *Neurology* 36:647–652, 1986.

19. Loong SC, Seah CS: Comparison of median and ulnar sensory nerve action potentials in the diagnosis of the carpal tunnel syndrome. *J Neurol Neurosurg Psychiat* 34:750–754, 1971.

20. Mavor H, Shiozawa R: Antidromic digital and palmar nerve action potentials. *Electroenceph Clin Neurophysiol* 30:210–221, 1971.

21. Melvin JL, Johnson EW, Duran R: Electrodiagnosis after surgery for carpal tunnel syndrome. *Arch Phys Med* 49:502, 1968.

22. Melvin JL, Burnett CN, Johnson EW: Median nerve conduction in pregnancy. *Arch Phys Med* 50:75, 1969.

23. Smith J: Radial nerve conduction in patients with carpal tunnel syndrome. *Appl Neurophysiol* 44:363–367, 1981.

24. Thomas JE, Lambert EH, Cseuz KA: Electrodiagnostic aspects of the carpal tunnel syndrome. *Arch Neurol* 16: , 1967.

25. Wongsam PE, Johnson EW, Weinerman JD: Carpal tunnel syndrome: use of palmar stimulation of sensory fibers. *Arch Phys Med Rehabil* 64:16–19, 1983.

6

Special Techniques in Electrodiagnosis

SUSAN L. HUBBELL

Several electrodiagnostic techniques that are being increasingly used in clinical electromyographic practice are presented in this chapter. Included are electrodiagnostic techniques for the facial nerve, phrenic nerve, spinal wave stimulation, F wave, and special pediatric considerations.

FACIAL NERVE

Paralysis of the muscles of facial expression is a sign of compromise of the facial nerve. The facial nerve is vulnerable to compromise in several areas along its course. It passes through the pons where various pontine lesions can produce peripheral facial palsy. In the area of the cerebellopontine angle it can be injured by an acoustic neuroma. It enters the internal auditory meatus and then runs anterolaterally until it reaches the geniculate ganglion where it curves posteriorly and inferiorly into the facial canal. This interosseous segment is the presumed site of the lesion in Bell palsy. It emerges from the stylomastoid foramen, gives off a branch to the posterior belly of the digastric and stylohyoid muscles, passes through the center of the parotid gland, and divides into its terminal branches.

Causes of facial paralysis include idiopathic (Bell palsy), parotid tumor, angle tumor, cholesteatoma, other middle ear diseases, trauma (basal skull fracture, surgical), generalized peripheral neuropathy (diabetes, Guillain-Barré syndrome), and herpes zoster (Ramsey-Hunt syndrome).

Electromyography of the muscles of facial expression, facial nerve conduction studies, and the electrically elicited blink reflex are helpful in localizing and evaluating the severity of the facial nerve pathology.

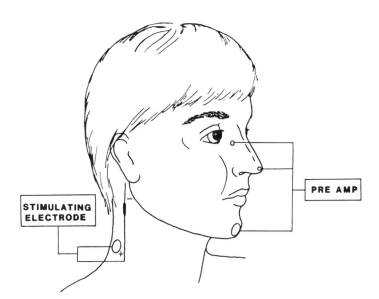

Figure 6.1. Electrode placement for facial nerve study recording from nasalis muscle.

Method for Nerve Conduction Studies

The facial nerve is best stimulated just below the ear and anterior to the mastoid process (Fig. 6.1) either with a needle electrode or standard surface stimulator. The recording electrode should be placed over the muscle to be studied. Muscles frequently used are the frontalis, orbicularis oculi, mentalis, and nasalis. Surface recording over the orbicularis oris may be confusing due to the volume-conducted masseter response, particularly in severe facial nerve injuries. The reference electrode is placed over the nose with the ground on the chin or forehead (see Fig. 6.1).

Normal Values

Latencies are felt to be abnormal if they are greater than 3.4 + .8 msec (14, 15) or greater than 4.1 msec (5).

Comparison of the amplitude of the evoked response side to side is useful in determining the extent of axon loss. It is also helpful to compare the amount of stimulus intensity needed to elicit the response side-to-side.

Distal excitability is normal for 3–4 days after injury, but is lost by the end of the first week if the nerve has degenerated.

BLINK REFLEX

Eliciting the blink reflex enables one to evaluate both the facial and trigeminal nerves. The examiner stimulates the supraorbital nerve (trigeminal nerve) and picks up evoked responses over the orbicularis oculi muscles (facial nerve). With a two-channel instrument, one should simultaneously pick up evoked responses from both orbicularis oculi muscles during stimulation of one supraorbital nerve. Two responses (R_1 and R_2) should be seen from the orbicularis oculi muscle ipsilateral to the stimulus. One response should be seen from the contralateral orbicularis oculi.

The R_1 or early response is felt to represent a pontine reflex, following a disynaptic pathway from the main sensory nucleus to the ipsilateral face. It is more stable than R_2 with repeated trials and is more sensitive for assessment of nerve conduction. It is abnormal in pathologic conditions involving the trigeminal and/or facial nerves, either central or peripheral.

The R_2 or late response is felt to represent a polysynaptic pathway via the spinal nucleus to the facial nuclei bilaterally, thus involving the pons and lateral medulla. It is essential to the differentiation of afferent from efferent pathway involvement. A lesion of the trigeminal nerve results in bilaterally slowed R_2 responses with stimulation on the affected side and bilaterally normal R_2 responses with stimulation on the unaffected side. A lesion of the facial nerve results in a normal R_2 on the unaffected side with stimulation on either side. The R_2 response on the affected side is abnormal with stimulation on either side.

Method for Recording

Stimulation is done using a surface stimulator or needle electrode at the supraorbital notch (Fig. 6.2). One can also use a glabellar tap with a reflex hammer attached via a microswitch to the stimulator. With this method, the R_1 response is elicited bilaterally.

A set of active and reference electrodes is placed over each orbicularis oculi muscle, with one set plugged into each preamplifier of a two-channel instrument. (If a two-channel instrument is not available, one must perform two recordings for the right stimulation and two for the left). The ground is placed on the chin. A minimum of eight responses should be obtained for each side, and the shortest latencies obtained should be recorded.

Normal Values

In adults R_1 latency should be less than 13.0 msec, and the side-to-side difference should be less than 1.2 msec (5). The R_2 should be less than 40 msec on the unilateral side and less than 41 msec on the con-

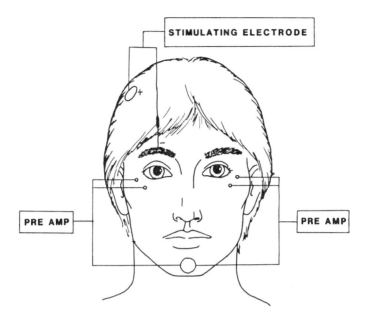

Figure 6.2. Blink reflex.

tralateral side with simultaneous latency difference of less than 5 msec. If the R_2 responses from the right and left stimulations are compared, the latency difference should be less than 7 msec.

PHRENIC NERVE STIMULATION

Evaluation of the phrenic nerve is valuable when decreased or absent diaphragmatic function is suspected in an individual suffering from respiratory distress. Clinical signs that are compatible with poor function of the diaphragm include increased respiratory distress in the supine position with improvement when in the upright position; inability to be weaned from the respirator after thoracic surgery, particularly open heart or mediastinal surgery; and inability of an individual with generalized peripheral polyneuropathy to be weaned from the respirator. Phrenic nerve stimulation is also useful with the high cervical quadriplegic patient, both in assessing the possibility of being able to wean him or her from the ventilator and in determining the feasibility of using an implanted phrenic nerve stimulator. Chest x-rays often show a high diaphragm on the side of a compromised phrenic nerve.

Phrenic nerve evaluation can be done with basic EMG instruments in the intensive care unit. Usually there is no significant interference

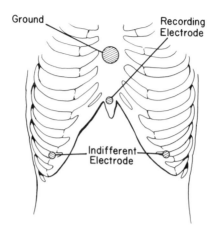

Figure 6.3. Recording electrode placement for phrenic nerve evaluation.

from the monitoring equipment and ventilator. It is helpful to turn off any florescent lights, radios, and other extraneous equipment.

Method

The recording electrodes are surface electrodes placed over the chest wall. MacLean (11) describes placement of the active electrode over the xiphoid process and the reference electrode over the intercostal space between the eighth and ninth ribs at the anterior axillary line. The ground is placed cephalad on the chest. (Fig. 6.3) Others have described placing both the active and reference electrode in the rib interspace.

Stimulation is through either surface or pin stimulation. The stimulation site is posterior to the sternocleidomastoid muscle at the level of the cricoid cartilage. When using the surface stimulator, it is necessary to push the stimulator slightly anteriorly and under the sternocleidomastoid muscle (Fig. 6.4). When using the monopolar needle to stimulate, the insertion site is posterior to the sternocleidomastoid at the level of the cricoid cartilage. The needle is inserted and advanced slightly anteriomedially (Fig. 6.5). The electomyographer should be aware of the pertinent anatomy in the area, particularly the carotid artery (Fig. 6.6).

Mean values and standard deviations using monopolar needle stimulation are 7.4 ± 0.6 msec for latency, with side-to-side difference of 0.08 ± 0.4 msec, as reported by MacLean and Mattioni (10) (Figs. 6.7 and 6.8).

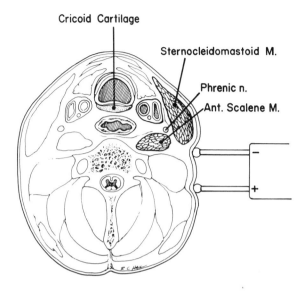

Figure 6.4. Surface stimulation for phrenic nerve conduction study.

SPINAL NERVE STIMULATION

Evaluation of the proximal portions of peripheral nerves by localized stimulus to the spinal nerve was introduced by MacLean and Taylor in

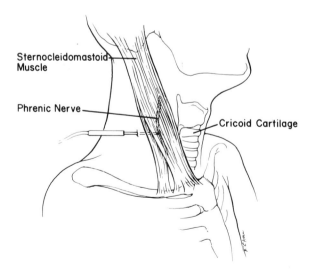

Figure 6.5. Needle electrode stimulation for phrenic nerve evaluation.

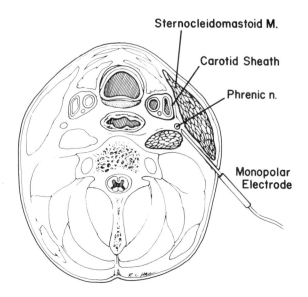

Figure 6.6. Anatomy for needle electrode stimulation in phrenic nerve evaluation.

1975 (11). They inserted a needle electrode into the cervical paraspinals and were able to depolarize the lower cervical roots. Since then the procedure has been refined to allow stimulation of spinal nerves from C5 to T1. MacLean in 1979 (8, 9) developed a standardized method for evaluating the lumbar and sacral plexuses individually.

Conduction across the brachial and lumbosacral plexuses can be evaluated by using the F wave, H reflex, or somatosensory evoked potentials (SEP). However, an abnormal value found using these methods may be due to pathology in the peripheral nerve, spinal cord, or intraspinal nerve roots, as well as in the plexus itself. Spinal nerve stimulation allows direct evaluation of the plexus. By stimulating proximally and distally to the plexus, one can localize the pathology to the plexus. This is helpful in evaluation of neurogenic thoracic outlet syndrome; compression of the plexus by mass lesions, such as enlarged lymph nodes or pelvic masses; radiation damage to the plexus; and traumatic plexus injuries.

Method

The cathode is a standard monopolar electrode, insulated throughout its length except for the exposed tip. The electrode should be 50–75 mm in length in the cervical region and 75 mm in the lumbosacral region. The anode is a standard surface electrode, taped to the skin

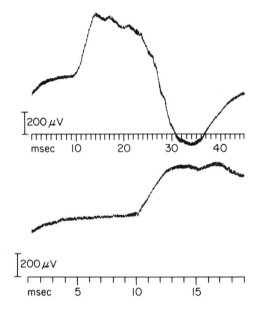

Figure 6.7. Normal response of the phrenic nerve with surface stimulation and recording electrodes.

opposite to the stimulating electrode. The electrode is inserted perpendicular to the skin and is advanced until the transverse process of the vertebra is touched (Fig. 6.9). If the electrode does not reach this depth, increased current will be required to obtain a response, with a resultant increase in patient discomfort.

The C5 and C6 spinal nerves are stimulated by inserting the electrode 1–2 cm lateral to the C5 spinous process (Fig. 6.10). The C8 and T1 spinal nerves are stimulated by inserting the electrode 1–2 cm lateral to the C7 spinous process (Fig. 6.11). The C6, C7, and C8 spinal nerves are evaluated at a site between the previous two electrodes.

Stimulation 2–3 cm lateral and slightly cephalad to the L4 spinous process results in depolarization of the L2, L3, and L4 spinal nerves (lumbar plexus) (Fig. 6.12). The sacral plexus can be studied by stimulating the L5 and S1 spinal nerves medial and slightly cephalad to the posterior superior iliac spine (Fig. 6.13).

Recording electrodes are placed over a muscle innervated by the spinal nerves being stimulated. The muscle selected should have as little overlapping innervation as possible. The active recording electrode is placed over the motor point of the muscle, and the reference is placed over an adjacent tendon or other electrically silent area. Examples of possible recording sites are:

CASE STUDY
63 y/o W/M for open heart surgery

PREOP

	R	L
• Latency (msec)	8.7	8.3
• Amplitude (μV)	600	500

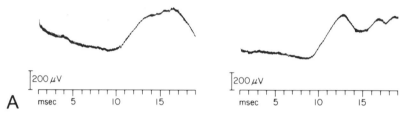

A

POSTOP

	R	L
• Latency (msec)	8.2	10.0
• Amplitude (μV)	400	50

• Left hemidiaphragm paralyzed on fluroscopy

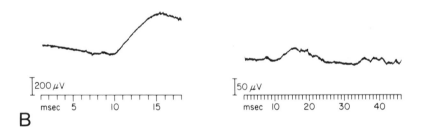

B

Figure 6.8. *A,* Preop studies before open heart surgery are normal. *B,* Postop study of the right phrenic nerve is normal, but the left phrenic nerve response is delayed and markedly decreased in amplitude.

• C5, C6: deltoid, biceps brachii
• C7, C8: triceps, extensor carpi radialis brevis, extensor digitorum communis
• C8, T1: abductor digiti minimi, abductor pollicis brevis
• L2, L3, L4: vastus medialis

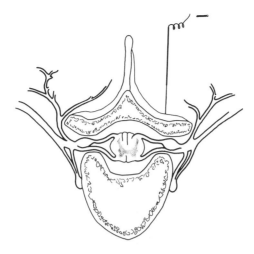

Figure 6.9. The electrode is inserted perpendicular to the skin and is advanced until the transverse process of the vertebra is touched.

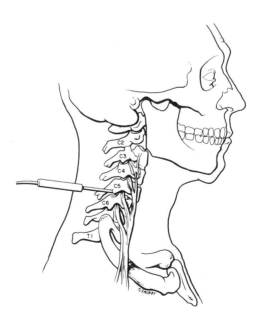

Figure 6.10. Stimulation site for the C5 and C6 spinal nerves is 1–2 cm lateral to the C5 spinous process. The needle electrode is inserted perpendicular to the frontal plane of the body.

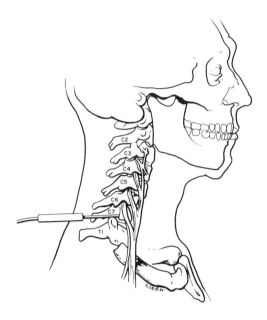

Figure 6.11. Stimulation site for the C8 and T1 spinal nerves is 1–2 cm lateral to the C7 spinous process with the monopolar needle electrode perpendicular to the frontal plane of the body.

- L5, S1: soleus (S1), abductor hallucis (S1), extensor digitorum communis (L5), peroneus longus (L5)

If a muscle is clinically weak and/or has abnormal insertional activity (i.e., positive waves or fibrillation potentials) or decreased number of voluntarily firing motor units on EMG examination, it would be prudent to select it as one of the muscles for recording purposes.

Isolation of an abnormality to the plexus can be done by stimulating the peripheral nerve distal to the plexus and subtracting the distal value from the proximal value. M-wave amplitude should also be observed proximal and distal to the suspected lesion as this can indicate the extent of neurapraxia versus more significant damage. This observation is particularly necessary when there is a suspicion of a lesion in the peripheral nerve distal to the plexus.

For evaluation of the lower trunk and medial cord, the ulnar nerve is stimulated in the axilla. The arm is abducted to 90°, and the stimulus is placed at a point 25 cm from the sternal notch.

The femoral nerve is stimulated just below the inguinal ligament and lateral to the femoral pulse to isolate the lumbar plexus (Fig. 6.12). A needle electrode can be used here, requiring much less current.

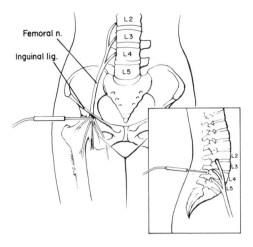

Figure 6.12. Stimulation site for the L2, L3, and L4 spinal nerves is 2–3 cm lateral and slightly cephalad to the L4 spinous process with the monopolar needle electrode perpendicular to the skin.

The sciatic nerve is stimulated to evaluate the sacral plexus. A needle electrode is inserted perpendicular to the skin at a gluteal skin fold halfway between the ischial tuberosity and the greater trochanter of the femur (Fig. 6.13).

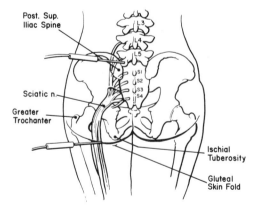

Figure 6.13. Stimulation site for the L5 and S1 spinal nerves is medial and slightly cephalad to the posterior superior iliac spine with the monopolar needle electrode perpendicular to the skin.

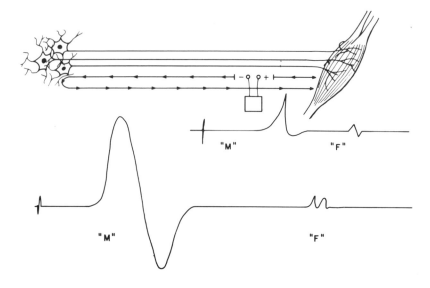

Figure 6.14. Schematic representation of F-wave pathway.

Normal Values

MacLean in his studies has found that comparing values from the two sides of the same patient is a more sensitive way of detecting abnormality than using a table of established normal values. He reports that a difference of more than 0.6, 0.7, or 0.9 msec for the brachial, lumbar, and sacral plexuses, respectively, should be considered abnormal.

F RESPONSE

The F wave allows the electromyographer to assess motor conduction along the proximal segments of nerves. It is a late muscle potential that results from the backfiring of antidromically activated anterior horn cells (Fig.6.14). The F response occurs after the direct or M response. Slowing of the F-wave latency indicates pathology along the nerve proximal to the stimulation site. Exact localization of the site of pathology requires concurrent use of standard nerve conduction techniques with the F response.

The F wave can be abnormal in most polyneuropathies, but is a most useful evaluation tool in patients with polyneuropathy primarily associated with proximal pathology, such as early Guillain-Barré syndrome (5–7).

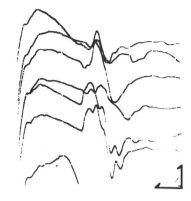

Figure 6.15. F waves in abductor pollicis brevis stimulating median nerve at elbow. Note M wave to the left of the screen. (Caliber: 5 msec, 200 μV.)

Method

The F wave study is usually done after standard distal nerve conduction studies are completed. Active, reference, and ground electrode placement is not changed. To shift to the F response study, one must adjust the sweep speed on the electromyograph to allow for a 20–50 msec latency, i.e., 5 or 10 msec/cm. The gain should be 200 μV/cm. One must study the M and F responses separately, using differing time bases and gains. The stimulator should be reversed so that the cathode is proximal. Supramaximal stimulation is used, and serial recordings are done at each stimulation point (Fig. 6.15). A minimum of ten identifiable F waves must be recorded. The minimal latency is measured, although maximal latency can be determined also and used as a measure of temporal dispersion (Table 6.1) (12). The F response can be elicited at several stimulation sites along each nerve. As the stimulation site moves proximally, the F wave latency should shorten.

Normal values are summarized in Tables 6.2 and 6.3.

Table 6.1. Methods of Evaluation of F Waves

Minimal latency
Min-max (chronodispersion)
Mean "F" latency
Number of F waves as compared to number of stimulations
Duration/amplitude of F
Frequency of similar F waves
Degree of polyphasicity

Table 6.2. F Waves in Normal Subjects[a]

Number of Nerves Tested	Site of Stimulation	F-Wave Latency to Recording Site	Difference between Right and Left	Central Latency[b] to and from the Spinal Cord	Difference between Right and Left	Conduction Velocity[c] to and from the Spinal Cord	F Ratio between Proximal and Distal Segment
		msec	*msec*	*msec*	*msec*	*msec*	
122 median nerves from 61 subjects	Wrist	26.6 ± 2.2 (31)[f]	0.95 ± 0.67 (2.3)[f]	23.0 ± 2.1 (27)[f]	0.93 ± 0.62 (2.2)[f]	65.3 ± 4.7 (56)[g]	
	Elbow	22.8 ± 1.9 (27)	0.76 ± 0.56 (1.9)	15.4 ± 1.4 (18)	0.71 ± 0.52 (1.8)	67.8 ± 5.8 (56)	
	Axilla[e]	20.4 ± 1.9 (24)	0.85 ± 0.61 (2.1)	10.6 ± 1.5 (14)	0.85 ± 0.58 (2.0)		
130 ulnar nerves from 65 subjects	Wrist	27.6 ± 2.2 (32)	1.00 ± 0.83 (2.7)	25.0 ± 2.1 (29)	0.84 ± 0.59 (2.0)	65.3 ± 4.8 (55)	
	Above elbow	23.1 ± 1.7 (27)	0.68 ± 0.48 (1.6)	16.0 ± 1.2 (18)	0.73 ± 0.52 (1.8)	65.7 ± 5.3 (55)	1.05 ± 0.09 (0.87–1.23)
	Axilla[e]	20.3 ± 1.6 (24)	0.73 ± 0.54 (1.8)	10.4 ± 1.1 (13)	0.76 ± 0.52 (1.8)		
120 peroneal nerves from 60 subjects	Ankle	48.4 ± 4.0 (56)	1.42 ± 1.03 (3.5)	44.7 ± 3.8 (52)	1.28 ± 0.90 (3.1)	49.8 ± 3.6 (46)	
	Above knee	39.9 ± 3.2 (46)	1.28 ± 0.91 (3.1)	27.3 ± 2.4 (32)	1.18 ± 0.89 (3.0)	55.1 ± 4.6 (46)	1.05 ± 0.09 (0.87–1.23)
118 tibial nerves from 59 subjects	Ankle	47.7 ± 5.0 (58)	1.40 ± 1.04 (3.5)	43.8 ± 4.5 (53)	1.52 ± 1.02 (2.6)	52.6 ± 4.3 (44)	
	Knee	39.6 ± 4.4 (48)	1.25 ± 0.92 (3.1)	27.6 ± 3.2 (34)	1.23 ± 0.88 (3.0)	53.7 ± 4.8 (44)	1.11 ± 0.11 (0.89–1.33)

[a]Reprinted from Argyropoulos CJ, et al: F-and M-wave conduction velocity in amyotrophic lateral sclerosis. *Muscle Nerve* 1:479, 1978.

[b]Central latency = F—M, where F and M are latencies of F-wave and M-response, respectively.

[c]Conduction velocity = 2D/(F—M—1), where D is the distance from the stimulus point to the C7 or T12 spinous process.

[d]F-ratio = (F—M—1)/2M with stimulation with the cathode on the volar crease at the elbow (median), 3 cm above the medial epicondyle (ulnar), just above the head of the fibula (peroneal), and in the popliteal fossa (tibial).

[e]F(A) = F(E) — M(E) + M(A), where F(A) and F(E) are latencies of F-wave with stimulation at the axilla and elbow, respectively, and M(A) and M(E) are latencies of the corresponding M-response.

[f]Upper limits of normal calculated as mean + 2 SD.

[g]Lower limits of normal calculated as mean − 2 SD.

Table 6.3. Comparison of F waves between Two Nerves in the Same Limb[a]

Site of Stimulation	F-Wave Latency to Recording Site			Central Latency[b] to and from the Spinal Cord		
	Median Nerve	Ulnar Nerve	Difference	Median Nerve	Ulnar Nerve	Difference
	msec	*msec*	*msec*	*msec*	*msec*	*msec*
Wrist	26.6 ± 2.3 (31)[c]	27.2 ± 2.5 (32)[c]	1.00 ± 0.68 (2.4)[c]	23.3 ± 2.2 (28)[c]	24.5 ± 2.4 (29)[c]	1.24 ± 0.75 (2.7)[c]
Elbow	22.9 ± 1.8 (26)	23.0 ± 1.7 (26)	0.84 ± 0.55 (1.9)	15.5 ± 1.4 (18)	16.0 ± 1.2 (18)	0.79 ± 0.65 (2.1)
	Peroneal Nerve	Tibial Nerve	Difference	Peroneal Nerve	Tibial Nerve	Difference
	msec	*msec*	*msec*	*msec*	*msec*	*msec*
Ankle	47.7 ± 4.0 (55)	48.1 ± 4.2 (57)	1.68 ± 1.21 (4.1)	43.6 ± 4.0 (52)	44.1 ± 3.9 (52)	1.79 ± 1.20 (4.2)
Knee	39.6 ± 3.7 (47)	40.1 ± 3.7 (48)	1.71 ± 1.19 (4.1)	27.1 ± 2.9 (33)	28.0 ± 2.7 (33)	1.75 ± 1.07 (3.9)

[a]Reprinted from Argyropoulos CJ, et al: F-and M-waves conduction velocity in amyotrophic lateral sclerosis. *Muscle Nerve* 1:479, 1978.
[b]Central latency = F—M, where F and M are latencies of F-wave and M-response, respectively.
[c]Upper limits of normal calculated as mean + 2 SD.

PEDIATRIC ELECTRODIAGNOSIS

When evaluating children, a careful history and physical examination are very important because they enable the examiner to plan the EMG carefully so that it can be completed expeditiously. It is neither desirable nor necessary to use anesthesia for the EMG examination. As a general rule, parents should not be present during the examination. However, the examiner will need the assistance of another person for children ages 2 to 6. The cooperation of children older than 6 can usually be obtained by explaining the procedure and their participation in it to them.

Equipment

A bare needle should be used as the reference electrode with a monopolar exploring electrode. For conduction studies, it may be necessary to use half-size EEG electrodes for recording or subcutaneous needle electrodes (these should *not* penetrate the muscle as that will not result in a compound evoked muscle action potential). For the stimulator, one can use either a small surface stimulator or a monopolar needle electrode as cathode, with a surface electrode placed underneath the proximal limb as the anode.

Needle EMG

The duration of the needle EMG examination should be abbreviated in children. Steps I and II should be done simultaneously. To examine muscles at rest, the electomyographer should place each muscle at its shortest length:

- Rectus femoris: Hyperflex hips and extend knee.
- Gastrocnemius: Plantarflex ankle and hyperflex knee.
- Biceps brevis: Flex elbow and supinate forearm.
- Pronator teres: Flex elbow and pronate forearm.

Steps III and IV require muscle contraction. In infants and uncooperative children the examiner may need to use reflexes and/or noxious stimuli to obtain muscle contractions.

Nerve Conduction Studies

Measurements must be done carefully as the small distances found in infants (6—8 cm) may introduce error. Mismeasurement of 1 cm will result in a 15% error. Motor nerve conduction velocity in newborns is about 50% of adults (2, 3) (Tables 6.4 and 6.5). Adult values are reached by age 4 (2, 3) (Fig. 6.16). Motor conduction in premature infants is inversely related to the degree of prematurity (3). Motor conduction velocity can be used to separate low weight term babies (dysmature)

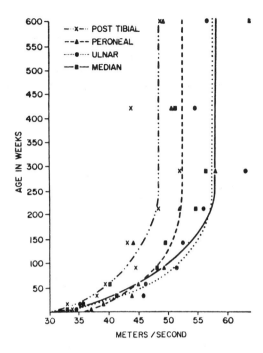

Figure 6.16. Curves demonstrating in children changes in motor nerve conduction velocities in ulnar, median, peroneal, and posterior tibial nerves, which all reach adult values at about 4 years of age. (From Baer RD, Johnson EW: Motor nerve conduction velocities in normal children. *Arch Phys Med Rehabil* 46:698–704, 1965.)

Table 6.4. Mean Motor Nerve Conduction Velocities Obtained for Children in Different Age Groups[a]

| Average Age of Group | Ulnar | Velocity in Meters/Second | | Posterior Tibial |
		Median	Peroneal	
5 (wks)	34.5 (11)[b]	33.1 (12)[b]	37.2 (6)[b]	34.3 (11)[b]
18 (wks)	35.4 (12)	35.8 (11)	39.1 (12)	32.7 (11)
34 (wks)	46.1 (12)	41.8 (12)	44.1 (12)	38.3 (12)
56 (wks)	46.7 (10)	40.4 (12)	46.7 (12)	39.8 (12)
88 (wks)	51.6 (12)	47.5 (12)	49.5 (12)	44.5 (12)
140 (wks)	52.4 (12)	49.4 (12)	44.2 (11)	43.1 (10)
210 (wks)	56.1 (12)	54.9 (12)	52.2 (12)	48.4 (12)

[a]Reprinted from Baer RD, Johnson EW: Motor nerve conduction velocities in normal children. *Arch Phys Med Rehabil* 46:698, 1965.
[b]Numbers in parenthesis refer to number of children in age group for whom nerve conduction velocity was determined.

from truly premature low weight babies (3, 13) (Tables 6.6 and 6.7 and Figs. 6.17–6.19). Distal motor latencies vary with the size of body part, as well as the degree of myelination.

Sensory conduction velocities should be calculated by dividing the distance by the latency minus .1 msec (latency of activation).

Table 6.5. Facial Nerve Conduction Delays in 78 Normal Children (Birth to 16 Years of Age)[a]

Age, Range	No. Subjects	Mean[b]	Range
		msec	msec
Newborn to 1 month	7	10.1	6.4–12.0
1 month to 1 year	13	7.0	5.0–10.0
1 to 2 years	16	5.1	3.6–6.3
2 to 3 years	7	3.9	3.8–4.5
3 to 4 years	6	3.7	3.4–4.0
4 to 5 years	7	4.1	3.5–5.0
5 to 7 years	10	3.9	3.2–5.0
7 to 16 years	12	4.0	3.0–5.0

[a]Reprinted from Waylonis G, Johnson EW: Facial nerve conduction delay. *Arch Phys Med* 41:539, 1960.
[b]Mean (3 years and over) = 3.9 msec.

Table 6.6. Motor Nerve Conduction Velocities of Premature Infants[a]

Days Prior to Estimated Day of Confinement	Weight	Ulnar	Peroneal
	gm		m/sec
−49	1553	16.5	14.5
−45	1830	21.4	16.7
−42	1985	20.2	15.4
−42	1434	16.8	13.7
−42	2180	19.1	15.1
−35	1829	18.6	23.3
−14	2276	22.5	18.7
−14	2119	21.5	22.2

[a]From Cerra D, Johnson EW: Motor nerve conduction velocities in premature infants. *Arch Phys Med Rehabil* 43:160, 1964.

Table 6.7. Motor Nerve Conduction Velocities of Low Birth Weight Term and Low Birth Weight Premature Infants[a]

Nerve	Eight Low Birth Weight Term Infants				Eleven Low Birth Weight Premature Infants			
	Birth	3 Months	6 Months	12 Months	Birth	3 Months	6 Months	12 Months
	m/sec	*m/sec*	*m/sec*	*m/sec*	*m/sec*	*m/sec*	*m/sec*	*m/sec*
Ulnar	29.5 ± 1.4[b]	34.66 ± 3.1	38.0 ± 3.7	45.2 ± 4.0	20.8 ± 3.9	29.18 ± 3.3	37.42 ± 4.6	43.5 ± 5.4
Median	28.87 ± 1.7	34.0 ± 3.8	37.4 ± 3.8	44.7 ± 3.6	20.55 ± 3.6	20.72 ± 3.8	39.13 ± 4.1	45.0 ± 3.2
Peroneal	30.0 ± 3.1	33.0 ± 1.6	37.0 ± 2.9	46.5 ± 4.6	18.91 ± 4.3	30.81 ± 3.8	37.4 ± 4.6	44.0 ± 4.8

[a]From Ruppert ES, Johnson EW: Motor nerve conduction velocities in low birth weight infants. *Pediatrics* 42:255, 1968.
[b]Values represent the mean and ± 1 standard deviation.

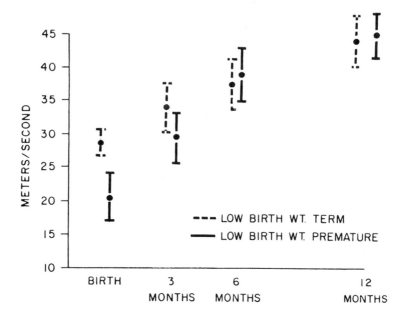

Figure 6.17. Conduction velocity in median nerve in infants. (From Ruppert ES, Johnson EW: Motor nerve conduction velocities in low birth weight infants. *Pediatrics* 42:255–259, 1968.)

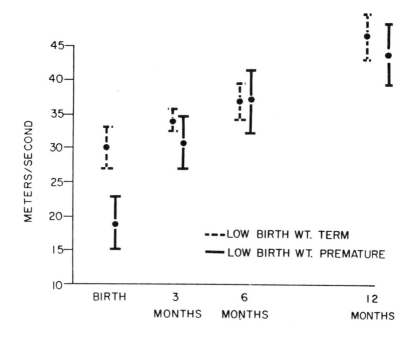

Figure 6.18. Conduction velocity in peroneal nerve in infants. (From Ruppert ES, Johnson EW: Motor nerve conduction velocities in low birth weight infants. *Pediatrics* 42:255–259, 1968.)

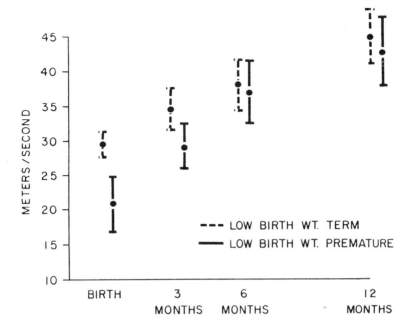

Figure 6.19. Conduction velocity in ulnar nerve in infants. (From Ruppert ES, Johnson EW: Motor nerve conduction velocities in low birth weight infants. *Pediatrics* 42:255–259, 1968.)

References

1. Argyropoulos CJ, Panayitopoulos CP, Scarpalezos S: F-and M-wave conduction velocity in amyotrophic lateral sclerosis. *Muscle Nerve* 1:479, 1978.
2. Baer RD, Johnson EW: Motor nerve conduction velocities in normal children. *Arch Phys Med Rehabil* 46:698–704, 1965.
3. Cerra D, Johnson EW: Motor nerve conduction velocity in premature infants. *Arch Phys Med Rehabil* 43:160–164, 1962.
4. Kimura J: Electrically elicited blink reflex in diagnosis of multiple sclerosis—review of 260 patients over a 7-year period. *Brain* 98:413, 1975.
5. Kimura J: Proximal versus distal slowing of motor nerve conduction velocity in the Guillain-Barré syndrome. *Ann Neurol* 3:344, 1978.
6. Kimura J, Butzer JF: F-wave conduction velocity in Guillain-Barré syndrome: assessment of nerve segment between axilla and spinal cord. *Arch Neurol* 32:524, 1975.
7. King D, Ashby C: Conduction velocity in the proximal segments of a motor nerve in the Guillain-Barré syndrome. *J Neurol Neurosurg Psychiat* 39:538, 1976.
8. MacLean IC: Nerve root stimulation to evaluate conduction across the lumbosacral plexus. Abstracts of Communications of the Sixth International Congress of Electromyography. Stockholm, Sweden, 1979, p 270.
9. MacLean IC: Nerve root stimulation to evaluate conduction across the brachial and lumbosacral plexuses. Third Annual Continuing Education Course, American Association of Electromyography and Electrodiagnosis, Philadelphia, September 25, 1980.
10. MacLean IC, Mattioni TA: Phrenic nerve conduction studies: a new technique and its application in quadriplegic patients. *Arch Phys Med Rehabil* 62:70, 1981.

11. MacLean IC, Taylor RS: Nerve root stimulation to evaluate brachial plexus conduction. Abstracts of Communications of the Fifth International Congress of Electromyography, Rochester, Minnesota, 1975, p 47.

12. Panayiotopoulos CP: F-chronodispersion: a new electrophysiologic method. *Muscle Nerve* 2:68–72, 1979.

13. Ruppert ES, Johnson EW: Motor nerve conduction velocities in low birth weight infants. *Pediatrics* 42:255–259, 1968.

14. Waylonis G, Johnson EW: Facial nerve conduction delay. *Arch Phys Med* 41:539–547, 1960.

15. Waylonis G, Johnson EW: Facial nerve conduction delay. *Arch Phys Med Rehabil* 45:539–541, 1964.

7

Electrodiagnosis of Radiculopathy

ERNEST W. JOHNSON

Suspected radiculopathy is the most frequent referral and diagnosis in most large EMG practices, both in-hospital and out-of-hospital. Over the years there have been many studies of EMG abnormalities in radiculopathy. It is widely recognized that fibrillation potentials in a particular root distribution are noted after the symptoms have been present for 3 weeks. These early abnormalities were studied usually in the anterior primary ramus distribution. Later, the importance of the EMG abnormalities in the posterior primary ramus and their earlier appearance than in the limb muscles began to be noted and reported. More recently, the late responses have been studied in radicular disease, e.g., prolonged H-reflex latency in S1 radiculopathy and a reduced number of F waves evoked in an appropriate muscle. Most recently studies have been conducted using central evoked potentials in radiculopathy. Yet, dermatomal stimulation in sensory evoked potentials remains controversial in the diagnosis of radiculopathy.

PRACTICAL ANATOMY FOR RADICULOPATHY

It is axiomatic that electrodiagnosis of a radiculopathy requires a thorough knowledge of surface and peripheral neuromuscular anatomy.

All muscles activating on the extremities are pluri-segmentally innervated, except the rhomboids, which receive motor fibers only from C5. Because the rest of the limb muscles have two or more nerve roots supplying them, it is useful to appreciate that the distribution of the motor axons from the roots generally occurs proximally to distally, anteriorly to posteriorly, and medially to laterally as the roots go cephalad to caudad.

Although there is considerable overlap superficially in the lumbar

229

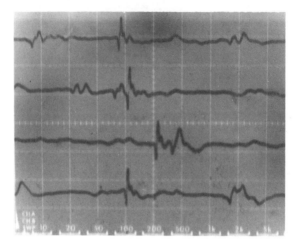

Figure 7.1. Recruitment interval (RI). Note that the first MU is firing at 10 Hz when the second unit begins to activate. RI = 100 msec, recruitment frequency = 10 Hz (Caliber: Each square = 10 msec, 500 µV.; Monopolar needle electrode in extensor digitorum longus.)

paraspinals, one usually can isolate the appropriate root level by deep penetration of the paraspinal muscle bulk by the electrode. Distribution of the lumbosacral root levels occurs directly lateral to the lumbar spinous processes. There is *no* S2 representation in the paraspinal muscles. The S2 anterior primary rami can be studied only by exploring the gluteus maximus, soleus, and intrinsic muscles of the foot.

S3/4 anterior primary rami can be investigated by exploring the external anal sphincter and the external urethral sphincter.

In the cervical paraspinals the root levels are quite caudal to the appropriate spinous process (Fig. 7.1). The most frequent cause of inability to find postprimary ramus abnormalities in cervical radiculopathy is the lack of needle exploration of the more caudal extent of the cervical paraspinal muscles.

Guides for Radicular Anatomy

In the lower extremity the only L4 motor distribution below the knee is to the anterior tibial muscle, and the only L5 motor distribution below the ankle is to the extensor digitorum brevis muscle.

In the upper extremity, the only C6 motor distribution below the elbow anteriorly and medially is to the pronator teres; anteriorly and laterally it is to the brachioradialis muscle. The only C6 motor distribution on the posterior aspect of the forearm below the elbow is to the extensor carpi radialis and supinator.

There is no C7 motor distribution below the wrist. Hand intrinsics

Table 7.1. Sequence of EMG Abnormalities in Radiculopathy

Days from Onset	Electrodiagnostic Abnormality
0	Reduced recruitment
	Reduced recruitment interval
	Prolonged H wave (S1) (7/8)
	Number of F waves reduced
	"Early" polyphasic MUP present
0 + 4	CMAP reduced in true weakness
0 + 7	Positive waves in paraspinal muscles
0 + 12–14	Positive waves in proximal limb muscle; fibrillation potentials in paraspinal muscles
0 + 18–21	All electrodiagnostic abnormalities are present
0 + 5–6 wk	Reinnervation MUP can be present
6 mo–1 yr	Increased amplitude of reinnervated MUPs

are supplied by C8 and T1, with the C8 more radialward and T1 more ulnarward.

CHRONOLOGY OF ELECTRODIAGNOSIS IN RADICULOPATHY (TABLE 7.1)

From the onset of the inflammation in the nerve root (and thus the radicular pain), several abnormalities are present on the EMG.

First, if the degree of weakness is significant (i.e., less than 4/5), it may be recognized as a reduced recruitment pattern on maximal contraction (see Chapter 1). However, if the weakness is minimal, the recruitment pattern may not be identified as reduced. Then, the electromyographer can, with a minimal contraction, identify a reduced recruitment interval (or increased recruitment frequency) (see Chapter 1) (Fig. 7.2).

Our study (12, 13) of early and mild L5 radiculopathy suggested a recruitment interval of 70–90 msec in the extensor digitorum longus as compared to a normal interval of 100–120 msec. It is best to compare the interval with that of the opposite uninvolved muscle in unilateral radiculopathy.

Also from the onset of radiculopathy, the H-reflex latency is prolonged in S1 radiculopathy (3). Our study as confirmed by others (20, 21) suggests that a latency difference from the uninvolved extremity of more than 1 msec is suggestive of S1 radiculopathy (Figs. 7.3 and 7.4).

In cervical radiculopathies, the H-reflex latency in the flexor carpi radialis can be useful in diagnosing C7 or C8 radiculopathies (Fig. 7.5). Prolongation of more than 1 msec (some say .8 msec) side to side is abnormal.

If weakness is substantial, the number of F waves evoked in a particular motor nerve in 12–16 stimulations can be reduced (perhaps

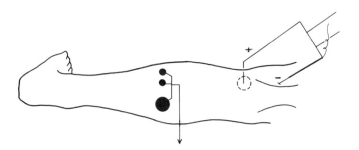

Figure 7.2. Electrode placement for H-reflex latency. Note that the recording electrode is over the soleus, and the stimulating electrode (needle) is over the tibial nerve in the lateral popliteal space.

evoking only 8–10 F-waves) if compared to the contralateral extremity (Fig. 7.6). In normal muscles, an F wave should be expected to occur with each stimulation.

After 7–8 days following the onset of radicular symptoms, positive sharp waves can be evoked in the posterior primary ramus distribution (paraspinal muscles). If this is the only finding in lumbosacral radiculopathy, the H-reflex latency determination can be used to differentiate the L5 and S1 radiculopathies because it is prolonged in the latter. Lumbosacral radiculopathies in most large series occur twice as often in L5 as in S1, and only about 5% occur in L4.

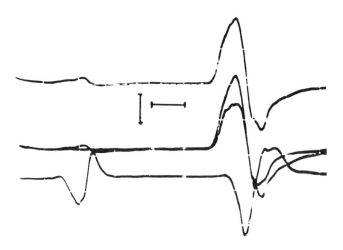

Figure 7.3. Prolonged H-reflex latency in S1 radiculopathy. *Top two traces,* Normal side. *Bottom trace,* S1 radiculopathy. (Caliber: 5 msec, 1 millivolt; stimulate the tibial nerve popliteal space; surface recording over soleus.)

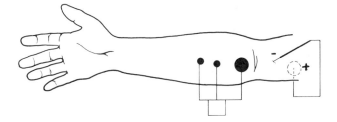

Figure 7.4. Electrode placement for H-reflex latency in flexor capri radialis. Note that the stimulating needle electrode (cathode) is over the median nerve. Anode is on the opposite side of arm.

By 13–14 days, positive waves can appear in the proximal limb muscles and fibrillation potentials in paraspinal muscles.

By 18–21 days, all muscles in a particular radiculopathy should have abnormalities, but not necessarily to the same degree.

The "Early" Polyphasic MUP

For some time clinical electromyographers have noted that polyphasic muscle unit potentials (MUPS) appear in the distribution of the involved root to a greater degree than normal early in the radiculopathy (Fig. 7.7).

We have described such a MUP and proposed a possible explanation: Whenever an inflamed motor nerve root is present, there exists the possibility of ephaptic activation of a neighboring axon by the volitionally activated one. This means that a second axon will generate a MUP

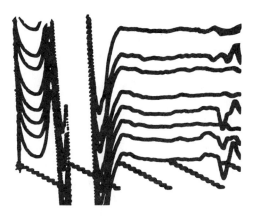

Figure 7.5. F waves in the soleus. Tibial nerve stimulation in S1 radiculopathy. Note that there are only five F waves in eight stimulations. (Caliber: Each slanted line = 10 msec. Height = 200 μV. Surface recording electrodes over soleus.)

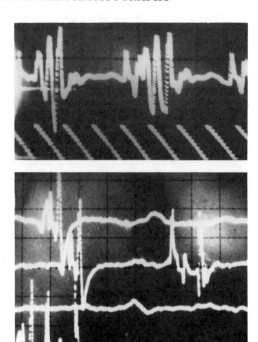

Figure 7.6. "Early" polyphasic MUP in acute radiculopathy. *Top,* Monopolar needle electrode in infraspinatus muscle in C6 radiculopathy. Duration of symptoms is 5 days. (Caliber: Each slanted line = 10 msec. Height = 200 μV.) *Bottom,* Monopolar needle electrode in extensor digitorum longus. Duration of symptoms is 10 days. (Caliber: Each slanted line = 10 msec. Height = 500 μV.)

synchronously but not simultaneously with the volitional MUP, resulting in a polyphasic MUP (actually 2 MUPs) being recorded by the needle electrode (Fig.7.8).

Note that the degree of polyphasicity is related to the difference in the conduction velocity between the two axons. These polyphasic MUPs can occur from the moment of onset of the inflammation in the nerve root.

After 4–5 days the muscles in the particular root distribution, if synchronously stimulated distally, will define the degree of neurapraxic weakness. Those axons that are undergoing Wallerian degeneration (i.e., dying) will no longer conduct, whereas those simply blocked neurapraxically at the inflamed root will conduct distal to the block and result in a compound muscle action potential (CMAP) representing the recoverable axons.

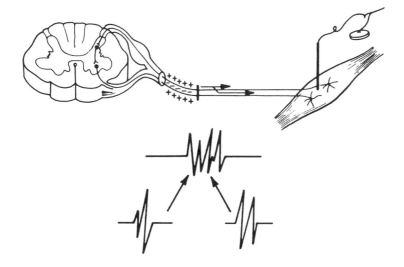

Figure 7.7. Hypothesis to explain "early" polyphasic MUP in acute radiculopathy.

M RESPONSE IN RADICULOPATHY

The CMAP of the weak muscle should be compared with a similar evoked CMAP from an uninvolved extremity (Fig. 7.9). The difference in the area under the negative spike reflects the degree of permanent axon loss (true weakness). Although the area under the negative spike is the best comparison, the amplitude of the CMAP is satisfactory. A reduction of 40% is compatible with adequate function in the weak muscle group.

This technique can give useful prognostic information to the managing physician as early as 4–5 days after onset and continuing on throughout the course of the radiculopathy. For example, if a patient has a foot drop clinically from an L5 radiculopathy, conventional EMG will indicate the diagnosis, but stimulation studies and analysis of the CMAP will yield the critical information of whether the foot drop weakness is neurapraxic or permanent. Similar changes occur in the sensory nerve action potential (Fig. 7.10).

As early as 4–6 weeks, if there is substantial axonal death, reinnervation potentials can appear that are long duration polyphasic MUPs. Later, some may appear as satellite potentials (Fig. 7.11).

Very late in radiculopathy, reinnervation potentials will be seen as synchronized MUPs of increased amplitude.

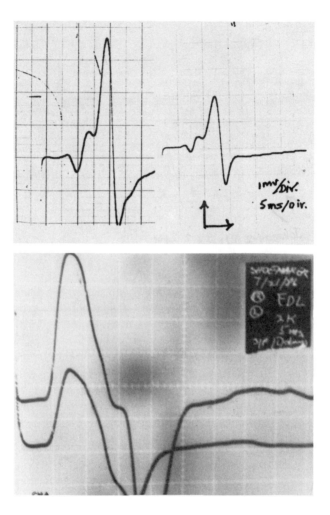

Figure 7.8. Reduced CMAP in acute radiculopathy. *Top,* Medial gastroc CMAP in S1 radiculopathy (R); normal extremity (L). (Caliber: On photo.) *Bottom,* Extensor digitorum longus CMAP in L5 radiculopathy (*Bottom trace*); normal extremity (*Top trace*). (Caliber: Square = 5 msec, 2 millivolts.)

H REFLEX IN S1 RADICULOPATHY

With surface electrodes over the soleus and tibial nerve stimulated in the popliteal space using 1.0 msec duration, low voltage, 0.5 Hz stimulation, the H reflex appears at 27–30 msec latency. Patients must be relaxed because mild contraction of the antagonist will inhibit the H reflex.

Amplitude of the H reflex is not a reliable parameter because it is influenced by many variables. The latency is the most sensitive and

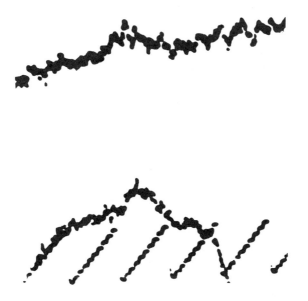

Figure 7.9. Antidromic SNAP Digit I in C6 radiculopathy. *Top trace,* Antidromic radial SNAP (Digit I). *Bottom trace,* Antidromic median SNAP (Digit I). (Caliber: Each slanted line = 1 msec. Height = 10 μV. Ring recording electrodes over Digit I 10 cm from stimulation.) Note that latencies are normal but amplitudes are reduced by over 100%.

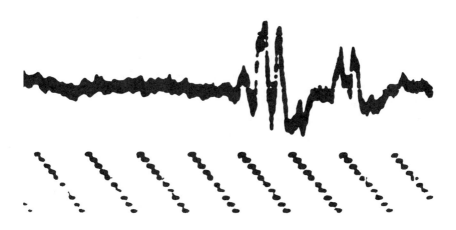

Figure 7.10. Polyphasic MUP in chronic radiculopathy. (Caliber: Each slanted line = 10 msec. Height = 200 μV. Monopolar needle electrode in infraspinatus.) Note that the satellite potential is 10 msec after major AP.

"H" REFLEX DIAGNOSTIC VALUE

Latency greater than 1 ms (than contralat) S.D. = 0.4 ms

Amplitude – **NO** Value

Absence of "H" reflex LESS important (facilitate with min. contr. of soleus)

Figure 7.11. Diagnostic value of H-reflex latency in S1 radiculopathy.

accurate indicator and has been used in diagnosis for more than 10 years. One standard deviation (SD) of variation between the right and left sides is .4 msec and so 3 SD = 1.2 msec. Any difference in latency greater than 1 msec is supportive of the diagnosis of S1 radiculopathy.

A formula may be used to predict the mean expected latency:

.46 × length in cm from medial malleolus to popliteal stimulation + .1 age in years + 9.14 constants = predicted mean latency.

If the side-to-side difference is less than 1 msec but greater than the predicted mean, one must do additional conduction studies. If the side-to-side difference is greater than 1 msec, S1 radiculopathy is probable (assuming the history, physical examination, and EMG are compatible) (Fig. 7.12).

The H reflex is useful in the following situations:

1. If EMG abnormalities on needle exam are limited to paraspinal muscles, then (a) a prolonged H-reflex latency suggests S1 radiculopathy or (b) if H latencies are normal side to side, then L5 radiculopathy is likely (95% of LS radiculopathies are L5 or S1);
2. If EMG abnormalities are inconclusive;
3. When radicular symptoms are present for only a few days;
4. If recurrent radiculopathy occurs in which paraspinal abnormalities are inconclusive.

Some investigators have used the interval latency time, i.e., onset of M wave to onset of the H reflex. This measurement removes some of the dilution that is present when measuring the H-reflex latency from the stimulation of the tibial nerve at the popliteal space to the onset of the H reflex. To reduce the dilution further, recently we have been stimulating the S1 spinal nerve and subtracting that time from the H-reflex latency (Fig. 7.13). In an average adult, this removes 14–15 msec from the overall H-reflex latency (Fig. 7.14).

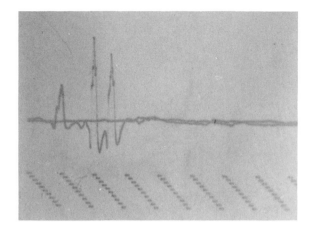

Figure 7.12. Late polyphasic in radiculopathy. Monopolar needle electrode in extensor digitorum longus. Status after 7 years following onset of radiculopathy. (Caliber: Each slanted line = 10 msec. Height = 200 µV.) Note that second trace did not include MUP.

A serendipitous observation with this S1 stimulation has been the frequency of a second action potential similar to the CMAP occurring 6–8 msec later (Fig. 7.15). We hypothesize this is the H wave responding to stimulation of the IA afferents at the S1 site (posterior superior iliac spine).

In individuals with S1 radiculopathy in which the H wave occurs later, perhaps 10–12 msec later, this technique provides a small loop

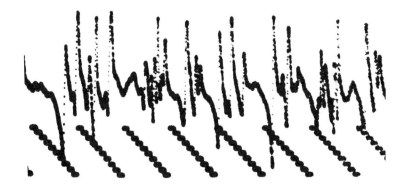

Figure 7.13. Complex repetitive discharge in posterior cervical muscles in C6 radiculopathy. (Caliber: Each slanted line = 10 msec. Height = 100 µV.) Monopolar needle electrode in cervical paraspinal at C6 level.)

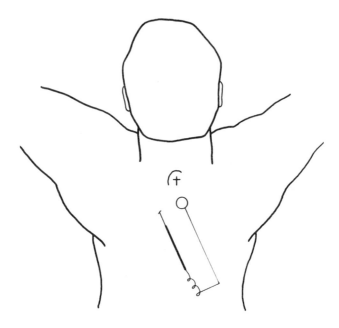

+ over tip of C7 Spinous Process

Figure 7.14. Needle electrode exploring appropriate level of cervical paraspinal muscles for C6 radiculopathy. Note the caudal extent of the position.

to investigate H-wave latency (Fig. 7.18). The H wave is facilitated by a longer duration of stimulation current (0.5–1 msec).

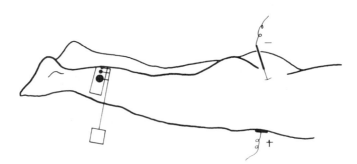

Figure 7.15. S1 spinal root stimulation. Monopolar needle electrode is inserted 1–2 cm medial to the posterior superior iliac spine. Anode is placed on the anterior trunk opposite the needle.

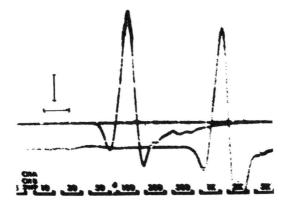

Figure 7.16. H wave and S1 M wave. *Top trace,* S1 spinal nerve M wave. *Bottom trace,* Tibial nerve H wave. (Caliber: 5 msec, 1 millivolt; Surface recording electrodes over soleus.)

ELECTROMYOGRAPHY AFTER MYELOGRAM OR LAMINECTOMY

EMG After Myelogram

EMG abnormalities in paraspinal muscles may result from a Pantopaque myelogram, but all abnormalities disappear by the fourth day. Recently, similar abnormalities were described after simple lumbar puncture (11). We have not confirmed this finding.

Postlaminectomy EMG

Electrodiagnostic findings may be confusing. Diffuse abnormalities (positive waves and fibrillation potentials) that are not diagnostically significant can occur in the paraspinal muscles along the scar. Localized EMG abnormalities at least 3 cm lateral to the scar and corresponding with the symptoms and physical findings can be diagnostically helpful. The paraspinals should be explored in postlaminectomy patients because doing so may be helpful in management and certainly would be an educational experience for the electromyographer. Findings in the distribution of the anterior primary rami may be equally confusing even when compared with preoperative findings.

CHRONIC RADICULOPATHIES

Evaluation of recurrent radiculopathy is a frequent and often difficult problem. Comparison with previous electrodiagnostic studies is most helpful.

If the previous radiculopathy is severe, one would expect the muscle fibers to atrophy. Thus, the fibrillation potentials would be small, in

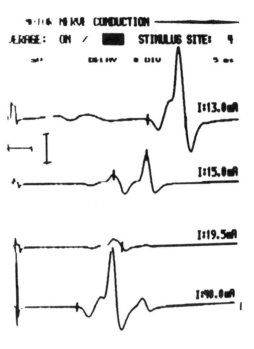

Figure 7.17. S1, H wave, and tibial H wave. *Top trace,* Beginning M wave to left and tibial H wave to right. *Second trace,* Small S1 direct M wave and S1 H wave. *Third trace,* Small S1 direct M wave. *Bottom trace,* Large direct S1 M wave. (Caliber: 5 msec, 1 millivolt.)

contrast with recent denervation, when the fibrillation potentials are larger. Reinnervation may have occurred, and thus the proportion of polyphasic MUPs will be increased (Fig. 7.17). These MUPs will also be increased in amplitude and duration. Reinnervation may occur as early as 5–6 weeks. Single fiber EMG may be useful to evaluate the progress of reinnervation.

Complex repetitive discharges may be recorded in chronic radiculopathies (Fig. 7.18). Stalberg has shown these to be activation of a denervated (or hyperirritable) muscle fiber that acts as a pacemaker by ephaptic transmission to neighboring denervated muscle fibers.

Radiculopathy in Chronic Neuropathies

In mild diabetic neuropathy, a radiculopathy may be the presenting symptom. Sudden onset of pain and atrophy of the thigh (unilaterally) in a diabetic patient traditionally were considered to be symptoms of a femoral neuropathy. With careful electrodiagnostic study, this syn-

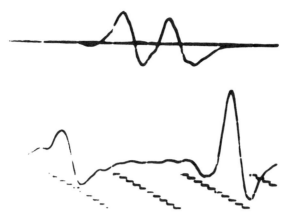

Figure 7.18. S1 spinal nerve stimulation direct and H wave. *Top trace,* First AP is the direct S1 stimulation, M. Second AP is the H wave. *Bottom trace,* H reflex wave occurring after tibial nerve stimulated at popliteal space. Note the M response beginning. (Caliber: Each slanted line = 10 msec. Height = 1 millivolt. Surface recording electrodes over soleus.)

drome has been shown to be multiple lumbar radiculopathy, e.g., L3/4. One explanation of the frequency of radiculopathies in diabetic patients (normal radiologic study) has been the dural root sleeve compromise of vulnerable nerves.

Radiculopathy occurs with the same frequency as other entrapment sites in generalized peripheral neuropathies and should always be considered in the differential diagnosis. H-reflex and F-wave latencies should be useful in making the diagnosis.

EVALUATION OF A POSSIBLE L5 RADICULOPATHY

Historical Features

When did pain begin? Classically it begins in the back; often a day or two later the radicular pain begins, most frequently in the buttocks.

Radicular pain is almost always in the lateral buttock and then the posterior thigh, calf, or lateral shin; often, it is present in the ankle or heel.

Pain is usually worst on sitting and is especially aggravated when driving a car; it is less while standing, and the least pain is experienced in the recumbent, side-lying position on a hard surface.

Physical Examination

	Reflex Reduced	Weakness
L4	Knee jerk reflex	Knee extensors weak
L5	Biceps femoris reflex	Toe extensors weak
S1	Ankle jerk reflex	Plantar flexors weak
C6	Biceps brachii reflex	Ext. sh. rotators weak
C7	Triceps reflex	Elbow extensors weak
C8	—	Wrist extensors weak

Electrodiagnosis

The patient is placed in the prone position over pillows. The examination should follow this sequence of steps:

1. Do needle study of paraspinals (bilateral).
2. Do needle study of weak limb muscles.
3. Determine recruitment interval (frequency). Compare with contralateral extremity muscle.
4. Determine H-reflex latency of both extremities.
5. Determine F waves: Number reduced in weak muscle (10–20).
6. Turn patient over (supine) and stimulate weak muscle; with surface record of CMAP, compare area under the negative spike of the CMAP of the involved and uninvolved extremities.

Suggested Muscles for CMAP Comparison

C5:	Deltoid
C6:	Infraspinatus
C7:	Triceps
C8:	Abductor pollicis brevis
T1:	Abductor digiti quinti
L4:	Anterior tibial or vastus medialis
L5:	Extensor digitorum longus
S1:	Medial gastrocnemius

SUMMARY

Electrodiagnostic techniques are essential to the diagnosis and management of radiculopathies from the onset of the radiculopathy, as well as after the traditional time period of 3 weeks postonset. They give information about the location and extent of the neurophysiologic dysfunction. Needle EMG techniques are necessary for all stages of the clinical course of radiculopathy; in addition, determination of the recruitment interval, H-reflex latency, and number of F waves and recognition of the "early" polyphasic MUP all give vital information.

References

1. Aminoff MJ, Goodin DS, Parry GJ, Barbaro NM, Weinstein PR, Rosenblum, ML: Electrophysiologic evaluation of lumbosacral radiculopathies: electromyography,

late responses, and somatosensory evoked potentials. *Neurology* 35:1514–1518, 1985.

2. Bonner FJ, Schmidt WH: Electromyography in disc disease. *Arch Phys Med Rehabil* 38-689, 1957.

3. Braddom RI, Johnson EW: Standardization of "H" reflex and diagnostic use in S1 radiculopathy. *Arch Phys Med Rehabil* 55:161, 1974.

4. Brazier MAB, Watkins AL, Michelsen JJ: Electromyography in differential diagnosis of ruptured cervical disc. *Arch Neurol Psychiat* 56:651, 1948.

5. Crue BL, Pudenz, RH, Sheldon CH: Observations on the value of clinical electromyography. *J Bone Joint Surg* 39A:492, 1957.

6. Fisher MA, Kaur D, Houchins J: Electrodiagnostic examination, back pain and entrapment of posterior rami. *Neurophysiology* 25:183–189, 1985.

7. Flax HJ, Berrios, R, Rivera D: Electromyography in the diagnosis of herniated lumbar disc. *Arch Phys Med Rehabil* 45:520, 1964.

8. Gough JG, Koepke GH: Electromyographic determination of motor root levels in erector spinal muscles. *Arch Phys Med Rehabil* 47:9, 1966.

9. Granger CV, Flanigan, S: Nerve root conduction studies during lumbar disc surgery. *J Neurosurg* 28:439, 1968.

10. Honet JC, Puri D: Cervical radiculitis: treatment and results in 82 patients. *Arch Phys Med Rehabil* 57:12, 1976.

11. Johnson EW, Melvin JL: Value of electromyography in lumbar radiculopathy. *Arch Phys Red Rehabil* 52:239, 1971.

12. Johnson EW, Stocklin R, LaBan MM: Use of electrodiagnostic examination in a university hospital. *Arch Phys Med Rehabil* 46:573, 1965.

13. Johnson EW, Burkhart JA, Earl WC: Electromyography in post laminectomy patients. *Arch Phys Med Rehabil* 53:407, 1972.

14. Johnson EW, Weber R, Mills P: Needle electrode stimulation in electromyography. *Arch Phys Med Rehabil* 58:520, 1977.

15. Johnson EW, Fletcher FR: Lumbosacral radiculopathy: review of 100 consecutive cases. *Arch Phys Med Rehabil* 62:321–323, 1981.

16. LaBan MM, Grant AE: Occult spinal metastases—early electromyographic manifestations. *Arch Phys Med Rehabil* 52:223, 1971.

17. Langstretch GF, Newcomer AD: Abdominal pain caused by diabetic radiculopathy. *Ann Intern Med* 86:166, 1977.

18. Mixter WJ, Barr JS: Rupture of the intervertebral disc with involvement of the spinal canal. *N Engl J Med* 211:210, 1934.

19. Peiris OA: Conduction in the fourth and fifth lumbar and first sacral nerve roots: preliminary communication. *NZ Med J* 80:502, 1974.

20. Schimsheimer RJ, Ongerboer BW, Visser DE, Kemp B: The flexor carpi radialis H-reflex in lesions of the sixth and seventh cervical nerve roots. *J Neurol Neurosurg Psychiat* 48:445–449, 1985.

21. Schuchmann JA: Evaluation of the H-reflex latency in radiculopathy. *Arch Phys Med Rehabil* 58:560, 1976.

22. Shea PA, Woods WW, Werden DH: Electromyography in diagnosis of nerve root compression syndrome. *Arch Neurol Psychiat* 64:93, 1950.

23. Treanor W: Diabetic polyradiculopathy: a syndrome in need of definition. *Arch Phys Med Rehabil* 55:593–595, 1974.

24. Troni W: The value and limits of the H reflex as a diagnostic tool in S1 root compression. *Neurophysiology* 23:471–480, 1983.

25. Weddell G, Feinstein B, Pattel RE: The electrical activity of voluntary muscle in man under normal and pathological conditions. *Brain* 67:178, 1944.

8

Peripheral Neuropathies

GEORGE H. KRAFT

Peripheral neuropathies present the most difficult differential diagnosis for electromyographers. The purpose of this chapter is to assist the electromyographer in sorting out the multiple conditions that can cause peripheral nerve dysfunction, so that the physician specializing in electrodiagnostic medicine can determine the likely etiology or etiologies of a neuropathy in a particular patient. These neuropathies are diseases causing dysfunction of peripheral nerve axons, their myelin sheaths, or both. Usually they are generalized and affect many nerves. They tend to be more severe in distal portions of extremities, especially in the feet and lower legs. Clinically, peripheral neuropathies generally produce impaired sensation, motor weakness, and hypo- or areflexia.

This chapter describes the nerve conduction and EMG abnormalities that occur in various peripheral neuropathies. It should be emphasized that an electroneuromyographic examination does not by itself give a diagnosis. However, electrophysiologic information about peripheral nerve function can help the electromyographer determine the most likely causes of a neuropathy. Not only is EMG important for making a diagnosis it is also necessary for determining an accurate prognosis and appropriate treatment.

There are two general categories of peripheral neuropathies: (a) diseases producing primary axonal degeneration, which may also cause secondary demyelination, and (b) diseases causing segmental demyelination, which, if extensive enough, may cause secondary axonal degeneration. In addition, some diseases may cause primary degeneration of both axon and myelin. Neuropathies can also be classified into four

The work described in this chapter was supported in part by Research Grants G008300076 and G008435053 from the National Institute of Disability and Rehabilitation Research (formerly the National Institute of Handicapped Research), Department of Education, Washington, DC.

Table 8.1. Categories of Peripheral Neuropathies

Hereditary neuropathies
Toxic neuropathies
  Heavy metals
  Organic compounds
  Drugs
Neuropathies associated with diseases
Idiopathic neuropathies

general etiologic categories: hereditary, toxic, those associated with disease, and idiopathic (Table 8.1).

Different peripheral neuropathies can also selectively affect different nerves or certain segments of nerves. For example, lead toxicity in adults classically produces greatest damage to the radial nerve. Some neuropathies have a predilection for motor nerves and others for sensory nerves. Although peripheral neuropathies generally produce the greatest dysfunction in distal portions of a nerve, some neuropathies (e.g., Guillain-Barré polyneuritis) may preferentially affect other segments during certain stages of disease.

NERVE CONDUCTION CHANGES IN PERIPHERAL NEUROPATHY

In the clinical recording of motor nerve conduction velocity, conduction of the fastest conducting fibers (A alpha) is measured. There is a linear relationship between the diameter of a myelinated fiber and its conduction velocity; as the diameter decreases, the conduction velocity decreases (159). Thus, in diseases in which there is loss of large diameter myelinated fibers or a reduction in diameter of all myelinated fibers, conduction velocity is generally slightly reduced. Amplitudes of evoked potentials are usually decreased, but temporal dispersion may be only minimal (Fig. 8.1).

Disorders of myelin are thought to reduce nerve conduction velocity in two ways. First, thinning of myelin itself slows conduction. Conduction remains saltatory until there is a conduction block, but the loss of current through a damaged internode increases the time required for the next internode to reach threshold, causing some decrease in conduction velocity (177). Second, conduction block can occur in severely demyelinated fibers as a result of the failure of an impulse to excite a node adjacent to a severely demyelinated internode (Fig. 8.1) (221). With pure loss of myelin, conduction velocity is moderately to markedly reduced, and temporal dispersion can be quite marked (Fig. 8.2) (146, 148). In the clinical setting, demyelinating neuropathies usually eventually affect all segments of the peripheral nerve, producing a

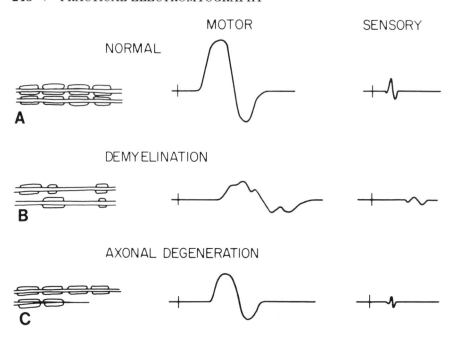

Figure 8.1. *A,* On the left is a schematic representation of two normal axons with normal myelin sheaths. These axons are oriented as if the cell bodys are to the left. Normal evoked motor and sensory potentials are demonstrated. *B,* In segmental demyelination, axis cylinders are preserved with random loss and attenuation of myelin internodes. In the diagram of the CMAP, the stimulus artifact is represented by the vertical line; note that there is an increased latency between the stimulus and the action potential. The action potential shows temporal dispersion and decreased amplitude. The compound SNAP also shows prolonged latency, temporal dispersion, and attenuation of amplitude. *C,* In axonal degeneration reduction in the diameter of the intact upper axis cylinder and dying-back of the lower axis cylinder are demonstrated; myelin may be unaffected except on the discontinuous axis cylinder. The motor and sensory nerve responses show slightly prolonged latencies with reduction in action potential amplitudes.

prolonged distal latency, as well as slowed conduction velocity (Fig. 8.3). Occasionally, however, selective areas of block occur, resulting in relatively normal distal latencies in the presence of striking proximal conduction slowing and temporal dispersion (Fig. 8.4).

In diseases in which both axonal degeneration and demyelination occur, a combination of the above findings is noted. Primary axonal diseases produce nerve dysfunction and slowing of conduction either throughout the length of the nerve or in the most distal portions; the exact pattern depends on the type of nerve dysfunction. Because of the great distance from the metabolic factory of the nerve cell body,

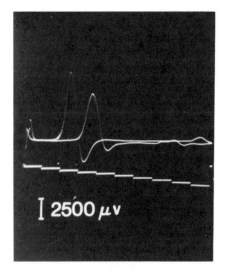
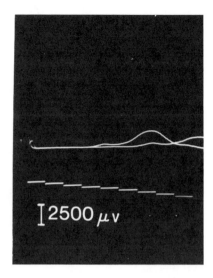

Figure 8.2. On the left are proximal and distal latencies from a guinea pig sciatic nerve 5 days after receiving peripheral nerve antigen. Conduction velocity was 59 m/sec. On the right is the response in the same nerve 22 days after receiving antigen. Note the marked prolongation of both proximal and distal latencies, the loss of amplitude, and the striking temporal dispersion. NCV was calculated to be 22 m/sec. The vertical bar indicates 2500 µV. Each horizontal step represents 1 msec.

nerve dysfunction and slowing of nerve conduction in neuronal atrophy are most pronounced in the distal portion of the lower extremity.

Demyelinating diseases, in contrast, may result in slowing of proximal nerve conduction during certain stages of disease, causing conduction abnormalities even in the nerve roots. Because the demyelination of different axons generally varies, the difference in conduction velocity between the fastest and the slowest fibers is greater the longer the distance over which the impulse is transmitted; consequently, temporal dispersion is more pronounced on proximal stimulation.

Certain nerve conduction techniques can be used to obtain information about conduction changes in a peripheral neuropathy. Conduction in the most proximal segments can be studied by means of the F wave, the H reflex, and somatosensory evoked potentials (SEPs.) Nerve conduction can be evaluated in proximal and distal segments of an extremity by using conventional NCV techniques. Distal latency measurements over a standard distance are useful (150), and residual latency determinations can give specific information about unique conduction characteristics in the most distal segments of nerve (133, 150).

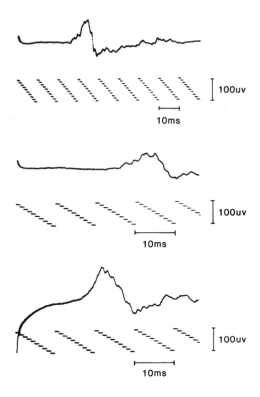

Figure 8.3. Peroneal motor nerve conduction studies 7 weeks following the on-set of Guillain-Barré syndrome in a 24-year-old woman. *Top* and *middle tracings* show the peroneal latency at different sweep speeds when stimulated below the fibular head. *Bottom tracings* show peroneal latency stimulated at the ankle. Note the marked reduction of CMAP amplitude and the temporal dispersion. Even though the amplitude is even lower on proximal stimulation, the duration of the M wave lengthens so the area under the negative (upgoing) phase is similar. The patient in whom this conduction was recorded had extensive fibrillation potentials in muscles innervated by the peroneal nerve. Conduction velocity was calculated to be 30 m/sec. Because all axons may not be able to be stimulated at all points, the M waves produced by proximal and distal stimulation may be made up of different populations of muscle fibers. For this reason, a good case can be made for repeating latencies at different distances, rather than a calculated NCV.

It is helpful to be able to record averaged nerve potentials to obtain information on sensory and mixed nerve conduction velocities; SEP recording permits the determination of proximal sensory nerve conduction values (224). Quantification of the compound muscle action potential (CMAP) is also useful (92).

Motor nerve conduction studies should be done using surface recording electrodes wherever possible. The M wave recorded by a surface

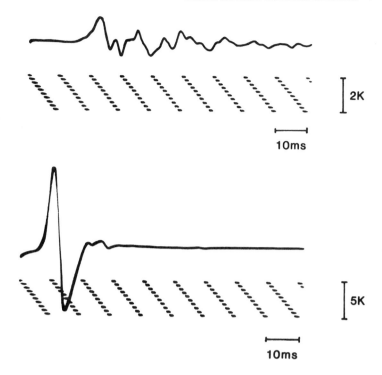

Figure 8.4. Tibial nerve conduction in a 30-year-old woman with a steroid-responsive polyneuropathy. This neuropathy was associated with a paucity of fibrillation potentials and a good response to prednisone. Note the relatively intact distal CMAP but marked temporal dispersion on stimulation at the popliteal fossa. NCV calculated to be 29 m/sec. This indicated a highly localized area of demyelination (between the popliteal fossa and ankle) with distal latency essentially normal. The excellent amplitude of the terminal latency also showed that little, if any, axonal degeneration had occurred.

electrode is a summation of nonsynchronous muscle fiber action potentials recorded from the entire muscle. The onset of this CMAP represents the earliest electrical response of the muscle and is produced by the first muscle fiber action potentials—regardless of where they are located in the muscle—innervated by the fastest conducting motor nerves. Therefore, the latency—defined as the onset of this M wave— is essentially the same over most of the surface of small distal muscles, but the amplitude will diminish as the distance between the generator and the recording electrode increases (41). In practice, then, regardless of where a surface electrode is placed, the latency is the same.

If a needle is used as the active recording electrode, the electrical activity recorded comes from only a small region around the needle tip. Consequently, the latency will vary as the needle is placed in different portions of the muscle. If it is close to the motor endplate area of a fast conducting axon, the latency will be short (approaching that recorded by a surface electrode). Conversely, if the needle is in a muscle fiber supplied by a slower conducting fiber and far from the endplate area, the electrical activity it "sees" will occur later. As a general statement, surface recording electrodes always measure the shortest latencies (121). Even though surface recorded amplitudes do vary with placement, needle recorded amplitudes vary more. Because amplitude measurements are also important in assessing nerve function, their quantification represents another reason to use surface electrodes.

However, there are three indications for using needle recording electrodes:

1. In a severe peripheral neuropathy where a satisfactory latency cannot be recorded using surface techniques—if only a few motor units are intact, the action potentials generated may not be sufficient to be recorded percutaneously. In such a situation, the only latency obtainable may be from needle recording.
2. If the muscle to be recorded must be isolated from an adjacent contracting muscle—an example of this is the measurement of a suprascapular nerve latency to the supraspinatus muscle. Stimulation of the suprascapular nerve produces some depolarization of cranial nerve XI and consequent contraction of the trapezius muscle. Because a needle records from a small territory, its use allows the necessary isolation (147).
3. To be sure of the localization of the responding muscle—because of the highly localizing qualities of needle recording, the muscle from which the action potential is recorded can be identified with certainty.

EMG CHANGES IN PERIPHERAL NEUROPATHIES

Needle EMG studies are an important component of the electrodiagnostic evaluation of peripheral neuropathies, although in mild peripheral neuropathies very little in the way of abnormalities may be seen. The most pronounced findings in a peripheral neuropathy are generally seen in the most distal muscles. The most subtle changes are an increase in polyphasicity and serration (several changes in direction, not crossing baseline) (152) of motor unit action potentials (MUAPs) and a slight increase in amplitude and duration of the action potentials. In more severe axonal neuropathies, fibrillation potentials and positive sharp waves are seen, and MUAPs are increased in amplitude, duration, and phasicity and are fewer in number. In severe acute axonal neuropathic conditions, positive sharp waves may occur as early as 10

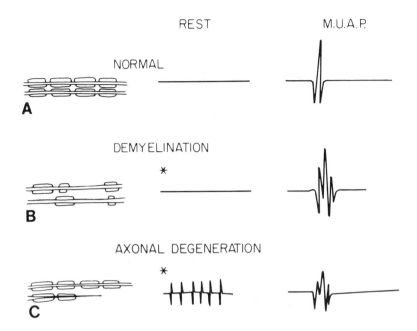

REST   M.U.A.P.

NORMAL

A

DEMYELINATION

*

B

AXONAL DEGENERATION

*

C

Figure 8.5. *A,* Schematic representation of two axons and their myelin sheaths is at the left. Orientation is as if the cell bodies are to the left. At rest no electrical activity is seen. *B,* Segmental demyelination is schematically represented. No fibrillation potentials are seen at rest, and voluntary MUAPs are serrated or polyphasic and have increased duration. *C,* Schematic axonal degeneration is shown at left. At rest fibrillation potentials are seen and voluntary MUAPs are polyphasic and have increased duration. Eventually, they will be increased in amplitude. On needle movement positive sharp waves are seen in axonal degeneration. Muscle may be irritable in demyelinating disease, and under some circumstance, trains of positive sharp wave-like potentials are seen.

days before fibrillations can be noted. In diseases producing segmental demyelination, fibrillation potentials are generally rare, although some positive sharp wave-like potentials may be noted (148) (Fig. 8.5).

In general, axonal neuropathies are likely to produce more polyphasicity of MUAPs than are demyelinating neuropathies. This is especially true if the neuropathy is severe and chronic (Fig. 8.6). In some muscles, strikingly serrated potentials are observed (Fig. 8.7). Changes are generally most pronounced in distal muscles. On the other hand, even in severe demyelinating neuropathies, only minimal polyphasicity is seen in MUAPs (Fig. 8.8).

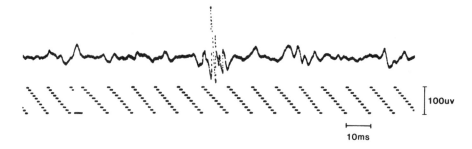

Figure 8.6. MUAP from the extensor digitorum communis of a patient with lead neuropathy. This action potential was recorded with a 28-gauge monopolar EMG needle. Note the increased number of phases.

HEREDITARY NEUROPATHIES (Tables 8.2, 8.3)

Charcot-Marie-Tooth Disease (Peroneal Muscular Atrophy, Hereditary Motor-Sensory Neuropathy I, HMSN I)

This autosomal dominant disorder, which is probably more common than generally appreciated, is now considered by most investigators to be a neuronal atrophy with secondary demyelination (73, 199). Studies by Brimijoin et al. (31) have demonstrated that an abnormality of axonal transport exists; they support the hypothesis that there is an inborn metabolic derangement in peripheral neurons that prevents substances essential for the development and maintenance of the cell from being properly synthesized, packaged, or transported. The cycle of demyelination and remyelination of atrophic fibers leads to onion-bulb formation. However, nerve graft studies suggest that the disease may be more complex, and they implicate some primary Schwann cell abnormalities (2).

Presenting symptoms usually begin in the first or second decade and consist of high arched feet and weakness of foot and lower leg muscles. Sensation is generally only minimally diminished. Peripheral nerves, especially the greater auricular nerve, are often large and palpable. Histologically many nerve fibers disappear, especially at the periphery. Sporadic cases may represent dominant inheritance with poor expressivity in one of the parents; NCVs in such a parent with subclinical disease should show abnormalities. An autosomal recessive form, clinically and electrodiagnostically identical to the dominant form, has been described in a family with a high consanguinity rate (111).

In addition to the motor and sensory abnormalities, studies have demonstrated minimal autonomic nerve (24, 32) and visual evoked potential (EP) (21) and auditory EP (93) abnormalities in some patients.

Table 8.2. Hereditary Neuropathies

Charcot-Marie-Tooth disease (HMSN I[a])
Hereditary motor-sensory neuropathy II (neuronal form of peroneal muscular atrophy)
Dejerine-Sottas disease (HMSN III)
Roussy-Lévy syndrome
Prednisone-responsive hereditary motor-sensory neuropathy
Hereditary sensory neuropathy
  Autosomal dominant
  Autosomal recessive
Hereditary compression neuropathy
Riley-Day syndrome
Friedreich ataxia
Spinocerebellar degenerations of adulthood
Familial spastic paraplegia (HSMN V)
Pelizaeus-Merzbacher disease
Refsum disease (HMSN IV)
Fabry disease
Metachromatic leukodystrophy
Krabbe leukodystrophy
Tangier disease
Abetalipoproteinemia
Primary familial amyloidosis
Acute intermittent porphyria
Giant axonal neuropathy

[a]Hereditary peripheral neuropathies affecting motor and sensory nerves have been classified as hereditary motor-sensory neuropathy (HMSN) Types I, II, III, IV, and V as listed above by the laboratory of P.J. Dyck at the Mayo Clinic. Additional, less common HMSNs have also been described.

Visual and auditory EP latencies were slightly prolonged. Somatosensory evoked potentials (SEPs) show essentially normal central conduc-

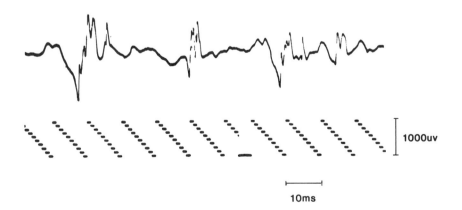

1000uv

10ms

Figure 8.7 Monopolar EMG recording of the anterior tibial muscle in a patient with hereditary motor-sensory neuropathy II. Note the serration of motor unit potentials.

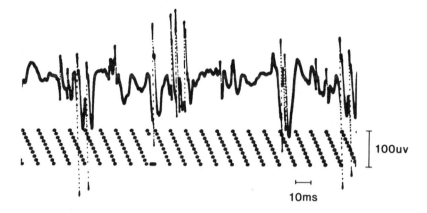

Figure 8.8. Representative MUAPs recorded with a monopolar needle in a patient with chronic steroid-responsive polyneuropathy (same patient whose nerve conductions are shown in Figure 8.4). Note the essential normality of the action potentials, with only a slight indication of increased serration.

tion, with any delay due to the slowing in the peripheral nervous system (129).

Conduction velocities of myelinated fibers are generally strikingly low, depending on the age of the patient and severity of the disease. Dyck and Lambert (69) reported that distal motor latencies averaged almost three times longer than normal and conduction velocities and CMAP amplitudes less than one-half the normal size. In reviewing our experience with Charcot-Marie-Tooth disease, we found residual latencies in the upper extremities to be approximately 2 SD above the mean, with some strikingly longer. Thus, although conduction slowing is generalized (163)—as opposed to that seen in acquired demyelinating neuropathies—it tends to be more severe in distal portions of nerves. We also studied the CMAP and found a highly significant difference between the integrated area under the M wave of normal adult males and those with Charcot-Marie-Tooth disease ($P < 0.001$) (92). Humberstone (123) states that the earliest conduction changes are a decrease in sensory nerve action potential (SNAP) amplitude and prolongation of sensory latency. Studies of F wave conduction velocity of the median and ulnar nerves show that proximal nerve segments are affected, but not as greatly as the more distal segments (138). One of the slowest motor nerve conduction velocities I have seen in an adult (7.8 m/sec in the ulnar nerve) was in a patient with Charcot-Marie-Tooth disease; most of his affected family members also had motor conduction velocities below 15 m/sec (Fig. 8.9).

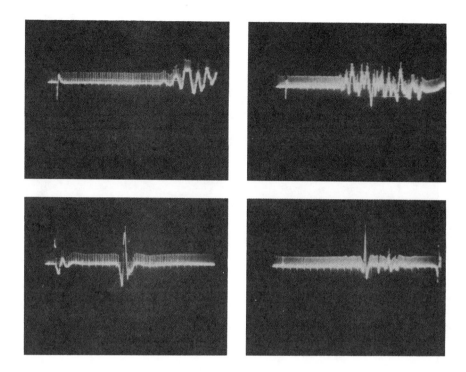

Figure 8.9. Motor nerve conduction latencies in the ulnar nerve of a patient with Charcot-Marie-Tooth Disease. The upper photographs show proximal latencies recorded with surface electrodes. Each vertical marking represents 0.5 msec. In the photograph in the upper right hand corner, sweep speed was reduced to demonstrate the striking temporal dispersion. The bottom photographs show latencies recorded with a needle recording electrode. On the left is the distal latency, on the right the proximal latency. Note that the muscle action potential can be more easily identified with a needle recording electrode but that temporal dispersion is less well demonstrated because action potentials are recorded only in the vicinity of the needle tip. Sensitivity of the upper photographs is five times that of the lower photographs and had to be increased that amount to demonstrate the take-off point of the action potential. Each vertical grid marking represents 200 μV in upper photos; 1000 μV in lower photos, NCV = 7.8 m/sec.

EMG changes may be widespread, but are especially marked in distal muscles of hands and feet. They consist of fibrillation potentials and positive sharp waves, as well as increased amplitude, duration, and polyphasicity of MUAPs firing in reduced number. In long-standing cases, complete neurogenic atrophy may have been present in the feet for so long that the muscles are electrically silent and show decreased insertional activity on needle movement.

Within families, NCVs in affected individuals are usually similar (36,

Table 8.3. Typical Nerve Conduction and Electromyographic Findings in Hereditary Neuropathies

Disease	Motor Nerve Conduction Velocity	Site of Maximum Nerve Conduction Velocity Slowing	Amplitude of Muscle Action Potential	Sensory Nerve Conduction Velocity	Amplitude of Sensory Action Potential	Electromyographic Findings	Other Useful Laboratory Tests
Charcot-Marie-Tooth disease	↓↓↓	Distal	↓↓↓	↓	↓↓↓	Fib.	Nerve biopsy
Hereditary motor-sensory neuropathy II	nl or ↓	None	↓↓	nl or ↓	↓↓↓	Fib.	Nerve biopsy
Dejerine-Sottas disease	↓↓↓	Distal	↓↓↓	Not obtainable	0	Fib.	Nerve biopsy
Roussy-Lévy syndrome	↓↓↓	Distal	↓↓↓	↓	↓↓↓	Fib.	Nerve biopsy
Prednisone-responsive HMSN	↓↓	General	↓↓	Not obtainable	0	Fib.	Nerve biopsy
Hereditary sensory neuropathy							
Dominant	→	None	nl	Not obtainable	0	nl	Nerve biopsy
Recessive	→	None	↓↓	Not obtainable	0	Fib	Nerve biopsy
Hereditary compression neuropathy	→	At sites of compression	→	→	→	Chronic neuropathic	
Riley-Day syndrome	→	None	nl	nl	↓↓↓	nl	SEP
Friedreich ataxia	→	General	→	Not obtainable	0	Fib.	SEP
Spinocerebellar degenerations of adulthood	→	General	→	↓	↓↓↓	Fib.	
Familial spastic paraplegia	→	Distal	→	→	↓↓↓	Fib.	SEP
Pelizaeus-Merzbacher disease	↓↓	General	↓↓	↓↓	↓↓	Fib.	
Refsum disease	↓↓	General	↓↓	↓↓	↓↓	Fib.	↑ serum phytanic acid
Fabry disease	→	Spotty	nl	→	→	nl	↓ alpha galactosidase
Metachromatic leukodystrophy	↓↓↓	General	↓↓	↓↓	↓↓	nl	↑ sulfatide in urine, specific enzyme assay, nerve biopsy

Table 8.3. Continued.

Disease	Motor Nerve Conduction Velocity	Site of Maximum Nerve Conduction Velocity Slowing	Amplitude of Muscle Action Potential	Sensory Nerve Conduction Velocity	Amplitude of Sensory Action Potential	Electromyographic Findings	Other Useful Laboratory Tests
Krabbe leukodystrophy	↓↓	General	↓↓	↓↓	↓↓	Fib.	Specific enzyme assay, nerve biopsy
Tangier disease	→	General	→	→	→	Fib.	↓ plasma high density lipoproteins
Abetalipoproteinemia	→	General	↓↓	→	↓↓↓	Fib.	↓ plasma low density lipoproteins, absence of apoprotein B, acanthocytosis
Primary amyloidosis	→	Distal	↓↓	→	↓↓↓	Fib.	Serum electrophoresis, nerve rectal biopsy
Acute intermittent porphyria	→	Proximal	↓↓	→	→	Fib.	↑ urine porphyrins
Giant axonal neuropathy	nl	General	nl	Not obtainable	0	Chronic neuropathic	Nerve biopsy

→ = low normal to slightly reduced
↓↓ = moderately low
↓↓↓ = extremely low

50) although occasionally, families have been reported in which some affected members have nerve conduction velocities unlike other affected members (247). This has been our experience and can make differentiation of HMSN I from HMSN II difficult (see below) (22, 35). Although it is not entirely clear when conduction slowing can first be detected, data indicate that affected individuals will show changes by the end of the first decade or earlier (106, 149).

We have evidence that the genetic pattern may be more complex. Some families show positive linkage of HMSN I to the Duffy blood group locus on Chromosome 1, whereas other families show no linkage (23). Neuropathy not linked to Duffy may have less severe slowing of motor nerve conduction velocities and less prominent onion-bulb formation on nerve biopsy.

Hereditary Motor-Sensory Neuropathy II, HMSN II (Neuronal Form of Peroneal Muscular Atrophy)

This dominantly inherited peripheral neuropathy is clinically similar to Charcot-Marie-Tooth disease, although less commonly seen. However, symptoms occur at a somewhat later age, and peripheral nerves are not enlarged. Electrodiagnostically, it differs strikingly because, in this disorder, peripheral nerve conduction velocities are in the low normal range or only minimally reduced; a common dividing line is above or below 38 m/sec (112). In more severely affected individuals, it may not be possible to obtain SNAPs, although, if they are obtained, distal latencies are generally normal (68).

As mentioned above in the section on Charcot-Marie-Tooth disease, it is sometimes difficult to determine whether a family should be placed in the HMSN I or HMSN II category because conduction velocities in affected family members may not be similar. Not infrequently they are not all on the same side of the 38 m/sec dividing line. This has led to the recommendation by Davis, Bradley, and Madrid that intermediate categories of HMSN be established. This suggestion calls for identification of (a) hypertrophic (NCV < 25 m/sec), (b) intermediate (NCV 25–45 m/sec), (c) neuronal sensorimotor (NCV > 45 m/sec), and (d) neuronal motor (NCV > 45 m/sec) forms of the disease (57).

Because NCVs may often be within the normal range, a very useful electrodiagnostic test is needle EMG, which shows positive sharp waves, fibrillation potentials, and an increase in MUAP phasicity or serration, especially in distal muscles of the feet (Fig. 8.7). In older patients, distal foot muscles may be fibrotic with decreased insertional activity. Another useful measure is the amount of current required for supramaximal stimulation. Whereas most nerves can be stimulated using 200 volts for 0.1 msec duration, peripheral nerves in patients with

HMSN II can often be depolarized only with maximal output of the stimulator.

The absence of decreased nerve conduction velocity may make early identification of children with HMSN II difficult. Clinical signs generally parallel the earliest electrodiagnostic changes.

Dejerine-Sottas Disease
(Hypertrophic Interstitial Neuropathy, HMSN III)

This recessively inherited disorder usually begins in infancy and is associated with marked onion-bulb formation caused by repeated demyelination and remyelination (67). Nerve conduction velocities are some of the lowest reported, being as low as 3–5 m/sec in the upper extremity. Distal latencies are often more than four times greater than normal, with the amplitude of the CMAP often 1/10 or 1/20 or normal. Frequently, no compound SNAP can be obtained (72). An abnormality of axonal flow has been reported, and the disease is considered to be a neuronal atrophy. Primary dysfunction of the Schwann cells may be present as well (68). A report of a marriage between two heterozygotes for CMT resulted in homozygote offspring with similar characteristics to the classic description of Dejerine-Sottas disease (137).

Roussy-Lévy Syndrome

In the peripheral nervous system, this disorder appears to be identical to Charcot-Marie-Tooth disease (231). However, essential tremor also occurs as part of the clinical syndrome (68). Nerve conduction and EMG findings are identical to those seen in Charcot-Marie-Tooth disease (153).

Prednisone-Responsive Hereditary Motor-Sensory Neuropathy

This is a recently described chronic, progressive neuropathy showing moderate to severely slowed motor nerve conduction velocities. Usually sensory nerve conductions cannot be obtained. EMG shows fibrillation potentials and increased amplitude, polyphasic MUAPs. The disorder clinically has the characteristics of a HMSN, but shows improvement on high doses (up to 120 mg/day) of prednisone. Cerebrospinal fluid proteins are elevated in most cases. Affected relatives generally show only mild disease. It is not clear whether the reported cases represent a specific type of HMSN or the concurrence of a chronic inflammatory demyelinating neuropathy and HMSN in the same patient (78).

Hereditary Sensory Neuropathy (Autosomal Dominant and Autosomal Recessive Types)

The autosomal dominant disease has its onset in the second or third decade, with lower extremity sensory deficit being the major clinical symptom. Motor nerve conduction velocities are in the low normal range, and SNAPs are generally not obtainable. The autosomal recessive disease is generally more severe and is present at birth or shortly thereafter. Motor conduction velocities are in the low normal range, but amplitude of the CMAP is abnormally low. Sensory conductions are unobtainable. EMG of distal muscles may show a few fibrillation potentials and signs of chronic denervation (203). Transplant studies indicate that the recessive type is a disease of axons, not Schwann cells (76).

Hereditary Compression Neuropathy (Hereditary Mononeuropathy Multiplex)

Patients with this disorder have an autosomal dominant inheritance of a propensity to develop multiple entrapment neuropathies of peripheral nerves. Frequently, a history of minor trauma to the nerve coincides with the onset of paresis. Partial or complete return is common, but not invariable. Motor conduction velocity in most nerves is in the low normal range in segments not affected, but nerves that have been repeatedly affected show slowing of conduction. Nerve conduction through areas of entrapment is slow. Needle EMG reveals neurogenic damage in distal muscles of the affected extremities (30, 59).

Riley-Day Syndrome (Familial Dysautonomia)

In this rare, recessively inherited disorder of nerve function in Jewish children presenting with insensitivity to pain, absence of tears, postural hypotension, and other autonomic signs and symptoms, motor nerve conduction velocity hovers around the lower limits of normal. Sensory conduction velocities may be unobtainable but, when they can be obtained, are in the normal range (33).

Friedreich Ataxia

This is perhaps the most common variety of spinocerebellar degeneration, and it is inherited in an autosomally recessive manner. Large nerve fibers (A alpha) are affected, whereas small fibers (A delta and C) are unaffected. Therefore, H reflexes should be abnormal. Sensory nerve conduction is either unobtainable or shows a strikingly diminished nerve action potential amplitude. Motor nerve conduction velocity and amplitude of evoked muscle action potential are either low normal or mildly reduced (70).

Spinocerebellar Degenerations of Adulthood

A number of kinship studies in this category have been reported (70). In the extensive autosomal dominant kinship reported by Ziegler et al. (270), nerve conduction studies showed mild slowing of both sensory and motor conduction velocity. EMG showed fibrillations and positive sharp waves in distal muscles in most patients. Observations in these degenerations indicate that there is marked loss of compound SNAP amplitude, with less marked prolongation of sensory latency, and only minimal decrease in motor nerve conduction velocity (20, 180).

Familial Spastic Paraplegia (HMSN V)

This autosomal dominant disease has been reported by Dyck (68) to produce borderline low motor nerve conduction velocities and diminished SNAPs, but McLeod and Morgan (181) found it to produce normal motor and sensory nerve conduction velocities. A large series reported by Harding and Thomas (113) confirms the former finding and emphasizes the clinical finding of increased muscle tone in the lower extremities. Needle electrode examination of the distal leg and foot muscles may show fibrillation potentials and increased size of the voluntary MUAPs (68).

Pelizaeus-Merzbacher Disease

This rare, sex-linked demyelinating disease of the central and peripheral nervous systems that affects male children can produce moderately slow motor and sensory nerve conductions with low amplitude responses. EMG may show fibrillations (168).

Refsum Disease (Heredopathia Atactica Polyneuritiformis, HMSN IV)

This rare, autosomal recessive disorder generally has, as its initial clinical presentation, night blindness; the age of onset is from childhood to early adult years. The clinical manifestations are pigmentary retinal degeneration, chronic polyneuropathy, and ataxia; the diagnosis is made by identifying elevated serum levels of phytanic acid. The pathology is an inborn error of metabolism causing an accumulation of phytanic acid. Accurate early diagnosis is mandatory because phytanic acid stems exclusively from exogenous sources, and the disease can be controlled and degeneration prevented by dietary modification. Both motor and sensory nerve conduction velocities are reduced, with the reduction sometimes very marked. The EMG examination may show evidence of denervation (222).

Fabry Disease (Angiokeratoma Corporis Diffusum)

This is a sex-linked recessive disease of boys and young men who present with painful burning sensations of the feet and legs. It is a storage disease in which stored glycosphingolipid (ceramide trihexose) is deposited in various tissues, producing a reddish-purple maculopapular rash, renal impairment, and symptoms of neuropathy. Diagnosis is made by assaying serum alpha-galactosidase and finding it reduced. Traditionally, both motor and sensory nerve conduction studies and EMG studies are normal, even though there is a loss of small peripheral sensory axons (201). More recent studies show spotty, mild slowing of nerve conduction (240).

Metachromatic Leukodystrophy (MLD)

This autosomal recessive disease begins in infancy with progressive central and peripheral nervous system symptoms starting as hypotonia. A variety also exists in which symptoms do not begin until early adult life. This is a disease of myelin lipids, and diffuse demyelination in the central and peripheral nervous system occurs.

Motor nerve conduction velocity is markedly reduced, especially in the infantile form, and is frequently below 20 m/sec (25). Occasionally, patients with this disorder may be misdiagnosed as having cerebral palsy; nerve conduction velocity studies are useful in differentiating these two diseases.

A central nervous system (CNS) disease with clinical resemblance (which must be differentiated from MLD) is infantile neuroaxonal dystrophy. This is an autosomal recessive disorder, producing the infantile onset of motor and corticospinal symptoms (hyperactive reflexes and Babinski sign). Motor nerve conduction velocity is normal in the early stages and mildly reduced in the later stages, in striking contrast to the dramatic nerve conduction velocity slowing in metachromatic leukodystrophy. Also in contrast, EMG shows the characteristic findings of distal denervation (66).

Krabbe (Globoid) Leukodystrophy

This is a very rapidly progressive form of leukodystrophy starting in early infancy. Both CNS and peripheral nervous system symptoms are prominent. Nerve conduction studies show motor conduction velocities to be only about one-half of what would be expected and distal latencies to be about double. EMG may show an increase in the number of polyphasic MUAPs with a few fibrillation potentials (117).

Tangier Disease

This is an extremely rare autosomal recessive storage disease producing tonsillar hypertrophy, hepatosplenomegaly, and severe motor and sensory peripheral neuropathy. Fibrillation potentials are seen on EMG, and nerve conduction veolcities show either mild slowing or normal conduction. Patients with this disorder have an extremely low concentration of high density lipoprotein, which causes cholesterol and cholesterol ester to accumulate in the reticuloendothelial system and in other tissues, including the peripheral nerves (214).

Abetalipoproteinemia

Patients with this autosomal recessive disease do not synthesize the precursor for the development of very low density lipoprotein, low density lipoprotein, and chylomicrons. They can be diagnosed by the absence of apoprotein B in plasma and acanthocytosis. The earliest symptoms are gastrointestinal and begin in infancy. Stocking-glove hypesthesia occurs. Nerve conduction velocities are moderately reduced (214), but with marked loss of compound sensory nerve and muscle action potential amplitudes (188). Early diagnosis is important, as a low fat diet and high doses of vitamins A and E retard disease progression (124).

Primary Familial Amyloidosis

Electrophysiologic changes in peripheral nerves, except for possible entrapment neuropathies, are rare in secondary amyloidosis. However, in autosomal dominant primary amyloidosis, conduction velocities in peripheral motor nerves frequently show borderline low nerve conduction velocities. There is loss of small fibers (A delta and C), with large fibers (A alpha) spared. Needle EMG may show typical changes of a mild peripheral neuropathy (8). The pathology is one of axonal damage, with distal sensory fibers affected first. Electrodiagnostic changes occur before the onset of clinical symptoms and are valuable, for purposes of genetic counseling, to identify the disease in a subject at risk (230).

Acute Intermittent Porphyria

Peripheral neuropathy is a symptom in almost 20% of patients with this disease; the majority of the neuropathies are either motor or mixed sensory and motor. Motor conduction velocities are moderately decreased in both upper and lower extremities, with reduction in amplitude of the CMAPs. Distal motor latencies are normal or only slightly prolonged. EMG shows fibrillation potentials in the acute stage (3). The

Table 8.4. Toxic Neuropathies

Heavy Metals	Drugs	Organic Compounds
Lead	Nitrofurantoin	Ethyl alcohol
Arsenic	(Furadantin)	N-hexane
Thallium	Diphenylhydantoin	Acrylamide
Mercury	(Dilantin)	Tri-ortho-cresyl phosphate
Antimony	Vincristine	Methyl-butyl-ketone
Gold	Isoniazide	Carbon disulfide
	Dapsone	Dichlorophenoxyacetic acid
	Corticosteroids	Ethylene oxide
	Sodium cyanate	
	Halogenated	
	hydroxyquinolines	
	Thalidomide	
	Hydralazine	
	Chloramphenicol	
	Disulfiram (Antabuse)	
	Heroin	
	LSD	
	Pyridoxine	
	Misonidazole	
	Amiodarone	
	Tetanus toxoid	

EMG data suggest an axonal neuropathy with abnormal findings first occurring proximally.

Giant Axonal Neuropathy

This rare, autosomal recessive disease presents in early childhood as a severe peripheral neuropathy. It is progressive and affects the CNS in the second decade. Clinically, tightly curled scalp hair is noted in most patients. The disease is named for the segmental ballooning of axons due to accumulation of large aggregates of neurofilaments (211). EMG data are limited, but sensory nerve responses have been reported as absent in the presence of normal motor nerve conduction studies. EMG shows long duration, large amplitude MUAPs (42).

TOXIC NEUROPATHIES (Table 8.4)

Heavy Metals (Table 8.5)

Lead

Lead toxicity classically occurs in children in the form of encephalopathy and in adults as a radial neuropathy. But the "classical" picture rarely holds true. Children with lead toxicity generally live in the poorer neighborhoods of large cities, whereas adults with lead toxicity usually work in occupations where they come in contact with lead-containing compounds, e.g., working with lead-storage batteries. The incidence of lead toxicity in children is considerably lower since the removal of lead from paints. Occasionally, there are still reports of lead toxicity in painters, workers in the lead industry, persons eating food stored in ceramic containers, and persons drinking lead-contaminated illicit alcohol (200). Diagnosis should be confirmed by finding elevated levels of lead in blood or urine, normochromic or hypochromic anemia, and the presence of lead lines in x-rays of long bones (161).

Lead neuropathy produces primarily motor symptoms. It can produce a more severe neuropathy in the upper extremities than in the lower, and it is not always symmetrical. In children, encephalopathy may be related to the acute ingestion of large amounts of lead, whereas the peripheral neuropathy seems to be related to prolonged ingestion of small amounts. Motor nerve conduction velocities with chronic lead neuropathy are mildly reduced (84). Fibrillations and positive sharp waves may be found in the weakest muscles.

In the adult with acute lead toxicity, slowing of nerve conduction takes several weeks to become maximal. Distal motor latencies appear to be prolonged more than conduction velocity is slowed; residual latencies are prolonged (200). Although slowing of nerve conduction velocity is not marked there can be a striking reduction in the amplitude of the evoked muscle action potential (200). Sensory conduction studies seem to be the most sensitive in detecting subclinical chronic lead toxicity (86). Although lead neuropathy in experimental animals has been shown to be a demyelinating disease (202) most likely resulting from direct injury to the Schwann cells related to endoneurial edema (195), the disorder in humans can have the electrodiagnostic appearance of axonal or motor neuron disease (28, 91).

Arsenic

Arsenic poisoning can result from household and agricultural accidents, as well as from industrial contact or poisoning. Persons may be exposed to arsenic in the smelting of nonferrous ores, particularly copper. Survival from severe arsenic poisoning is rare, but is now possible with supportive medical care and the use of British anti-Lewisite (161).

Nerve conduction changes in chronic arsenic toxicity seem to differ from those seen in acute toxicity. As is true with other heavy metal toxins, chronic arsenic exposure produces greater nerve degeneration distally. Yet, in acute toxicity the dysfunction is more diffuse. We have followed a patient for almost 3 years following arsenic ingestion and found maximal nerve conduction slowing to occur several weeks after ingestion. Slowing in the elbow-to-wrist and knee-to-ankle segments paralleled slowing of the distal latencies; residual latencies never become strikingly prolonged. Therefore, the toxic effect seems to be on

Table 8.5. Typical Nerve Conduction and Electromyographic Findings in Heavy Metal Neuropathies

Heavy Metals	Motor Nerve Conduction Velocity	Site of Maximum Nerve Conduction Velocity Slowing	Amplitude of Muscle Action Potential	Sensory Nerve Conduction Velocity	Amplitude of Sensory Action Potential	Electromyographic Findings	Other Useful Laboratory Tests
Lead	↓	Distal	↓↓	↓	↓↓	fib.	CBC ↑ lead in blood and urine, lead lines in long bones
Arsenic	↓	Distal	↓↓↓	↓	↓↓↓	fib.	↑ arsenic in urine, hair, nails
Thallium	↓	Distal	↓↓	↓	↓↓↓	fib.	↑ thallium in urine
Mercury	nl	Distal	nl	↓	↓↓	fib.	↑ mercury in urine
Antimony	Insufficient data						
Gold	↓	Distal	↓	↓	↓↓	fib.	

↓ = low normal to slightly reduced
↓↓ = moderately low
↓↓↓ = extremely low

all segments of nerve, with the longer nerves of the lower extremities most severely affected. Conduction was lost in the peroneal nerves at 3 weeks, although it was present at 2 weeks.

The lowest conduction velocities in the upper extremities that we obtained were between one-half and two-thirds of normal. There was a marked decrease in the amplitude of the evoked muscle response. At 146 weeks, the ulnar and median motor nerve conduction velocities returned to normal, but conduction never returned in the distal segments of the peroneal nerves. EMG revealed profuse fibrillation and positive sharp wave potentials in the affected distal muscles (206). These findings have been confirmed by others (194).

Arsenic neuropathy is an axonal neuropathy (233) that careful electrodiagnostic studies can identify in exposed individuals. The earliest findings in such patients are decreased amplitudes of compound sensory and muscle action potentials in the lower extremities (85).

Thallium

Toxicity from this metal is very rare. If seen, it is probably the result of ingestion of insecticides or rodenticides. The symptoms of toxicity are paresthesias, arthralgias, and alopecia. Thallium neuropathy is mainly sensory, and the pathology is primarily axonal degeneration (98). In mild cases conduction velocities are only slightly decreased, but the amplitude of the SNAP is markedly diminished (61). In severe cases, sensory nerve conduction is unobtainable, and fibrillation potentials are seen (164).

Mercury

Generally, the toxicity of mercury is industrially related. Neuropathy is rare, but when it occurs it tends to be mainly sensory and of the axonal type. Motor conduction velocities tend to be relatively normal, but sensory nerve conduction studies reveal amplitude reduction (4) and conduction deficit (48). Smaller diameter nerve fibers seem to be more affected. Distal fibrillations and large amplitude MUAPs can also be seen (4).

Antimony

Antimony intoxication can result in alopecia and weakness. However, although it has been considered to cause a peripheral neuropathy, it has not been determined for certain if the weakness is due to central or peripheral nerve dysfunction (98).

Gold

It is uncertain whether observed gold neuropathy is due to a direct toxic effect of the drug, an allergic reaction, or the underlying disease.

Axonal degeneration is the predominant pathologic change in nerves (162, 184). Attenuation of compound SNAP amplitude and distal fibrillation potentials would be expected.

Drugs (Table 8.6)

Nitrofurantoin (Furadantin)

As of the last decade, 137 cases of peripheral neuropathy attributed to Furadantin had been reported in the world's literature. Symptoms are sensory and motor, and recovery is related to the severity of symptoms and not to the dosage. Symptoms start, in most cases, within a month and a half following institution of Furadantin treatment (260).

The first report of electrophysiologic studies in this axonal neuropathy was by Honet (118) who reported generalized fibrillation potentials and positive sharp waves on EMG of both proximal and distal muscles of upper and lower extremities. He found it impossible to obtain motor nerve conduction in the peroneal, tibial, and median nerves of his patient, but was able to obtain moderately reduced ulnar and radial conduction velocities by using a needle recording electrode. In Furadantin neuropathy, the amplitude of the CMAPs is also diminished (100).

The effect on peripheral nerves is due to the drug's toxicity, rather than to underlying renal disease. Tool and Parrish (261) gave the usual therapeutic Furadantin dose and course (400 mg daily for 14 days) to 14 healthy volunteers. They reported very slight slowing of motor nerve conduction velocities (especially noticeable in some subjects), as well as slowing of mean sensory conduction velocity and slight prolongation of distal sensory latencies.

Diphenylhydantoin (Dilantin)

There is an increased incidence of peripheral neuropathy in epileptic patients with long-term use of Dilantin and other anticonvulsants (252). Clinically, the syndrome presents with a stocking hypesthesia and loss of deep tendon reflexes in the lower extremities. The toxic effects seem to be cumulative, and some studies have shown they are more likely to occur in patients who have been on anticonvulsant therapy more than 10 years.

Conduction velocities in areflexic patients are mildly slowed in the lower extremities and may be low normal in the upper extremities. EMG shows fibrillations and reduced numbers of voluntary action potentials in affected muscles (167). In patients who have been on Dilantin for more than 10 years but who have no clinical signs of neuropathy some subtle electrical abnormalities may be present. Eisen et al. (80) found that slightly under 20% of these asymptomatic patients showed conduction slowing in peroneal motor nerves, distal median motor

Table 8.6. Typical Nerve Conduction and Electromyographic Findings in Drug Neuropathies

DRUGS	Motor Nerve Conduction Velocity	Site of Maximum Nerve Conduction Velocity Slowing	Amplitude of Muscle Action Potential	Sensory Nerve Conduction Velocity	Amplitude of Sensory Action Potential	Electromyographic Findings	Other Useful Laboratory Tests
Nitrofurantoin	↓↓	General	↓↓	↓↓	↓↓	Fib.	
Diphenylhydantoin	→	Distal	→	→	↓↓	Fib.	
Vincristine	→	General	↓↓↓	→	↓↓↓	Fib.	
Isoniazid	→	Distal	→	→	↓↓	Fib.	
Dapsone	nl	None	→	nl	↓↓	nl	
Corticosteroids	→	General	→	→	→	Fib.	
Sodium cyanate	→	General	→	↓↓	↓↓	nl	
Halogenated hydroxyquinolines	nl	None	nl	nl	nl	nl	SEP
Thalidomide	nl	Distal	nl	→	↓↓↓	Fib.	
Hydralazine	nl	Distal	nl	→	→	nl	
Chloramphenicol	nl	None	nl	nl	↓↓	nl	
Disulfiram	→	Distal	↓↓↓	→	↓↓	Fib.	
Heroin	nl	Distal	→	nl	↓↓	Fib.	
LSD	nl	Distal	→	nl	↓↓	Fib.	
Pyridoxine	nl	Distal	nl	Not obtainable	0	nl	SEP
Misonidazole	nl	None	nl	nl	→	Fib.	
Amiodarone	→	Distal	→	→	→	Fib.	
Tetanus toxoid	↓↓	General	↓↓	Unobtainable	0	Fib.	

nerves, or distal median sensory fibers. (Caution is advised in using motor or sensory conduction velocities from distal portions of the median nerve, especially in a chronic neuropathic disease, as criteria for the presence of a peripheral neuropathy because of the frequency of conduction slowing at points of pressure in chronic neuropathies.) In general, motor findings predominated over sensory ones. They also tested the H reflex and found it to be minimally prolonged in patients who had the most severe distal slowing. This finding suggests that the pathology that was present tended to be most marked in the distal portion of nerve. Recent studies have shown that during Dilantin intoxication slowing in NCV can occur in both sensory (243) and motor (170) nerve fibers. These changes are reversible on drug reduction or elimination.

Vincristine

Vincristine can cause peripheral neuropathy that produces a minimal reduction in motor nerve conduction velocity. However, the amplitude of both the evoked motor response and the sensory response can fall dramatically to only 10 or 20% of normal (162). Distal latencies are essentially unchanged (232). H reflexes are prolonged early in the toxicity state because early pathology is caused by a dying-back of large diameter myelinated afferents from the muscle spindle (A alpha). Needle EMG shows fibrillation potentials in affected muscles with reduced numbers of voluntary action potentials. As would be expected from these electrodiagnostic studies, vincristine produces a generalized primary axonal degeneration.

Isoniazide (INH, Isonicotinic Acid Hydrazide)

Isoniazide clinically produces more severe sensory symptoms than motor symptoms, and these are limited almost exclusively to the legs. Isoniazide toxicity is predominantly axonal (100). It first affects the distal portions of the longest nerve fibers and then slowly spreads centripetally (97). The EMG shows evidence of denervation in severely affected muscles; nerve conduction should be only mildly reduced distally, with the greatest nerve change reduction in amplitude of the compound SNAP.

Dapsone

Dapsone is a sulfone that has, in recent years, come to be used for dermatologic conditions other than leprosy. There have been cases of axonal disease reported that were presumably produced by this drug. Motor and sensory conduction velocities and latencies were normal, but the amplitude of the M response was reduced. EMG showed fibrillations and a neuropathic pattern of action potentials in affected muscles (105).

Corticosteroids

It is not commonly recognized that corticosteroids can produce disease of the peripheral nerves. Administration of high doses of prednisone in rabbits has been reported to produce segmental demyelination in peripheral nerves. A study in humans with chronic obstructive lung disease (COPD) showed motor nerve conduction velocity in both upper and lower extremities to be reduced approximately 10% when compared to controls with the same clinical disorder but who were not receiving steroids (6). The severity was proportional to the dose and duration of steroid therapy.

Sodium Cyanate

Since the early part of the 1970s, when it was first noted that sodium cyanate inhibits sickling of erythrocytes in vitro with no toxicity to the erythrocyte, this compound has received increasing attention as a possible treatment for sickle cell disease. Early studies showed relative lack of toxicity, and the compound was tried clinically. In 1974, two patients undergoing this treatment were identified as having developed motor and sensory peripheral neuropathies while on the drug. The severity of the neuropathy seemed to be related to the duration of treatment, as well as the dosage. In patients in whom the neuropathy developed, some improvement was noted several weeks after cessation of sodium cyanate. Slowing of nerve conduction was more pronounced in sensory fibers than in motor nerves and in the lower extremities than in the upper. Slowing appeared to affect the nerve in a rather diffuse manner so that the abnormal prolongation of the distal latency was about equal to the slowing of nerve conduction velocity in more proximal nerve segments. In addition to the two patients who presented obvious clinical signs of neuropathy, some electrodiagnostic evidence of alteration of peripheral nerve function was seen in 16 of 27 asymptomatic patients receiving the drug (212).

Needle EMG of muscles in affected patients showed fibrillation potentials and reduced voluntary motor unit potentials, thereby indicating the presence of axonal degeneration. It seems prudent that any patient who receives the drug during future clinical studies should be evaluated with periodic nerve conduction velocity determinations to detect early reversible neuropathy (212).

Halogenated Hydroxyquinolines (Clioquinal)

A variety of case reports have suggested that these drugs are potentially neurotoxic when given in high doses over an extended period of time. The drug can cause subacute myelo-optico-neuropathy (SMON), with symptoms of toxicity: optic nerve atrophy, myelopathy, and, traditionally, polyneuropathy (131). Although the drugs have previously been considered to produce peripheral axonal degeneration, there is only limited neurophysiologic confirmation (19). Somatosensory evoked potentials (SEPs) have been shown to be useful in this toxicity state by demonstrating delayed central conduction (241).

Thalidomide

Although this drug is no longer available, it is thought to have produced irreversible axonal degeneration in some cases. Conduction studies have shown motor nerve conduction velocities to be unaffected and SNAPs to be reduced in amplitude or absent (162).

Hydralazine (Apresoline)

Whether the sensory neuropathy produced by this drug is a direct effect of the medication or due to the pyridoxine deficiency produced by the drug is unclear (162). The amplitude of the sensory action potential is reduced.

Chloramphenicol (Chloromycetin)

Relatively mild sensory symptoms in the feet, preceded by optic neuritis, have been reported. This finding has been seen only in patients with impaired renal function who have been taking the drug and is most likely due to impaired drug excretion (162). SNAP amplitude is diminished.

Disulfiram (Antabuse)

This drug, which is used in the treatment of chronic alcoholism, is converted enzymatically to carbon disulfide, the agent that may produce the neurotoxicity (see section on carbon disulfide under organic compounds below) (7). Even though peripheral neuropathy is associated with chronic alcoholism, disulfiram is itself neurotoxic, and the neuropathy is dose-related. The pathology is a neurofilamentous axonopathy that is potentially reversible (190). Motor nerve studies show a reduction in conduction velocity and in the amplitude of the CMAP. Sensory conductions may be unobtainable, and EMG shows signs of denervation (162, 204).

Heroin

DiBenedetto has reported motor and sensory nerve conduction velocities to be normal and sensory potential amplitudes to average only one-half the normal size in a group of heroin users (62). In several users there were also reduced amplitudes and temporal dispersion of the

CMAP. Subsequent reports have been infrequent (165), and the extent to which other causes of neuropathy (e.g., nutritional) have been excluded in these reports is unclear.

Lysergic Acid Diethylamide (LSD)

Evidence of axonal degeneration has been described in LSD users. Sensory amplitudes were approximately one-half of normal, but other parameters were within normal limits (62). Again, other coexisting causes of neuropathy must be excluded.

Pyridoxine (Vitamin B₆)

Megadoses of this vitamin (up to 5 gm/day) have been reported to produce a profound sensory neuropathy (234). The neuropathy is at least partially reversible on cessation of B_6. Although motor nerve conduction studies are normal, peripheral sensory responses are unobtainable. SEPs show only low amplitude proximal limb responses, with no central responses. Clinical improvement is associated with return of cord and scalp responses (234).

Misonidazole

This radiosensitizing antitumor drug has been reported to produce an axonal neuropathy. NCVs are not affected, but amplitude of the compound SNAP is reduced. Fibrillations are noted in EMG (186).

Amiodarone

This antiarrhythmia drug is reported to cause a peripheral neuropathy in 10% of patients. Both motor and sensory nerve conductions are slowed distally, and EMG shows fibrillations (172).

Tetanus Toxoid

There have now been over a dozen reports of sensory-motor polyneuropathy associated with multiple tetanus toxoid injections given over a relatively short period of time. Electrodiagnostic studies have been limited, but suggest axonal loss, as well as demyelination. Distal EMG can show fibrillations, unobtainable sensory NCVs, and slow motor NCV (223).

Organic Compounds (Table 8.7)

Ethyl Alcohol

The most important organic compound neuropathy is alcoholic neuropathy, which is most likely due to primary ethinolic toxicity plus nutritional deficiency. It is an insidious mixed motor and sensory disorder with symptoms occurring first in the legs. Symptoms are worst

Table 8.7. Typical Nerve Conduction and Electromyographic Findings in Organic Compound Neuropathies

Compounds	Motor Nerve Conduction Velocity	Site of Maximum Nerve Conduction Velocity Slowing	Amplitude of Muscle Action Potential	Sensory Nerve Conduction Velocity	Amplitude of Sensory Action Potential	Electromyographic Findings	Other Useful Laboratory Tests
Ethyl alcohol	↓	General	↓	↓	↓↓		
N-hexane	↓↓	Distal	↓	↓↓	↓↓↓	Fib.	
Acrylamide	↓	Distal	↓	↓↓	↓↓↓	Fib.	
Tri-ortho-cresyl phosphate	↓	Distal	↓↓	↓	↓↓	Fib.	
Methyl-butyl-ketone	↓	Distal	↓	↓	↓↓	Fib.	
Carbon disulfide	↓	Distal	↓↓	↓	↓↓	Fib.	
Dichlorophenoxy acetic acid	nl	Distal	↓	↓	↓↓	Fib.	
Ethylene oxide	↓	Distal	↓↓	↓	↓↓	Fib.	

↓ = low normal to slightly reduced
↓↓ = moderately low
↓↓↓ = extremely low

in the distal muscles of the extremities. They often start with burning of the feet or painful paresthesias and cramps. Even in severe cases gross slowing of motor conduction velocity is rare; conduction is rarely reduced more than 20%. Compound SNAP amplitude is decreased, and sensory nerve conduction may be slightly more reduced than motor. The earliest finding is this decrease in amplitude, with distal amplitude reduced more than proximal amplitude (26, 43, 44).

Using a variety of electrophysiologic techniques to evaluate nerve function in alcoholic neuropathy, Blackstock et al. (26) documented only very minimal reduction in maximal motor conduction velocity but much more marked slowing of minimum conduction velocity (small myelinated nerve fibers). They also noted a prolongation of the H reflex.

Our experience with alcoholic neuropathy and analysis of recent data also indicates that motor nerve conduction velocities in both upper and lower extremities are only minimally reduced and that residual latencies are not prolonged. Unlike diabetic neuropathy where there is a predilection to subclinical carpal tunnel syndrome, no abnormally prolonged distal median latency was observed. Thus, the pattern of involvement of motor nerves in alcoholic neuropathy is one of only very minimal conduction slowing, equally affecting both proximal and distal segments of nerve.

EMG studies show numerous fibrillations, especially in distal muscles. Voluntary MUAPs are reduced in number, are polyphasic, and have an increased amplitude. Single fiber EMG studies show increased fiber density (257). These data, as well as results of quantitative electrophysiologic investigation and histologic studies, indicate that the primary lesion is axonal degeneration (14).

N-Hexane

N-hexane is an organic solvent widely used in printing and in commercial glues. There have been reports of a "dying-back" polyneuropathy in persons exposed to this compound in industrial adhesives and in "glue sniffers" (99, 208, 262). Clinically, an insidious, symmetrical stocking-glove sensory-motor disturbance develops several months after exposure to the substance, and recovery requires many months. Recovery is relatively complete in mild cases and is partial in severe cases.

In the reported cases, motor nerve conduction velocities and distal motor latencies in the upper extremities average about two-thirds of normal (262). Lower extremity motor nerve conduction velocities are reduced about the same degree. Sensory conduction velocities are either unobtainable or in the same range as motor velocities. EMG shows fibrillation potentials of an acute neuropathic process.

Acrylamide

This is an important neuropathy because of the large-scale production of acrylamide by the chemical industry and use in experimental animals to produce a pure dying-back neuropathy (245). These studies have revealed the following information about dying-back neuropathies: (a) Toxicity is related to the volume of the nerve cell (the long, large diameter sensory fibers to the feet have the largest volume and are affected first), (b) a minimum time is required for toxic effects (15 days for acrylamide), and (c) toxicity occurs beyond a fixed distance from the cell bodies (distal lower extremities for acrylamide); above this point peripheral nerve cross-section is preserved. Motor nerve conduction velocities are either normal or just below normal limits, but lower extremity distal latencies are prolonged. SNAPs are either reduced in amplitude or absent with prolongation of distal latency (120). In chronic or severe cases fibrillation potentials are seen on EMG.

Tri-ortho-cresyl Phosphate (TOCP, Jacaica Ginger Paralysis)

TOCP has probably produced the greatest number of cases of toxic neuropathy in humans. In 1929 and 1930, alcoholic extracts of ginger and rum contaminated with TOCP were used as alcoholic drinks, causing many thousands of cases of neuropathy by the end of 1930. Contamination of cooking oil with TOCP has also produced several major episodes of neuropathy, the largest in Morocco in 1959 affecting about 10,000 people. An excellent review of these epidemics has recently been published (191).

TOCP causes a dying-back distal degeneration of axons. In the recovery phase, when distal axonal regeneration has occurred, fairly normal conduction velocities are recorded with prolonged terminal latencies (97). Data from primates indicate that in the acute phase the conduction velocity does not fall; however, the amplitude of the CMAP potential decreases steadily until at about 40 days it is approximately 10% of normal. Needle EMG shows fibrillation potentials in distal muscles (116). Clinical studies from an outbreak in Sri Lanka in 1977–1978 show fibrillations on EMG and marked prolongation of distal motor latencies, with more moderate slowing of motor nerve conduction (236). Sensory nerve studies were not done during the acute stage.

Methyl-butyl-ketone (MBK)

A dying-back peripheral neuropathy caused by MBK was first identified in 1973 among the workers of a coated fabric plant. Motor and sensory distal latencies were usually prolonged and nerve conduction velocities either normal or only moderately reduced. Needle EMG showed numerous fibrillation and positive sharp wave potentials in distal muscles (5).

Carbon Disulfide

This industrial solvent can produce peripheral axonopathy. It is thought to be the toxic metabolite responsible for disulfiram neurotoxicity (see section on disulfiram under drugs above). Electrodiagnostic findings occur predominantly in distal segments of nerve. Nerve conduction slowing and amplitude reduction are most pronounced in distal sensory fibers (263). Denervation in distal muscles can be seen in more severe cases (120).

Dichlorophenoxyacetic Acid

This widely used compound in herbicides has produced several reported cases of peripheral axonopathy. EMG shows denervation, but nerve conduction velocity is not slowed (120).

Ethylene Oxide

Peripheral neuropathy from this gas, which is used to sterilize heat-sensitive materials in health facilities, was first reported in 1979 (103). Since then, other cases in hospital sterilizer workers have been reported (88). The neuropathy produced is an insidious motor-sensory axonopathy in distal lower extremities. EMG shows fibrillation potentials, and NCV is characterized by low amplitude motor and sensory responses, with moderate conduction slowing.

PERIPHERAL NEUROPATHIES ASSOCIATED WITH DISEASES
(Tables 8.8 and 8.9)

Diabetes Mellitus

Diabetic neuropathy, in all of its varied forms, is the most common neuropathy associated with a particular disease. There are at least eight different clinical syndromes: diabetic polyneuropathy (the typical "diabetic neuropathy"), diabetic mononeuropathy, diabetic amyotrophy, thoracolumbar neuropathy, painful neuropathy, hypoglycemic neuropathy, neuropathy of uncontrolled diabetes and autonomic neuropathy. Diabetic neuropathy is common among diabetic patients. In a classic study, Mulder et al. (193) found that one-third of an unselected group of diabetic patients had polyneuropathy and one-sixth had mononeuropathy, usually at the common sites of nerve entrapment—the median nerve at the wrist, the peroneal nerve at the fibular head, and the ulnar nerve at the elbow.

Diabetic *polyneuropathy* can be present even with good diabetic con-

Table 8.8. Diseases associated with Peripheral Neuropathies

Diabetes Mellitus	Chronic liver disease
Polyneuropathy	Thermal burns
Uncontrolled diabetic neuropathy	Diphtheria
Mononeuropathy	Leprosy
Amyotrophy	Herpes zoster
Thoracoabdominal neuropathy	Thiamine (vitamin B₁) deficiency
Painful neuropathy	Riboflavin (vitamin B₂) deficiency
Hypoglycemic neuropathy	Pyridoxine (vitamin B₆) deficiency
Autonomic neuropathy	Pernicious anemia (vitamin B₁₂) deficiency
Chronic renal insufficiency	Malnutrition
Carcinoma	Postgastrectomy state
Plasma cell dyscrasias	Tropical (nutritional) ataxia
Multiple myelomia	Chronic obstructive pulmonary disease
Waldenstrom macroglobulinemia	(COPD)
Other monoclonal gammopathies	Polycythemia vera
Primary nonfamilial amyloidosis	Gout
Osteosclerotic myeloma	
Rheumatoid arthritis	
Sjogren syndrome	
Scleroderma	
Systemic lupus erythematosus	
Cranial arteritis	
Hypothyroidism	
Mononeuropathy	
Polyneuropathy	
Polyarteritis nodosa	
Sarcoidosis	
Lymphomas	
Systemic	
Focal	
Cryoglobulinemia	

trol. Although good control is necessary for optimal maintenance of peripheral nerve function (101), rigorous control achieves no further benefit (238). In general, the more severe the clinical signs of neuropathy, the greater the slowing of nerve conduction. Three factors tend to affect the electrodiagnostic findings adversely: (a) older age, (b) more severe diabetes, and (c) longer duration of diabetes (34).

Mulder et al. (193) reported that peroneal motor conduction measurement was a more sensitive indicator of diabetic polyneuropathy than upper extremity motor nerve evaluation. About the same time, Downie and Newell (65) presented data indicating that sensory nerve conduction and evoked potential amplitude decrements were also very sensitive detectors of diabetic neuropathy. The most sensitive indicators of diabetic polyneuropathy of generally available electrodiagnostic techniques are compound SNAP amplitudes (198) and peroneal and median NCVs (109). Reduction in nerve conduction velocity seems to be greatest in distal segments of peripheral nerves (34). Buchthal et al.

Table 8.9. Typical Nerve Conduction and Electromyographic Findings in Peripheral Neuropathies Associated with Diseases

Disease	Motor Nerve Conduction Velocity	Site of Maximum Nerve Conduction Velocity Slowing	Amplitude of Muscle Action Potential	Sensory Nerve Conduction Velocity	Amplitude of Sensory Action Potential	Electromyographic Findings	Other Useful Laboratory Tests
Diabetes mellitus Polyneuropathy	↓↓	General	→	↓↓	↓↓	nl	↑ urine and blood glucose
Mononeuropathy	↓↓	Local blocks	↓↓	↓↓	↓↓	Fib.	Same as above
Amyotrophy	nl	Nerves to thigh muscles	↓↓	nl	nl	Fib.	Same as above
Hypoglycemic neuropathy	nl	Nerves of upper extremities	→	nl	→	Fib.	↓ blood glucose
Uncontrolled	↓↓	General	→	↓↓	↓↓	nl	↓ urine and blood glucose
Thoracoabdominal	nl	None	→	nl	nl	Fib.	
Painful neuropathy	nl	None	→	nl	nl	Fib.	
Renal insufficiency	↓↓	General	→	↓↓	↓↓	Fib.	↑ blood urea and creatinine
Carcinoma	nl	General	→	→	↓↓↓	Fib.	
Plasma cell dyscrasias							
Multiple myeloma	→	General	→	→	↓↓	Fib.	Serum electrophoresis
Waldenstrom macroglobulinemia	→	General	→	→	→	Fib.	Same as above
Monoclonal gammopathies	→	Distal	→	nl	nl	Fib.	Serum electrophoresis
Primary non familial amyloidosis	→	General	→	nl	nl	Fib.	Same as above
Osteosclerotic myeloma	↓↓	General	→	→	nl	Fib.	Same as above

↓ = low normal to slightly reduced
↓↓ = moderately low
↓↓↓ = extremely low

Table 8.9. Continued.

Disease	Motor Nerve Conduction Velocity	Site of Maximum Nerve Conduction Velocity Slowing	Amplitude of Muscle Action Potential	Sensory Nerve Conduction Velocity	Amplitude of Sensory Action Potential	Electromyographic Findings	Other Useful Laboratory Tests
Rheumatoid arthritis	↓	Segmental	↓	↓	↓	Fib.	↑ sed rate + rheumatoid factor
Sjogren syndrome	↓	Segmental	↓	↓	↓	Fib.	↓ salivation
Scleroderma	↓	Segmental	↓	↓	↓	Fib.	
Systemic lupus erythematosus	Insufficient data						+ L.E. prep.
Cranial arteritis	Insufficient data						↑ sed rate
Hypothyroidism Mononeuropathy	nl	Carpal Tunnel	↓	nl	↓	Fib.	↓ PBI
Polyneuropathy	nl	Distal	↓	↓↓	↓↓	nl	↓ T₄
Polyarteritis	↓	Segmental	↓	↓	↓	Fib.	Sed rate, nerve biopsy
Sarcoidosis	↓	Facial nerve	↓	↓	↓	Fib.	+ Kveim reaction
Lymphoma Systemic	↓	General	↓	↓	↓↓↓	Fib.	CBC
Focal	↓	Local infiltrates	↓	↓	↓↓	Fib.	CBC
Cryoglobulinemia	↓	Distal	↓	↓↓	↓↓	Fib.	+ cryoglobulins
Chronic liver disease	↓	General	↓	↓↓	↓↓	Fib.	Abnormal liver function tests
Thermal burns	↓	General	↓↓	↓	↓↓↓	nl.	
Diphtheria	↓↓	Distal	↓↓	↓↓	↓↓	Fib.	Nerve biopsy
Leprosy	↓	Segmental; where nerve is enlarged	↓	↓	↓↓	Fib.	Biopsy—skin or nerve
Herpes zoster	nl	Same root level as cutaneous	↓	nl	↓	Fib.	
Thiamine deficiency	↓↓	Distal	↓↓	↓↓	↓↓	Fib.	

Table 8.9. Continued.

Disease	Motor Nerve Conduction Velocity	Site of Maximum Nerve Conduction Velocity Slowing	Amplitude of Muscle Action Potential	Sensory Nerve Conduction Velocity	Amplitude of Sensory Action Potential	Electromyographic Findings	Other Useful Laboratory Tests
Riboflavin deficiency	↓	Distal	↓	↓	↓↓	Fib.	
Pyridoxine deficiency	↓	Distal	↓	↓	↓↓	Fib.	
Pernicious anemia	nl	Distal	nl	↓	nl	nl	+ Schilling test, SEP
Malnutrition	↓	General	↓	↓	↓	nl	
Postgastrectomy	nl	None	nl	nl	↓	nl	
Tropical ataxis	↓↓	Lower extremities	↓	↓↓	↓	nl	
COPD	nl	General	↓	nl	↓↓	Fib.	
Polycythemia vera	↓	Distal	↓	↓	↓	Fib.	
Gout	↓	Distal	↓	↓	↓	nl	

↓ = low normal to slightly reduced
↓↓ = moderately low
↓↓↓ = extremely low

(37) have suggested that an increase in temporal dispersion of the sensory potential (prolonged duration and irregular shape) is the earliest sign of diabetic neuropathy; it can be observed even when conduction along the fastest fibers and the amplitude of the potential are still within the normal range.

Among less available techniques, Rondinelli and Stolov have reported that an approach, utilizing a computer-assisted multivariate analysis of multiple parameters (latency, amplitude, and NCV for median [motor and sensory], peroneal, and sural nerves) can more reliably differentiate diabetic (nerves) from normal nerves (226). Using computer-derived distributions of conduction velocities in peripheral nerves, Dorfman et al. have shown a shift toward lower conduction velocity distribution in diabetic nerves, even in the presence of normal conventional NCVs (54, 64).

Motor nerve conduction velocity decrements correlate strikingly with diabetic complications. This may be because of direct osmotic damage to various organ tissues by an accumulation of sorbitol and fructose in tissues freely permeable to glucose, as a result of glucose escaping glycolytic breakdown because of high glucose levels (83). Patients who have normal or only slightly reduced conduction velocities tend to have few diabetic complications, but those who have marked reduction in conduction velocities generally have multiple and severe complications. We reviewed information on 100 diabetics who had had their conduction velocities determined from 1 to 8 years previously and found that patients who had died since the prior determination (44%) had had conduction velocities that had been considerably lower than the group of diabetics who had survived. The former had had a mean peroneal motor conduction velocity of 27.1 m/sec, whereas the surviving group had had a mean of 35.9 m/sec. Both had shown low normal ulnar motor values (151, 244).

Electrodiagnostic identification of neuropathy in diabetic children under age 5 is negligible. However, over age 5 conduction slows with age, especially in the peroneal nerve; 48% of older children who have had diabetes longer than 5 years have abnormal motor nerve conductions (81). Motor nerves in the lower extremities are involved even when sensory nerves in the upper extremities are normal.

Both axonal degeneration and segmental demyelination can occur in diabetic neuropathy (259). Current information supports the hypothesis that diabetes can primarily affect both the axon and Schwann cell in the development of polyneuropathy. The disease can produce a distal, length-dependent axonopathy and also segmental demyelination, which is independent of axon loss and which can even produce onion-bulb formations (34, 248). Single fiber EMG studies have shown that diabetic fiber density may not differ significantly from normal and that there is a low incidence of jitter; this indicates that the primary nerve dysfunction in diabetic polyneuropathy is produced by demyelination (257). We have reviewed our data on patients with diabetic polyneuropathy, including those with markedly reduced conduction velocities, and found that residual latencies in the ulnar nerve were normal and those of the peroneal nerve close to normal. This indicates that the conduction deficit is comparable in middle and distal segments of nerve. We also noted that the residual latency of the median nerve tended to be prolonged, indicating, as did the study of Mulder et al. (193), that many patients with diabetic polyneuropathy are subject to subclinical carpal tunnel syndrome. F-wave studies in diabetics show conduction slowing in the most proximal segments of nerve (52). Thus, the pattern of nerve conduction change in diabetic polyneuropathy is moderate slowing of comparable degree in both proximal and distal segments, with conduction more affected in the lower extremities. Sensory studies seem to be more sensitive than motor studies for detection of early polyneuropathy in adults.

EMG studies of diabetic polyneuropathy generally show few, if any, fibrillation potentials. Voluntary MUAPs are generally close to normal in configuration, amplitude, and duration, but may be reduced in number (244,257). When abnormalities are present they generally demonstrate increased serration (Fig. 8.4) or minimal polyphasicity (Fig. 8.3). The refractory period between two nerve stimuli has been reported to be prolonged in diabetic patients prior to the development of significant changes in conduction velocity (219).

SEPs show a slowing of spinal conduction through the posterior columns in a significant percentage of diabetic adults (104) and children (53). In a group of diabetic adults, cord conduction was 39.4 ± 13.3 m/sec. (versus 54.2 ± 10.5 m/sec in controls) (104). SEP supraspinal conduction appears not to be slowed, although visual evoked potentials in diabetics have been reported to be prolonged (218).

A rapid, clear-cut increase in conduction velocity results from adequate treatment of *uncontrolled diabetic neuropathy* following either initial diagnosis or an episode of ketoacidosis. Guyton (107) showed an 8 m/sec improvement in peroneal nerve conduction velocity over a 10-hour period following recovery from diabetic coma. Gregersen (102) followed recently diagnosed diabetics treated with insulin for 8–35 days and found conduction velocities in the peroneal nerve to increase as much as 10 m/sec, generally within the first week. These results have been confirmed by other studies in other motor nerves (39, 266).

Diabetic *mononeuropathy* at sites of entrapment generally affects one or two peripheral nerves and can occur either in association with polyneuropathy or in the absence of it. Mulder et al. (193) reported the peroneal nerve to be the most commonly involved. Signs of peroneal conduction deficit were seen in about 12% of diabetic individuals; symptoms and findings are similar to those commonly seen in crossed-leg palsy. Median nerve compression at the wrist and ulnar nerve compression at the elbow were reported to occur with less frequency (193). However, our recent experience indicates that over one-half of diabetic patients may have asymptomatic subclinical carpal tunnel syndrome if diagnosed on the basis of prolonged median nerve residual latencies in the presence of normal ulnar residual latencies (150). Another form of neuropathy may be Bell palsy. In a series of patients with this facial neuropathy, almost 40% were diabetic. Diabetic patients had a predilection for development of the nerve lesion distal to the chorda tympani, which was not seen in patients whose glucose was normal (209).

Diabetic *amyotrophy* is a clinical syndrome consisting of pain in muscles of the thigh associated with sudden weight loss and an absence of sensory symptoms. The onset of symptoms may be fairly rapid, and clinical improvement, once optimal diabetic management is achieved, can be prompt. This condition may occur in patients in whom no polyneuropathy is seen. Fibrillation potentials and positive sharp waves are commonly encountered in affected muscles, as contrasted to their paucity in diabetic polyneuropathy, and nerve conduction velocities are not usually decreased. EMG is abnormal in muscles of the thigh and lower paraspinals (63). Peroneal F-wave studies demonstrate a greater degree of slowing in proximal than distal segments of lower extremity nerves (47).

A similar syndrome can affect other parts of the body in diabetics (18). If primarily in the upper back, chest, or abdomen, the conditions can be termed *thoracoabdominal neuropathy* (136, 250). If primarily in the sacral roots or feet, the syndrome can be termed *painful neuropathy* (9,156). This latter syndrome can occur in the presence of completely normal nerve conduction studies (9). It has been suggested that the term "diabetic polyradiculopathy" might be used for these latter three conditions. They have in common the presence of pain, fibrillations on EMG, no peripheral NCV slowing and, unlike diabetic polyneuropathy, little correlation with other diabetic complications. Interestingly, the syndrome is thought not to occur in the cervical region.

Hypoglycemic peripheral neuropathy is very rare and is associated with various types of hyperinsulinism, including insulin-secreting islet cells adenomas of the pancreas. It is a motor-sensory neuropathy with greater involvement of nerves of the upper extremities. Fibrillations can occur in distal hand muscles, with little or no motor nerve conduction slowing until late in the disease (56). At times, it may mimic motor neuron disease (192).

Studies suggest that specific treatment of diabetic neuropathy may be possible. Aldose reductase inhibition (to reduce the accumulation of sorbitol and fructose in peripheral nerves) has been shown to be of limited effectiveness in improving NCV in diabetics (83, 128). Cerebral ganglioside administration has also been reported to increase the amplitudes of compound sensory nerve and muscle action potentials in diabetic patients, although NCV or latency was not affected (improvement was also noted in alcoholic neuropathy) (16).

Chronic Renal Insufficiency

The neuropathy of renal failure is of specific interest to electromyographers. Dialysis judged to be adequate by many blood chemistry standards may not be adequate to arrest peripheral neuropathy. Therefore, since the early reports by Jebsen and co-workers at the University of Washington (119, 127, 256) of the value of motor nerve conduction velocity determinations in monitoring uremic neuropathy, NCVs have been used as part of the evaluation process of adequate hemodialysis. These investigators showed that inadequate dialysis resulted in decreased motor NCVs and adequate dialysis resulted in improved conduction velocities.

The neuropathy of chronic renal disease is both motor and sensory; both motor and sensory NCVs are equally slowed (126). It is generally believed that patients with chronic renal disease can have subclinical neuropathy detected by slowing of nerve conduction in the absence of signs of clinical neuropathy (127). Although symptoms are more pronounced in the lower extremities, the degree of conduction slowing is approximately equal in nerves of the arms and legs (119). In cases of severe neuropathy, NCVs in the rage of 20 m/sec may be seen in the peroneal nerve, and NCVs in the range of 30 m/sec may be seen in nerves of the upper extremities.

Changes in nerve conduction have been reported to be statistically no different in terminal segments of peripheral nerves than in midextremity segments (27). Terminal latencies are not significantly prolonged when compared to proximal conduction (207). Residual latencies are not prolonged in most patients whom we have studied, although in some patients (11% in ulnar nerve, 22% in median nerve), they are prolonged. Amplitudes of compound SNAPs (49, 192) and H-reflex latencies (1, 108) are the most sensitive indicators of uremic neuropathy.

A single episode of dialysis seems to have no effect on NCV (127). In the past, patients occasionally showed an explosive and rapidly progressive peripheral neuropathy during the first weeks of hemodialysis, although this is much more uncommon now with improved dialysis techniques. Increase in conduction velocity with adequate dialysis is slow, and abnormalities may never completely revert to normal. Because of this slow change, some question the capability of conduction studies to monitor dialysis (75). With successful renal transplantation, complete reversal of neuropathy can occur (255).

EMG in patients with uremic neuropathy shows fibrillation potentials in the most paretic distal muscles and MUAPs that may initially be normal but that decrease in number and grow larger in amplitude later in the disease (71, 257).

Thiele and Stalberg found that fiber density and jitter in uremic neuropathy did not differ significantly from normal, indicating that uremic neuropathy has characteristics more in common with a demyelinating than an axonal lesion (257). However, others have found abnormal jitter (143). Dyck et al. (71), on the basis of in vitro compound action potential studies, quantitative histologic and teased-fiber studies, and electron microscopy on nerves from two patients, felt that there is evidence that the site of primary disease is the neuron, resulting in degeneration of the axis cylinder and secondary demyelination. Recent studies have shown a complex picture of a variety of neuropathies occurring in chronic renal failure—acute axonal neuropathy, a predominantly demyelinative neuropathy, and a progressive axonal neuropathy with secondary segmental demyelination—probably resulting from the complex effects of renal failure on the metabolism of peripheral neurons, myelin, and Schwann cells (229). Unlike some of the hereditary neuropathies all nerve fibers can be affected.

One of the significant aspects of uremic neuropathy is that it predisposes the uremic patient to other types of superimposed neuropathies. Carpal tunnel syndrome (110) and severe neuropathy from diabetes (189) are more likely to occur in end-stage renal disease.

Our data indicate that in most patients there is no predilection for preferential distal conduction slowing. However, in approximately one-fifth of our patients, preferential distal slowing, which seems to occur in chronic axonal disease, was prominent. It may be that acute uremic neuropathy has different characteristics from chronic uremic neuropathy.

Among less common electrodiagnostic tests, the relative refractory period is prolonged in about one-half of patients with chronic renal failure (169). SEPs are not commonly studied in end-stage renal disease, but do show slowing of spinal, but not cortical, conduction (227).

Carcinoma

The main symptoms of carcinomatous neuropathy, due to the remote effect of tumors, are generally sensory. When there is motor involvement as well, distal muscles may show fibrillations and a reduction in number of MUAPs, with an increased number of polyphasic potentials. Motor NCVs are minimally reduced. Compound SNAPs may be markedly reduced in amplitude, and NCVs are minimally reduced (40). Terminal latencies may be slightly prolonged in some patients with normal conduction velocities (179).

Pathologic changes in peripheral nerve are inflammation and degeneration of dorsal root ganglia and degeneration of posterior roots and posterior columns of the spinal cord (122). Sural nerve biopsies may show immune deposits of immunoglobulin M, C_3, and $C1_q$ in the inner laminae of the perineurium and around endoneural capillaries (205). Rarely, in leukemias, direct infiltration into nerve can produce neuropathy with slow conduction velocities (249).

Plasma Cell Dyscrasias

In the last few years a number of new paraproteinemias have been recognized and studied as causes of peripheral neuropathies. Paraproteins are immunoglobulins produced by a clone of neoplastic plasma cells proliferating abnormally.

The best known of the plasma cell dyscrasias is *multiple myeloma.* Clinically, the neuropathy associated with it is typically a painful sensory-motor polyneuropathy. Electrophysiologically, the picture is heterogeneous, with evidence of both axonal and myelin dysfunction (134). NCVs in both upper and lower extremities are mildly reduced, as are amplitudes of upper and lower extremity sensory action potentials. Midextremity and terminal segments are equally affected (265).

There are only a few published reports of electrodiagnostic studies in *Waldenstrom's macroglobulinemia* and too little data for a complete understanding of the associated neuropathy. The several studies that have been published report motor nerve conduction to vary from normal to minimally slowed. Fibrillations have been reported in clinically affected muscles (182).

Peripheral neuropathy has also been described in association with other *monoclonal gammopathies.* Most commonly, an IgM is produced, which can be an antibody to a major myelin-associated glycoprotein and cause active demyelination (187, 246). Investigators have shown the production of axonal damage by the paraprotein (90, 239) or primary damage to both myelin and axon (197, 216). The electrodiagnostic hallmark of this heterogeneous category is prolongation of distal latencies to a greater degree than NCV is slowed (increased residual latency) (134).

Primary nonfamilial amyloidosis is also associated with gammopathy (130). NCVs are generally normal in this group, but fibrillations may be seen, suggestive of axonal degeneration (134).

Osteosclerotic myeloma shows the greatest degree of NCV slowing of this group and most closely fits the pattern of a pure demyelinating disease (134).

The significance of the plasma cell dyscrasias is that they may explain the cause of many acquired peripheral neuropathies. In a series from the Mayo Clinic, 10% of the unknown neuropathies were found to be associated with paraproteinemia (135). Diagnosis of these conditions and delineation from other neuropathies are important as they may be treatable with immunosuppressants (55).

Rheumatoid Arthritis

Neuropathy may be seen in as many as 10% of patients with rheumatoid arthritis; it varies in severity from a mild distal sensory neuropathy to acute episodes of mononeuropathy multiplex. The pathogenesis is the vasculitis associated with rheumatoid arthritis that produces axonal damage (213). In patients with marked neuropathy, fibrillation potentials may be seen on EMG.

The most commonly encountered peripheral nerve disease in rheumatoid arthritis is considered by many to be entrapment neuropathy of the median nerve at the wrist (51). However, Herbison et al. (115) have presented data that indicate that, although carpal tunnel syndrome occurs in rheumatoid arthritis, it may not be seen any more frequently than in an age-matched population. Furthermore, many patients with rheumatoid arthritis who have symptoms of a carpal tunnel syndrome may have normal nerve latency studies; their symptoms are probably due to rheumatoid synovitis and not carpal tunnel syndrome.

Sjogren Syndrome

The neuropathy of this disease seems to be identical to that of rheumatoid arthritis and occurs in about 10% of patients with the disease. It is a nonhomogeneous neuropathy, most likely caused by vasculitis (213). NCV is slightly reduced in affected nerves, distal latencies are prolonged, and compound SNAPs are reduced in amplitude. EMG of paretic muscles shows signs of denervation (132).

Scleroderma

Peripheral neuropathy is an extremely rare complication of scleroderma. Histologic sections of affected nerves look similar to nerves from patients with rheumatoid neuropathy, and it might be expected that nerve conduction and EMG changes would be similar (51).

Systemic Lupus Erythematosus

Progressive symmetrical ascending sensory-motor neuropathy is a rare complication of systemic lupus erythematosus. Cases of mononeuropathy multiplex have also been reported. However, sufficient studies have not yet been done to outline the EMG pattern of lupus neuropathy (10, 51).

Cranial Arteritis

Peripheral neuropathy has been described in association with giant cell arteritis and may manifest itself either as a symmetrical polyneuropathy or as mononeuropathy multiplex. Adequate data are not available to determine nerve conduction and EMG changes in this disease (51).

Hypothyroidism

Two types of neuropathy occur in hypothyroidism. The most common type is *carpal tunnel syndrome*. It is felt that increased amounts of acid mucopolysaccharides, which normally constitute the bulk of the ground substance of extracellular connective tissue, effectively diminish the space available to the median nerve as it passes through the carpal tunnel. Symptoms of the carpal tunnel syndrome of myxedema can, however, usually be successfully treated with hormonal therapy. If a patient can be made to remain euthyroid, abnormally prolonged distal motor latency in the median nerve may return to normal (17).

The second type of neuropathy in hypothyroidism is diffuse *peripheral neuropathy*. Conduction in motor and sensory fibers of peripheral nerves may be slow, especially in distal segments. These findings may also be improved with good medical management (17). Fincham and Cape (87) studied motor and sensory nerve conduction in a group of myxedematous patients and found amplitudes of sensory action potentials to be reduced and sensory nerve conduction velocities to be slow; motor nerve conduction was less affected. Histologic studies can identify segmental demyelination, in some cases with onion-bulb formation (242).

Polyarteritis Nodosa

Clinical neuropathy in polyarteritis is common and starts out as a sensory-motor mononeuropathy multiplex that becomes a symmetrical polyneuropathy at a later stage. The pathology of the neuropathy is an acute arteritis, which accounts for the initial segmental symptoms that involve small arteries in segments of nerve. The later polyneuropathy is probably due to the coalescence of multiple segments of nerve lesions. NCV in affected nerves is decreased, and EMG of affected muscles shows signs of denervation (166).

Sarcoidosis

Peripheral neuropathy is an extremely rare complication of this disease and generally occurs only in the facial nerve, although polyneuropathy has been described (196). Fluctuating and remitting cranial nerve palsies may occur (''polyneuritis cranialis''), which clinically are indistinguishable from idiopathic Bell palsy. Needle EMG generally shows fibrillations in affected muscles (173).

The polyneuropathy produces NCV slowing, especially in the lower extremities, loss of amplitude of compound SNAPs, and fibrillations and other EMG signs of denervation (196). Both axonal and demyelinating changes are seen on nerve section.

Lymphomas (Hodgkin's Disease, Lymphosarcoma, Reticulum Cell Sarcoma, Follicular Lymphoma)

Sensory neuropathies and sensory-motor neuropathies have been described in lymphomas. The neuropathy may be either acute, subacute, or chronic; some are relapsing and remitting. One-third of the patients with lymphomas show a mild reduction in motor NCVs (183). The neuropathy may be due either to a direct infiltration of tumor cells or remote effects of tumor. Histopathologic changes in various stages of disease may show both segmental demyelination and axonal degeneration. During acute exacerbations, low conduction velocities can decrease even further (29). The mechanisms may be similar to polyneuropathies in carcinoma and plasma cell dyscrasias (see above).

Cryoglobulinemia

Peripheral neuropathy is a rare complication of this disorder. EMG may show denervation changes in affected muscles. Motor conduction velocities are minimally slowed, and it may not be possible to obtain sensory action potentials (46, 182).

Chronic Liver Disease

Peripheral neuropathy can be seen in a variety of disorders producing chronic liver disease: chronic alcoholism, infectious mononucleosis, acute intermittent porphyria, periarteritis nodosa, secondary amyloidosis, celiac disease, and certain intoxications.

Electrophysiologic abnormalities have been reported in from 14 to 68% of patients with chronic liver disease. Abnormalities consist of slowing of motor nerve conduction velocities (a slowing that can be quite marked in some patients), fibrillations in affected muscles, increase in sensory latency, and reduction in the amplitude of the SNAP (11, 141, 237). Careful exclusion of all patients with liver disease who may have other causes for peripheral neuropathy (e.g., alcoholism and diabetes) may reveal very few peripheral neuropathies caused by liver disease alone without other explanations. In addition, there is a distinct disease clinically similar to Guillain-Barré syndrome associated with acute viral hepatitis (11).

Thermal Burns

Henderson et al. (114) reported a 15% incidence of polyneuropathy in a large series of patients on a burn unit. The electrophysiologic abnormality that was reported was a reduction in motor nerve conduction velocity. In general, neuropathy was found to develop approximately 9 weeks after the burn and to be unrelated to the severity of the burn. One-half of the patients recovered spontaneously with discontinuation of antibiotics. The authors considered the neuropathy most likely to be due to antibiotics used in treatment. However, only a few antibiotics have been clearly identified as producing peripheral polyneuropathies; some of the nerve dysfunctions may have been directly related to some unknown toxic effect of the burn.

Diphtheria

Corynebacterium diphtheriae produces an exotoxin that causes segmental demyelination of peripheral nerves. Diphtheritic neuropathy produces mixed sensory and motor symptoms and does not generally occur until 8 weeks after onset of illness. There are only a few case reports in the literature of conduction studies in humans. One indicates that motor conduction velocities at their nadir may be markedly reduced and, with clinical improvement, can return to normal (178). Another case report suggests that, in the late stage, even when conduction velocities have returned to normal, distal latencies may still be prolonged (142).

We have had the opportunity to study a patient recovering from diphtheria who, upon discharge from the hospital, developed generalized weakness. Nerve testing showed low normal motor conduction velocities with prolonged distal latencies and decreased amplitude, temporally dispersed CMAPs. EMG showed fibrillation potentials and positive sharp waves in affected muscles. Most information on changes in nerve conduction in diphtheria have been obtained from experimental animals, but it may be that, in some cases, human diphtheria causes axonal degeneration, as well as demyelination.

Leprosy

The neuropathy of leprosy is a patchy, predominantly cutaneous neuropathy, affecting different nerves in a spotty manner (210). In general, conduction slowing occurs through areas where nerves are swollen and palpable, and proximal and distal conduction are normal. The ulnar nerve is often involved earlier and more extensively than other nerves. Distal latencies are frequently prolonged, and CMAPs are temporally dispersed and decreased in amplitude. Sensory conduction studies may be difficult to obtain; where they can be obtained, they generally show a reduction in amplitude of the SNAP. EMG may show changes of denervation. Short duration, polyphasic, low amplitude potentials suggestive of myopathy have also been reported. Signs of denervation are most frequently seen in the orbicularis oris muscle (228).

Herpes Zoster

Five percent of the patients with clinical herpes zoster have zoster-induced motor nerve involvement at the same root level as their sensory lesion. This condition always follows cutaneous zoster. Fibrillation potentials are always present in affected muscles, including those innervated by the posterior primary division of the spinal nerve. Voluntary MUAPs are compatible with a neuropathic disease. Motor and sensory conduction values are generally normal (258).

Thiamine (Vitamin B₁) Deficiency

Thiamine deficiency causes a distal sensory-motor neuropathy, more pronounced in the lower extremities. In animals, thiamine deficiency causes degenerative changes of nerves of the feet commonly seen in dying-back polyneuropathies (217). The largest and longest nerve fibers are the first to degenerate; if the deficiency is prolonged, small nerve fibers degenerate as well (264). Nerve conduction and EMG studies have been carried out in thiamine-deficient rats. It has been found that motor nerve velocities decrease to nearly half the normal value and that this decrease is associated with a decrease in amplitude of the evoked muscle response. Experimental studies have shown that electrical stimulation of peripheral nerves causes release of thiamine and that a thiamine antagonist impairs the conductivity of peripheral nerves. Therefore, nerve conduction might be altered in thiamine deficiency without having significant histologic changes in peripheral nerve (264). EMG shows fibrillations in affected muscles (155).

It is difficult to study thiamine deficiency in humans because of the rarity of the deficiency occurring without a deficiency of other vitamins as well. Consequently, there is a paucity of pathologic and electrical information on changes in peripheral nerves in humans. However, a pathologic study by Takahashi and Nakamura (253) in nine patients showed axonal degeneration of large myelinated fibers to be the major change.

Riboflavin (Vitamin B₂) Deficiency

A deficiency of riboflavin is possibly related to the etiology of Strachan's syndrome: painful neuropathy, amblyopia, and orogenital dermatitis. Extensive pathologic or electrodiagnostic data are not available in this disease, but it is postulated to be a dying-back neuropathy that is expected to show the EMG and NCV changes associated with such a condition (264). Painful paresthesias or burning feet can occur in the absence of the other components of Strachan's syndrome and may respond favorably to riboflavin injections. Lai and Ransome (158) reported such a case. Burning feet may also occur with alcoholic neuropathy, diabetes, beri-beri, or pellagra.

Pyridoxine (Vitamine B$_6$) Deficiency

It is thought that deficiency of pyridoxine is responsible for the neurologic aspects of pellagra, whereas the other manifestations of this deficiency state—dermal lesions and gastrointestinal symptoms—are probably due to lack of niacin. The distribution of the neuropathy is a stocking-glove motor-sensory loss. Pathologic sections of peripheral nerve show degeneration of myelin sheaths in early cases, although in advanced pellagra, Wallerian degeneration is evident (264). EMG might be expected to show a picture of axonal degeneration in advanced deficiency states.

Much has been written about pyridoxine deficit as a cause of carpal tunnel syndrome (or, at least, the reversibility of the syndrome by pyridoxine administration). We have shown that patients with carpal tunnel syndrome do not have deficits of pyridoxine metabolism, but that many patients with neuropathy do (38). Considering the neurotoxicity of megadoses of pyridoxine (234), added caution must be used in replacement therapy (see pyridoxine under toxic neuropathies above).

Pernicious Anemia (Vitamin B$_{12}$ Deficiency)

Because of the posterior column lesion of pernicious anemia, the clinical identification of polyneuropathy is often difficult. Mayer evaluated 53 patients with vitamin B$_{12}$ deficiency and found that nerve conduction abnormalities were present only when patients had neurologic signs (176). They consisted mainly of conduction slowing in distal sensory fibers and prolongation of the H reflex. The amplitude of the sensory action potential, motor nerve conduction in the lower and upper extremities, and proximal sensory conduction were all normal. Because of disease in posterior columns, lower extremity SEPs are abnormal (154).

Malnutrition

Inadequate fetal and infant nutrition is associated with decreased NCVs (95,225). It appears that nutrition before age 12 months is especially critical to the development of normal peripheral nerve myelination, and early nutritional deficits may have a long-term effect, causing a marked NCV deficit (225). Even in adults, persistent neurologic deficit can occur from prolonged periods of severe malnutrition (96).

To study the acute effect of nutritional deficit, NCVs were determined in a group of patients who fasted from 14 to 28 days and received no vitamin supplements. Motor conduction velocities in the upper and lower extremities and sensory latencies in the upper extremities were found to be statistically unchanged during the period of fasting, even though approximately one-fourth of the patients developed paresthesias (174).

Postgastrectomy State

Symptoms of peripheral neuropathy are common in patients following gastrectomy, but electrodiagnostic studies of postgastrectomy patients with symptoms of peripheral neuropathy have not been reported to reveal nerve conduction or EMG abnormalities (268). More recently, a syndrome of mostly proprioceptive neuropathy has been reported following gastric partitioning (175).

Tropical (Nutritional) Ataxia

This disease is endemic in certain parts of Africa and is thought to be due to a vitamin deficiency. Others have speculated that it may be due to chronic cyanide intoxication from diets of cassava plants prepared in a particular way. Histologically, peripheral nerves show segmental demyelination with relative sparing of axons. Motor nerve conduction velocities are markedly decreased in the lower extremities and normal or mildly decreased in the upper extremities. Only occasionally are fibrillation potentials noted in paretic muscles (267).

Chronic Obstructive Pulmonary Disease (COPD)

On careful testing, many patients with COPD are found to have a reduction of amplitude of compound SNAP that is occasionally associated with distal lower extremity fibrillations (82). These changes are not seen in age-matched smokers.

Polycythemia Vera

A significant percentage of patients with polycythemia vera have distal sensory symptoms that are caused by axonal degeneration. Distal lower extremity sensory nerve amplitudes are reduced and latencies prolonged (269).

Gout

The neuropathy occasionally seen in hyperuricemia may be due to this disease and not be secondary to other disorders. The electrodiagnostic changes due to distal axonopathy (reduced amplitude of compound SNAP) worsen as uric acid levels increase (60).

Table 8.10. Idiopathic Neuropathies

Guillain-Barré syndrome
Chronic polyradiculoneuropathy
Steroid-responsive polyneuropathy
Fisher syndrome
Shoulder girdle neuropathy

IDIOPATHIC NEUROPATHIES (Tables 8.10 and 8.11)

Guillain-Barré Syndrome (Idiopathic Polyradiculoneuritis, Landry-Guillain-Barré-Strohl Syndrome)

The Guillain-Barré syndrome is a disorder in which nerve conduction studies and EMG can be of great value in confirming the diagnosis, identifying the segments of diseased nerve, and determining prognosis. However, there are a number of reports of the electrodiagnostic findings in this disease, some showing little change in nerve conduction in the presence of severe weakness, leading to the conclusion by some that there is no correlation between clinical symptoms and nerve conduction studies (58).

The explanations for this lack of correlation are that pathologic changes do not occur equally in all parts of a peripheral nerve at the same time and that the segment studied may not be the segment producing the neurologic defect. The first area of dysfunction is generally the nerve root, followed shortly by dysfunction of the terminal portion of the nerve (144). Radiculitis is generally associated with the most profound clinical weakness, and NCVs in standard segments tested may be normal. Later, as clinical strength improves, a centrifugal pattern of demyelination may develop, and successively more distal nerve segments may show slowing of conduction velocity. Most of the conduction studies in the Guillain-Barré syndrome have not been serial evaluations, but have been single determinations in patients with a variety of stages of disease. This has led to a lack of appreciation by many of the pattern of nerve conduction changes in Guillain-Barré polyneuritis.

The pathologic changes in peripheral nerve consist of mononuclear cell infiltration and segmental demyelination in the motor and sensory roots, eventually involving the entire length of the neuraxis. Probably because lesions are spotty (163), there is a greater probability of dysfunction and a greater preponderance of clinical signs in distal muscles, reflecting the greater probability that, the longer the individual axon at risk, the more likely it is to be affected at one of more points along its course. Axonal degeneration can occur in severe cases and has traditionally been considered to be secondary to the inflammatory process

Table 8.11. Typical Nerve Conduction and Electromyographic Findings in Idiopathic Neuropathies

Disease	Motor Nerve Conduction Velocity	Site of Maximum Nerve Conduction Velocity Slowing	Amplitude of Muscle Action Potential	Sensory Nerve Conduction Velocity	Amplitude of Sensory Action Potential	Electromyographic Findings	Other Useful Laboratory Tests
Guillain-Barré syndrome	↓↓	Spotty centrifugal	↓↓	↓↓	↓↓	+/− fib.	F Wave, H reflex
Chronic polyradiculoneuropathy	↓↓	General	↓↓	nl	↓↓↓	Fib.	
Steroid-responsive polyneuropathy	↓↓	Spotty	↓↓	→	→	nl	
Fisher syndrome	nl	none	nl	nl	↓→	nl	
Shoulder girdle neuropathy	→	Nerves to shoulder	↓↓	nl	nl	Fib.	

↓ = low normal to slightly reduced
↓↓ = moderately low
↓↓↓ = extremely low

associated with demyelination. The mononuclear inflammatory process in the peripheral nervous system may persist in low grade fashion for months and years after clinical recovery (12).

Early studies by Cerra and Johnson (45) showed that motor NCV determinations were helpful in the diagnosis of Guillain-Barré syndrome by showing slowing of conduction in midextremity segments of peripheral nerves. Lambert and Mulder (160) showed that, during the first 3 weeks of illness, 61% of patients diagnosed as having the Guillain-Barré syndrome had slowing of motor nerve conduction in one or more peripheral nerves and an additional 25% had temporal dispersion of the CMAP.

But what of the 14% of patients showing no abnormalities of conduction velocity or terminal latency? If the demyelinating process starts in the nerve roots, radicular nerve conduction velocity should be reduced in the early stages of the disease before conduction slowing occurs in more distal segments. Kimura et al. (139) measured F wave conduction velocities in ten patients with Guillain-Barré syndrome during the first 4 weeks after onset of symptoms and found them to be slow in eight out of ten patients. F-wave slowing was approximately 20 m/sec slower than normal, whereas conduction slowing that was observed at that time in more distal segments was much less pronounced. Similarly, Lachman et al. (157) studied patients with Guillain-Barré syndrome within 6 weeks of the onset of symptoms and found the H reflex in the lower extremity and F response to the abductor pollicis brevis muscle to be prolonged in all of seven patients tested. In two of these patients, routine motor and sensory conductions in distal nerve segments were normal. King (140) has also reported F-wave latencies to be prolonged in all patients with Guillain-Barré syndrome, even though distal conduction velocity was within the normal range. In our experience, late responses in the early stages of Guillain-Barré syndrome are either prolonged or unobtainable and represent the best of conventional electrophysiologic tests to make an early diagnosis.

In addition to the radicular conduction slowing that occurs during the earliest part of the disease, there is also an early slowing in the terminal axons, as noted by Lambert and Mulder (160), producing a prolongation of the distal latency (125, 139, 235). Conventional NCVs may be normal when radicular and terminal latency studies demonstrate slowed conduction (79). We have reviewed our electrodiagnostic data of Guillain-Barré polyneuritis and found, after the onset phase of disease, many of the distal latency measurements of the median, ulnar, and peroneal nerves to be the longest we have observed in any disease. We have recorded distal motor latencies up to 34 msec in the peroneal nerve, 30 msec in the median nerve, and 18 msec in the ulnar nerve.

Longitudinal studies of changes in nerve conduction in the Guillain-

Barré syndrome are useful in understanding the pattern of development of the nerve lesion and helping the electromyographer interpret the findings. Such data in the literature are limited. In a classic paper, Bannister and Sears (15) reported the serial changes in nerve conduction recorded from one patient starting 12 days after the onset of illness. At that time, the patient was almost totally paralyzed, but had motor nerve conduction velocity in the low-normal range. The distal motor latency that was measured over a relatively short distance (6 cm) was 5.0 msec. On subsequent examination, the patient was clinically stronger, but the distal motor latency became even more prolonged and motor conduction velocity in the forearm decreased slightly. It was not possible to record any sensory response until the 50th day, at which time the patient had made marked recovery; the distal sensory latency was prolonged (8.0 msec), sensory conduction velocity slow (20 m/sec), and the sensory action potential very low in amplitude. McQuillen and Gorin (185) studied three patients during recovery and found forearm motor conduction velocities to continue to decrease from 2 to 17 weeks after the point of minimum strength had occurred; as conduction velocity fell further, strength returned. Cerra and Johnson (45) also noted that recovery of nerve conduction velocity lags behind the return of clinical strength.

We have studied serial motor nerve conduction velocities over a 17-week period in a 19-year-old male with Guillain-Barré syndrome (Table 8.12). The discrepancy between early clinical improvement and continued deterioration of nerve conduction in mid and distal portions of the extremities can be noted. The pattern is spotty; as conduction is one segment improves, another may worsen. Overall, there is a tendency for a centrifugal movement of dysfunction and improvement (Fig. 8.10). Distal latency prolongation, NCV slowing and attenuation, and temporal dispersion of the CMAP can be quite marked (Fig. 8.3). Note in this figure that even though the amplitude of the proximal muscle action potential is lower than the distal (because of temporal dispersion) the area under the negative portion of the M wave is the same proximally and distally (Fig. 8.3). What must be stressed is the importance of studying multiple nerves in a patient with Guillain-Barré polyneuritis, because any one segment or any one particular nerve might be normal while other segments might be abnormal (94, 215).

The best indicator of prognosis in the Guillain-Barré syndrome is needle EMG. Patients requiring the longest time to recover demonstrate fibrillation potentials and positive sharp waves in paretic muscles (79). In a study of 50 patients, Ramon and Taori (220) have shown that the presence of profuse fibrillation potentials within the first 4 weeks of illness, with or without associated nerve conduction deficits,

Table 8.12. Guillain-Barré Syndrome in a 19-Year-Old Male

Time after Onset	Motor Nerve	Conduction Velocity	Distal Motor Latency	Strength
		m/sec	*m/sec*	
6 weeks	R Ulnar-distal	52.2	4.5	Started to
	R Peroneal-distal	31.5	9.0	improve
11 weeks	R Ulnar-distal	43.1	7.3	Much improved
	R Peroneal-distal	37.1	13.5	
	R Median-distal	40.7	11.2	
	R Median-proximal	32.4		
12 weeks	R Ulnar-distal	40.8	6.4	Continued
	R Ulnar-proximal	38.5		improvement
	L Median-distal	43.0	9.5	
	L Median-proximal	38.9		
	L Ulnar-distal	43.7	6.5	
	L Ulnar-proximal	38.5		
	L Peroneal-distal	31.1	12.6	
17 weeks	R Ulnar-distal	45.8	4.3	Almost normal
	R Ulnar-proximal	45.7		
	L Median-distal	46.1	6.5	
	L Median-proximal	53.9		
	R Peroneal-distal	52.9	7.7	
	L Ulnar-distal	54.8	11.5	
	L Ulnar-proximal	41.4		

a condition seen in approximately one-third of their patients, is associated with poor prognosis and pronounced residual deficits.

It is not clear why nerve dysfunction should occur in nerves of Guillain-Barré patients where there is little inflammation. Asbury has noted little inflammatory reaction in terminal segments of peripheral nerves with this disease (139—see Asbury's comments, p. 61). Why, then, is there such striking prolongation of distal motor latency? Is it because radicular inflammation affects the most distant part of the neuraxis, or is it because histologic material has not been studied when terminal latencies were prolonged? Also, why are there classically more motor than sensory symptoms (79)? Arnason (10) has pointed out that there is no preferential histologic involvement of motor over sensory roots.

There are many unanswered questions about idiopathic polyneuritis, but a pattern of nerve conduction and EMG changes can be established. During the first month, there is a great likelihood of finding conduction changes in the most proximal segments followed shortly thereafter by changes in the distal latencies. Later, when recovery may be occurring clinically, midextremity conduction velocities may decrease even further. An absence of fibrillation potential and positive sharp waves indicates a good prognosis.

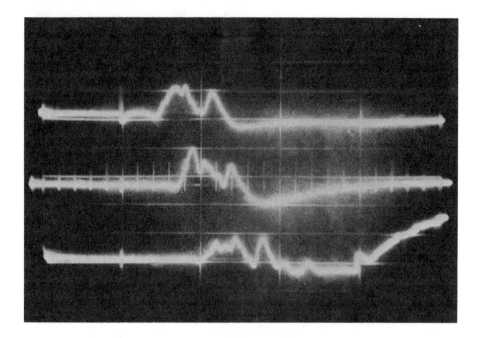

Figure 8.10. Left median motor studies of a 19-year-old patient with Gullain-Barré polyneuritis 12 weeks after onset of disease. (Caliber: Each vertical division = 1000 µV: each major horizontal division = 20 msec.) All latencies were recorded with surface electrodes. *Top,* distal latency. *Middle,* latency at antecubital fossa: *Lower,* latency from the supraclavicular point of stimulation. Note the low amplitude, temporally dispersed muscle action potential. Proximal NCV is 38.9 m/sec; distal NCV is 43.0 m/sec.

Chronic Polyneuropathy (Chronic Inflammatory Polyradiculoneuropathy)

This term can be applied to an idiopathic polyradiculoneuropathy having either a steady (no improvement by 6 months) or progressive course or to a recurring polyneuropathy producing a stepwise progression of symptoms. Dyck et al. (74) have reported a series of 53 patients meeting these criteria, with nerve biopsy showing segmental demyelination. Prognosis was poor; complete recovery occurred only occasionally, although patients were followed an average of 7.5 years. Most of the pathologic changes occurred in the spinal roots and proximal portions of nerves.

Chronic polyradiculoneuropathy seems to be characterized by diffusely slow motor conduction velocities and difficulty in obtaining any SEPs. EMG of severely involved muscles shows signs of denervation. Amplitudes of CMAPs are low, and distal latencies are only minimally prolonged. When sensory conduction velocities can be obtained they are essentially normal. Tasker and Chutorian (254) reported results of electrodiagnostic studies in 16 children with chronic polyneuritis of childhood (persisting longer than 1 year), and they also found decreased NCVs and EMG signs of denervation. Most are nonsteroid responsive.

Steroid-Responsive Polyneuropathy

There is a form of chronic polyradiculoneuropathy that can, at least to a degree, be favorably influenced by corticosteroids. This steroid-responsive polyneuropathy seems to be characterized neurophysiologically predominantly by nerve conduction abnormalities, with a paucity of fibrillation potentials (13). In our experience, the NCV changes show a strikingly spotty pattern of slowing, with distal latencies often relatively normal (Fig. 8.4) and showing highly localized areas of conduction abnormalities. EMG can show minimal increases in polyphasicity of MUAPs (Fig. 8.8). Steroid responsiveness of a peripheral neuropathy can also indicate a neuropathy with a specific etiology (i.e., lymphoma or leukemia) and mandates evaluation to rule out the cause.

Fisher Syndrome

Miller Fisher syndrome is considered to be a variant of idiopathic polyneuritis in which external ophthalmoplegia and ataxia also occur (89). Electrodiagnostic studies generally show little or no conduction abnormalities in peripheral nerves, although areflexia and peripheral weakness are present (251).

Idiopathic Shoulder Girdle Neuropathy (Brachial Neuritis)

Symptoms of this disease classically start with an acute, sharp pain in one shoulder, invariably mistaken for bursitis, followed several days later by a dull ache. About the same time, the patient notices shoulder weakness, which is followed by atrophy of specific muscles of the shoulder girdle. Sensory loss, if present, is less striking. In one-third of the patients, both shoulders are involved, with symptoms developing in the second shoulder hours to days after the first.

The most commonly affected nerves are the suprascapular nerve to the supraspinatus muscle, the suprascapular nerve to the infraspinatus muscle, and the axillary nerve to the deltoid muscle. The 11th cranial nerve can also be involved. Branches of other peripheral nerves are also occasionally affected, including nerves of the lower extremities (145, 171). If sensory loss is present, it is almost always in the distribution of the axillary, radial, or cutaneous nerves of the forearm.

Motor nerve conduction velocities from Erb's point to the elbow and from the elbow to the wrist, as well as terminal latencies, are normal when recorded to unaffected muscles. However, latencies from Erb's point to paretic shoulder muscles and terminal latencies to paretic distal muscles are slightly prolonged, have reduced amplitude, and show temporal dispersion (147). The conduction dysfunction parallels the severity of clinical involvement. In completely denervated muscles that have started to reinnervate, latencies can be extremely long (171). This is caused by markedly reduced conduction in the small diameter, poorly myelinated, newly regenerated terminal twigs. Frequently there is a marked disparity between severity of involvement of two muscles supplied by the same nerve, e.g., supraspinatus and infraspinatus. EMG shows fibrillation potentials in affected muscles.

AN APPROACH TO THE ELECTRODIAGNOSTIC STUDY OF PERIPHERAL NEUROPATHIES

More electrodiagnostic information can be obtained from a patient with a peripheral neuropathy than simple determination of conventional NCVs. The physician practicing electrodiagnostic medicine now has the capability of determining peripheral NCV in different segments of nerve: root, proximal extremity, distal extremity, and terminal. With the development of SEPs, more complete studies of proximal peripheral nerve conduction are possible. Using careful techniques, determination of differences in conduction along as short as 1-cm segments is possible. Separate information about conduction velocities in motor and sensory fibers is also useful.

NCV is very slow if demyelination is present in a segment, but only moderately slow if axonal degeneration has occurred. If only demyelination is occurring, the area of the M wave should be in the normal range, although it may be temporally dispersed. If axonal loss is present, the amplitude of both the compound sensory nerve and muscle action potentials is decreased and the area of the M wave reduced. If the neuropathy is evolving, serial conduction studies can provide even more information. Needle EMG yields additional data unobtainable from any type of conduction study and can confirm the degree of axonal loss and regeneration.

At the initial sorting-through process, several groupings should be made. First, most toxic neuropathies generally produce their earliest and greatest effect on the distal portion of the largest diameter axons; cells with the largest volume tend to be most vulnerable (233). The process is generally axonal degeneration. Therefore, the earliest electrodiagnostic change is reduction of amplitude of compound SNAPs and distal fibrillations—all occurring first in the legs and feet.

Hereditary neuropathies often manifest themselves first in motor symptoms, again most severe distally in the legs. The striking electrodiagnostic finding in many of these, in contradistinction to the toxic neuropathies, is reduction in motor NCV. Neuropathies associated with various systemic diseases often show a mixed picture of both axonal and demyelinating disease.

The electromyographer should be familiar with the various electrophysiologic patterns of peripheral nerve dysfunction seen in different peripheral neuropathies and be able to identify conditions compatible with the electrodiagnostic observations. As a starting point, Tables 8.3, 8.5-8.7, 8.9 and 8.11 tabulate the motor and sensory NCV, motor and sensory evoked potential amplitude, site of motor NCV slowing, and EMG findings reported from the studies of the diseases discussed in this chapter. By reviewing this chapter and other sources, additional electrodiagnostic information may be obtained.

As the sorting-through process continues, certain neuropathies can be excluded because they do not fit the electrophysiologic pattern, whereas others will be seen to be compatible with the electrodiagnostic findings. For example, NCVs may be very helpful in differentiating the Guillain-Barré syndrome from chronic polyradiculoneuropathy. In the former, terminal motor latency prolongation is striking and sensory nerve conduction is slow, whereas, in the latter condition, motor nerve conduction is equally reduced in midextremity and terminal segments and, if obtainable, the sensory NCV may be normal. As another example, Charcot-Marie-Tooth disease can be differentiated from HMSN II by the marked slowing of motor nerve conduction in the former.

How many times has an electromyographer been asked to identify the cause of a peripheral neuropathy in an alcoholic patient with diabetes? This may not be possible with a high degree of certainty, but in general, a paucity of fibrillation potentials with fairly substantial motor and sensory conduction slowing would favor diabetic neuropathy, whereas fibrillations, marked reduction in amplitude of compound SNAPs, and only minimal nerve conduction slowing would favor alcoholic neuropathy.

Of the patients with a peripheral neuropathy, approximately half of the neuropathies are associated with an identifiable disease that can cause it (135). In the remaining half—the cryptogenic neuropathies—what are the possible explanations? In a large series from the Mayo Clinic, intensive evaluations of previously undiagnosed neuropathies revealed HMSNs accounted for 42% (77). Thus, study of other family members may add additional information. At the same institution, data have also been presented suggesting that 10% of cryptogenic neuropathies have monoclonal serum proteins, which may account for the neuropathy (135). Thus, serum protein electrophoresis is necessary in evaluation of these neuropathies.

At the conclusion of the sorting-through process, the electromyographer will have compiled those peripheral neuropathies compatible with the electrodiagnostic observations. This list will be shortened by historical, clinical, and other laboratory data, and final diagnostic impressions can then be made.

In summary, this chapter is intended to be a comprehensive but practical guide to peripheral neuropathies from the electromyographer's viewpoint. Nerve conduction and EMG techniques should become even more useful in the identification and evaluation of peripheral neuropathies as additional techniques (e.g., SEPs, H- and F-wave studies, and residual latencies) enter into the electromyographer's armamentarium. It is hoped that this chapter can help the electromyographer identify what studies to do, understand how to interpret them, and learn how best to use information obtained to evaluate a patient with a peripheral neuropathy.

References

1. Ackil AA, Shahani BT, Young RR: Sural nerve conduction studies and late responses in children undergoing hemodialysis. *Arch Phys Med Rehabil* 62:487–491,1981.
2. Aguayo A: Experimental studies of demyelinating neuropathies. *AAEE Course*, 1980.
3. Albers JW, Robertson WC, Daube J: Electromyographic findings in porphyric neuropathy. *Arch Phys Med Rehabil* 57:595, 1976.
4. Albers JW, Cavender GD, Levine SP, Langolf GD: Asymptomatic sensorimotor polyneuropathy in workers exposed to elemental mercury. *Neurology* 32:1168–1174, 1982.
5. Allen N, Mendell JR, Billmaier D, Fontaine RE: An outbreak of a previously undescribed toxic polyneuropathy due to industrial solvent. *Trans Am Neurol Assoc* 99:74–79, 1974.
6. Ansari KA: Steroids and motor nerve conduction velocity. *Neurology* 20:396, 1970.
7. Ansbacher LE, Bosch EP, Cancilla PA: Disulfiram neuropathy: a neurofilamentous distal axonopathy. *Neurology* 32:424–428, 1982.
8. Araki S, Mawatari S, Ohta M, Nakajima A, Kuroiwa Y: Polyneuritic amyloidosis in a Japanese family. *Arch Neurol* 18:593–602, 1968.
9. Archer AG, Watkins PJ, Thomas PK, Sharma AK, Payan J: The natural history of acute painful neuropathy in diabetes mellitus. *J Neurol Neurosurg Psychiat* 46:491–499, 1983.
10. Arnason BGW: Inflammatory polyradiculoneuropathies. In Dyck PJ, Thomas PK, Lambert EH (eds): *Peripheral Neuropathy*, vol 2 Philadelphia, WB Saunders, 1975, pp 1110–1148.
11. Asbury AK: Hepatic neuropathy. In Dyck PJ, Thomas PK, Lambert EH (eds): *Peripheral Neuropathy*, vol 1. Philadelphia, WB Saunders, 1975, pp 993–998.
12. Asbury AK, Arnason BG, Adams RD: The inflammatory lesion in idiopathic polyneuritis: its role in pathogenesis. *Medicine* 48:173–215, 1969.
13. Austin JH: Recurrent polyneuropathies and their corticosteroid treatment. With five-year observations of a placebo-controlled case treated with corticotropin, cortisone and prednisone. *Brain* 81:157–192, 1958.
14. Ballantyne JP, Hansen S, Weir A, Whitehead JRG, Mullin PJ: Quantitative electrophysiological study of alcoholic neuropathy. *J Neurol Neurosurg Psychiat* 43:427–432, 1980.

15. Bannister RG, Sears TA: The changes in nerve conduction in acute idiopathic polyneuritis. *J Neurol Neurosurg Psychiat* 25:321–328, 1962.
16. Bassi S, Albizzati MG, Calloni E, Frattola L: Electromyographic study of diabetic and alcoholic polyneuropathic patients treated with gangliosides. *Muscle Nerve* 5:351–356, 1982.
17. Bastron JA: Neuropathy in diseases of the thyroid. In Dyck PJ, Thomas PK, Lambert EH (eds): *Peripheral Neuropathy,* vol 1. Philadelphia, WB Saunders, 1975, pp 999–1011.
18. Bastron JA, Thomas JE: Diabetic polyradiculopathy. Clinical and electromyographic findings in 105 patients. *Mayo Clin Proc* 56:725–732, 1981.
19. Baumgartner G, Gawel MJ, Kaeser HE, Pallis CA, Rose FC, Schaumburg HH, Thomas PK, Wadia NH: Neurotoxicity of halogenated hydroxyquinolines: clinical analysis of cases reported outside Japan. *J Neurol Neurosurg Psychiat* 42:1073–1083, 1979.
20. Bennett R, Ludvigson P, DeLeon G, Berry G: Large-fiber sensory neuropathy in autosomal dominant spinocerebellar degeneration. *Arch Neurol* 41:175–178, 1984.
21. Bird T, Griep E: Pattern reversal visual evoked potentials. Studies in Charcot-Marie-Tooth hereditary neuropathy. *Arch Neurol* 38:739–742, 1981.
22. Bird T, Kraft G: Charcot-Marie-Tooth disease: data for genetic counseling relating age to risk *Clin Gene* 14:43–49, 1978.
23. Bird T, Ott J, Giblet E, Chance P, Sumi S, Kraft G: Genetic linkage evidence for heterogeneity in Charcot-Marie-Tooth neuropathy (HMSN Type I). *Ann Neurol* 14:679–684, 1983.
24. Bird T, Reenan A, Pfeifer M: Autonomic nervous system function in genetic neuromuscular disorders. *Arch Neurol* 41:43–46, 1984.
25. Bischoff A: Neuropathy in leukodystrophies. In Dyck PJ, Thomas PK, Lambert EH (eds): *Peripheral Neuropathy,* vol 1. Philadelphia, WB Saunders, 1975, pp 891–913.
26. Blackstock E, Rushworth G, Gath D: Electrophysiological studies in alcoholism. *J Neurol Neurosurg Psychiat* 35:326–334, 1972.
27. Blagg CR, Kemble F, Taverner D: Nerve conduction velocity in relationship to the severity of renal disease. *Nephron* 5:290–299, 1968.
28. Boothby JA, deJesus PV, Rowland LP: Reversible forms of motor neuron disease. *Arch Neurol* 31:18–23, 1974.
29. Borit A, Altrocchi PH: Recurrent polyneuropathy and neurolymphomatosis. *Arch Neurol* 24:40–49, 1971.
30. Bosch E, Chui H, Martin M, Cancilla P: Brachial plexus involvement in familial pressure-sensitive neuropathy: electrophysiological and morphological findings. *Ann Neurol* 8:620–624, 1980.
31. Brimijoin S, Capek P, Dyck P: Axonal transport of dopamine-B-hydroxylase by human sural nerves in vitro. *Science* 180:1295, 1973.
32. Brooks A: Abnormal vascular reflexes in Charcot-Marie-Tooth disease. *J. Neurol Neurosurg Psychiat* 43:348–350, 1980.
33. Brown J, Johns R: Nerve conduction in familial dysautonomia (Riley-Day syndrome). *JAMA* 201:118–120, July, 1967.
34. Brown MJ, Asbury AK: Diabetic neuropathy. *Ann Neurol* 15:2–12, 1984.
35. Brust J, Lovelace R, Devi S: Clinical and electrodiagnostic features of Charcot-Marie-Tooth syndrome. *Acta Neurol Scand* 58 (suppl 68): 5–141, 1978.
36. Buchthal F, Behse F: Peroneal muscular atrophy (PMA) and related disorders. I. Clinical manifestations as related to biopsy findings, nerve conduction and electromyography. *Brain* 100:41–66, 1977.
37. Buchthal F, Rosenfalck A, Behse F: Sensory potentials of normal and diseased nerves. In Dyck PJ, Thomas PK and Lambert EH (eds): *Peripheral Neuropathy,* vol 1. Philadelphia, WB Saunders, 1975, pp 492–464.

38. Byers C, DeLisa J, Frankel D, Kraft G: Pyridoxine metabolism in carpal tunnel syndrome, with and without peripheral neuropathy. *Arch Phys Med Rehabil* 65:712–716, 1984.

39. Campbell IW, et al: Peripheral and autonomic nerve function diabetic ketoacidosis. *Lancet* 2:167–169, 1976.

40. Campbell MJ, Paty DW: Carcinomatous neuromyopathy: 1. Electrophysiologic studies. An electrophysiological and immunological study of patients with carcinoma of the lung. *J Neurol Neurosurg Psychiat* 37:131–141, 1974.

41. Carpendale MTF: Conduction time in the terminal portion of the motor fibers of the ulnar, median and peroneal nerves in healthy subjects and in patients with neuropathy. MS Thesis, University of Minnesota, 1956.

42. Carpenter S, Karpati G. Andermann F, Gold R: Giant axonal neuropathy. A clinical and morphologically distinct neurological disease. *Arch Neurol* 31:312–316, 1974.

43. Casey EB, LeQuesne PM: Electrophysiological evidence for a distal lesion in alcoholic neuropathy. *J Neurol Neurosurg Psychiat* 35:624–630, 1972.

44. Casey EB, LeQuesne PM: Alcoholic neuropathy. In Desmedt JE (ed): *New Developments in Electrophyography and Clinical Neurophysiology*, vol 2. Basel, S Karger, 1973, pp 279–285.

45. Cerra D, Johnson EW: Motor nerve conduction velocity in "idiopathic" polyneuritis. *Arch Phys Med Rehabil* 42:159–163, 1961.

46. Chad D, Pariser K, Bradley WG, Adelman LS, Pinn VW: The pathogenesis of cryoglobulinemic neuropathy. *Neurology* 32:725–729, 1982.

47. Chokroverty S: Proximal nerve dysfunction in diabetic proximal amyotrophy. Electrophysiology and electron microscopy. *Arch Neurol* 39:403–408, 1982.

48. Cinca I, Dumitrescu I, Onaca P, Serbanescu A, Nestorescu B: Accidental ethyl mercury poisoning with nervous system, skeletal muscle, and myocardium injury. *J Neurol Neurosurg Psychiat* 43:143–149, 1979.

49. Codish SD, Cress RJ: Motor and sensory nerve conduction in uremic patients undergoing repeated dialysis. *Arch Phys Med Rehabil* 52:260–263, 1971.

50. Combarros O, Calleja J, Figols J, Cabello A, Berciano J: Dominantly inherited motor and sensory neuropathy Type I. *J Neurol Sci* 61:181–191, 1983.

51. Conn DI, Dyck PJ: Angiopathic neuropathy in connective tissue disease. In Dyck PJ, Thomas Pk and Lambert EH (eds): *Peripheral Neuropathy*, Vol 1. Philadelphia, WB Saunders, 1975, pp 1149–1165.

52. Conrad B, Aschoff JC: The diagnostic value of the F-wave latency. *Proc 5th Int'l Cong EMG Clin Neurophys*. Rochester. MN, September 1975.

53. Cracco J, Castells S, Mark E: Spinal somatosensory evoked potentials in juvenile diabetes. *Ann Neurol* 15:55–58, 1984.

54. Cummins KL, Dorfman LJ: Nerve fiber conduction velocity distributions: studies of normal and diabetic human nerves. *Ann Neurol* 9:67–74, 1981.

55. Dalakas MC, Engel WK: Polyneuropathy with monoclonal gammopathy: studies of 11 patients. *Ann Neurol* 10:45–52, 1981.

56. Danta G: Hypoglycemic peripheral neuropathy. *Arch Neurol* 21:121–132, 1969.

57. Davis, C, Bradley W, Madrid R: The peroneal muscular atrophy syndrome. Clinical, genetic, electrophysiological and nerve biopsy studies. I. Clinical, genetic and electrophysiological findings & classification. *J Genet Hum* 26:311–349, 1978.

58. DeJesus PV: Landry-Guillain-Barré-Strohl syndrome: neuronal disorder and clinico-electrophysiological correlation. *Electromyogr Clin Neurophysiol* 14:115–132, 1974.

59. DeWeerdt C, Staal A, Went L: Erfelijke compressie-neuropathie (Hereditary compression neuropathy): Een classificatieprobleem bij erfelijke neurologische ziekten. *Ned Tijdschr Geneeskd* 114:1648–1654, 1970.

60. Delaney P: Gouty neuropathy. *Arch Neurol* 40:823–824, 1983.
61. DiBenedetto M: Evoked sensory potentials in peripheral neuropathy. *Arch Phys Med Rehabil* 53:126–131, 1972.
62. DiBenedetto M: Electrodiagnostic evidence of subclinical disease states in drug abusers. *Arch Phys Med Rehabil* 57:62–66, 1976.
63. Donovan WH, Sumi SM: Diabetic amyotrophy—a more diffuse process than clinically suspected. *Arch Phys Med Rehabil* 57:397–403, 1976.
64. Dorfman LJ, Cummins KL, Reaven GM, Ceranski J, Greenfield MS, Doberne L: Studies of diabetic polyneuropathy using conduction velocity distribution (DCV) analysis. *Neurology* 33:773–779, 1983.
65. Downie AW, Newell DJ: Sensory nerve conduction in patients with diabetes mellitus and controls. *Neurology* (Minneap) 11:876–882. 1961.
66. Duncan C, Strub R, McGarry P, Duncan D: Peripheral nerve biopsy as an aid to diagnosis in infantile neuroaxonal dystrophy. *Neurology* 20:1024–1032, 1970.
67. Dyck P: Experimental hypertrophic neuropathy. *Arch Neurol* 21:73–95, 1969.
68. Dyck P: Inherited neuronal degeneration and atrophy affecting peripheral motor sensory and autonomic neurons. In Dyck P, Thomas P, Lambert E (eds): *Peripheral Neuropathy*, vol 1. Philadelphia, WB Saunders, 1975, pp 825–867.
69. Dyck P, Lambert E: Lower motor and primary sensory neuron diseases with peroneal muscular atrophy. I. Neurologic, genetic and electrophysiologic findings in hereditary polyneuropathies. *Arch Neurol* 18:603, 1968a.
70. Dyck P, Ohta M: Neuronal atrophy and degeneration predominantly affecting peripheral sensory neurons. In Dyck, P, Thomas P and Lambert E (eds): *Peripheral Neuropathy, vol 1*. Philadelphia, WB Saunders, 1975, pp 791-824.
71. Dyck PJ, Johnson WJ, Lambert EH, O'Brien PC: Segmental demyelination secondary to axonal degeneration in uremic neuropathy. *Mayo Clin Proc* 46:400–431, 1971.
72. Dyck P, Lambert E, Sanders K, O'Brien P: Severe hypomyelination and marked abnormality of conduction in Dejerine-Sottas hypertrophic neuropathy: myelin thickness and compound action potential of sural nerve in vitro. *Mayo Clin Proc* 46:432–436, 1971.
73. Dyck P, Lais A, Offord K: The nature of myelinated nerve fiber degeneration in dominantly inherited hypertrophic neuropathy. *Mayo Clin Proc* 49:34–39, 1974.
74. Dyck PJ, Lais AC, Ohta M, Bastron JA, Ohazaki H, Groover RV: Chronic inflammatory polyradiculoneuropathy. *Mayo Clin Proc* 50:621–637, 1975.
75. Dyck PJ, Johnson WJ, Lambert EH, O'Brien PC, Daube JR, Oviatt KF: Comparison of symptoms, chemistry, and nerve function to assess adequacy of hemodialysis. *Neurology* 29:1361–1368, 1979.
76. Dyck P, Lais A, Sparks M, Oviatt K, Hexum L, Steinmuller D: Nerve xenografts to apportion the role of axon and Schwann cell in myelinated fiber absence in hereditary sensory neuropathy, Type II. *Neurology* 29:1215–1221, 1979.
77. Dyck PJ, Oviatt KF Lambert EH: Intensive evaluation of referred unclassified neuropathies yields improved diagnosis. *Ann Neurol* 10:222–226, 1981.
78. Dyck P, Swanson C, Low P, Bartleson J, Lambert E: Prednisone-responsive hereditary motor and sensory neuropathy. *Mayo Clin Proc* 57:239–246, 1982.
79. Eisen AA, Humphreys P: The Guillain-Barré syndrome: a clinical and electrodiagnostic study of 25 cases. Arch Neurol 30:438–443, 1974.
80. Eisen AA, Woods JF, Sherwin AL: Peripheral nerve function in long-term therapy with diphenylhydantoin. *Neurology* (Minneap) 24:411–417, 1974.
81. Eng GD, Hung W, August GP, Smokvina MD: Nerve conduction velocity determinations in juvenile diabetes: Continuing study of 190 patients. *Arch Phys Med Rehabil* 56:1–5, 1976.

82. Faden A, Mendoza E, Flynn F: Subclinical neuropathy associated with chronic obstructive pulmonary disease. Possible pathophysiologic role of smoking. *Arch Neurol* 38:639–642, 1981.

83. Fagius J, Jameson S: Effects of aldose reductase inhibitor treatment in diabetic polyneuropathy—a clinical and neurophysiological study. *J Neurol Neurosurg Psychiat* 44:991–1001, 1981.

84. Feldman RG, Haddow J, Kopito L, Schwachman H: Altered peripheral nerve conduction velocity: chronic lead intoxication in children. *Am J Dis Child* 125:39–41, 1973.

85. Feldman RG, Niles CA, Kelly-Hayes M, Sax DS, Dixon WJ, Thompson DJ, Landau E: Peripheral neuropathy in arsenic smelter workers. *Neurology* 29:939–944, 1979.

86. Fiaschi AF, DeGrandis D, Ferrari F: Correlations between neurophysiological and histologic findings in subclinical lead neuropathy. *Proc 5th Int'l Cong EMG Clin Neurophys*, Rochester, MN, September, 1975.

87. Fincham RW, Cape CA: Neuropathy in myxedema: a study of sensory nerve conduction in the upper extremities. *Arch Neurol* 19:464–466, 1968.

88. Finelli PS, Morgan TF, Yaar I, Granger CV: Ethylene oxide-induced polyneuropathy. A clinical and electrophysiologic study. *Arch Neurol* 40:419–422, 1983.

89. Fisher M: An unusual variant of acute idiopathic polyneuritis (syndrome of ophthalmoplegia, ataxia and areflexia). *N Eng J Med* 255:57–65, 1956.

90. Fitting JW, Bischoff A, Regli F, DeCrousaz G: Neuropathy, amyloidosis, and monoclonal gammopathy. *J Neurol Neurosurg Psychiat* 42:193–202, 1979.

91. Fullerton PM, Harrison MJG: Subclinical lead neuropathy in man. *Electroenceph Clin Neurophysiol* 27:718, 1969.

92. Gans B, Kraft G: M Response quantification: a technique. *Arch Phys Med Rehabil* 62:376–380, 1981.

93. Garg B, Markand O, Bustion P: Brainstem auditory evoked responses in hereditary motor-sensory neuropathy: Site of origin of Wave II. *Neurology* 32:1017–1019, 1982.

94. Gassel MM; Test of nerve conduction to muscles of shoulder girdle as aid in diagnosis of proximal neurogenic and muscular disease. *J Neurol Neurosurg Psychiat* 27:200–205, 1964.

95. Ghosh S, Vaid K, Mohan M, Maheshwari MC: Effect of degree and duration of protein energy malnutrition on peripheral nerves in children. *J Neurol Neurosurg Psychiat* 42:760–763, 1979.

96. Gill GV, Bell DR: Persisting nutritional neuropathy amongst former war prisoners. *J Neurol Neurosurg Psychiat* 45:861–865, 1982.

97. Gilliat RW: Recent advances in the pathophysiology of nerve conduction. In Desmedt JE (ed): *New Developments in Electromyography and Clinical Neurophysiology*, vol 2. Basel, S Karger, 1973, pp 2–18.

98. Goldstein NP, McCall JT, Dyck PJ: Metal neuropathy. In Dyck PJ, Thomas PK, Lambert EH (eds): *Peripheral Neuropathy*, vol 1. Philadelphia, WB Saunders, 1975, pp 1227–1262.

99. Gonzalez EG, Downey JA: Polyneuropathy in a glue sniffer. *Arch Phys Med Rehabil* 53:333–337, 1972.

100. Goodgold J, Eberstein A: *Electrodiagnosis of Neuromuscular Diseases*. Baltimore, Williams & Wilkins, 1972, pp 157–205.

101. Graf RJ, Halter JB, Halar E, Porte D: Nerve conduction abnormalities in untreated maturity-onset diabetes: relation to levels of fasting plasma glucose and glycosylated hemoglobin. *Ann Intern Med* 90:298–303, 1979.

102. Gregersen G: Variations in motor conduction velocity produced by acute changes of the metabolic state in diabetic patients. *Diabetologia* 4:273–277, 1968.

103. Gross JA, Haas ML and Swift TR: Ethylene oxide neurotoxicity: Report of four cases and review of the literature. *Neurology* 29:978–982, July 1979.

104. Gupta PR, Dorfman LJ: Spinal somatosensory conduction in diabetes. *Neurology* 31:841–845, 1981.

105. Gutmann L, Martin JD, Welton W: Dapsone motor neuropathy—an axonal disease. *Proc 5th Int'l Cong EMG Clin Neurophys*, Rochester, MN, September, 1975.

106. Gutmann L, Fakadej A, Riggs J: Evaluation of nerve conduction abnormalities in children with dominant hypertrophic neuropathy of the Charcot-Marie-Tooth type. *Muscle Nerve.* 6:515–519, 1983.

107. Guyton JD: The effects of changes in carbohydrate metabolism on motor nerve conduction velocity. MSc thesis, Ohio State University, 1961.

108. Halar EM, Brozovich FV, Milutinovic J, Inouye VL, Becker VM: H-reflex latency in uremic neuropathy: correlation with NCV and clinical findings. *Arch Phys Med Rehabil* 60:174–177, 1979.

109. Halar EM, Graf RJ, Halter JB, Brozovich FV, Soine TL: Diabetic neuropathy: a clinical, laboratory and electrodiagnostic study. *Arch Phys Med Rehabil* 63:298–303, 1982.

110. Halter SK, DeLisa JA, Stolov WC, Scardapane D, Sherrard DJ: Carpal tunnel syndrome in chronic renal dialysis patients. *Arch Phys Med Rehabil* 62:197–201, 1981.

111. Harding A, Thomas P: Autosomal recessive forms of hereditary motor and sensory neuropathy. *J Neurol Neurosurg Psychiat* 43:699–678, 1980.

112. Harding A, Thomas P: The clinical features of hereditary motor and sensory neuropathy Types I and II. *Brain* 103:259–280, 1980.

113. Harding A, Thomas P: Peroneal muscular atrophy with pyramidal features. *J Neurol Neurosurg Psychiat* 47:168–172, 1984.

114. Henderson B, Koepke GH, Feller I: Peripheral polyneuropathy among patients with burns. *Arch Phys Med Rehabil* 52:149–151, 1971.

115. Herbison GJ, Teng CS, Martin JH, Ditunno JF, Birtwell WM, Tourtellote CD: Peripheral neuropathy in rheumatoid arthritis. Paper presented at American Academy of PM&R Annual Meeting, August 23, 1970.

116. Hern JEC: Tri-ortho-cresyl phosphate neuropathy in the baboon. In Desmedt JE (ed): *New Developments in Electromyography and Neurophysiology*, vol 2. Basel, S Karger, 1973, pp 181–187.

117. Hogan GR, Gutmann L, Chou SM: The peripheral neuropathy of Krabbe's (globoid) leukodystrophy. *Neurology* (Minneap) 19:1094–1100, 1969.

118. Honet JC: Electrodiagnostic study of a patient with peripheral neuropathy after nitrofurantoin therapy. *Arch Phys Med Rehabil* 48:209–212, 1967.

119. Honet JC, Jebsen RH, Tenckhoff HA, McDonald JR: Motor nerve conduction velocity in chronic renal insufficiency. *Arch Phys Med Rehabil* 47:647–652, 1966.

120. Hopkins A: Toxic neuropathy due to industrial agents. In Dyck PJ, Thomas PK and Lambert EH (eds): *Peripheral Neuropathy*, vol 1. Philadelphia, WB Saunders, 1975, pp 1207–1226.

121. Horning M, Kraft G, Guy A: Latencies recorded by intramuscular needle electrodes in different portions of a muscle; variation and comparison with surface electrodes. *Arch Phys Med Rehabil* 53:206–211, 1972.

122. Horwich MS, Cho L, Porro RS, Posner JB: Subacute sensory neuropathy: a remote effect of carcinoma. *Ann Neurol* 2:7–19, 1977.

123. Humberstone P: Nerve conduction studies in Charcot-Marie-Tooth disease. *Acta Neurol Scand* 48:176–190, 1972.

124. Illingworth DR, Connor WE, Miller RG: Abetalipoproteinema: report of two cases and review of therapy. *Arch Neurol* 37:659–662, 1980.

125. Isch F, Isch-Treussard C, Jesel M: Diagnostic and prognostic value of the electromyographic findings in polyradiculoneuritis. *Electroenceph Clin Neurophysiol* 23:387, 1967.

126. Jebsen RH, Tenckhoff H: Comparison of motor and sensory nerve conduction velocity in early uremic polyneuropathy. *Arch Phys Med Rehabil* 50:124–126, 1969.

127. Jebsen RH, Tenckhoff H, Honet JC: Natural history of uremic polyneuropathy and effects of dialysis. *N Engl J Med* 277:327–333, 1967.
128. Jedzewitsch RG, Jaspan JB, Polonsky KS, Weinberg CR, Halter JB, Halar E, Pfeifer MA, Vukadinovic C, Bernstein L, Schneider M, Liang KY, Gabbay KH, Rubenstein AH, Porte D Jr: Aldose reductase inhibition improves nerve conduction velocity in diabetic patients. *N Engl J Med* 308:119–125, 1983.
129. Jones S, Halliday A: Subcortical and cortical somatosensory evoked potentials: characteristic waveform changes associated with disorders of the peripheral and central nervous system. In Courjon J, Mauguier F, Revol M (eds): *Clinical Applications of Evoked Potentials in Neurology*. New York, Raven, 1982, pp 313–320.
130. Julien J, Vital C, Vallat JM, Lagueny A, Ferrer X, Deminiere C, Leboutet MJ, Effroy C: IgM demyelinative neuropathy with amyloidosis and biclonal gammopathy. *Ann Neurol* 15:395–399, 1984.
131. Kaeser HE, Wuthrich R: Zur frage der neurotoxizitat der oxychinoline. *Dtsch med Wschr* 95:1685–1688, 1970.
132. Kaltreider HB, Talal N: The neuropathy of Sjogren's syndrome. Trigeminal nerve involvement. *Ann Intern Med* 70:751–762, 1969.
133. Kaplan P: Sensory and motor residual latency measurements in healthy patients and patients with neuropathy. *J-Neurol Neurosurg Psychiat* 39:338–340, 1976.
134. Kelly JJ: The electrodiagnostic findings in peripheral neuropathy associated with monoclonal gammopathy. *Muscle Nerve* 67:504–509, 1983.
135. Kelly JJ, Kyle RA, O'Brien PC, Dyck PJ: Prevalence of monoclonal protein in peripheral neuropathy. *Neurology* 31:1480–1483, 1981.
136. Kikta DG, Breuer AC, Wilbourn AJ: Thoracic root pain in diabetes: the spectrum of clinical and electromyographic findings. *Ann Neurol* 11:80–85, 1982.
137. Killian J, Kloepfer H: Homozygous expression of a dominant gene for Charcot-Marie-Tooth neuropathy. *Ann Neurol* 5:515–522, 1979.
138. Kimura J: F-wave velocity in the central segment of the median and ulnar nerves: a study in normal subjects and in patients with Charcot-Marie-Tooth disease. *Neurology* (Minneap) 24:539–546, 1974.
139. Kimura J, Butzer JF, Van Allen MW: F-wave conduction velocity between axilla and spinal cord in the Guillain-Barré syndrome. *Trans Am Neurol Assoc* 99:52–62, 1974.
140. King D: Conduction velocity in the proximal segments of motor nerves in the Guillain-Barré, syndrome. *Proc 5th Int'l Cong EMG Clin Neuropshy*. Rochester, MN, September 1975.
141. Knill-Jones RP, Goodwill CJ, Dayan AD, Williams R: Peripheral neuropathy in chronic liver disease: clinical, electrodiagnostic and nerve biopsy findings. *J Neurol Neurosurg Psychiat*, 35:22–30, 1972.
142. Kocen RS, McDonald WI, Frengley JD: Nerve conduction studies in a patient with diptheritic neuropathy. *Proc 5th Int'l Cong EMG Clin Neurophys*. Rochester, MN, September 1975.
143. Konishi T, Nishitani H, Motomura S: Single fiber electromyography in chronic renal failure. *Muscle Nerve* 5:458–461, 1982.
144. Kraft GH: Experimental allergic neuritis: A model of idiopathic (Guillain-Barré) polyneuritis. *Arch Phys Med Rehabil* 49:490–501, 1968.
145. Kraft GH: Multiple distal neuritis of the shoulder girdle: an electromyographic clarification of "paralytic brachial neuritis". *Electroenceph Clin Neurophysiol* 27:722, 1969.
146. Kraft G: Serial motor nerve latency and electromyographic determinations in experimental allergic neuritis. *Electromyography* 1:61–74, 1971.

147. Kraft G: Axillary, musculocutaneous and suprascapular nerve latency studies. *Arch Phys Med Rehabil* 53:383–387, 1972.
148. Kraft G: Serial nerve conduction and electromyographic studies in experimental allergic neuritis. *Arch Phys Med Rehabil* 56:333–340, 1975.
149. Kraft G, Bird T: Nerve conduction velocities in children with Charcot-Marie-Tooth disease. *Muscle Nerve.* 5:567, 1982.
150. Kraft G, Halvorson G: Median nerve residual latency: normal value and use in diagnosis of carpal tunnel syndrome. *Arch Phys Med Rehabil* 64:221–226, 1983.
151. Kraft GH, Guyton JD, Huffman JD: Follow-up study of motor nerve conduction velocities in patients with diabetes mellitus. *Arch Phys Med Rehabil* 51:207–209, 1970.
152. Kraft G, Daube J, DeLisa J, Goodgold J, Jablecki C, Lambert E, Simpson J, Struppler A, Wiechers D: *A Glossary of Terms used in Clinical Electromyography.* Rochester, MN, American Association of Electromyography and Electrodiagnosis, 1980.
153. Kriel R, Cliffer K, Berry J, Sung J, Bland C: Investigation of a family with hypertrophic neuropathy resembling Roussy-Lévy syndrome. *Neurology* (Minneap): 24:801–809, 1974.
154. Krunholz A, Weiss HD, Goldstein PJ, Harris KC: Evoked responses in vitamin B_{12} deficiency. *Ann Neurol* 9:407–409, 1981.
155. Kunze K, Muskat E: Thiamine deficiency neuropathy in rats. *Electroenceph Clin Neurophysiol* 27:721, 1969.
156. Kvinesdal B, Molin J, Froland A, Gram LF: Imipramine treatment of painful diabetic neuropathy. *JAMA* 251:13:1727–1730, 1984.
157. Lachman T, Shahani BT, Young RR: Late responses as diagnostic aids in Landry-Guillain-Barré syndrome. *Arch Phys Med Rehabil* 57:600, 1976.
158. Lai CS, Ransome GA: Burning-feet syndrome. Case due to malabsorption and riboflavine responding. *Br Med J* 2:151–152, 1970.
159. Lambert E, Dyck P: Compound action potentials of sural nerve in vitro in peripheral neuropathy. In Dyck P, Thomas P, Lambert E (eds): *Peripheral Neuropathy,* vol 1. Philadelphia, WB Saunders, 1975, pp 427–441.
160. Lambert EH, Mulder DW: Nerve conduction in the Guillain-Barré syndrome. *Am Assoc Electromyogr Electrodiag* 10:13, 1963.
161. Landrigan PJ: Occupational and community exposures to toxic metals: Lead, cadmium, mercury and arsenic. *Wes J Med* 6:531–540, 1982.
162. LeQuesne PM: Neuropathy due to drugs. In Dyck P, Thomas PK, Lambert EH (eds): *Peripheral Neuropathy,* vol 1. Philadelphia, WB Saunders, 1975, pp 1263–1280.
163. Lewis, R, Sumner A: The electrodiagnostic distinctions between chronic familial and acquired demyelinative neuropathies. *Neurology* (New York) 32:592–596, 1982.
164. Limos LC, Ohnishi A, Suzuki N, Kojima N, Yoshimura T, Goto I, Kuroiwa Y: Axonal degeneration and focal muscle fiber necrosis in human thallotoxicosis: histopathological studies of nerve and muscle. *Muscle Nerve* 5: 698–706, 1982.
165. Loizou LA, Boddie HG: Polyradiculoneuropathy associated with heroin abuse. *J Neurol Neurosurg Psychiat* 41:855–857, 1978.
166. Lovelace RE: Mononeuritis multiplex in polyarteritis nodosa. *Neurology* (Minneap) 14:434–442, 1964.
167. Lovelace RE, Horwitz SJ: Peripheral neuropathy in long-term diphenylhydantoin therapy. *Arch Neurol* 18:69–77, 1968.
168. Lovelace RE, Johnson WG, Martin J: Peripheral nerve involvement and carrier detection in Pelizaeus-Merzbacher disease. *Arch Phys Med Rehabil* 57:600. 1976.

169. Lowitzsch K, Gohring U, Hecking E, Kohler H: Refractory period, sensory conduction velocity and visual evoked potentials before and after haemodialysis. *J Neurol Neurosurg Psychiat* 44:121–128, 1981.
170. Marcus DJ, Swift TR, McDonald TF: Acute effects of phenytoin on peripheral nerve function in the rat. *Muscle Nerve* 4:48–50, 1981.
171. Martin WA, Kraft GH: Shoulder girdle neuritis: a clinical and electrophysiological evaluation. *Mil Med* 139:21–25, 1974.
172. Martinez-Arizala A, Sobol SM, McCarty GE, Nichols BR, Rakita L: Amiodarone neuropathy. *Neurology* 33:643–645, 1983.
173. Matthews WB: Sarcoid neuropathy. In Dyck PJ, Thomas PK and Lambert EH (eds): *Peripheral Neuropathy,* vol 1. Philadelphia, WB Saunders, 1975, pp 1199–1206.
174. Mattson RH, Lecocq RF: Nerve conduction velocities in fasting patients. *Neurology* 18:335–339, 1968.
175. May WE: Nutritional sensory neuronopathy. An emerging new syndrome. *Arch Neurol* 41:559–560, 1984.
176. Mayer RF: Peripheral nerve function in vitamin B_{12} deficiency. *Arch Neurol* 13:355–362, 1965.
177. McDonald W: Experimental neuropathy. In Desmedt J (ed): *New Developments in Electromyography and Clinical Neurophysiology,* vol. 2. Basel, S Karger, 1973, pp 128–144.
178. McDonald WI, Kocen RS: Diptheritic neuropathy. In Dyck PJ, Thomas PK, Lambert EH (eds): *Peripheral Neuropathy,* vol 1. Philadelphia, WB Saunders, 1975, pp 1281–1300.
179. McLeod JC: Carcinomatous neuropathy. In Dyck PJ, Thomas PK, Lambert EH (eds): *Peripheral Neuropathy,* vol 1. Philadelphia, WB Saunders, 1975, pp 1301–1313.
180. McLeod J, Evans W: Peripheral neuropathy in spinocerebellar degenerations. *Muscle Nerve.* 4:51–61, 1981.
181. McLeod JG, Morgan JA: Nerve conduction studies in spinocerebellar degenerations. *Proc 5th Int'l Cong EMG Clin Neurophys* Rochester, MN, September, 1975.
182. McLeod JG, Walsh JC: Neuropathies associated with paraproteinemias and dysproteinemias. In Dyck PJ, Thomas PK, Lambert EH (eds): *Peripheral Neuropathy,* vol 1. Philadelphia, WB Saunders, 1975, pp 1012–1029.
183. McLeod JG, Walsh JC: Peripheral neuropathy associated with lymphomas and other reticuloses. In Dyck PJ, Thomas PK, Lambert EH (eds): *Peripheral Neuropathy,* vol 1. Philadelphia, WB Saunders, 1975, pp 1314–1325.
184. McLeod JG, Walsh JC: Little JM: Sural nerve biopsy. *Med J. Aust* 2:1092–1096, 1969.
185. McQuillen MP, Gorin FJ: Serial ulnar nerve conduction velocity measurements in normal subjects and in patients with idiopathic polyneuritis. *Neurology* 18:285, 1968.
186. Melgaard B, Hansen HS, Kamieniecka Z, Paulson OB, Pedersen AG, Tang X, Trojaborg W: Misonidazole neuropathy: a clinical electrophysiological, and histologic study. *Ann Neurol* 12:10–17, 1982.
187. Melmed C, Frail D, Duncan I, Braun P, Danoff D, Finlayson M, Stewart J: Peripheral neuropathy with IgM kappa monoclonal immunoglobulin directed against myelin-associated glycoprotein. *Neurology* 33:1397–1405, 1983.
188. Miller RG, Davis CJF, Illingworth DR, Bradley W: The neuropathy of abetalipoproteinemia. *Neurology* 30:1286–1291, 1980.
189. Mitz M, DiBenedetto M, Klingbeil GE, Melvin JL, Piering W: Neuropathy in end-stage renal disease secondary to primary renal disease and diabetes. *Arch Phys Med Rehabil* 65:235–238, 1984.
190. Mokri B, Ohnishi A, Dyck PJ: Disulfiram neuropathy. *Neurology* 31:730–735, 1981.

191. Morgan JP: The Jamaica ginger paralysis. *JAMA* 248:1864–1868, 1982.
192. Mulder DW: Motor neuron disease. In Dyck PJ, Thomas PK and Lambert EH (eds): *Peripheral Neuropathy*, vol 1. Philadelphia, WB Saunders, 1975, pp 759–770.
193. Mulder DW, Lambert EH, Bastron JA, Sprague RG: The neuropathies associated with diabetes mellitus: a clinical and electromyographic study of 103 unselected diabetic patients. *Neurology* (Minneap) 11:275–285, 1961.
194. Murphy MJ, Lyon LW, Taylor JW: Subacute arsenic neuropathy: clinical and electrophysiological observations. *J Neurol Neurosurg Psychiat* 44:896–900, 1981.
195. Myers RR, Powell HC, Shapiro HM, Costello MI, Lampert PW: Changes in endoneurial fluid pressure, permeability, and peripheral nerve ultrastructure in experimental lead neuropathy. *Ann Neurol* 8:392–401, 1980.
196. Nemni R, Galassi G, Cohen M, Hays AP, Gould R, Singh N, Bressman S, Gamboa ET: Symmetric sarcoid polyneuropathy: analysis of a sural nerve biopsy. *Neurology* (New York) 31:1217–1223, 1981.
197. Nemni R, Galassi G, Latov N, Sherman WH, Olarte MR, Hays AP: Polyneuropathy in nonmalignant IgM plasma cell dyscrasia: a morphological study. *Ann Neurol* 14:43–54, 1983.
198. Noel P: Diabetic neuropathy. In Desmedt JE (ed): *New Developments in Electromyography and Neurophysiology*, vol 2. Basel, S Karger, 1973, pp. 318–352.
199. Nukada H, Dyck P, Karnes J: Thin axons relative to myelin spiral length in hereditary motor and sensory neuropathy, Type I. *Ann Neurol* 14:6:648–655, 1983.
200. Oh SJ: Lead neuropathy: case report. *Arch Phys Med Rehabil* 56:312–317, 1975.
201. Ohnishi A, Dyck PJ: Loss of small peripheral sensory neurons in Fabry disease. *Arch Neurol* 31:120–127, 1974.
202. Ohnishi A, Schilling K, Brimijoin WS, Lambert EH, Fairbanks VF, Dyck PJ: Lead neuropathy (1) Morphometry, nerve conduction, and choline acetyltransferase transport: new finding of endoneurial edema associated with segmental demyelination. *J Neuropath Exp Neurol* 36:499–518, 1977.
203 Ohta M, Ellefson R, Lambert E, Dyck P: Hereditary sensory neuropathy, Type II. Clinical, electrophysiologic, histologic and biochemical studies of a Quebec kinship. *Arch Neurol* 29:23–37, 1973.
204. Olney RK, Miller RG: Peripheral neuropathy associated with disulfiram administration. *Muscle Nerve* 3:172–175, 1980.
205. Ongerboer de Visser BW, Feltkamp-Vroom TM, Feltkamp CA: Sural nerve immune deposits in polyneuropathy as a remote effect of malignancy. *Ann Neurol* 14:261–266, 1983.
206. O'Shaughnessy E, Kraft GH: Arsenic poisoning: long term follow-up of a nonfatal case. *Arch Phys Med Rehabil* 57:403–406, 1976.
207. Panayiotopoulos CP, Lagos G: Tibial nerve H-reflex and F-wave studies in patients with uremic neuropathy. *Muscle Nerve* 3:423–426, 1980.
208. Paulson GW, Waylonis GW: Polyneuropathy due to N-hexane. *Arch Intern Med* 136:880–882, 1976.
209. Pecket P, Schattner A: Concurrent Bell's palsy and diabetes mellitus: a diabetic mononeuropathy? *J Neurol Neurosurg Psychiat* 45:652–655, 1982.
210. Pedley JC, Harman DJ, Waudby H, McDougall AC: Leprosy in peripheral nerves: histopathological findings in 119 untreated patients in Nepal. *J Neurol Neurosurg Psychiat* 43:198–204, 1980.
211. Pena SD: Giant axonal neuropathy: an inborn error of organization of intermediate filaments. *Muscle Nerve* 5:166–172, 1982.
212. Peterson CM, Tsairis P, Ohnishi A, Lu YS, Grady R, Cerami A, Dyck PJ: Sodium cyanate induced polyneuropathy in patients with sickle-cell disease. *Ann Intern Med* 81:152–158, 1974.

213. Peyronnard JM, Charron L, Beaudet F, Couture F: Vasculitic neuropathy in rheumatoid disease and Sjogren syndrome. *Neurology* 32:839–845, 1982.
214. Pleasure DE: Abetalipoproteinemia and Tangier disease. In Dyck PJ, Thomas PK and Lambert EH (eds): Peripheral Neuropathy, vol 1. Philadelphia, WB Saunders, 1975, pp 928–941.
215. Pleasure DE, Lovelace RE, Duvoisin RC: The prognosis of acute polyradiculoneuritis. *Neurology* (Minneap) 18:1143–1148, 1968.
216. Powell HC, Rodriguez M, Hughes RAC: Microangiopathy of vasa nervorum in dysglobulinemic neuropathy. *Ann Neruol* 15:386–394, 1984.
217. Prineas J: Peripheral nerve changes in thiamine-deficient rats: an electron microscope study. *Arch Neurol* 23:541–548, 1970.
218. Puvanendran K, Devasthasan G, Wong PK: Visual evoked responses in diabetes. *J Neurol Neurosurg Psychiat* 46:643–647, 1983.
219. Rajeswaramma V, Perez S, Miglietta O: The refractory period of the sensory fibers of the median nerve in normal and diabetic patients. *Arch Phys Med Rehabil* 54:595, 1973.
220. Raman PT, Taori GM: Prognostic significance of electrodiagnostic studies in the Guillain-Barré syndrome. *J Neurol Neurosurg Psychiat* 39:163–170, 1976.
221. Rasminsky M, Sears T: Saltatory conduction in demyelinated nerve fibers. In Desmedt J (ed): *New Developments in Electromyography and Clinical Neurophysiology*, vol 2. Basel, S Karger, 1973, pp 158–165.
222. Refsum S: Herodopathia atactica polyneuritiformis (Refsum's Disease): Clinical and genetic aspects of Refsum's disease. In Dyck PJ, Thomas PK, Lambert EH (eds). *Peripheral Neuropathy*, vol 1. Philadelphia, WB Saunders, 1975, pp 868–890.
223. Reinstein L, Pargament JM, Goodman JS: Peripheral neuropathy after multiple tetanus toxoid injections. *Arch Phys Med Rehab* 63:332–334, 1981.
224. Robertson W, Lambert E: Measurement of sensory nerve conduction velocity in children using cerebral evoked potentials. *Arch Phys Med Rehabil* 57:603, 1976.
225. Robinson RO, Robertson WC Jr: Fetal nutrition and peripheral nerve conduction velocity. *Neurology* 31:327–329, 1981.
226. Rondinelli RD, Stolov WC: Electrodiagnosis of diabetic polyneuropathy: a multivariate analytical approach. *Muscle Nerve.* 7:537,1983.
227. Rossini PM, Treviso M, DiStefano E, DiPaolo B: Nervous impulse propagation along peripheral and central fibres in patients with chronic renal failure. *Electroenceph Clin Neurophysiol* 56:293–303, 1983.
228. Sabin TD and Swift TR: Leprosy. In Dyck PJ, Thomas PK and Lambert EH (eds): *Peripheral Neuropathy*, vol 1. Philadelphia, WB Saunders, 1975, pp 1166–1198.
229. Said G, Boudier L, Selva J, Zingraff J, Drueke T: Different patterns of uremic polyneuropathy: clinicopathologic study. *Neurology* 33:567–574, 1983.
230. Sales Luis ML: Electroneurophysiological studies in familial amyloid polyneuropathy—Portuguese type. *J Neurol Neurosurg Psychiat* 41:847–850, 1978.
231. Salisachs, P, Findley L, Codina M, Torre P, Martinez-Lage J: Data on three of the original patients of Roussy and Lévy (1926). *Muscle Nerve* 5:663–664, 1982.
232. Sandler SG, Tobin W, Henderson ES: Vincristine-induced neuropathy: a clinical study of fifty leukemic patients. *Neurology* (Minneap) 19:367–374, 1969.
233. Schaumburg HH, Spencer PS: Toxic neuropathies. *Neurology* 29:429–431, 1979.
234. Schaumberg H, Kaplan J, Windebank A, Vick N, Rasmus S, Pleasure D, Brown MJ: Sensory neuropathy from pyridoxine abuse. A new megavitamin syndrome. *N Engl J Med* 309:8:445–448, 1983.
235. Schneider C, Dumrese C: Le syndrome de Guillain-Barré: etude clinique et electromyographique de 36 observations. *Schweiz med Wschr 104:393–400, 1974.*
236. Senanayake N: Tri-cresyl-phosphate neuropathy in Sri Lanka: a clinical and neu-

rophysiological study with a three year follow up. *J Neurol Neurosurg Psychiat* 44:775-780, 1981.

237. Seneviratne KN, Peiris OA: Peripheral nerve function in chronic liver disease. *J Neurol Neurosurg Psychiat* 33:609-614, 1970.

238. Service FJ, Daube JR, O'Brien PC, Zimmerman BR, Swanson CJ, Brennan MD, Dyck PJ: Effect of blood glucose control on peripheral nerve function in diabetic patients. *Mayo Clin Proc* 58:283-289, 1983.

239. Sherman WH, Latov N, Hays AP, Takatsu M, Nemni R, Galassi G, Osserman EF: Monoclonal IgM$_k$ antibody precipitating with chondroitin sulfate C from patients with axonal polyneuropathy and epidermolysis. *Neurology* 33:192-201, 1983.

240. Sheth K, Swick H: Peripheral nerve conduction in Fabry disease. *Ann Neurol* 7:319-323, 1980.

241. Shibasaki H, Kakigi R, Ohnishi A, Kuroiwa Y: Peripheral and central nerve conduction in subacute myelo-optico-neuropathy. *Neurology* 32:1186-1189, 1982.

242. Shirabe T, Tawara S, Terao A, Araki S: Myxoedematous polyneuropathy: a light and electron microscopic study of the peripheral nerve and muscle. *J Neurol Neurosurg Psychiat* 38:241-247, 1975.

243. Shorvon SD, Reynolds EH: Anticonvulsant peripheral neuropathy: a clinical and electrophysiological study of patients on single drug treatment with phenytoin, carbamazepine or barbiturates. *J Neurol Neurosurg Psychiat* 45:620-626, 1982.

244. Skillman TG, Johnson EW, Hamwi GJ, Driskill HJ: Motor nerve conduction velocity in diabetes mellitus. *Diabetes* 10:46-51, 1961.

245. Spencer PS, Schaumburg HH: A review of acrylamide neurotoxicity Part I. Properties, uses and human exposure. *Can J Neurol Sci* 12:143-150, 1974.

246. Steck AJ, Murray N, Meier C, Page N, Perruisseau G: Demyelinating neuropathy and monoclonal IgM antibody to myelin-associated glycoprotein. *Neurology* 33:19-23, 1983.

247. Streib E, Sun S, Kimberling W, Smith S: Hypertrophic form of peroneal muscular atrophy (PMA): unusual nerve conduction results. *Muscle Nerve* 7:32-34, 1984.

248. Sugimura K, Dyck PJ: Sural nerve myelin thickness and axis cylinder caliber in human diabetes. *Neurology* 31:1087-1091, 1981.

249. Sumi SM, Farrell DF, Knauss TA: Lymphoma and leukemia manifested by steroid-responsive polyneuropathy. *Arch Neurol* 40:577-582, 1983.

250. Sun SF, Streib EW: Diabetic thoracoabdominal neuropathy: clinical and electrodiagnostic features. *Ann Neurol* 9:75-79, 1981.

251. Swick HM: Pseudointernuclear ophthalmoplegia in acute idiopathic polyneuritis (Fisher's syndrome). *Am J Opthal* 77:725-728, 1974.

252. Swift TR, Gross JA, Ward LC, Crout BO: Peripheral neuropathy in epileptic patients. *Neurology* 31:826-831, 1981.

253. Takahashi K, Nakamura H: Axonal degeneration in beriberi neuropathy. *Arch Neurol* 33:836-841, 1976.

254. Tasker WG, Chutorian AM: Chronic polyneuritis of childhood. *Neurology* (Minneap) 18:302, 1968.

255. Taylor N, Halar EM, Tenckhoff H, Marchioro TL, Masock AJ: Effects of renal transplantation on motor nerve conduction velocity. *Arch Phys Med Rehabil* 53:227-231, 1972.

256. Tenckhoff HA, Boen FST, Jebsen RH, Spiegler JH: Polyneuropathy in chronic renal insufficiency. *JAMA* 192:91-94, 1965.

257. Thiele B, Stalberg E: Single fiber EMG findings in polyneuropathies of different aetiology. *J Neurol Neurosurg Psychiat* 38:881-887, 1975.

258. Thomas JE, Howard FM: Segmental zoster paresis—a disease profile. *Neurology* (Minneap) 22:459-466, 1972.

259. Thomas PK and Eliasson SG: Diabetic neuropathy. In Dyck PJ, Thomas PK and Lambert EH (eds): *Peripheral Neuropathy,* vol 1. Philadelphia, WB Saunders, 1975, pp 956-981.
260. Toole JF, Gergen JA, Hayes DM, Felts JH: Neural effects of nitrofurantoin. *Arch Neurol* 18:680-687, 1968.
261. Toole JF, Parrish ML: Nitrofurantoin polyneuropathy. *Neurology* (Minneap) 23:554-559, 1973.
262. Towfighi J, Gonatas NK, Pleasure D, Cooper HS, McCree L: Glue sniffer's neuropathy. *Neurology* (Minneap) 26:238-243, 1976.
263. Vasilescu C: Motor and sensory nerve conduction velocity in chronic carbon disulfide poisoning. *Proc 5th Int'l Cong EMG Clin Neurophys.* Rochester, MN, September, 1975.
264. Victor M: Polyneuropathy due to nutritional deficiency and alcoholism. In Dyck PJ, Thomas PK, Lambert EH (eds): *Peripheral Neuropathy,* vol 1. Philadelphia, WB Saunders, 1975, pp 1030-1066.
265. Walsh JC: The neuropathy of multiple myeloma: an electrphysiological and histological study. *Arch Neurol* 25:404-414, 1971.
266. Ward JD, Fisher DJ, Barnes CG, Jessop JD, Baker RWR: Improvement in nerve conduction following treatment in newly diagnosed diabetics. *Lancet* 428-431, 1971.
267. Williams AO, Osuntokun BO: Peripheral neuropathy in tropical (nutritional) ataxia in Nigeria. *Arch Neurol* 21:475-492, 1969.
268. Williams JA, Hall GS, Thompson AG, Cooke WT: Neurological disease after partial gastrectomy. *Br Med J* 3:210-212, 1969.
269. Yiannikas C, McLeod JG, Walsh JC: Peripheral neuropathy associated with polycythemia vera. *Neurology* (New York) 33:139-143, 1983.
270. Ziegler D, Schimke R, Kepes J, Rose D, Klinkerfuss G: Late onset ataxia, rigidity and peripheral neuropathy. *Arch Neurol* 27:52-66, 1972.

9

Neuromuscular Junction

IAN C. MACLEAN

In 1936, Dale was awarded the Nobel prize in medicine for proposing and elucidating the mechanism of neuromuscular transmission. It was the first time that synaptic transmission of any kind had been shown to be chemically mediated. During the ensuing half-century, much has been learned about how the junction works, and many diseases have been discovered that affect its function. Electrodiagnostic studies can be very helpful in detecting and characterizing these diseases.

STRUCTURE AND FUNCTION OF THE NEUROMUSCULAR JUNCTION

Distally, the motor axon branches into a number of terminal endings. Normally, up to 2–3% of muscle fibers have multiple innervation, but, in general, there is only one terminal branch and one junction per muscle fiber. The junctional apparatus (Fig. 9.1) includes a nerve terminal, a motor endplate (an extension of the muscle fiber membrane) and a synaptic cleft of about 400-500 Å that separates the two. The endplate forms a trough or groove that envelopes the nerve terminal.

The presynaptic terminals contain mitochondria, cytoskeletal elements, and vesicles filled with acetylcholine (ACh) molecules. The postsynaptic membrane has extensive infoldings and consequently a much larger surface area than the nerve terminal it envelopes. In this membrane, largely clustered on the crests of the postjunctional folds are receptor sites that interact with ACh released from the nerve terminal. Schwann cell processes do not extend into the synaptic cleft.

Acetylcholine Storage

The size of the vesicles in the nerve terminal is quite uniform, each containing about 10,000 molecules of ACh. From a functional standpoint, vesicles are stored either for immediate release or as backup to the immediately available store (44). In response to depolarization of the nerve terminal, some vesicles transfer from the unavailable store to the immediately available store and, in the process, form what has

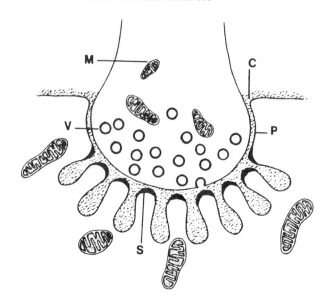

Figure 9.1 Simplified, schematic representation of the junctional apparatus: *M*-mitochondium, *V*-synaptic vesicle, *C*-synaptic cleft, *D*-postsynaptic membrane, *S*-receptor site.

been referred to as the mobilization store. The rate of mobilization is a function of the frequency of depolarization of the nerve terminal and of the degree of depletion of the immediately available store.

Miniature Endplate Potentials

In the presynaptic membrane, there are active sites at which exocytosis of vesicles has been observed (40). When this occurs, the contents of the vesicle are released into the synaptic cleft, a *quantal emission*. (Spontaneous nonquantal release also occurs from cytoplasmic ACh leaking through the nerve terminal membrane (47).) In the resting state, there is a random release of quanta of ACh once every 5 or more seconds. As ACh is released, it is diffused across the synaptic cleft. Some is hydrolyzed in the process by acetylcholinesterase (AChE), but the remainder reacts with receptor sites (ACh-Rs) on the postjunctional membrane. This reaction causes, at that site, a sudden permeability of the membrane to sodium, potassium, and other cations. Little or no change in permeability of the endplate to anions is produced. The resulting low amplitude membrane excitations, which are on the order of close to 1 millivolt, are known as *miniature endplate potentials* (MEPPs). When first observed in the early 1950s by Fatt and Katz (31), the phenomenon was referred to as "biological noise."

When an EMG needle is introduced into the innervation zone, the mechanical disturbance induces high frequency quantal emissions (85). Because the resulting monophasic potentials are recorded from the extracellular space, they have a negative spike that is 200 μV or less (usually 5–20 μV), a fraction of the actual transmembrane potential. The amplitudes of the spikes are variable because the MEPPs occur randomly in overlapping time sequences so that their potentials summate. The sound heard via the speaker system is referred to as a "seashell murmur."

Quantal Liberation by Nerve Impulse

A single depolarization of a presynaptic terminal results in the release of a large number of quanta almost simultaneously. This occurs in response to a voltage-dependent influx of calcium into the nerve terminal (21). The amount of ACh released in response to a nerve impulse can be increased or decreased by increasing or decreasing, respectively, the extracellular calcium concentration, but the actual release mechanism within the nerve terminal triggered by the influx of calcium is unknown. It is known, however, that the process requires about 500 microsec, although the calcium returns to the extracellular space within about 200 microsec.

Only one-half to two-thirds of the ACh released by a nerve impulse into the synaptic cleft reaches the receptor sites on the postsynaptic membrane. The remainder is destroyed in transit as it diffuses from the nerve terminal membrane to the receptor sites, a process that takes about 50 microsec. The remainder of the ACh binds briefly to the ACh-Rs (about 100-200 microsec). It is then released and, except for some recombining of ACh with ACh-Rs, thus prolonging the endplate current (46), it is destroyed. The breakdown of ACh is by hydrolysis mediated via AChE.

Endplate Potential

The multiquantal release induced by depolarization of the presynaptic terminal leads to a local depolarization of the postsynaptic membrane, known as the endplate potential (EPP). The quantal nature of the EPP with each quantal step related (though nonlinearly) to a MEPP can be shown experimentally (25), but because of the enormous emission associated with the nerve impulse, the quantal composition is not normally revealed.

The endplate potential was first shown by Gopfert and Schaefer in 1938 (33) and was subsequently elucidated by Fatt and Katz more than a decade later (31). It is nonpropagated, spreads simply by the cable properties of the muscle fiber, and so is decreased progressively in space and time, becoming nearly depleted at 3–4 mm from the endplate. It has no refactory period. An excitation that occurs before total decay from a previous excitation will result in summation along the whole length of the electronic extension of the EPP.

The Muscle Fiber Action Potential

The resting transmembrane potential of a muscle fiber is approximately 90 millivolts with an intracellular negativity. As depolarization at the endplate proceeds, the potential difference becomes smaller until it reaches a critical threshold, and a propagated action spike develops along the length of the muscle fiber. This muscle fiber action potential spreads in both directions from the endplate and triggers a mechanical contraction. Until sufficient internal negativity is restored, the muscle fiber remains refactory to a subsequent multiquantal emission.

The time sequence of neuromuscular transmission is of interest. Following the arrival of the nerve impulse, no electrical change is seen in the muscle fiber for about 0.5–0.8 msec. Another 0.5 msec is required for the EPP to reach the threshold of excitation of the muscle fiber. These findings are totally consistent with the chemical nature of transmission at the neuromuscular synapse.

Synthesis of Acetylcholine

Although ACh can be synthesized elsewhere in the motoneuron (15), the primary site is the axon terminal. Choline and acetyl coenzyme A combine to form ACh. The reaction is catalyzed by the enzyme choline acetyltransferase, a substance synthesized in the motoneuron cell body and transported to the axon terminal.

The main source of choline for this process is from the degradation of ACh in the synaptic cleft. Choline is actively transported across the terminal membrane, a mechanism accelerated by depolarization of the axon terminal. This transport system can be blocked experimentally by hemicholinium (26).

Thus, ACh in the nerve terminal becomes its own main source for replenishment. To summarize, it is released into the synaptic cleft following a nerve impulse and is hydrolyzed by AChE, either before or after reacting with receptor sites on the postsynaptic membrane. Also, some leakage of cytoplasmic (nonquantal) ACh occurs spontaneously, unrelated to the arrival of an impulse at the nerve terminal (47). Choline, a product of the degradation, is then actively transported across the terminal membrane of the axon where it combines with acetyl coenzyme A to reform ACh. A simplified, schematic outline of synaptic transmission is presented in Figure 9.2.

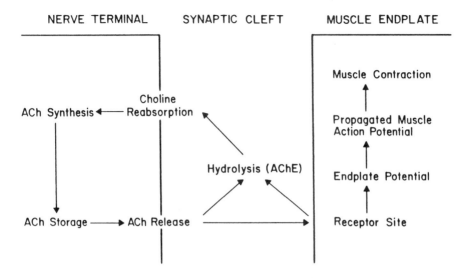

Figure 9.2 Summary of the process of synaptic transmission.

Quantal Liberation during Repetitive Nerve Impulses

The amount of ACh released from a nerve terminal with each depolarization varies considerably during repetitive nerve impulses (43). It changes during the initial volley and adjusts to a relatively steady state that depends on the frequency of the volleys. These changes in quantal content are reflected in a wide range of EPP amplitudes, but at normal neuromuscular junctions, the EPP exceeds by two to four times the threshold amplitude necessary to achieve a propagated muscle fiber action potential. This has been referred to as the *safety factor of neuromuscular transmission* and accounts for why, under normal physiologic circumstances, no failure of transmission occurs.

Two main factors influence the magnitude of a quantal emission. One is the number of synaptic vesicles in the immediately available store; the other is the ease of release of ACh from the vesicles into the synaptic cleft. Ease of release is related to accumulation of calcium in the nerve terminal in conjunction with a nerve impulse.

When a single nerve volley causes a quantal emission, the immediately available store is reduced. Because replacement from the mobilization store takes 5–10 sec, nerve impulses arriving less frequently than one every 10 sec will be unaffected by changes in the immediately available store. Alternatively, volleys at rates faster than one every 5 sec will progressively deplete the immediately available store until mobilization achieves an equilibrium between depletion and replenishment.

The influx of calcium that accompanies each nerve volley facilitates quantal emission. Because 100–200 msec are required to complete the diffusion of calcium from the nerve terminal, impulse intervals of less than 100–200 msec (i.e., rates of greater than 5–10 Hz) result in accumulation of calcium in the terminal.

As an example, for purposes of explanation only, if 1000 quanta were present in the immediately available store, an initial nerve impulse might cause the release of 150 quanta (or 15%), leaving 850 quanta. A second impulse 500 msec later with the same ease of release as the first would produce an emission of 15% of the 850 remaining quanta or approximately 130. However, if the second volley followed the first after only 50 msec, calcium accumulation within the nerve terminal would increase the ease of release and might result in a larger emission than occurred with the first volley, even though the immediately available store was less.

Postactivation Facilitation and Exhaustion

When a nerve fires repetitively at any rate within the physiologic range, mobilization of ACh occurs that tends to replenish quanta released from the immediately available store. When the nerve stops firing, mobilization of ACh continues for several seconds, filling the immediately available store in excess of its resting state. An impulse arriving at the nerve terminal during this period will release quanta sufficient to produce an EPP amplitude greater than a single EPP elicited during the preactive resting state. This phenomenon is known as *postactivation facilitation.* Following this period, a single nerve impulse produces an EPP amplitude that is smaller than a single EPP elicited during the preactive resting state. This phenomenon, known as *postactivation exhaustion,* is best observed 2–4 minutes after the repetitive nerve volley. Its mechanism is unknown.

ELECTRODIAGNOSTIC TECHNIQUES IN THE CLINICAL LABORATORY

With single fiber electromyography one can evaluate single fiber potentials; with standard needle electromyography, one can analyze compound motor unit potentials; and with nerve stimulation, maximum compound muscle action potentials; (CMAPs) can provide information about whole muscles or groups of muscles. These techniques do not reveal or measure EPPs, but rather postsynaptic muscle fiber action potentials.

Anticholinesterase medication should be terminated, if clinically safe, at least 4–6 hours before electrophysiologic testing. Terminating it 12–24 hours before is preferable. Doing so decreases the drug-induced interference with degradation of ACh at the receptor sites.

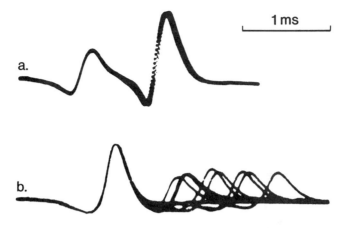

1 ms

a.

b.

Figure 9.3. Single fiber electromyography showing *A*, normal single fiber action potential pairs and *B*, very large jitter in a patient with myasthenia gravis.

Single Fiber Electromyography (SFEMG)

This technique is described in more detail in Chapter 10. It is a method of measuring intervals between the occurrence of action potentials of two or more individual muscle fibers of the same motor unit resulting from a single nerve volley. A random variation of the interval of less than 50 microsec occurs normally, but in disorders that affect the neuromuscular junction this interval, known as *jitter*, tends to increase. As jitter increases, intermittent failure of transmission occurs, a phenomenon called *blocking* (Fig. 9.3).

The standard needle electrode examination and nerve stimulation studies reveal abnormalities of neuromuscular transmission only when blocking occurs. SFEMG is therefore more sensitive in detecting abnormality, because it recognizes an abnormal increase in jitter before blocking occurs. However, because abnormal jitter can be found in conditions not in the category of diseases of neuromuscular transmission, SFEMG cannot be relied on by itself as a diagnostic tool.

Needle Electrode Examination

Perhaps the easiest test for detecting a neuromuscular transmission defect is evaluation of the motor unit action potential (MUAP) by insertion of a standard needle electrode into a muscle (38). The patient is then asked to maintain a minimal voluntary contraction, and the firing series of a single motor unit is observed and recorded. In theory, if every muscle fiber of the motor unit depolarizes with each nerve impulse and if the needle is absolutely stationary within the motor unit

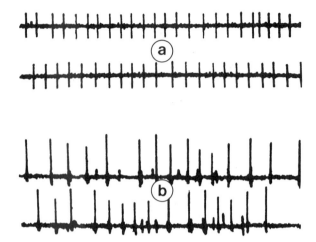

Figure 9.4. Single motor unit potential firing repetitively under voluntary control: *A*, Stable amplitude of a potential of a normal subject. *B*, Fluctuating amplitude of a potential of a patient with myasthenia gravis.

territory, then the amplitude, duration, and configuration of each successive action potential of the same motor unit will be identical. In practice, a variation of up to 5% in amplitude can occur normally. With disorders of neuromuscular transmission, individual motor unit potentials can fluctuate in amplitude during repetitive firing (Fig. 9.4).

Single Supramaximal Stimulation

Several investigators have evaluated the muscle response to a single supramaximal nerve stimulation in relation to abnormality of neuromuscular transmission (38,61). Although the amplitude is clearly below normal range in patients with myasthenic syndrome and a few with myasthenia gravis, the value of this test by itself is very limited. Supplemental studies are virtually always required to confirm a diagnosis, and it therefore should be used only to raise the electromyographer's index of suspicion that an abnormality may exist. One's time and effort are more fruitfully spent on other parts of the examination.

Repetitive Stimulation

Various methods of stimulating nerves repetitively and recording responses from muscle have been developed and are gradually being scrutinized and standardized for more accurate interpretation in the diagnosis of neuromuscular transmission defects (6,61). In 1895, Jolly (45) described a technique of observation of muscle fatigue during repetitive electrical stimulation. The method was crude by present stand-

---

Table 9.1 The Technique for Repetitive Stimulation

Select the nerve-muscle combination(s) to be studied.
Apply electrodes.
Establish supramaximal stimulation.
Determine how potentials should be displayed.
Choose the appropriate frequency of stimulation.
Evoke potentials repetitively.
Perform exercise testing as indicated.
Analyze results.

---

ards, but it was based on sound principles and the conclusions he was able to reach were remarkable for his time. The method continues to generate interest (59), although it is no longer widely used. Today, as a result of the development of electronic equipment that can accurately record the parameters of evoked CMAPs, it is possible to demonstrate slight deviations from normal muscle responses. To accomplish this, the electromyographer must pay careful attention to the details of the procedure, or confusing and erroneous results may be obtained.

The specific steps to achieve accurate results in repetitive stimulation studies are outlined in Table 9.1 and presented below. During testing, the muscle being studied should be kept between 35°C and 37°C. Cooler temperatures increase the safety factor for neuromuscular transmission and may obscure abnormalities that might otherwise be detected. The effect of temperature on myasthenic neuromuscular block has been amply demonstrated (6).

Step 1: Selection of Area to be Studied

Repetitive stimulation can be performed on any combination of nerve and muscle that is anatomically available. For instance, it is technically very simple to stimulate the ulnar nerve at the wrist and record from the hypothenar muscles of the hand. Although it may be desirable to stimulate the third cranial nerve and record from the extraocular muscles, this is technically impossible with present methods. Therefore, one must choose nerve-muscle combinations that are accessible. The recording electrode must be placed near the motor point to permit recording of a large, well-synchronized potential with initial negative deflection. Stimuli should be square wave pulses of 50-500 microsec.

There are advantages and disadvantages to the use of each nerve-muscle system that might be studied. The degree of technical difficulty must be considered, because it is a factor directly related to reliability of results. The yield of abnormality is also a factor. It can be higher at one site than another depending on the disease process. Thus, the decision as to which nerve-muscle combination to use must be based on clinical judgment.

Perhaps the most commonly examined combination is stimulation of the ulnar nerve at the wrist with the response recorded from the hypothenar muscles. This may be the simplest test to perform, and the response is technically highly reliable. Also, it is a site that is accessible to study under ischemic conditions. However, it is often less involved by the disease process than proximal sites. The median nerve-thenar test is similar, but may be technically less desirable, because movement of the hand in response to stimulation may be more difficult to avoid.

Although it is often preferable to use a proximal nerve-muscle combination, proximal sites tend, in general, to be technically more difficult to study and can be more painful. A proximal nerve-muscle system that largely avoids these problems is accessory-trapezius (19). This combination is highly recommended because the yield is comparable to other proximal sites, such as brachial plexus-infraspinatus or brachial plexus-deltoid, but the technique is much simpler and the discomfort to the patient is less.

Other useful combinations in the upper limb are median (at elbow)-flexor carpi radialis and musculocutaneous (at axilla)-biceps. The latter is not easy from a technical standpoint and requires some practice to perform.

In the lower limb, a combination that is technically easy to use is peroneal-anterior tibial. If a more proximal group is desired, femoral-quadriceps is possible.

When bulbar symptoms predominate and electrophysiologic abnormalities have not been detected in the limbs, the facial nerve can be used with surface electrodes over frontalis, orbicularis oculi, or other facial muscles.

Step 2: Application of Electrodes/Avoidance of Movement

To avoid serious error, one must be certain that both the stimulating and recording electrodes are securely fastened to the patient in a manner that eliminates movement between the electrodes and the nerve or muscle underlying them. If surface electrodes are used, the skin should be clean and dry; alcohol or other solvent is useful. Only the smallest dot of electrode paste should be used for each site to avoid extension of the paste beyond the diameter of the electrode. Each electrode should be secured to the skin with ample adhesive tape; Velcro straps or similar devices are not adequate for this purpose.

Some investigators feel that, to avoid errors, short subcutaneous needle electrodes should be used to record from the muscle. If these

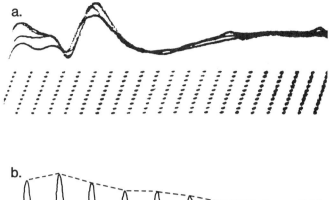

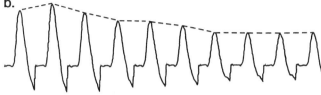

Figure 9.5. Repetitive stimulation at 2 Hz showing spurious decremental responses in normal subjects: *A*, Facial nerve to nasalis due to movement of the recording electrode. *B*, Median nerve to thenar muscles due to movement of the recording electrode. Note erratic display (highlighted by *dotted line*) resulting from faulty technique. When superimposed as in *A*, note that the baseline fluctuates, as well as the AP.

are used, care must be taken to avoid piercing the muscle with the needle, because only a few motor units will be recorded, rather than the CMAP. Also, each stimulation will cause movement of the tip of the electrode, thereby negating the recording.

For nerve stimulation, needle electrodes can also be used. With the tip of the cathode in close proximity to the nerve, only very small amounts of current are required; but if the needle is not correctly placed, local muscle contraction in the area of the electrode can easily cause the needle to shift. This can result in a change from supra- to submaximal stimulation of the nerve and lead to errors in interpretation. Whether needle or surface electrodes are used, they should not be held by hand.

In this step of the procedure, emphasis must be on immobilizing the limb being examined and anchoring the electrodes in relation to that limb so as to minimize movement between electrodes and the underlying nerves and muscles. Doing so will avoid spurious alterations in recorded responses that might be misconstrued as electrophysiologic abnormality (Fig. 9.5).

Step 3: Establishment of Supramaximal Stimulation

With each stimulus, adequate current must pass through the nerve to depolarize all the motor axons in the nerve trunk being stimulated. To determine the desired intensity, the current is increased gradually. When the first motor axon is depolarized, a threshold response is recorded; as the intensity becomes greater, the CMAP increases. When the current intensity is just sufficient to depolarize all the motor nerve fibers, the evoked potential reaches its maximum. For the purpose of these studies, it is necessary always to have this maximal evoked response to ensure a constant standard input to all neuromuscular junctions. To be certain this response occurs with each stimulus, the current intensity is increased at least 25–50% above that required for a maximal response. Periodically throughout the course of the examination, the electromyographer must determine that the stimulus has remained supramaximal.

Step 4: Selection of Frequency and Duration of Stimulation

The range of frequency of repetitive stimulation generally considered for use in detecting defects in neuromuscular transmission by electrophysiologic determinations is 1–50 Hz. (Higher frequencies may be more suitable for evaluating mechnical parameters of muscle contraction.) The recovery cycle following a single stimulus is such that, at 1-Hz stimulation, many patients with mild to moderate myasthenia gravis do not show a defect, whereas at 10 Hz, a facilitation of quantal ejection can confuse or obscure a typical myasthenic decrement. Therefore, Desmedt (18) has advocated 3-Hz stimulation to maximize decremental responses, and there is general agreement that 2–3 Hz is optimum. To avoid long-term activity-dependent alterations in the level of neuromuscular block, these trains of stimuli are applied at intervals of not less than 30 sec.

Repetitive stimulation at rates of 10–50 Hz can be used to reveal abnormality in diseases that respond to facilitation, such as the myasthenic syndrome of Lambert-Eaton or botulism intoxication. However, rapid repetitive stimulation is usually unnecessary and should be avoided whenever possible, because patient discomfort increases with increasing frequency of stimulation. A more comfortable method of inducing facilitation is to have the patient produce a maximum voluntary contraction for 10 sec in the muscle or muscle group being studied. The response to a single supramaximal stimulus immediately after exercise is compared to the response resulting from the same stimulus applied in the resting state before exercise. An increase in the post-exercise response of a few percent can be seen normally, but a marked increase is indicative of abnormality.

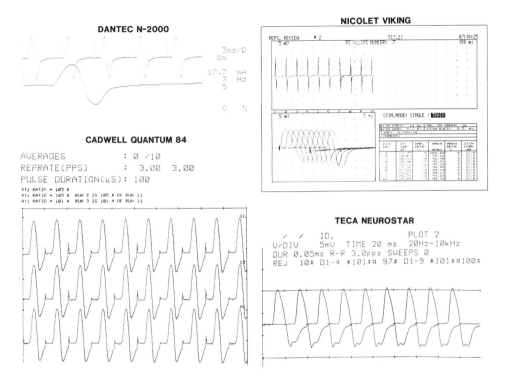

Figure 9.6. Printout displays from commercially available electromyographic equipment showing records elicited from normal subjects by repetitive stimulation.

Step 5: Determination of Mode of Display

The muscle response to repetitive nerve stimulation can be displayed and recorded in various ways. However, there are a few basic requirements. First, the display must separate each response sequentially so that amplitudes and configurations of the evoked potentials can be compared (Fig. 9.6). Second, if consecutive responses are to be evaluated manually, rather than electronically, there must be a method of permanently recording the responses so that time can be devoted to accurate measurements of the potentials. It is not sufficient to estimate alterations that may appear transiently during a brief sweep across an oscilloscope.

Step 6: Evaluation of the Evoked Potentials

With the safety factors that exist in the normal individual to preserve neuromuscular transmission at the maximum, there should never be a decrement, at least theoretically, that would not be considered abnormal. However, in practice, decrements as large as -8% occur in normal subjects during slow repetitive stimulation (1–5 Hz), so it is generally considered that a -10% decrement is required before abnormality can be established. With rapid repetitive stimulation (10–50 Hz), incremental responses are usually noted in normal subjects and may be as great as 40% (61). However, this increase is due to synchronization, and the area under the evoked potential curve does not change. To calculate percentage change, increase or decrease, a comparison is made between the amplitude of the first evoked CMAP (P1) and the amplitude of a subsequent CMAP (Ps) in the same train of responses, according to the following formula:

$$\% = \frac{100(Ps - P1)}{P1}$$

In myasthenia gravis, the maximum decrement occurring with slow repetitive stimulation usually occurs at the fourth to sixth potential. When rapid repetitive stimulation is used for studying the Lambert-Eaton syndrome, maximum facilitation may not occur for several seconds. Therefore, the initial potential might be compared to the two-, three-, or four hundredth potential.

True increments and decrements occur smoothly in a geometrical progression from one evoked potential to the next. If alterations in amplitude occur erratically, there is a technical error in performance of the procedure. The results must be discarded, the source of error eliminated, and the procedure repeated.

Step 7: Performance of Exercise Testing

The tests of repetitive stimulation described above are performed first on rested muscle. The muscle is then exercised. The duration of exercise is adjusted to the clinical picture and results of electrodiagnostic testing at that point. The exercise is always a maximal voluntary isometric contraction. Patients do not find this difficult to maintain for 15–20 sec, but when 1–2 minutes of exercise are required, they are best divided into 20-sec periods with intervals of not more than 5 sec. A more standardized method of exercise can be achieved with repetitive stimulation, but this is probably unnecessary and the discomfort to the patient makes it difficult to justify.

Step 8: Performance of Exercise under Ischemia

If efforts to this point have been unsuccessful in revealing an abnormality of neuromuscular transmission, the combination of ischemia plus exercise may expose an occult defect in patients who are suspected of having myasthenic gravis. In normal subjects, ischemia without exercise does not produce a decrement, and the combination of ischemia plus exercise does not cause a significant decrement.

To perform the test, a sphygmomanometer cuff is placed on the arm and inflated above systolic pressure. Exercise followed by electrical stimulation is done as in *Step 7* above. Because the ischemic limb becomes cold quickly, an infrared lamp should be used during the test to maintain warmth and avoid missing an abnormal response. Although ischemia limits the procedure to the distal limb muscles, a number of nerve-muscle combinations are possible and should be tried before reporting a negative result.

Summary of the Procedure for Repetitive Stimulation

If the patient has been taking drugs that affect neuromuscular transmission, these drugs should be discontinued for at least 4–6 hours prior to the examination and, if tolerated by the patient, for 12–24 hours or more.

Recording and stimulating electrodes must be applied with great care to avoid movement during the procedure relative to underlying structures. Whether using surface electrodes or subcutaneous needles or wires, the key is to avoid movement.

When a stimulus in the approximate range of 150% of maximal has been established, repetitive stimulation is initiated. For diseases that are characterized by a decrementing neuromuscular block, stimulation of 2–3 Hz before and after exercise is recommended. It is then repeated every 30 sec for 3–5 minutes. In the absence of abnormality, the procedure is repeated under ischemic conditions.

If a decrement is induced, an attempt to repair the defect can be made by producing facilitation with a 10-sec period of exercise. The additional information gained in this step can add weight to the interpretation of results.

In selected cases of diseases characterized by neuromuscular facilitation, repetitive stimulation at 10-50/sec can be tried. However, if facilitation in response to voluntary exercise can be documented, rapid repetitive stimulation may not be necessary.

SPECIAL STUDIES

Microelectrode Studies

Evaluation of the endplate region of the muscle fiber by microelectrodes has become a very fruitful method of analyzing pathophysiologic mechanisms of neuromuscular transmission. Classical techniques for recording intracellular electrical events are used.

A number of parameters can be monitored. The number of quanta released by a nerve impulse can be calculated, as well as the rate of random release and the rate at which quanta can be mobilized for release. The store of readily available quanta can be ascertained. The response of the postsynaptic membrane to a single quantum can be measured, and the sensitivity of the membrane to iontophoretically applied ACh can be estimated.

The typical microelectrode findings have been established for myasthenia gravis, myasthenic syndrome, and other better known disorders of the neuromuscular junction, such as botulinum intoxication. Microelectrode techniques, however, do not lend themselves to widespread use, and, in fact, are only available in a very limited number of laboratories. They seem likely to be most useful for research purposes and for illuminating previously unrecognized disorders of a neuromuscular transmission.

Curare Test

For many years curare has been known to accentuate the symptoms of myasthenia gravis and has been used to reveal a decremental response to repetitive stimulation that could not otherwise be detected. Because patients suffering from this disease show an exquisite sensitivity to the drug, very small doses can sometimes lead to respiratory arrest. Arrangements for management of this situation must therefore be available during the testing period. To avoid systemic administration of the drug, a regional curare test (41) has been devised by which, after application of a sphygmomanometer cuff above systolic pressure, 0.2 mg d-Tubocurarine in 20 ml of 0.9% NaCl is injected intravenously into the forearm. This is followed by repetitive stimulation under ischemic conditions. The test is designed to produce decremental responses in patients with myasthenia gravis but not in normal subjects.

Mechanical Responses

The well-known phenomenon of progressive weakness during exercise in patients with myasthenia gravis can be recorded by simple ergometry, but more quantitative methods for recording mechanical responses to electrical stimulation have been described (74).

Forces produced during isometric contractions can be recorded in a number of ways using pressure transducers or strain gauge devices. During repetitive stimulation in normal subjects, there is a successive increase in force known as the *staircase phenomenon*. In patients with myasthenia gravis, the staircase potentiation tends to be diminished, although there is no serious discrepancy between amplitudes of CMAPs and simultanously recorded forces of isometric contraction. Explanation of the staircase mechanism is still open to question, as is the possibility of abnormality of the contractile process in myasthenia gravis.

Table 9.2. Diseases that Impair Neuromuscular Transmission

Disease	Presynaptic Defect	Postsynaptic Defect	Pre-and Postsynaptic
Myasthenia gravis		X	
Lambert-Eaton myasthenic syndrome	X		
Botulism	X		
Envenomation			
Elapid snakes		X	
Black and brown widow spiders	X		
Ticks	X		
Drugs			
Chloroquin	X		
Lincomycin			X
Polymyxins			X
Tetracyclines		X	
Congenital neuromuscular syndromes			
AChE deficiency, small nerve terminals, and reduced ACh release	X		
Slow-channel syndrome		X	
Impaired ACh synthesis (familial infantile myasthenia)	X		
ACh-R deficiency		X	
Other neuromuscular syndromes			
Neurogenic abnormalities (e.g., ALS)	X		
Muscular dystrophies	X		
Myotonic disorders		X	
McArdle syndrome		X	

DISORDERS OF NEUROMUSCULAR TRANSMISSION

The causes of abnormal neuromuscular transmission are many (Table 9.2). Some disorders impair the function of the nerve terminal and are classified as presynaptic disorders. Others affect the muscle endplate and are therefore postsynaptic. Still others induce combined pre- and postsynaptic abnormalities.

When muscle weakness is minimal, fluctuating, or localized, electrodiagnostic procedures can frequently be helpful. Even in syndromes that appear to be easily recognized, electrical studies add weight to the diagnosis, provide objective documentation, and offer a monitoring method for following the course of the disease.

Myasthenia Gravis

Autoimmune myasthenia gravis is a disease characterized by weakness that increases with muscular effort and improves with rest. Any striated muscle group may be affected. Typically, there is ptosis of the eyelids and diplopia. Weakness of the face, neck, and limbs is also common, and other signs and symptoms, such as dysarthria and difficulty chewing, may also be present. The patient is most functional in the morning and worsens as the day progresses. Asymmetry is common. Spontaneous remissions and exacerbations are characteristic. Symptoms may begin at any age, usually in the second through fourth decades. Females have a peak incidence in the early thirties and a predominance overall of about 2:1. The peak incidence for males is in the late fifties.

Various clinical types of myasthenia gravis were classified by Osserman (60). Although his groupings remain firmly entrenched, they have been extended to reflect the more recent understanding of the heterogeneous nature of the disease (11).

It is now accepted that the defect in autoimmune myasthenia gravis is postsynaptic and that the primary abnormality is the destruction of endplate receptors by antibodies directed against the receptor proteins (63). The loss of receptor sites was established through the use of α-bungarotoxin (a snake venom that combines selectively and irreversibly with the active sites of ACh receptors) that was labeled with radioactive iodine. By measuring the quantity of the bound radioactive label, the number of receptor sites per junction was determined (30). A striking loss of receptors was noted in patients with myasthenia gravis, and this was later confirmed both by toxin-binding assays (34) and by quantitative measurements of ACh sensitivity (2).

A large percentage of patients with myasthenia gravis have antireceptor antibodies in their sera. However, there is a group of patients, including some patients with recent onset acquired autoimmune myasthenia and some with the ocular form, who lack detectable antibodies. This group also includes patients who probably do not have an autoimmune basis for their disease. Whether or not antireceptor antibodies are present, electrophysiologic studies preceding serum assay are useful to exclude neuromuscular disease that may mimic myasthenia. The usefulness of various laboratory techniques in the diagnosis of myasthenia gravis has been reported (48).

Muscle weakness, the clinical hallmark of all diseases that impair the function of the neuromuscular junction, is the result of blocking of transmission of the electrical impulse from nerve terminal to muscle fiber because depolarization at the endplate is insufficient to reach threshold. In myasthenia gravis, the amplitude of the depolarization is reduced because a decreased number of receptor sites diminishes the possibility of interaction of ACh and receptor molecules, even though quantal emission from the nerve terminal remains normal. Miniature endplate potentials are abnormally small; this in turn reduces the amplitude of the endplate spike, thus narrowing the safety margin for neuromuscular transmission.

In myasthenia gravis, the typical electrophysiologic abnormality is a decremental response of the CMAP amplitude to repeated stimuli at a rate of 2–3 Hz (16). Usually, there is an initial decrement until the fourth to sixth potential; then a transient increase is followed by a second, more slowly progressive decrease. The initial decrement should be 8–10% before being considered abnormal, and it must be reproducible. Because the neuromuscular junction requires about 12 sec to recover from a single shock, and more time is needed for recovery from multiple stimuli, the muscle must be rested at least 15 sec before repeating the tests. A 30-sec interval between repetitive stimulation studies is the standard minimum in the clinical laboratory.

Tests are continued through the period of postactivation exhaustion, which requires 10–15 min for recovery.

The evaluation of how exercise affects the response of myasthenic muscle to slow repetitive stimulation (1–5 Hz) is very helpful in assessing patients with myasthenia gravis. If there is a decremental response before exercise, a 10-sec voluntary tetanic contraction of the muscle will reveal postactivation facilitation by partially or completely repairing of the decrement when the study is repeated immediately after the contraction. About 2–4 minutes after the contraction, postactivation exhaustion results in a decrement that is more marked than it had been in the well-rested muscle. To maximize this effect, a 1–2 minute voluntary tetanic contraction is usually optimal. Thus, it is useful to test the muscle first at rest, then immediately after a 10-sec period of exercise, and finally, at 2, 3, and 4 minutes after 1–2 minutes of exercise (Fig. 9.7). The response returns to its pre-exercise state about 10–15 minutes after the 1-to-2-minute period of exercise.

Several muscles, proximal and distal, should be examined. The distal muscles are usually easier to test, but the proximal muscles tend to have a higher yield of abnormality and larger decremental responses.

Repetitive stimulation at 10–50 Hz may or may not induce an initial decrement, but often results in an incremental response, usually less than 30%, but sometimes greater than 40–50%. It should be noted also that, even at rates of 1–5 Hz, incremental responses can be found (55, 57). However, the more typical decremental findings of myasthenia gravis are usually detectable in other muscles or in the same muscles at other times.

SFEMG is more sensitive in detecting pathophysiology in myasthenia

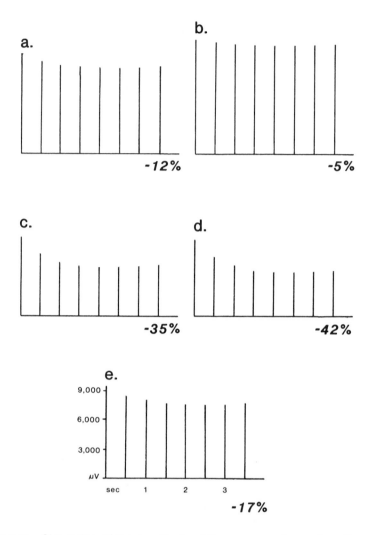

Figure 9.7. Simulation of the amplitude of the compound muscle action potentials following repetitive supramaximal nerve stimulation in moderately severe myasthenia gravis. *A*, before exercise; *B*, immediately after exercise; *C*, 2 minutes after exercise; *D*, 4 minutes after exercise; and *E*, 8 minutes after exercise.

gravis than the repetitive stimulation studies (48) because no abnormality occurs in the latter until blocking of neuromuscular transmission occurs, whereas SFEMG detects abnormal jitter that precedes blocking. However, SFEMG must never be used as the sole criterion for determining the diagnosis because increased jitter is observed in neuropathies, anterior horn cell disorders, and some myopathies as well.

Because routine EMG delineates these problems, it should be an integral part of the evaluation of a patient suspected of having myasthenia gravis.

A useful method of establishing that a reproducible decremental response is not spurious but is due to an impairment of neuromuscular transmission is to administer edrophonium chloride (Tensilon) to the patient and then to check for a repair of the decrement. The technique is the same as is used clinically for detecting a postinjection increase in strength (73). Although this is a strongly confirmatory test when the decrement is repaired, it is not usually required for the diagnosis.

Several other tests have been reported as helpful in diagnosing myasthenia gravis. Some of these include increasing postactivation exhaustion by ischemia (20), the regional curare test combined with repetitive stimulation studies (41), repetitive stapedius reflex testing (76), and electronystagmography (8).

Lambert-Eaton Myasthenic Syndrome

The Lambert-Eaton myasthenia syndrome (LEMS) was first described in 1956 (51). Its link to carcinoma, particularly small cell carcinoma of the lung, was evident from the start, but many cases have subsequently been reported, mainly in women, that are unassociated with carcinoma.

The clinical presentation (39) is of weakness, predominantly proximal, especially in the pelvic girdle and thighs. As the condition progresses, weakness and easy fatigability can be profound. Aching of the thighs occurs, muscle stretch reflexes disappear, and dryness of the mouth develops. Some patients note paresthesia, dysphagia, or impotence. In a few the condition is complicated by ptosis, diplopia, and dysarthria. The syndrome tends to occur after the age of 40, but has been reported as early as age 9. There is a male predominance of about 1.5:1.

The abnormality is presynaptic, and the characteristic defect (25) is a very low number of quanta being released in response to a nerve action potential, even though available stores of ACh are normal. MEPP amplitudes are normal, whereas EPP amplitudes are so diminished that they often fail to reach threshold.

It seems that LEMS is an autoimmune phenomenon. It has been demonstrated (52) that the defect in neuromuscular transmission can be transferred to mice via the IgG fraction of plasma from patients with LEMS. Also, a decrease in the number of active zones for ACh release at the presynaptic membrane of the nerve terminal has been documented (32), which is presumably the result of antibodies directed at the protein components of the active sites.

In LEMS, because facilitation of neuromuscular transmission occurs

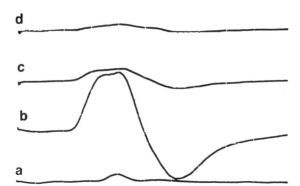

Figure 9.8 Lambert-Eaton myasthenic syndrome: single supramaximal stimulus (ulnar-hypothenar) *A*, at rest, *B*, immediately after 10 sec exercise, *C*, 15 sec after exercise, *D*, 30 sec after exercise.

during voluntary contraction, the condition is well advanced before the patient begins to perceive weakness. Therefore, even those patients with mild symptoms have easily detectable electrophysiologic abnormalities. With the muscle at rest, a single supramaximal stimulus evokes only a very low amplitude CMAP. Immediately after a maximum-effort, voluntary contraction of 10 sec duration, the amplitude evoked by a single shock increases 2–19 times (mean 6 times) (50). (The incremental response sometimes seen in myasthenia gravis under the same conditions never exceeds two times the amplitude of the initial potential.) The size of the response then decreases rapidly toward the resting state over the next 15-30 sec after exercise (Fig. 9.8).

At stimulation rates of 1–5 Hz, decremental responses are seen very much as in myasthenia gravis. Also, there is a postactivation exhaustion at 2–4 minutes. The key difference between the two diseases at these slow rates of stimulation is the striking facilitation of 200% or more in LEMS immediately following exercise. This is similar to the facilitation seen with single stimuli before and after exercise.

Rapid rates of stimulation (20–50 Hz) are very effective in demonstrating the facilitation phenomenon in LEMS (Fig. 9.9) and can be used to characterize further (49) the abnormal increment detected by 10 sec of a voluntary maximum muscle contraction. However, rapid stimulation is quite uncomfortable and usually unnecessary.

When a conventional needle electrode is inserted into a muscle, single motor unit potentials are seen to vary in shape and amplitude from moment to moment. At times, the repetitive firing of a motor unit can induce a progressive facilitation of its own action potential.

The increase of jitter and blocking detected by SFEMG (7) is more

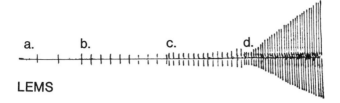

Figure 9.9. Lambert-Eaton myasthenia syndrome: repetitive supramaximal stimulation of the median nerve at *A*, 5 Hz, *B*, 10 Hz, *C*, 20 Hz, and *D*, 40 Hz recording from thenar muscles.

pronounced than in myasthenia gravis. Also, the facilitation of neuromuscular transmission that occurs at high rates of firing of the motor unit causes the jitter to revert toward normal.

The electrophysiologic abnormalities in LEMS can be detected in any muscle, distal as well as proximal, with equal facility. Also, the findings do not vary from one limb to another. Therefore, it is not necessary to study a large number of muscles distally and proximally, as it is in myasthenia gravis.

Botulism

Botulism is a syndrome caused by various toxins elaborated by the bacterium *Clostridium botulinum,* an ubiquitous anaerobic spore-former that causes human pathology under three circumstances. The first is by ingestion of the toxin through poisoned food, usually improperly home-canned vegetables in which unkilled organisms thrive in the anaerobic environment. The second circumstance occurs when the organism continues its life cycle within ischemic tissue in a wound. This may be difficult to diagnose if the wound is not obvious, because the symptoms can be confused with myasthenia gravis or some other neuromuscular disease. The third way in which the toxin affects humans was not recognized until 1976 (65). It occurs when the clostridium spore colonizes the large intestine and, by releasing the toxin slowly, produces gradually progressive weakness. This syndrome is known as infant botulism because it only happens during the first year of life.

Symptoms of botulism (66, 79) result from blockage at parasympathetic and skeletal neuromuscular junctions. Dryness of the mouth and difficulty focusing visually to a near point are very common complaints. The latter difficulty is often interpreted by the patient as dizziness or blurred vision. Other symptoms include photophobia, constipation (although nausea, vomiting, and diarrhea may occur early in food botulism), difficulty with urination, dysphagia, dysphonia, dysarthria, and diplopia. Generalized weakness develops gradually and is most evident in the neck flexors and proximally in the upper limbs. Ventilatory insufficiency is manifested by tachypnea and/or dyspnea. In infant botulism, constipation may be the first sign, followed over 2 or 3 days by the loss of the ability to suck strongly. Hypotonia then becomes manifest, followed by respiratory insufficiency.

The main physiologic abnormality in botulism (75) is a blocking of quantal release of ACh from the nerve terminals. In addition, quantal size is low normal, and the number of available quanta in the nerve terminal is abnormally low. Intracellular microelectrode studies demonstrate a small reduction in MEPP amplitude and a marked decrease in MEPP frequency. However, quantal reactions with the postsynaptic membrane remain completely normal.

Clinical electrophysiologic testing demonstrates the abnormality in several ways (9, 14, 36). Amplitudes of CMAPs evoked by a single supramaximal stimulus tend to be in the low normal range or smaller and can be less than a millivolt. Immediately following a 10-sec tetanic muscle contraction, the amplitude of a single muscle action potential may reveal considerable facilitation, but not to a degree comparable to that seen in Lambert-Eaton myasthenic syndrome. Although some patients can provide a voluntary contraction, a tetanic electrical nerve stimulus must be used for infants and for those patients who are very weak. Interestingly, facilitation in botulism, unlike in LEMS, lasts several minutes. Slow repetitive stimulation does not induce a decremental response as it does in LEMS. Nerve conduction remains completely normal.

On needle electrode examination, motor unit potentials are low in amplitude and fibrillation can be seen, presumably because blocking at the nerve terminal is so complete and irreversible that the muscle fiber is effectively denervated. Recovery occurs through collateral sprouting of intramuscular nerve fibers and the re-establishment of new neuromuscular junctions (22). SFEMG reveals abnormal jitter that improves as the firing rate of the motor unit increases.

Envenomation

Several animal toxins have their effect at the neuromuscular junction. Neuromuscular blockade by the venoms of elapid snakes has been extensively studied (54). The mechanism is binding of the toxin to the active sites of ACh-Rs on the postsynaptic membrane. Cobra toxin in particular has been shown to reproduce in rats all the typical features of human myasthenia gravis (69).

Venoms from the black widow spider and the brown recluse have diffuse stimulating effects on the central and peripheral nervous systems. At the neuromuscular junction, the mechanism is presynaptic and results in excessive release of ACh. Black widow venom causes persistent release (42); release associated with brown recluse venom is discontinuous (16).

Certain species of ticks elaborate a salivary toxin that produces a syndrome of generalized weakness. Depending on the species, the pathologic mechanism may inhibit release of ACh indirectly by impairing conduction in neuron terminals (58) or may produce its inhibiting effect directly by interfering with the presynaptic physiology normally triggered by the nerve impulse (13). The clinical electrophysiology associated with tick paralysis has been described (10, 78).

Toxins from the scorpion, as well as the bee, wasp, and hornet, have been implicated in having an effect on the neuromuscular junction. However, the clinical disturbance in humans is not prominent.

Drug-Induced Neuromuscular Syndromes

Morbidity and even mortality can result from drug-induced disorders of neuromuscular transmission. Because these unusual but well-documented syndromes (4) are potentially reversible by discontinuance of the drug, the importance of recognizing them is readily apparent.

The most common manifestation of drug-induced neuromuscular blockade is postoperative respiratory depression, but syndromes that mimic myasthenia gravis are well known. Furthermore, drugs that impair neuromuscular transmission can unmask such disorders as myasthenia gravis that are not clinically manifest, presumably because the safety factor for neuromuscular transmission has not been reduced into a symptomatic range before administration of the drug.

A few of the possible mechanisms of drug-induced blockade are known. One is the inhibition of ACh release by interference with propagation of the nerve action potential at the terminal. Chloroquin (81) and lincomycin (68) are offenders of this type. Another mechanism is postsynaptic blockade at the receptor site by polymyxins and tetracyclines (86), among other drugs. Other drugs, such as propranolol (84), have been shown to interfere both pre- and postsynaptically.

A drug that can cause a myasthenic picture clinically without itself affecting the neuromuscular junction is D-penicillamine. It impairs neuromuscular transmission through an immunologically mediated reaction directed against the endplate.

Congenital Neuromuscular Syndromes

These syndromes are unrelated to transient neonatal myasthenia in infants born to mothers with myasthenia gravis. There are at least four congenital myasthenic syndromes (27), but because possibilities for a much wider range of related diseases exist, it is likely that other genetic myasthenic syndromes await discovery. One syndrome, familial infantile myasthenia, is often distinguished from congenital myasthenia, but this separation is disputed (72). Familial autoimmune myasthenia gravis has recently been reported for the first time (62).

Congenital Endplate Acetylcholinesterase Deficiency, Small Nerve Terminals, and Reduced ACh Release

Only one case of this syndrome has been reported (28). The patient presented with weakness and fatigability of all muscles at birth. When seen at age 15, he had intermittent ptosis and generalized weakness that did not respond to edrophonium or neostigmine. On EMG, individual motor unit potentials varied in amplitude from moment to moment. Decremental amplitudes of CMAPs were noted in response to repetitive nerve stimulation at 2 Hz. Single nerve stimuli resulted in repetitive muscle twitches. The latter, plus lack of response to anticholinesterase medication, was attributed to AChE deficiency. Intracellular microelectrode studies revealed a low frequency of MEPPs and low quantal release following nerve stimulus, both of which were felt to be associated with smallness of nerve terminals that averaged one-fourth to one-third of normal size.

Slow-Channel Syndrome, an Abnormality of ACH-Rs

This syndrome has been studied in six patients: five from two families and one sporadic case (29). Inheritance appears to be autosomal dominant. Onset can begin in infancy, but is variable chronologically. Weakness and wasting of scapular and forearm muscles are sometimes accompanied by involvement of ocular, masticatory, facial, and cervical muscles. A single nerve stimulus evokes repetitive muscle action potentials in all muscles tested. Because there is no AChE deficiency, this phenomenon has been explained by a prolonged open time of the ACh-R ion channels. Clinically involved muscles show a decremental response to repetitive nerve stimulation.

Syndrome of Assumed Abnormality of ACh Synthesis

This syndrome has been reported by several authors (1, 12, 35, 37, 67), and is, or appears to be, the single disease entity often called familial infantile myasthenia. The inheritance is probably autosomal recessive. It is noted soon after birth and is characterized by intermittent ptosis and opthalmoparesis, easy fatigability, and difficulty feeding. Episodic apnea has been reported following crying, vomiting, and febrile illness and occasionally is fatal. Marked weakness results from exercise; recovery of strength follows 10–20 minutes of rest. Symptoms improve with age, although severe respiratory exacerbations can continue into early adult life. Electrophysiologically, a decremental response at 2-Hz stimulation can be found in weak muscles or in other muscles following a few minutes of sustained exercise. (In infants, a sustained muscle contraction can be achieved by 10 Hz stimulation.) The findings are similar to those detected in studies of normal muscle treated with hemicholinium (an inhibitor of choline uptake by the nerve terminal).

Congenital ACh-R Deficiency

This syndrome may be less than clearly defined in that not all cases show a reduction in ACh-Rs (53, 56, 82). It presents with findings similar to autoimmune myasthenia gravis, although no serum antibodies to ACh-R are present. As in autoimmune myasthenia gravis, neuromuscular transmission fails because a reduction in functioning ACh-Rs results in decreased MEPP amplitudes. This in turn reduces the EPP's safety factor.

Miscellaneous Neuromuscular Syndromes

In a number of neuromuscular diseases, failure of neuromuscular transmission may result from pathology that does not directly affect the neuromuscular junction. Abnormalities may be due to impaired excitability of nerve terminals or muscle fibers or to other secondary effects.

Neurogenic Abnormalities

Electrophysiologic disturbances suggesting impairment of neuromuscular transmission are well documented in diseases that affect the motor neuron. Amyotrophic lateral sclerosis (5, 17, 77) and a spectrum of peripheral polyneuropathies (80) are particularly well studied. Sites of malfunction likely to account for observed abnormalities are (a) junctions undergoing degeneration, (b) immature junctions resulting from collateral sprouting or nerve regeneration, and (c) impaired conduction in newly formed terminal nerve endings. The first two may be associated with smaller stores of ACh available for release and impaired ACh release mechanisms. They probably are responsible for decremental responses seen at stimulus frequencies of 3 Hz or less. In decremental responses that occur at frequencies exceeding 10 Hz, all three sources probably play a role.

In addition to decremental responses, postactivation facilitation and exhaustion may be detected (Fig. 9.10). Motor unit potentials may vary in amplitude from moment to moment, and SFEMG may reveal increased jitter and blocking. Electrophysiologic abnormalities are more likely to be found in weaker muscles and when the disease is actively progressive, rather than chronic.

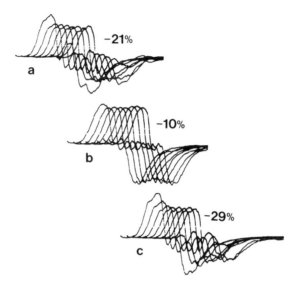

Figure 9.10 Amyotrophic lateral sclerosis: repetitive supramaximal stimulation of the peroneal nerve at 2 Hz, recording from a severely denervated anterior tibialis *A*, before exercise, *B*, immediately after 30 sec exercise, *C*, 2 minutes after exercise.

Muscular Dystrophies

Decremental responses, increased jitter, and impulse blocking occur in limb-girdle, facioscapulohumeral, and especially Duchenne muscular dystrophies. Although they are primary muscle diseases, it is well recognized that these conditions are associated with muscle fiber denervation and reinnervation (21). Thus, it seems likely that the comments offered in the preceding section to explain abnormalities of neuromuscular transmission in neurogenic disease apply also to the muscular dystrophies.

Myotonic Disorders

Repetitive stimulation results in decremental amplitudes of the M wave in myotonic dystrophy, myotonia congenita, and paramyotonia (3). Decrements do not begin early in the train of stimuli and do not plateau as they do in myasthenia gravis. They can be evoked by direct muscle stimulation, which is consistent with a postjunctional defect. Repetitive stimulation causes repetitive firing, then inexcitability, and later a return of excitability of the sarcolemmal membrane. Increasing frequencies of stimulation are associated with increasing decrements.

This is a depolarization block. In paramyotonia congenita, cooling of the rested muscle increases the decrement.

Periodic Paralysis

The amplitude of the CMAP evoked by a single supramaximal nerve stimulus is abnormally small in proportion to the degree of muscle weakness (7). Repetitive stimulation may produce an incremental response that decreases during rest.

McArdle Syndrome

During exercise, glycogen is not converted to lactic acid because there is a deficiency of myophosphorylase (23). Firmness of the muscle develops that is not correlated with electrical activity of the muscle membrane; that is, an electrically silent contracture develops. This phenomenon can be reproduced by rapid repetitive stimulation during which time a gradually decreasing CMAP is recorded.

Diseases of the Central Nervous System

Reports of progressive muscle weakness during exercise followed by recovery with rest in patients with encephalitis have been reviewed (19), but this phenomenon has not been systematically studied electrodiagnostically. Similar symptoms have been recognized in some patients with multiple sclerosis, and electrophysiologic studies (24, 64, 83) support these findings with the demonstration of decremental responses, increased jitter, and fluctuation of motor unit potential amplitudes. Improvement with administration of anticholinesterase medication has also been documented. The pathophysiologic mechanism remains uncertain, but it has been postulated that the defect is the result of abnormality in the peripheral motor neuron.

References

1. Albers JW, Faulkner JA, Dorovini-Zis K, Barald KF, Must RE, Ball RD: Abnormal neuromuscular transmission in an infantile myasthenic syndrome. *Ann Neurol* 16:28-34, 1984.
2. Albuquerque EX, Rash JE, Mayer RF, Satterfield JR: An electrophysiological and morphological study of the neuromuscular junctions in patients with myasthenia gravis. *Exp Neurol* 51:536-563, 1976.
3. Aminoff MJ, Layzer RB, Satya-Murti S. Faden AI: The declining electrical response of muscle to repetitive nerve stimulation in myotonia. *Neurology* 27:812-816, 1977.
4. Argov Z, Mastaglia FL: Disorders of neuromuscular transmission caused by drugs. *N Engl J Med 301:409-413, 1979.*
5. Bernstein LP, Antel JP: Motor neuron disease: decremental responses to repetitive nerve stimulation. *Neurology* 31:202-204, 1981.
6. Borenstein S. Desmedt JE: New diagnostic procedures in myasthenia gravis. In Desmedt JE (ed): *New Developments in Electromyography and Clinical Neurophysiology,* Vol 1. Basel, S Karger, 1973, pp 350–374.

7. Campa JF, Sanders DB: Familial hypokalemic periodic paralysis: local recovery after nerve stimulation. *Arch Neurol* 31:110-115, 1974.

8. Campbell MJ, Simpson E. Crombie AL, Walton JN: Ocular myasthenia and evaluation of tensilon tonography and electronystagmography as diagnostic tests. *J Neurol Neurosurg Psychiat* 33:639-646, 1970.

9. Cherington M: Electrophysiologic methods as an aid in diagnosis of botulism: a review. *Muscle Nerve* 5:S28–S29, 1982.

10. Cherington M, Snyder R: Tick paralysis, neurophysiologic studies. *N Engl J Med* 278:95-97, 1968.

11. Compston DAS, Vincent A, Newsom-Davis J, Batchelor JR: Clinical, pathological, HLA antigen and immunological evidence for disease heterogeneity in myasthenia gravis. *Brain* 103:579-601, 1980.

12. Conomy JP, Levinsohn M, Fanaroff A: Familial infantile myasthenia gravis: a cause of sudden death in young children. *J Pediatr* 87:428-430, 1975.

13. Cooper BJ, Spence I: Temperature-dependent inhibition of evoked acetylcholine release in tick paralysis. *Nature* 263:693-695, 1976.

14. Cornblath DR, Sladky JT, Sumner AJ: Clinical electrophysiology of infantile botulism. *Muscle Nerve* 6:448-452, 1983.

15. Decino P: Transmitter release properties along regenerated nerve processes at the frog neuromuscular junction. *J Neurosci* 1:308-317, 1981.

16. DelCastillo J, Pumplin DW: Discrete and discontinuous action of brown widow spider venom on the presynaptic nerve terminals of frog muscle. *J Physiol* (Lond) 252:491-508, 1975.

17. Denys EH, Norris FH Jr: Amyotrophic lateral sclerosis: impairment of neuromuscular transmission. *Arch Neurol* 36:202-205, 1979.

18. Desmedt JE: The neuromuscular disorder in myasthenia gravis. In Desmedt JE (ed): *New Developments in Electromyography and Clinical Neurophysiology*, vol 1. Basel, S Karger, 1973, pp 241-305.

19. Desmedt JE, Borenstein S: Regeneration in Duchenne muscular dystrophy. *Arch Neurol* 33:642-650, 1976.

20. Desmedt JE, Borenstein S: Double-step nerve stimulation test for myasthenic block: sensitization of post-activation exhaustion by ischemia. *Ann Neurol* 1:55-64, 1977.

21. Dodge FA Jr. Miledi R, Rahamimoff R: Strontium and quantal release of transmitter at the neuromuscular junction. *J Physiol* (Lond) 200:267-283, 1969.

22. Duchen LW: An electronmicroscopic study of the changes induced by botulism toxin in the motor endplate of slow and fast skeletal muscle fibers of the mouse. *J Neurol Sci* 14:47-60, 1971.

23. Dyken ML, Smith DM, Peak RL: An electromyographic diagnostic screening test in McArdle's disease and a case report. Neurology 17:45-50, 1967.

24. Eisen A, Yufe R, Trop D, Campbell I: Reduced neuromuscular transmission safety factor in multiple sclerosis. *Neurology* 28:598-602, 1978.

25. Elmqvist D, Lambert EH: Detailed analysis of neuromuscular transmission in a patient with myasthenic syndrome sometimes associated with bronchogenic carcinoma. *Mayo Clin Proc* 43:689-713, 1968.

26. Elmqvist D, Quastel DMJ: Presynaptic action of hemicholinium at the neuromuscular junction. *J Physiol* 177:463-482, 1965.

27. Engel AG: Myasthenia gravis and myasthenic syndromes. *Ann Neurol* 16:519-534, 1984.

28. Engel AG, Lambert EH, Gomez MR: A new myasthenic syndrome with endplate acetylcholinesterase deficiency, small nerve terminals, and reduced acetylcholine release. *Ann Neurol* 1:315-330, 1977.

29. Engel AG, Lambert EH, Mulder DM, Torres CF, Sahashi K, Bertorini TE, Whitaker JN: A newly recognized congenital myasthenic syndrome attributed to a prolonged open time of the acetylcholine-induced ion channel. *Ann Neurol* 11:553-569, 1982.

30. Fambrough DM, Drachman DB, Satyamurti S: Neuromuscular junction in myasthenia gravis: decreased acetylcholine receptors. *Science* 182:293-295, 1973.
31. Fatt P, Katz B: Spontaneous subthreshold activity at motor nerve endings. *J Physiol* (Lond) 117:109-128, 1952.
32. Fukunaga H, Engel AG, Osame M, Lambert EH: Paucity of presynaptic membrane active zones in Lambert-Eaton myasthenic syndrome. *Muscle Nerve* 5:686-697, 1982.
33. Gopfert H, Schaefer H: Uber den direkt und indirekt erregten Aktionsstrom und das Funktion der motorischen endplatte. *Pflugers Arch Ges Physiol* 239:597-619, 1938.
34. Green DPL, Miledi R, Vincent A: Neuromuscular transmission after immunization against acetylcholine receptors. *Proc Roy Soc Lond* [Biol] 189:57-68, 1975.
35. Greer M, Schatland M: Myasthenia gravis in the newborn. *Pediatrics* 26:101-108, 1960.
36. Gutmann L, Pratt L: Pathophysiologic aspects of human botulism. *Arch Neurol* 33:175-179, 1976.
37. Hart Z, Sahashi K, Lambert EH, Engel AG, Linstrom JM: A congenital, familial myasthenic syndrome caused by a presynaptic defect of transmitter resynthesis or mobilization (Abstract). Neurology (NY) 29:556, 1979.
38. Harvey AM, Masland RL: A method for the study of neuromuscular transmission in human subjects. *Bull Johns Hopkins Hosp* 68:81-93, 1940.
39. Henriksson KG, Nilsson O, Rosen I, Schiller HH: Clinical, neurophysiological and morphological findings in Eaton-Lambert syndrome. *Acta Neurol Scand* 56:117-140, 1977.
40. Heuser JE, Reese TS, Dennis MJ, Jan Y, Evans L: Synaptic vesicle exocytosis captured by quick freezing and correlation with quantal transmitter release. *J Cell Biol* 81:275-300, 1979.
41. Horowitz SH, Jenkins G, Kornfeld P, Papatestas AE: Regional curare test in evaluation of ocular myasthenia. *Arch Neurol* 32:83:88, 1975.
42. Howard BD, Gundersen CB Jr: Effects and mechanisms of polypeptide neurotoxins that act presynaptically. *Ann Rev Pharmacol Toxicol* 20:307-336, 1980.
43. Hubbard JI: Repetitive stimulation at the mamalian neuromuscular junction, and the mobilization of transmitter. *J Physiol* 169:641-662, 1963.
44. Hubbard JI: Microphysiology of vertebrate neuromuscular transmission. *Physiol Rev* 53:674-725, 1973.
45. Jolly F: Uber Myasthenia Gravis pseudoparalytica. *Berl Klin Wschr* 32:1-7, 1895
46. Katz B. Miledi R: The binding of acetylcholine to receptors and its removal from the synaptic cleft. *J Physiol* 231:549-574, 1973.
47. Katz B, Miledi R: Transmitter leakage from motor nerve endings. *Proc Roy Soc Lond* [Biol] 196:59-72, 1977.
48. Kelly JJ, Daube JR, Lennon VA, Howard FM Jr, Younge BR: The laboratory diagnosis of mild myasthenia gravis. *Ann Neurol* 2:238-242, 1982.
49. Lambert EH: Defects of neuromuscular transmission in syndromes other than myasthenia gravis. *Ann NY Acad Sci* 135:367-384, 1966.
50. Lambert EH, Rooke ED: Myasthenic state and lung cancer. In Brain WR, Norris FH Jr (eds): *The Remote Effects of Cancer on the Nervous System.* New York, Grune & Stratton, 1965, pp 67-80.
51. Lambert EH, Eaton IM, Rooke ED: Defect of neuromuscular conduction associated with malignant neoplasm. *Am J Physiol* 187:612-613, 1956.
52. Lang B. Newsom-Davis J, Wray D, Vincent A, Murray N: Autoimmune etiology for myasthenic (Eaton-Lambert) syndrome. *Lancet* 2:224-226, 1981.
53. Lecky BRF, Morgan-Hughes JA, Murray NMF, Landon DN, Wray D, Prior C: Congenital myasthenia: further evidence of disease heterogeneity. *Muscle Nerve* 9:233-242, 1986.

54. Lee CY: Chemistry and pharmacology of polypeptide toxins in snake vernoms. *Ann Rev Pharmacol* 12:265-286, 1972.
55. Mayer RF, Williams IR: Incrementing responses in myasthenia gravis. *Arch Neurol* 31:24-26, 1974.
56. Morgan-Hughes JA, Lecky BRF, Landon DN, Murray NMH: Alterations in the number and affinity of junctional acetylcholine receptors in a myopathy with tubular aggregates: a newly recognized receptor defect. *Brain* 104:279-295, 1981.
57. Mori M, Takamori M: Hyperthyroidism and myasthenia gravis with features of Eaton-Lambert syndrome. *Neurology* 26:882-887, 1976.
58. Murnaghan M: Conduction block of terminal somatic motor fibers in tick paralysis. *Can J Biochem Physiol* 38:287-295, 1960.
59. Oh SJ, Nichihira T, Sarala PK: The diagnostic value of the Jolly test: reappraisal. Presented at the 23rd annual meeting of the AAEE, San Diego, 1976.
60. Osserman KE: *Myasthenia Gravis.* New York, Grune & Stratton, 1958, pp 79-80.
61. Ozdemir C, Young RR: The results to be expected from electrical testing in the diagnosis of myasthenia gravis. *Ann NY Acad Sci* 274:203-222, 1976.
62. Pascuzzi RM, Sermas A, Phillips LH II, Johns TR: Familial autoimmune myasthenia gravis and thymoma: occurrence in two brothers. *Neurology* (Minneap) 36:423-427, 1986.
63. Patrick J, Lindstrom J: Autoimmune response to acetylcholine receptor. *Science* 180:871-872, 1973.
64. Patten BM, Hert A, Lovelace R: Multiple sclerosis associated with defects in neuromuscular transmission. *J Neurol Neurosurg Paychiat* 35:385-394, 1972.
65. Pickett J, Berg B, Chaplin E, Brunstetter-Schafer M-A: Syndrome of botulism in infancy: clinical and electrophysiologic study. *N Engl J Med* 295:770-772, 1976.
66. Rapoport S, Watkins PB: Descending paralysis resulting from occult wound botulism. *Ann Neurol* 16:359-361, 1984.
67. Robertson WC Jr, Chun RWM, Kornguth SE: Familial infantile myasthenia. *Arch Neurol* 37:117-119, 1980.
68. Rubbo JT, Gergis SD, Sokoll MD: Comparative neuromuscular effects of lincomycin and clindamycin. *Anesth Analg* (Cleve) 56:329-332, 1977.
69. Stayamurti S, Drachman DB, Slone F: Blockade of acetylcholine receptors: a model of myasthenia gravis. *Science* 187:955-957, 1975.
70. Schumm F, Stohr M: Accessory nerve stimulation in the assessment of myasthenia gravis. *Muscle Nerve* 7:141-151, 1984.
71. Schwartz MS, Stalberg E: Myasthenic syndrome studied with single fiber electromyography. *Arch Neurol* 32:815–818, 1975.
72. Scoppetta C, Casali C, Piantelli M: Congenital myasthenia gravis. *Muscle Nerve* 5:493, 1982.
73. Seybold ME: The office tensilon test for ocular myasthenia gravis. *Arch Neurol* 43:842-843, 1986.
74. Slomic A, Rosenfalck A, Buchthal F: Electrical and mechanical response of normal and myasthenic muscle. *Brain Res* 10:1-74, 1968.
75. Spitzer N: Miniature endplate potentials at mammalian neuromuscular junctions poisoned by botulism toxin. *Nature New Biol* 237:26-27, 1972.
76. Stalberg E: Clinical electrophysiology in myasthenia gravis. *J Neurol Neurosurg Psychiat* 43:622-633, 1980.
77. Stalberg E, Schwartz MS, Trontelj JV: Single-fiber electromyography in various processes affecting the anterior horn cell.*J Neurol Sci* 24:403-415, 1975.
78. Swift TR, Ignacio OJ: Tick paralysis: electrophysiologic studies. *Neurology* (Minneap) 25:1130-1133, 1975.

79. Terranova W, Palumbo JN, Breman JG: Ocular findings in botulism type B. *JAMA* 241:475-477, 1979.

80. Thiele B, Stalberg E: Single-fiber electromyography findings in polyneuropathies of different etiology. *J Neurol Neurosurg Psychiat* 38:881-889, 1975.

81. Vartanian GA, Chinyanga HM: The mechanism of acute neuromuscular weakness induced by chloroquine. *Can J Physiol Pharmacol* 50:1099-1103, 1972.

82. Vincent A, Cull-Candy SG, Newsom-Davis J, Trautman A, Molenaar PC, Polak RL: Congenital myasthenia: endplate acetylcholine receptors and electrophysiology in five cases. *Muscle Nerve* 4:306-318, 1981.

83. Weir A, Hansen S, Ballantyne JP: Motor unit potential abnormalities in multiple sclerosis: further evidence for a peripheral nervous system defect. *J Neurol Neurosurg Psychiat* 43:999-1004, 1980.

84. Werman R, Wislicki L: Propranolol, a curariform and cholinomimetic agent at the frog neuromuscular junction. *Comp Gen Pharmacol* 2:69-81, 1971.

85. Wiederholt WC: "End-plate" noise in electromyography. *Neurology* (Minneap) 20:214-224, 1970.

86. Wright JM, Collier B: The site of the neuromuscular block produced by polymyxin B and rolitetracycline. *Can J Physiol Parmacol* 54:926-936, 1976.

10

Single Fiber Electromyography

DAVID O. WIECHERS

Single fiber electromyography (SFEMG) is a technique that was developed by Jan Ekstadt and Erik Stalberg in the mid-1960s (2, 5). This technique records the electrical depolarization of single muscle fibers and thus enables the microphysiology of an individual motor unit to be studied. The clinical applications of the technique have been further developed by Stalberg (21).

In the mid-1970s there was a mystique about SFEMG. Many electromyographers ventured to Sweden to study and learn the technique directly from Stalberg and then returned to the United States to teach other interested physicians. Yet, SFEMG seemed too complicated for practical applications. First, the required modifications of standard EMG recording systems were expensive. Second, in order to be time effective, SFEMG analysis had to be performed by computer, which necessitated the development of software programs and hardware modifications of general-purpose computers. Third, many American electromyographers were unfamiliar with the use of the trigger-and-delay device to analyze motor unit action potentials (MUAPs), a technique that was critical to SFEMG application. Consequently, few electromyographers developed expertise and the test was unavailable in most medical centers in this country.

Fortunately, in the mid-1980s, there have been significant practical improvements in the clinical use of SFEMG. The use of a trigger-and-delay device for MUAP analysis is now a routine part of the standard clinical examination. Dedicated computer-based EMG instruments now commercially available make SFEMG analysis so simple, with some programs even allowing for the immediate cancellation of any portion of poorly recorded data, that with practice most electromyographers can now competently perform SFEMG. And, in addition to its obvious di-

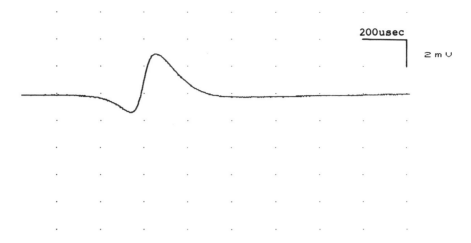

Figure 10.1. Recording of a single muscle fiber discharge.

agnostic value, the technique of SFEMG can also improve the skill of the electromyographers' performance of the routine EMG examination by acclimating them to the examination of the repetitive discharge of individual MUAPs in the analysis of MUAP stability.

SINGLE FIBER RECORDING

In SFEMG, the action potential of a single muscle fiber is recorded from a concentric needle electrode with a 25-μM diameter recording surface (4). The recording surface is placed on the cutting side of the needle shaft approximately 4 mm from its point. This positioning of the recording surface minimizes damage to the muscle fiber from which the recording is made. The single muscle fiber discharge is recorded as a biphasic spike with an initial positive deflection and a duration of less than 1 msec (Fig. 10.1). (7) The amplitude of the potential is dependent not only upon the fiber diameter but more importantly on the proximity of the recording surface to the active muscle fiber (Fig. 10.2). Normal amplitude varies from 200 μV to 7 millivolts. The primary goal of SFEMG recordings—to determine the variation in time between the depolarization of two single fibers that receive the impulse from the same motor neuron (22)—is achieved by positioning the electrode manually to record from two single muscle fibers, both of which belong to the same motor unit.

This variation in time is referred to as *jitter* and reveals information about

1. Impulse transmission in the terminal axon below its branching site;

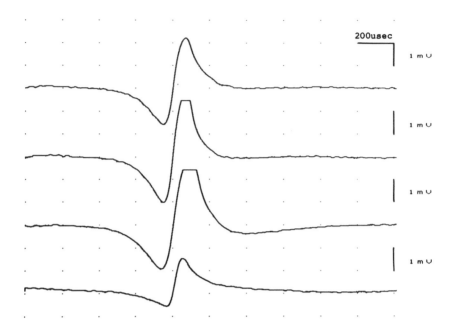

Figure 10.2. Recordings made from the same single fiber demonstrating the great variability in amplitude due to the difficulty in holding the electrode perfectly still during recordings.

2. Impulse transmission across the neuromuscular junction;
3. Impulse transmission along the muscle fiber membrane to the recording electrode.

In addition to the study of the microphysiology of an individual motor unit, SFEMG can also provide information about the anatomic arrangement of muscle fibers within a motor unit. By inserting the electrode into a minimally contracting muscle and manipulating this SFEMG electrode to record the nearby electrical activity, in 70% of insertions only one single fiber discharge is recorded. In approximately 25% of random muscle insertions the SFEMG electrode records two muscle fibers belonging to the same motor unit. Recordings that repetitively demonstrate many single fiber discharges belonging to the same motor unit imply an abnormally increased density of fibers. This "fiber density" determination is the second direct clinical application of this technique.

Recording System

The SFEMG electrode with its 25 μM recording surface has a high impedance, and the recording amplifier must have a corresponding high

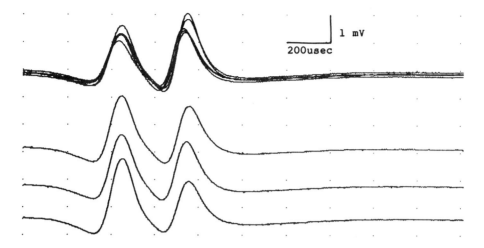

Figure 10.3. A pair of single fiber discharges locked in time to each other and therefore belonging to the same motor unit. Top recording is the superimposition of five discharges with normal jitter.

input impedance of approximately 100 megohms. Today, this high input impedance is generally a standard feature on most modern instruments. Another essentially standard feature is a trigger-and-delay device that is necessary to study the SFEMG potential, just as it is with routine MUAP recordings. The frequency response necessary to study the waveforms of single fiber potentials with their rapid rise times is 2 Hz to 20 KHz (7). The single fiber electrode records from a hemisphere of 250–350 μM in diameter. Single fiber potentials outside of this recording area produce unwanted fluctuations of the baseline. By raising the low frequency response, most of these unwanted baseline fluctuations are removed. Therefore, with routine SFEMG recordings the frequency response utilized is 500 Hz to 20 KHz.

Techniques

The techniques of SFEMG requires some practice before the electromyographer uses it clinically. The patient and examiner should be comfortably positioned. The SFEMG electrode is inserted perpendicular to the direction of the muscle fibers. The patient is then requested to provide a minimal voluntary contraction of the muscle. When a single fiber discharge is recorded, the electrode is manipulated within the muscle to attempt to find and record a second single fiber discharge (Figure 10.3). It is frequently helpful to insert the electrode through the muscle to be examined and then to slowly withdraw it. To be certain that the second single fiber discharge recorded belongs to the same motor unit as the first fiber, the following criteria must be met:

1. A rise time of the positive to negative spike of less than 300 microsec;
2. An amplitude of greater than 200 μV;
3. Second fiber is locked in time to the first potential.

The third criterion means that the second potential is only seen in association with the first potential. If the first potential stops firing and the second potential continues to fire at a steady rate that is not influenced by the first potential, then the second potential probably belongs to another motor unit. Similarly, if the second potential is seen only when the first potential is firing, then these potentials most likely belong to the same motor unit. Even though the recording surface is on the cutting side of the needle, the muscle fiber being recorded may occasionally be injured, especially if a hook or barb develops on the tip of the needle. The result of the damage to the recorded fiber is the generation of a second potential that is monophasic in a positive direction with longer duration and rise time than that of a normal single fiber potential. This "false-double potential" or "injured fiber" potential may cause the inexperienced examiner to think that this is a second single fiber discharge belonging to the same motor unit. With increased rates of discharge this false-double potential will have abnormal variability in its appearance following the original fiber's discharge. These potentials are not acceptable recordings for analysis.

Fiber Density

Information about the architecture of the motor unit can be gained by systematically recording from different areas of a muscle and recording the mean of the number of muscle fibers of a motor unit that fall within the 250 μM–350 μM diameter hemisphere recording area of the SFEMG electrode. This technique is referred to as *fiber density* (25). Twenty recordings, usually made from four skin insertions, are systematically performed. The electrode is inserted perpendicular to the direction of the muscle fibers and is then manipulated manually to maximize the amplitude of the first fiber recorded. Other single muscle fibers belonging to the same motor unit are now counted if their amplitudes are greater than 200 μV and they have rise times of less than 300 microsec. Normally, in about 70% of insertions only one muscle fiber is recorded. In about 25% of recordings two fibers are seen, and occasionally three fibers are recorded. Fiber density is expressed as the mean of the number of muscle fibers belonging to one motor unit when recordings are made from 20 different locations in one muscle. Normal

Table 10.1 Normal Fiber Density and Jitter Values in Patients Younger than 60 Years of Age

Muscle	Upper Limit Individual Paired Jitter	Upper Limit Mean Jitter of 20 Recordings	Upper Limit Fiber Density
	microsec	*microsec*	
Extensor digitorum communis	55	34	1.5
Biceps	35	30	1.4
Deltoid	35	30	1.4
Frontalis	45	30	1.8
Tibialis	75	50	1.7

fiber density varies from muscle to muscle, but is usually less than 1.8 (Table 10.1).

Jitter

Recording the time interval between discharges of the same single muscle fiber potential as its motor neuron fires repetitively reveals the *interdischarge interval* (IDI) of that individual fiber or the rate of firing of the motor unit. When recording potentials from two single muscle fibers belonging to the same motor unit, the time between depolarization of the two different fibers or the *interpotential interval* (IPI) can be determined. Jitter is defined as the variation of the IPI with consecutive discharges of the motor unit (6). There are three sites where motor unit transmission can alter the jitter. The "three determinants of jitter" of transmission are

1. In the distal axon below the branching sites;
2. Across the neuromuscular junction;
3. Along the muscle fiber membrane to the recording electrode.

Jitter is expressed statistically as the mean of the consecutive differences (MCD) of the IPIs with 50–200 consecutive discharges of the motor unit. The jitter or MCD is expressed in microseconds. When making recordings the rate of motor unit discharge with voluntary contraction by the patient should be kept as constant as possible and between 10–20 Hz. It is helpful to have a rate meter that the patient can see for feedback. If the rate of motor unit firing (IDI) fluctuates significantly, an artificial increase in the MCD can result. This increase is due to a change in the speed of conduction down the muscle fiber being altered by a previous or conditioned depolarization (14). When the IPI is influenced by the previous IDI, the IPIs should be sorted according to the preceding IDI in increasing order. The mean of the now sorted consecutive differences (MSD) is calculated. If the MCD/MSD value is greater than 1.25, then the MCD has been influenced by variations in the IDIs, and the MSD is the more correct expression of jitter. The longer the duration of the IPI, the greater is the effect of fluctuations in the IDI; therefore, recordings with an interspike interval greater than 4 msec are not routinely used for jitter analysis. Because of the time required to record and measure the IPI on paper and calculate the MCD by hand, jitter is calculated almost exclusively by computer (1).

Recordings can be analyzed immediately or stored on magnetic tape and analyzed later. When recording data on tape for later analysis, a small amount of jitter may be added by the tape recording system. This nonbiologic jitter must be taken into consideration for analysis.

The IPI can easily be determined with a two-trigger system. The first trigger is set on the first single fiber discharge, and the second trigger is set on the second single fiber discharge. The computer then takes a time measurement from a clock or counter started by the first trigger and stopped by the second trigger; this is the IPI. The differences between the consecutive IPIs are calculated by the computer, and the mean is determined (MCD). Methods for off-line analysis give greater flexibility of analysis. Off-line 50–100 consecutive discharges can be stored and displayed. The examiner can then discard falsely triggered or poor recordings. The acceptable discharges are then redisplayed and the IPIs marked for the computer. Although the error margin is less off-line, analysis is more time consuming. For statistical purposes at least 20 recordings are made from each muscle. With computer-assisted calculations, 20 motor units or 40 motor endplates can be analyzed, and the whole examination and analyses can be performed in less than 2 hours.

In normal muscle with repetitive discharge of the motor unit, variation in the IPI occurs that represents the normal variation in the chemically mediated neuromuscular transmission. This normal jitter is in the range of 10–30 microsec. Normal jitter varies from muscle to muscle. Normal jitter values are given in Table 10.1.

On occasion the MCD recorded on-line between two fibers is less than 5 microsec or less than 10 microsec when analyzed off-line (3). This variability is too small for neuromuscular transmission time, and these potentials are most likely from the same single fiber that has split or has a bud. Split fibers are frequently seen in weightlifters and in patients with myopathic conditions (11). These potentials are not used for jitter determination or fiber density measurements (Figure 10.4).

The second fiber may, in as frequent as 1 out of 20 recordings, appear to jitter around two different means. This flip-flop phenomenon occurs when the IPIs have a bimodal distribution; it is called *bimodal jitter* (26). This jumping back and forth of the potential occurs in short

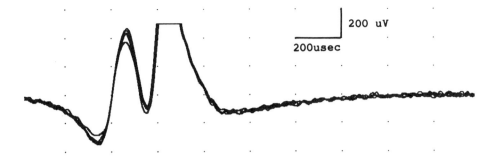

Figure 10.4. Split fiber recording with jitter less than 5 microsec.

and longer intervals. Short jumps of less than 250 microsec are frequently seen in normals and in reinnervated muscles. Longer jumps are most frequently seen in reinnervation. These recordings should not be used for jitter determination.

In each recording the duration between single fiber components can vary. The duration of the recording is the time between the baseline crossing of the first single fiber component to the baseline crossing of the last single fiber component of that recording complex. The normal duration is usually less than 4 msec, but is frequently so short that the second fiber appears to be riding on the downward slope of the first fiber. If the duration of the recording is divided by the number of intervals between fibers or by the number of fibers minus one, the *mean interspike interval* (MISI) is obtained. In normal muscle the MISI is usually less than 0.7 msec.

Blocking

When recording abnormal jitter that is usually greater than 80–90 microsec, the impulse transmission to the second fiber is occasionally so impaired that the transmission fails (Figure 10.5). The recording then demonstrates an intermittent disappearance of the second fiber with repetitive motor unit discharge. The presence of this severe abnormality when there is failure of transmission is called *blocking* (18, 20). The site of blocking of transmission can occur at any of the three determinants of jitter. If only two fibers are recorded and one blocks, it is not possible to determine where in the distal motor unit the transmission failure has occurred. When three or more single muscle fibers are present in one recording, two or more of the fibers can block consistently as a pair or group. When this blocking in pairs or groups of fibers occurs, the transmission failure is most probably in the terminal axon

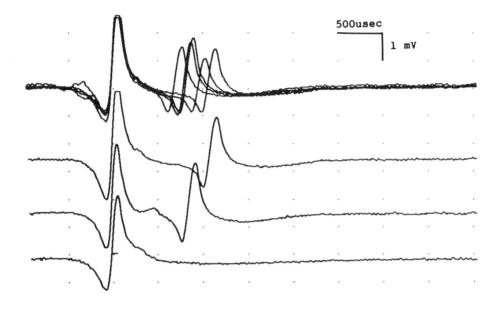

Figure 10.5. Recording from a patient with myasthenia gravis. Top recording is the superimposition of five discharges with increased jitter. Bottom recording demonstrates failed transmission of the impulse to the second fiber or blocking.

supplying that pair or group of fibers. This blocking of fibers as a group is referred to as *neurogenic blocking.*

Reporting

The microphysiology of individual motor units is studied with SFEMG. Because the physiology of the muscle as a whole is not revealed with SFEMG, routine concentric or monopolar recordings are always performed before SFEMG in order to establish or rule out pathologic processes that can produce transmission abnormalities. Fiber density determinations are made first. In this manner the examiner is not biased by the need to find pairs for jitter analysis. Fiber density results also give helpful information as to which of the three determinants of jitter may be the site of transmission abnormalities. After the fiber density is determined, at least 20 recordings from different areas are made for jitter calculations from each muscle examined. If a pair of single muscle fibers demonstrates an increase in jitter, it is not known whether the abnormalities are in the transmission to the first or second fiber. Therefore, when studying 20 recordings, 40 motor endplates are analyzed, ideally from 20 different motor units. First, the percentage of normal recordings is reported. Next, the percentage of recordings demonstrating mild transmission abnormalities as demonstrated by an increase in jitter is reported. Finally, the percentage of recordings with a severe transmission abnormality as demonstrated by blocking is reported. One abnormal recording in 20 is acceptable for a muscle to be classified as normal. If all the recordings are normal but there remains a high index of clinical suspicion that a disease process exists, then a second muscle is examined.

SINGLE FIBER EMG IN PATHOLOGIC CONDITIONS

Disorders of Neuromuscular Transmission

The current major clinical application of SFEMG is to aid in the early diagnosis of myasthenia gravis (12, 13, 16, 19, 23). Routine EMG testing for myasthenia depends on the demonstration of a fall in the CMAP to repetitive stimulation. A decrement of approximately 10% between the first and fourth response is considered abnormal in most laboratories. This falling response to repetitive stimulation is based upon the occurrence of failed transmission or blocking in at least 10% of all the muscle fibers within the muscle. Such a response obviously only occurs in the presence of a significant amount of disease and in retrospect is why repetitive stimulation techniques have been frequently normal in patients with obvious clinical disease.

The presence of 1 recording with an abnormal increase in jitter in 20 is acceptable in a normal muscle. If two recordings are abnormal, this is considered an abnormal study. The presence and distribution of abnormal motor endplates vary with the degree of clinical involvement. The muscles with the greatest clinical involvement usually demonstrate the greatest SFEMG abnormalities (Figure 10.6). As a rule, normal strength muscles in patients with myasthenia gravis demonstrate abnormalities in jitter in some recordings, but not necessarily blockings. The extensor digitorum communis is the muscle most frequently studied. Most patients with early symptoms of myasthenia have increased jitter in 40–50% of recordings. Sanders and Howard have an ongoing study of SFEMG in myasthenia and have stressed the importance of also calculating the mean value of the MCD of all 20 recordings. Currently, in 316 SFEMG studies in patients with myasthenia gravis, 233 were abnormal by both criteria or by having more than two individual recordings with increased jitter and an abnormal mean jitter value, and 34 patients were abnormal by only one criterion. In their experience, about 8% of patients will demonstrate an abnormality only in mean jitter.

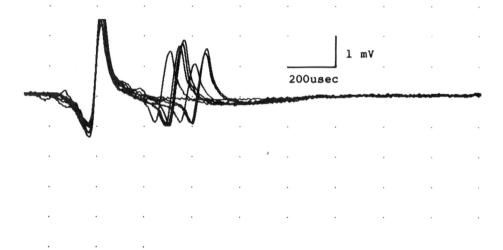

Figure 10.6. Superimposed recording of increased jitter in a myasthenic patient. In one of the discharges the second fiber is blocked as demonstrated by the straight baseline running through the recording of the second fiber.

Patients with ocular myasthenia have the fewest abnormalities. Approximately 60% of patients who have purely ocular myasthenia have abnormalities in the extensor digitorum communis. If the frontalis is studied, 85% of patients with ocular myasthenia demonstrate an increase in jitter (19).

Patients need not stop their anticholinesterase medications before examination. Jitter abnormalities are increased by an increased rate of motor unit discharge and an increasing temperature. Edrophonium injected during an abnormal recording usually stops any blocking and reverts the increased jitter back toward normal.

Jitter values are also greatly increased in the Lambert-Eaton myasthenic syndrome. As would be expected, the degree of blocking and jitter decreases with an increased discharge rate. Extremely large jitter values have been reported at low frequencies of motor unit discharge in myasthenic syndrome. It is this effect of activity that is the main difference between the jitter of myasthenia gravis and that of Lambert-Eaton syndrome.

Neuropathic Disorders

All that jitters and blocks is not myasthenia. During the early stages of reinnervation, abnormalities of impulse transmission are present (8,

28, 29). Transmission failures frequently occur at the branching site of the reinnervating terminal axon sprout. Transmission failure at the site where a new axon sprout leaves the axon to supply several muscle fibers is the origin of "neurogenic" blocking. Conduction down this initially unmyelinated terminal sprout is slowed, crossing the immature, newly developed neuromuscular junction may be difficult, and, a site of increased jitter and blocking. With time and maturation of these reinnervation structures the blocking stops and the jitter reverts to normal. Fiber density, as expected, is increased in reinnervated muscles. When the neurogenic compromise is mild and a only one-time event, such as a peripheral or root level nerve injury, the local reinnervation of deinnervated muscle fibers by unaffected neighboring motor units will be complete (8, 28). When the compromise is severe, more muscle fibers are deinnervated than can be reinnervated by the surviving motor units and transmission may never stabilize.

SFEMG is then of great value in routine clinical practice in determining whether reinnervation following nerve compromise is completed or ongoing. The presence of active reinnervation (blocking and increased jitter and increasing fiber density) in a muscle, the nerve of which was partially compromised 4 to 5 years ago, adds confirmation to the clinical impression of a second (now new) injury to that same peripheral or root level nerve. Using SFEMG as an aid in the diagnosis of recurrent root level nerve compromise may be its greatest value in everyday clinical practice (28).

Disorders affecting the motor neuron with resultant reinnervation by terminal axon sprouting demonstrate various increases in fiber density, jitter, and blocking. If the disease process is slow, as in juvenile progressive spinomuscular atrophy, there is a large increase in fiber density, very little blocking, and increased jitter. If the process of motor neuron loss is rapid, as in amyotrophic lateral sclerosis, then the fiber density is mildly increased with a marked presence of blocking and increased jitter. In rapidly advancing ALS, the blocking is so pronouced that it becomes difficult to find a single stable fiber to use for triggering.

In certain neuropathic conditions, late onset of motor unit abnormalities may occur (29). Recordings from previously compromised and now normal-strength or grade G (4/5 MRC) muscles in patients 22–60 years postpoliomyelitis demonstrate an increasing frequency of transmission abnormalities. The percentage of recordings demonstrating increased jitter and blocking seems to increase with the time since recovery from poliomyelitis. The exact etiology of these SFEMG abnormalities is unknown, but most likely relates to an inability of the reinnervated motor unit to supply all of its muscle fibers metabolically after having been overworked for the past 30–40 years. Whether or

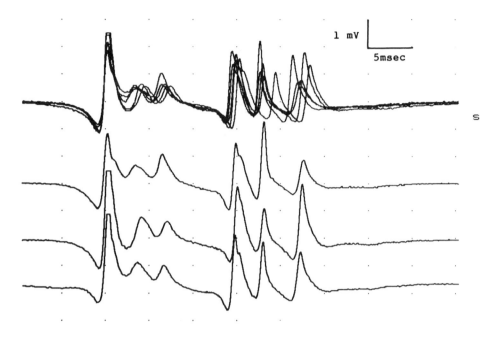

Figure 10.7. Abnormal jitter in a patient now 50 years postpolio.

not this same process of late changes in the motor unit occurs in other neuropathic conditions remains to be determined (Figure 10.7).

Patients with peripheral neuropathies have an increase in jitter and blocking. Transmission abnormalities may be occurring in the terminal axon. Reinnervation by terminal axon sprouting occurs to some degree in most of these disorders, making it difficult to localize specifically the site of SFEMG abnormalities.

Myopathic Disorders

Various SFEMG abnormalities are found in almost all of the muscular dystrophies (10, 15, 24). As with neuropathic disorders, the SFEMG abnormalities are not specific for a certain type of myopathy, but reflect the underlying pathophysiology. Abnormalities vary with the time course of the disease, again reflecting the changes with time of the pathophysiology. Fiber density is increased in most forms of muscular dystrophy. In facioscapulohumeral (FSH) and limb-girdle muscular dystrophy, fiber density is only mildly increased. However, in the Duchenne and Becker varieties of dystrophy, increased fiber density is most prominent with values that are two to three times normal. As the patient approaches end-stage disease the fiber density falls back toward

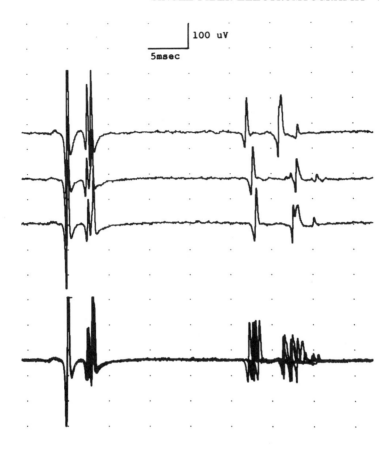

Figure 10.8 Recording from a teenage boy with Becker dystrophy.

normal, but remains elevated. Recordings from Duchenne and Becker varieties often reveal potentials with 5 to 6 single fiber components and not uncommonly 16 components. The duration of these components is usually approximately 10 msec, but durations of 40–50 msec are not uncommon (Figure 10.8).

The increase in fiber density in myopathic disorders may be the result of several factors. With fiber atrophy, the amplitude of the spike would be recorded over a smaller area. This shrinkage or compacting of the motor units together would not in itself explain the increased fiber density. It is more likely that it occurs as a result of innervation of regenerated muscle fibers from satellite cells or the reinnervation of segments of muscle fibers that were deinnervated due to segmental muscle cell necrosis. Fiber splitting would result in an increase in fiber density, as would ephaptic activation of adjacent muscle fibers. There may also be some terminal axon abnormalities. In the dystrophies, the duration between single muscle fiber discharges or the interspike intervals is prolonged. Normally, the MISI is 0.2–0.7 msec. In Duchenne dystrophy, the value is 1.0 to 1.5 msec and longer.

Jitter is increased in about 25% of recordings in Duchenne dystrophy, but only about 5–10% of recordings demonstrate blocking. The jitter in myopathic conditions is very dependent upon the IDI; therefore, the MSD is commonly the more correct value. Split fibers and nearby fibers recruited by ephaptic activation have values less than 5 microsec and, with standard voluntary activated recordings, comprise 5% of recordings. When electrical nerve stimulation is used at a constant rate to remove jitter produced by variation of the rate of activation or the IDI, almost 30% of recordings demonstrate these very low jitter values. This implies that fiber splitting and ephaptic activation of muscle fibers in dystrophies are much more common than originally thought (11). Jitter values are increased in limb-girdle and FSH dystrophy in about 50% of recordings, with blocking occurring in about 10% of recordings. Abnormalities in polymyositis and other inflammatory myopathies vary greatly and tend to reflect the activity and extent of the disease process (9). Just as in the other myopathies, abnormalities in inflammatory myopathies can vary from muscle to muscle, reflecting the extent of pathologic involvement.

Future Applications

The ability of SFEMG to record from a single muscle fiber of a motor unit has opened the door to new concepts of studying the motor unit. Several research techniques of quantitative analysis of MUAPs and "macro" EMG are based on SFEMG. "Macro EMG" is a technique used to study the depolarizations of all the muscle fibers belonging to a motor unit (17). A SFEMG recording is used to trigger and subsequently average the data obtained by a 15 mm macrorecording electrode. This technique of triggering and averaging results in an electrical summation of all the muscle fibers of the motor unit containing the triggering single fiber discharge. The use of SFEMG as a trigger also for the random selection of MUAPs in quantitative analysis is under investigation. Future clinical applications of these and other research techniques that are based on SFEMG will, no doubt, be forthcoming.

References

1. Antoni L, Stalberg E, Sanders D: Automated analysis of neuromuscular jitter. *Comput Prog Biomed* 16:175, 1983.
2. Ekstedt J: Human single muscle fiber action potentials. *Acta Physiol Scand* 61 (suppl 226):1, 1964.
3. Ekstedt J, Stalberg E: Abnormal connections between skeletal muscle fibers. *Electroenceph Clin Neurophysiol* 27:607, 1969.

4. Ekstedt J, Stalberg E: How the size of the needle electrode lead-off surface influences the shape of the single muscle fiber action potential in electromyography. *Comput Prog Med* 3:204, 1973.
5. Ekstedt J, Stalberg E: Single fiber electromyography for the study of the microphysiology of the human muscle. In Desmedt JE (ed): *New Developments in Electromyography and Clinical Neurophysiology*, vol 1. Basel, Karger, 1973, p. 84.
6. Ekstedt J, Nilsson G, Stalberg E: Calculation of the electromyographic jitter. *J Neurol Neurosurg Psychiat* 37:526, 1974.
7. Gath I, Stalberg E: Frequency and time domain characteristics of single muscle fiber action potentials. *Electroenceph Clin Neurophysiol* 39:371, 1975.
8. Hakelius L, Stalberg E: Electromyographical studies of free autogenous muscle transplant in man. *Scand J Plast Reconstr Surg* 8:211, 1974.
9. Hendriksson K, Stalberg E: The terminal innervation pattern of polymyositis: a histochemical and SFEMG study. *Muscle Nerve* 1:3, 1978.
10. Hilton-Brown P, Stalberg E: The motor unit in muscular dystrophy, a single fiber and scanning EMG study. *J Neurol Neurosurg Psychiat* 46:981, 1985.
11. Hilton-Brown P, Stalberg E, Trontelj J, Mihelin M: Causes of the increased fiber density in muscular dystrophies studied with single fiber EMG during electrical stimulation. *Muscle Nerve* 8:383, 1985.
12. Sanders D, Howard J: Single fiber EMG in the diagnosis of myasthenia gravis. *Muscle Nerve* 4:253, 1981.
13. Sanders D, Howard J, Johns T: Single fiber electromyography in myasthenia gravis. *Neurology* 29:68, 1979.
14. Stalberg, E: Propagation velocity in human muscle fibers in situ. *Acta Physiol Scand* 70 (suppl 287): 1, 1966.
15. Stalberg, E.: Electrogenesis in human dystrophic muscle. In Roland (ed): *Pathogenesis of Human Muscular Dystrophies.* Proceedings of 5th International Conference of the Muscular Dystrophy Association. Amsterdam-Oxford, Excerpta Medica, 1977, p 570.
16. Stalberg E: Clinical electrophysiology in myasthenia gravis. *J Neurol Neurosurg Psychiat* 43:522, 1980.
17. Stalberg E: Macro EMG, a new recording technique. *J Neurol Neurosurg Psychiat* 43:475, 1980.
18. Stalberg E, Ekstedt J: Single fiber EMG and microphysiology of the motor unit in normal and diseased human muscle. In Desmedt JE (ed): *New Developments in Electromyography and Clinical Neurophysiology*, vol 1. Basel, S Karger, 1973, p. 113.
19. Stalberg E, Sanders D: Electrophysiological tests of neuromuscular transmission. In Stalberg E, Young (eds): *Clinical Neurophysiology*. Boston, Butterworths, 1981, p 88.
20. Stalberg E, Thiele B: Transmission block in terminal nerve twigs: a single fiber electromyographic finding in man. *J Neurol Neurosurg Psychiat* 35:52, 1972.
21. Stalberg E, Trontelj J: *Single Fiber Electromyography*. Working U.K., Mirvalle Press, 1979.
22. Stalberg E, Ekstedt J, Broman A: The electromyographic jitter in normal human muscles. *Electroenceph Clin Neurophysiol* 31:429, 1971.
23. Stalberg E, Ekstedt J, Broman A: Neuromuscular transmission in myasthenia gravis studied with single fiber electromyography. *J Neurol Neurosurg Psychiat* 37:540, 1974.
24. Stalberg E, Trontelj J, Janko M: Single fiber EMG findings in muscular dystrophy. In Hausmanova-Petrusenicz, Tedrzejowska (eds): *Structure and Function of Nor-*

mal and Diseased Muscle and Peripheral Nerve. Warsaw, Polish Medical Publishers, 1974, p 185.

25. Thiele B, Stalberg E: Fiber density of the motor unit in the extensor digitorum communis muscles in man. *J Neurol Neurosurg Psychiat* 37:874, 1975.
26. Thiele B, Stalberg E: The bimodal jitter: a single fiber electromyographic finding. *J Neurol Neurosurg Psychiat* 37:403, 1974.
27. Thiele B, Stalberg E: Single fiber EMG findings in polyneuropathies of different etiology. *J Neurol Neurosurg Psychiat* 38:881, 1975.
28. Wiechers D: Single fiber electromyography with a standard monopolar electrode. *Arch Phys Med Rehab* 66:47, 1985.
29. Wiechers D, Hubbell S: Late changes in the motor unit after acute poliomyelitis. *Muscle Nerve* 4:524, 1981.

11

Somatosensory, Brainstem, and Visual Evoked Potentials

RANDALL L. BRADDOM

The use of evoked potential studies in clinical practice has grown dramatically over the past decade. Evoked potential studies have now developed from being just a laboratory curiosity to a practical clinical tool, as a great body of research has documented their value in the diagnosis of numerous conditions affecting both the peripheral and central nervous systems. Evoked potential studies are particularly helpful in demonstrating abnormalities in *sensory* function, even in cases having a normal or equivocal clinical sensory examination. They can help delineate the location of central nervous system (CNS) disease that in some instances cannot be localized by any other method. They also can be used to document changes in a patient's status over time (15).

There are three evoked potential studies in general use: pattern shift visual evoked potentials (PSVEP or VEP), brainstem auditory evoked potentials (BAEP or BAER), and somatosensory evoked potentials (SEP). These studies give reproducible wave morphologies, latencies, and amplitudes that usually allow a clear separation of normal from abnormal. This chapter is intended to be a "first look" at these three studies.

GENERAL PRINCIPLES OF EVOKED POTENTIAL STUDIES

Instrumentation

The evoked potential apparatus should meet at least the *minimum* standards suggested by the American Electroencephalographic Society (AES) (1) and the Evoked Potentials Committee of the American Association of Electromyography and Electrodiagnosis (AAEE-EPC) (41). The common mode signal rejection, averaging, filtering, and overall amplification of the amplifiers must be highly sophisticated. Because evoked potentials are of very low amplitude, amplification capacity must be up to 500,000 times the original signal input. The common mode rejection ratio should be at least 80 dB (10,000 to 1). The noise level of the amplifier should not exceed 3 μV (RMS) at a bandwidth of 0.1 to 5,000 Hz. A wide selection of signal filtration settings should be available from at least 0.1 to 5000 Hz.

Digital averaging capacity is required because these evoked potentials generally cannot be seen without averaging. The averager must have at least 80 microsec/data point/channel to monitor the incoming signal adequately. There should be at least 250 addresses of memory for each channel, with the capacity to average up to 4000 trials. The sweep analysis time should be variable from 10 msec to 100 sec.

Although evoked potential studies can be done with a single channel, it is preferable and more efficient to have at least four channels. Multiple channels allow the simultaneous study of the evoked potential at various sites. A system for obtaining a hard copy of the results should be available.

Electrode Placement

The most common recording electrode in use is the surface EEG cup electrode, which may have a pinhole in the top. A monopolar EMG pin can be used as a recording electrode if the insulation is scraped from the distal 1 cm of the shaft—the small surface area usually exposed on a monopolar pin is insufficient (15). Needle electrodes can be applied to the patient much more quickly than surface electrodes and are the only practical electrode choice for some locations, such as the external ear canal. Needle electrodes are more painful and are not practical for prolonged monitoring because of their tendency to fall out.

Because evoked potentials are extremely small in amplitude, *extreme care must be used in applying the electrodes.* Surface cup electrodes should be applied with a suitable electrode paste after careful preparation of the skin with an abrasive compound, such an Omni Prep®. The cleansing preparation should remove all oil, dirt, and the outermost layer of epithelium to reduce the impedance between the patient and the electrode. The electrode can be attached with collodion for prolonged monitoring or with nonadhesive electrode paste for routine studies.

Poor electrode application is the most common reason for a poor evoked potential study. Only when the impedance between the electrode and the skin is less than 5000 Ohms and preferably less than 3000 Ohms is the surface electrode adequately applied. Needle electrodes usually have higher impedance and may be used with an impedance of up to 7000 Ohms. Most commercially available instruments have the built-in capacity to measure electrode impedance directly. The common mode rejection capacity of the amplifier deteriorates if the amplifier/electrode impedance ratio decreases because of high electrode impedance (88). No currently available evoked potential apparatus will give satisfactory results when electrodes are applied incorrectly.

When electrodes are applied to the head, the International Ten-Twenty System of electrode site placement is used (53). This system is widely used for electroencephalography and has been adapted for use in evoked potentials. The 10-20 system is so named because the commonly used electrode sites are placed either 10% or 20% of the total distance between landmarks on the skull (Fig. 11.1).

Polarity

One of the most confusing aspects facing both the beginner and the veteran electromyographer is the assignment of polarity. There is no absolute consensus about how evoked potentials should be recorded in terms of polarity, and the AES has chosen not to set a standard in this regard (1).

Chiappa recommends that the polarity be identified with a statement, such as "the relative positivity of an electrode produces an upward deflection (15)". The term "relative" is used because if a signal voltage is $+50$ μV at the active electrode and $+30$ μV at the reference, the result will be a positive deflection of $+20$ μV. Actually in this case both electrodes are "positive." Switching the polarity of two electrodes being used to record an evoked potential does not change the result, except to present its mirror image.

Electromyographers and electroencephalographers have generally adopted the convention of having negativity in the electrode attached to lead one of the instrument produce an upward deflection. Most evoked potential investigators have adopted the practice of negativity being upward, unless the major waves of interest are mainly positive. In that case they often reverse the electrodes to make the major waves of interest "upright." Until a standard convention is adopted, investigators should be able to recognize evoked potential shapes, regardless of the polarity setting. In the following sections that describe the three most commonly used evoked potential studies, the electrode positions and polarities used are those most commonly seen in the literature.

Standardization

There is no single method of doing evoked potential studies, just as there is no single universally recognized method of doing peripheral nerve conduction studies. Each laboratory should standardize its tech-

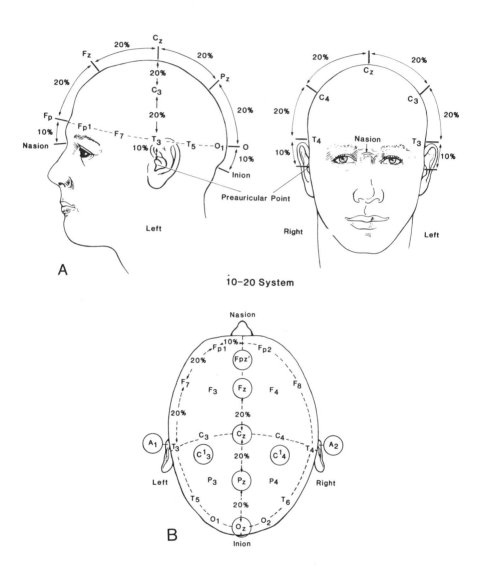

Figure 11.1. *A,* International 10-20 System of Electrode Placement. This system was designed for EEG, but with minor modification is useful for evoked potential studies. The system is based on four anatomic landmarks: the nasion, inion, and bilateral preauricular points. The distances are in 10% or 20% segments. *B,* The most common electrode sites for evoked potential studies are circled.

niques in terms of electrode type and location, evoked potential apparatus used, filter and averager settings, and even environmental conditions, such as temperature, noise, and light level. All of these factors affect the values that are obtained in evoked potential studies. The AAEE Committee on Evoked Potentials (41) reports that it is acceptable to use the normal values of another laboratory provided that the same testing conditions are used for at least 20 normal subjects and 95% of this subset of normal values fall within the normal range of the reference laboratory. Otherwise, each laboratory *must standardize a set of normal values* with a sufficient number of subjects.

An evoked potential study should be done at least twice for each stimulus condition to make certain that the results are reproducible. It is better to compare duplicate studies, rather than to do a single study with a very high number of average responses. Stolov (88) points out that increasing the number of averages from 100 to 1000 actually improves the amplitude ratio only 3.2 times. Increasing the number of repetitions from 1000 to 2000 improves the signal to noise ratio only 1.4 times. Consequently, it is better to average 500 responses twice than 1000 responses once. If the results are confusing, it is good practice to do a dry run in which the procedure is followed in the usual manner, except that the stimulus is not applied to the patient. Doing so will detect interfering potentials that are being averaged, but that are not due to the stimulus.

Stolov (88) and Lueders (62) point out that the best recording of evoked potentials occurs when the noise level is low, the filter band is relatively narrow, and the stimulus is adequate to provide the highest amplitude of the evoked potential. The noise is kept low by relaxing the patient and using as electrically clean an environment as possible. Depending on the type of study, it may or may not be appropriate to have the patient sleep, because sleep can give interfering EEG potentials in some cases. The stimulus for each type of study should be carefully adjusted to give the highest amplitude responses.

In the interpretation of evoked potential studies one should concentrate on the potentials that are routinely present in normals (15). A wave that is present only in occasional normals cannot be relied on for clinical interpretation. Consequently, many frequently seen waves— for example, waves VI and VII in brainstem auditory evoked potential studies—are generally not very useful in clinical interpretation because they are not uniformly present in normals.

Nomenclature

Because the study of evoked potentials is relatively new, there is of yet no standardized method of naming the waveforms. Two basic methods of nomenclature are in use. One method simply numbers the waveforms in sequence. For example, the commonly seen waves in brainstem auditory evoked potential studies (BAEPs) are generally numbered as Roman numerals I through VII. The other method is to label each individual wave by its usual polarity and latency to the peak of the wave. The largest waveform in the pattern-shift visual evoked response (PSVEP) is commonly called P100 because of its relative positivity and its usual latency of approximately 100 msec. The main advantage of this method is that it provides a descriptive label. Its disadvantage is that the wave name (P100) may be confused with the actual patient data result. The practice of placing a line over the number, as in P100 to denote the name of a potential rather than a value, is gaining popularity (27).

A standard method of labeling and reporting the parameters of the waves should be developed in each laboratory to minimize confusion. In some cases it may be necessary to describe the waves that are seen, rather than use any standard nomenclature. Over the next decade a standard nomenclature will probably emerge, either by common usage in the literature or by the edict of an internationally recognized body.

Wave Measurements

The latency and amplitude of evoked potentials are commonly measured and recorded. The latency is usually more helpful clinically than the amplitude. The absolute latency is always measured from the stimulus onset to the peak of the wave.

Measurement of the wave amplitude is currently being done in three ways. Perhaps the most common method is to report the amplitude as the voltage difference from the peak of the wave to the maximum point of the immediately following opposite polarity. Another popular technique is to record the amplitude from the baseline to the peak of the wave. The third and least used technique is to calculate the area under the entire wave curve. Amplitudes are usually more variable than latencies and are most helpful when compared from side to side in the same patient.

SOMATOSENSORY EVOKED POTENTIAL STUDIES

Somatosensory evoked potential studies (SEPs) are becoming increasingly popular because of a growing variety of important clinical uses. They are used to investigate focal lesions situated along the SEP pathway, including peripheral nerve lesions, brachial plexus problems, root dysfunction, and other lesions in the CNS. The safety of scoliosis and other spinal surgery seems to be improved by the use of SEP intraoperative monitoring. SEPs have also become particularly useful in the diagnosis of multiple sclerosis, as well as other common CNS diseases.

Evoked potentials were first noted over the scalp after median nerve stimulation by Dawson in 1947 (23). Stimulation of lower extremity nerves was also found to evoke potentials over the spine (6) and scalp (92). SEPs seem to follow the posterior columns pathway and, as are the BAEP and the VEP, are sensory system studies. One of the advantages of SEPs for studying the sensory system is that the CNS has a built-in amplifier effect. Consequently, it is possible in many cases to record a SEP from stimulation of a peripheral sensory nerve when a sensory nerve action potential (SNAP) cannot be recorded (37).

The SEP pathway seems to follow the classical posterior columns sensory pathway. The stimulus for a SEP study must excite the largest myelinated afferent fibers in the peripheral nerve. The response pathway is from the peripheral nerve to the dorsal column sensory fibers, the cell bodies of which lie in the dorsal root ganglion. The response then travels in the ipsilateral posterior columns to synapse in the dorsal column nuclei (nucleus cuneatus and nucleus gracilis). The second CNS fiber in the pathway crosses in the medial lemniscus to the ventral posterior lateral (VPL) nucleus of the thalamus. After a synapse in the thalamus, the third CNS fiber in this pathway goes to the cortex. Generally, SEP abnormalities are associated with disorders of touch, vibration, and conscious proprioception (joint position) (15). Giblin (37) found a good correlation between SEP abnormalities and abnormalities in position and passive joint movements in patients with spinal cord and brainstem lesions. The SEPs were normal in patients who had abnormalities only in pain and temperature sensation (37).

General Methodology

There are many factors to consider in SEP methodology. Hundreds of articles on SEPs have been published, and few have used exactly the same methods. Recently, attempts have been made to standardize at least the most common SEP studies. The American Electroencephalographic Society recently published guidelines for doing SEP studies (1). These guidelines are similar to those adopted by the Evoked Potentials Committee of the American Association of Electromyography and Electrodiagnosis (AAEE-EPC) (41).

The general requirements of the apparatus for SEPs follow the guidelines described in the first section of this chapter. Four channels are needed for routine clinical work, and six or more channels are useful for investigative work and special clinical problems. The stimulus must be delivered to the patient through an isolation transformer apparatus to minimize the shock artifact. The stimulating electrodes may be either of the surface or needle type. Surface electrode stimulation is done with a bipolar apparatus that usually consists of a pair of electrodes attached to a plastic bar. The electrodes can be taped over the appropriate extremity nerve. The skin should be prepared to reduce the skin-electrode impedance.

The AAEE-EPC recommends that the stimulus be a 200-to-300-microsec rectangular pulse at sufficient intensity to produce a visible muscle twitch (assuming stimulation of a mixed nerve) (41). Either a constant current or constant voltage stimulator may be used. There is some argument in the literature regarding the optimal stimulus intensity. Lueders (64) reports that the stimulus intensity should be the sum of the motor threshold plus the sensory threshold. Eisen (30) reports that the SEP is not enhanced by increasing the stimulus intensity beyond that level that produces the smallest visible muscle twitch. Stimulus frequency should be 4–7 Hz and preferably not an integral of 60.

Stimulus frequencies faster than 10 Hz begin to suppress the SEP response because of the recovery curve that starts to affect SEP amplitudes when the stimulus interval drops below 100 msec (12). Bilateral stimuli may be used simultaneously.

Methodology for Upper Extremity Studies

A number of montages have been suggested in the literature for recording SEPs from stimulation of upper extremity mixed nerves. The median nerve is the most commonly used upper extremity nerve. Most authors recommend viewing these SEPs with Erb's point-noncephalic, scalp-neck, scalp-noncephalic, and scalp-scalp montages.

One montage should be selected to demonstrate clearly the Erb's point[a] potential (EP) generated by the brachial plexus. It is important to demonstrate EP because it can be used not only for peripheral nerve conduction velocities but also as a "reference potential" for timing SEPs through the CNS (15). The best recording site is in the supraclavicular fossa where the least stimulus produces a hand twitch. It is generally about 2 cm above the midpoint of the clavicle (15). This recording site may need to be adjusted if necessary to register the EP of greatest amplitude. The AAEE-EPC recommends that the EP be evaluated with a montage of EP1-EP2 (41) (Fig. 11.2). This is a convenient montage because both supraclavicular fossa sites are usually used for a bilateral upper extremity nerve SEP study and require electrode placements there anyway.

The montage for channel 2 in upper extremity studies should compare SEP activity in the scalp and neck. The AAEE-EPC recommends C5S-Fz (or C2S-Fz) (41). C2S and C5S represent sites over the dorsal

---

[a]Editor's Note: Although convention dictates Erb point as supraclavicular electrode placement, Erb's point is, by definition, at the tip of the C6 vertebral transverse process—well above actual electrode placement.

spines of the C2 and C5 vertebrae, respectively. The scalp-neck montage looks at SEP activity in the upper cervical cord and brainstem. The scalp-neck montage usually gives N9, N11, and N13 potentials (Fig. 11.2), with N13 the most frequently seen.

Channel 3 is used by most investigators for a scalp-noncephalic montage. The AAEE-EPC recommends C3'-EPC and C4'-EPC (EPC is the contralateral EP site) (41). C3' and C4' are 2 cm posterior to C3 and C4, respectively (Fig. 11.1). The scalp-noncephalic montage gives P9, P11, and P13-14 (Fig. 11.2).

Channel 4 is used by most investigators as a scalp-scalp montage. The AAEE-EPC recommends C3'-Fz or C4'-Fz (41). This gives N20 (some authors call it N19) (Fig. 11.2).

The resulting SEPs should be analyzed for the presence or absence of the usual waves. Figure 11.2 shows the ideal median nerve SEP results, and Figure 11.3 shows results that are more typically seen in routine clinical practice. These potentials should be seen in normals: EP, N13, P13-14, and N20. EP, N13, and N20 are the most easily elicited and the most commonly used for interpretation in clinical practice. Waves N9, N11, P9, and P11 should also be noted when present (41). The amplitudes and interpeak latencies should be measured for the major waves. The absolute latencies vary in different patients, but the interpeak latencies are usually similar (Table 11.1).

The peripheral conduction velocity can be determined by measuring from the point of stimulus (assumed to be under the cathode of the stimulator) to the Erb's point recording site and dividing this distance by the latency of EP. The height, age, and gender of the patient should be recorded.

SEPs can also be obtained by the stimulation of sensory nerves or the skin of a sensory dermatomal area. The responses that result from sensory nerve or dermatomal area stimulation have lower amplitudes than those from mixed nerves. Chiappa (15) reports that electrical stimuli of approximately three times the intensity of sensory threshold produce scalp SEPs that are usually about half the size of SEPs seen after the stimulation of mixed nerves. The conduction velocity from stimulation of sensory nerves or skin dermatomes is slightly slower than with stimulation of mixed nerves. This is due to the use of Type II fibers, rather than the Type IA fibers in mixed nerves (111). Skin dermatomal and sensory nerve stimulation studies are further described in the section on radiculopathy.

Methodology for Lower Extremity Studies

There is much variability in the methodology suggested in the literature for lower extremity SEPs. For tibial nerve studies the AAEE-EPC recommends a scalp-scalp montage, two spine-spine montages, and a

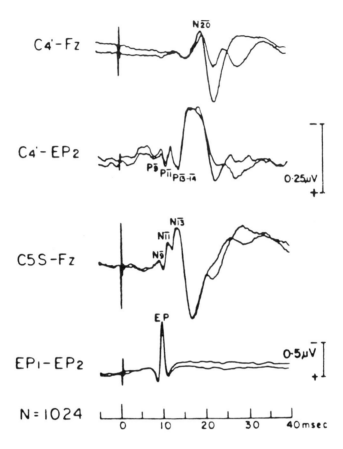

Figure 11.2. Short latency SEPs to left median nerve stimulation at the wrist in a 24-year-old man. Stimulus consisted of monophasic square waves of 200 microsec duration repeated at 5.4/sec. Muscle twitch causing abduction of the thumb was observed. (Reprinted with permission from AES:Guidelines for clinical evoked potential studies. *J Clin Neurophysiol* 1:3, 1984.)

lower extremity montage (41). This gives four channel montages of popliteal fossa (PF)-medial surface of knee; L3S-4 cm rostral; T12S-4 cm rostral, and Cz'-FPz'. Cz' is 2 cm posterior to Cz, and FPz' is midway between Fz and FPz (Fig. 11.1). T12S and L3S are over the dorsal spines of T12 and L3, respectively. The PF site is over the tibial nerve in the popliteal fossa. The tibial nerve is stimulated at the ankle. A band ground electrode should be placed around the calf.

These montages for the tibial nerve consistently give the following responses in normal individuals that need to be observed and measured (Fig. 11.4). The tibial nerve potential in the popliteal fossa is usually

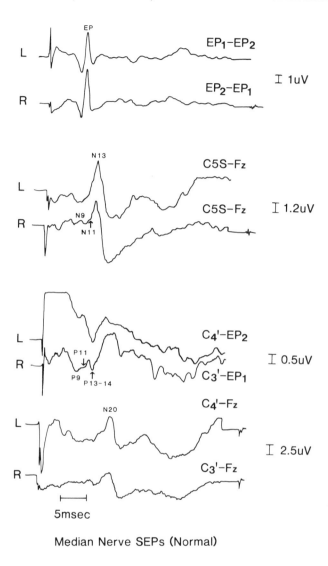

Median Nerve SEPs (Normal)

Figure 11.3. Normal SEPs to median nerve stimulation in a 43-year-old woman. Averages of 500 sweeps using TECA TD 20.

designated as the PF potential. The spine components usually seen are the L3 potential in the L3S-4 cm rostral montage and T12 in the T12S-4 cm rostral montage. The scalp components are generally P37 and N45.

The absolute latencies of PF, L3, T12, and P37 potentials should be measured. The following body measurements should be made:

Table 11.1. Normal Data for Median Nerve SEPs from 50 Subjects[a]

Parameter	Mean	SD	Mean + 3SD	Min	Max
Absolute latency (msec)					
EP	9.7	0.76	12.0	7.9	11.2
P/N13	13.5	0.92	16.3	11.5	15.6
N19	19.0	1.02	22.1	16.7	21.2
P22	22.0	1.29	25.9	19.1	25.2
Interwave latency					
EP-P/N13	3.8	0.45	5.2	2.7	4.5
EP-N19	9.3	0.53	10.9	7.8	10.4
EP-P22	12.3	0.86	14.9	10.0	15.0
P/N13-N19	5.5	0.42	6.8	4.7	6.8
Left-right latency differences					
EP	0.2	0.20	0.8	0.0	0.9
EP-P/N13	0.2	0.17	0.7	0.0	0.6
EP-N19	0.2	0.21	0.8	0.0	0.8
EP-P22	0.3	0.24	1.0	0.0	1.1
P/N13-N19	0.3	0.25	1.1	0.0	1.1
Amplitudes (μV)[b]					
EP	3.0	1.86	8.6	0.5	8.6
P/N13	2.3	0.87	4.9	0.8	4.4
N19	1.0	0.56	2.7	0.1	2.7
P22	2.2	1.10	5.5	0.5	5.5
Left-right amplitude difference (%) $[(abs(a-b))/((a+b)/2)] \times 100$					
N19	41.7	33.14	141.1	0.0	144.4
P22	25.7	21.23	89.4	0.0	90.4

[a]Reprinted with permission from Chiappa KH: *Evoked Potentials in Clinical Medicine.* New York, Raven Press, 1983.

[b]Amplitudes measured from baseline to peak for the Erb's point potential, P/N13 and N19 peak to P22 peak for P22 amplitude. Stimulus duration 0.2 msec, rate 5 Hertz.

1. The distance between the stimulating cathode and the PF recording electrode;
2. The distance between the cathode and the L3S and T12S electrodes;
3. The distance between the Cz' electrode and both L3S and T12S electrodes.

The following latency measurements should be made: (a) latency of PF, (b) latencies of L3 and T12, and (c) latency of P37.

The following conduction velocities should be calculated: (a) the peripheral nerve conduction velocity from the stimulating cathode to PF and also from the cathode to L3 and (b) the conduction velocity from the spine to the scalp. This calculation is made by subtracting the latencies of the L3 and T12 spine potentials from P37 and dividing these differences into the corresponding distances. The nerve conduction velocity from L3S to T12S is usually too variable in normals to be clini-

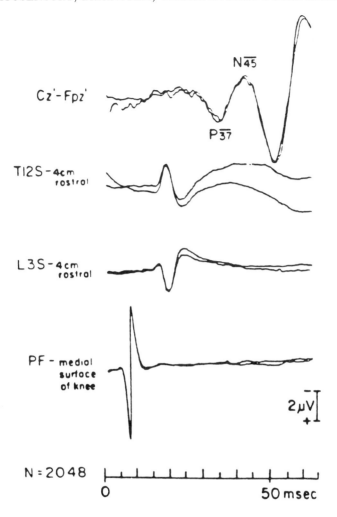

Figure 11.4. Short latency SEPs to right tibial nerve stimulation at the ankle in a 24-year-old man. Stimulus consisted of monophasic square pluses of 200 microsec duration repeated at 5.4/second. Muscle twitch caused plantar flexion of the toes. (Reprinted with permission from AES:Guidelines for clinical evoked potential studies. *J Clin Neurophysiol* 1:3, 1984.)

cally useful (41). Normal values for tibial and other lower extremity nerve SEPs have been reported by numerous investigators (15, 30).

For a common peroneal nerve study, the AAEE-EPC recommends scalp-scalp and three spine-spine montages. These are Cz'-FPz', T6S-4 cm rostral, T12S-4 cm rostral, and L3S-4 cm rostral. The common peroneal nerve is stimulated just distal to the knee. The spine derivations

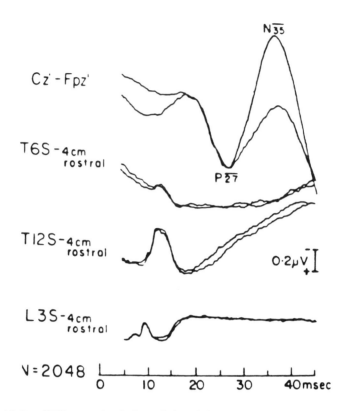

Figure 11.5. SEPs to stimulation of the right common peroneal nerve at the knee in a 20-year-old normal woman. Stimulus consisted of monophasic square pulses of 200 microsec duration repeated at 7/second. Muscle twitch caused plantar flexion and eversion of the foot. (Reprinted with permission from AES: Guidelines for clinical evoked potential studies. *J Clin Neurophysiol* 1:3, 1984.)

should show L3, T12, and T6 spinal potentials. The scalp-scalp derivations should give the components P27 and N35 (Fig. 11.5). The amplitudes of the major components of the SEP from stimulation of the peroneal nerve at the knee are generally lower than those from stimulating the tibial nerve at the ankle (41).

Lower extremity sensory nerves and skin dermatomal areas can also be stimulated. These studies generally give much smaller amplitudes than those from mixed nerves. It is often very difficult to obtain the spinal potentials that result from stimulation of lower extremity sensory nerves, but scalp potentials are usually present. The conduction velocities from stimulation of lower extremity sensory nerves and skin dermatomal areas are generally somewhat lower than from the lower extremity mixed nerves (see section on radiculopathy).

Factors affecting Normal Results

A number of factors affect SEP study results. The absolute latencies of SEPs are longer in premature than in full-term infants (20), decrease further over the first 2 years of life, and decline in absolute latency until reaching adult values from 5 (20) to 8 years of age (25). Absolute SEP latencies increase slowly with age in adults in a manner analogous to the slowing of peripheral nerve conduction. There is some evidence that the natural decline in conduction velocity with age occurs more rapidly in peripheral nerves than in CNS neurons (24). Interpeak SEP latencies show only minor changes with age. Women have slightly shorter central conduction times than men (38). The exact reasons for this difference are still speculative.

Body size makes a great difference in the absolute latency of SEPs because of the obvious distance factors. Most of the difference in body size for upper extremity SEPs can be largely ignored if latencies are measured in relation to Erb's potential. The effect of body size is much greater with lower limb testing, and a correction for body height must be used for both the absolute latencies and the conduction time from the lower cord to the cerebrum (15). The suggested methodology of the AAEE-EPC (4) resolves most of the body size problems by converting absolute latencies to nerve conduction velocities.

Body temperature has much more of an effect on peripheral than central nerve conduction velocity. The temperature factor can largely be ignored if studies are made in reference to EP in the upper extremity and to the lumbar potential in the lower extremity.

Drugs do not generally affect the SEP values. Hume et al. (52) found no relationship between the blood levels of phenobarbitol in comatose patients and the upper limb SEP central conduction times. Anesthetic agents may have an effect on SEP amplitudes (see sections on intraoperative monitoring).

Peripheral neuropathies also affect the absolute latencies of SEPs. The severity and type of this effect are a function of whether the peripheral neuropathy is of the axonal or demyelinating type. Demyelinating lesions produce very prolonged absolute latencies. Diseases affecting the myelin of peripheral nerves may or may not affect the myelinated pathways of the CNS. Axonal neuropathy reduces the amplitude of EP and cerebral SEPs, but does not generally affect the latency.

Clinical Uses of Somatosensory Evoked Potentials

SEPs are useful in testing the peripheral nervous system (nerves and roots), as well as the posterior column sensory tract pathway in the CNS. Additional uses will undoubtedly be described in the future, but Aminoff (2) and others are beginning to call for a more cautious and critical use of SEP studies. Some of the most frequent current clinical uses of SEPs are outlined below.

Use of SEPs for Peripheral Nerve Problems

In some peripheral neuropathy cases, it is possible to see SEPs when the sensory nerve action potential (SNAP) is unrecordable (37) due to amplification of the peripheral nerve volley in the CNS (30). The sensory nerve conduction velocity can be determined when SNAPs are unrecordable by stimulating a sensory nerve at two sites and subtracting the latencies of corresponding scalp-recorded SEPs. In peripheral nerve lesions, the presence of SEPs indicates that the nerve has axonal continuity, even if SNAPs are unrecordable.

Proximal neuropathy, such as in Guillain-Barré syndrome, can produce SEP changes even when peripheral nerve conduction is still normal (15). Brown et al. (10) reported changes in SEPs, such as prolonged EP-P/N13 conduction time, when peripheral conductions were still normal in 25% of their Guillain-Barré cases. McLeod et al., however (68), found this change in only 1 of 14 cases. With further refinement, SEP studies may be a very useful addition to our current methods of studying proximal nerve conduction, such as the F-wave, H-reflex, and spinal nerve root stimulation techniques (see Chapter 9.).

SEPs can be used in peripheral nerve entrapment cases and show particular promise for studying the lateral femoral cutaneous nerve. This nerve is difficult to study with standard nerve conduction techniques (12), but may be more amenable to SEP studies. Eisen (30) presented a case of meralgia paresthetica in which stimulation of the lateral femoral cutaneous nerves gave a P40 of 31.8 msec on the unaffected side and 39.1 msec on the affected side. A similar case has been presented by Stolov (89).

SEP studies can also be used to assess slowing of central conduction when peripheral conduction is normal, which has been reported in vitamin B_{12} deficiency (59). SEP studies have shown that some common peripheral neuropathies also have slowing of central conduction. This has been reported in diabetes (42), Guillain-Barré syndrome (67), Charcot-Marie Tooth disease (45), and other conditions (15).

Use of SEPs in Brachial Plexopathy

SEP studies are potentially helpful in the diagnosis of brachial plexopathy (1, 30). Conventional studies of brachial plexopathy look for abnormal muscle membrane irritability and a reduction in the number of voluntary motor units firing in the muscles innervated by the affected nerves. Recording SNAPs of the appropriate nerves is also important. Usually, the major diagnostic problem in brachial plexopathy is determining whether any part of the plexus is in anatomic discontinuity and may be amenable to surgery. If the EMG shows any voluntary motor units, then the corresponding motor part of the brachial plexus must be in anatomic continuity even if it is severely bruised, stretched, or entrapped. If the EMG shows no voluntary activity, the nerves may still be anatomically continuous. Because SEP studies are sensory in nature, they can only imply that motor fibers are anatomically continuous.

The SEP in some instances can help assess whether the preganglionic portion of a sensory root is pulled off the spinal cord in traumatic brachial plexopathy. If a SNAP is present, the corresponding sensory fibers must be intact to the dorsal root ganglion, but a preganglionic lesion may still be present. If a SNAP is absent, the lesion is postganglionic. SEPs are particularly likely to be helpful in looking at sensory root function if the stimulation is segment specific, rather than using a large multisegmented nerve, such as the median or tibial nerve. Studies using large multisegmental nerves have not been more than 50–75% accurate in separating preganglionic from postganglionic lesions (7, 56). Eisen (30) and others (15) have had more accurate results using segmental nerve stimulation to isolate the affected sensory root. The absence of a SEP in the presence of a SNAP is good evidence of a preganglionic sensory root injury, such as root avulsion.

Use of SEPs in Thoracic Outlet Syndrome

Thoracic outlet syndrome (TOS) has been described by many authors, and many tests have been devised to aid in its diagnosis. The obvious cases of TOS generally involve weakness and sensory loss in the C8 and T1 distribution, wasting of the intrinsic muscles of the hand, prolongation of the ulnar nerve F-wave latencies to hand intrinsic muscles, and an abnormal EMG (see Chapter 4). Many other patients with symptoms suggestive of TOS presumably have primarily a vascular abnormality with no neurologic deficit. A recent study (96) of 12 patients with cervical ribs and symptoms suggestive of TOS showed that only those with a neurologic deficit had an abnormal SEP study. Only two patients had an abnormal SEP without also having abnormal EMG and

Table 11.2. Results of Segmental Sensory Stimulation[a]

Cutaneous Nerve	Stimulation Site	Segment	Latency to N20 or P40 (MEAN,SD)
			msec
Musculocutaneous	Forearm	C5	17.4 (1.2)
Median	Thumb	C6	22.5 (1.1)
Median	Adjoining surfaces of index and middle fingers	C7	21.2 (1.2)
Ulnar	Little finger	C8	22.5 (1.1)
Lateral femoral cutaneous	Thigh	L2	31.8 (1.8)
Saphenous	Knee	L3	37.6 (2.0)
Saphenous	Ankle	L4	43.4 (2.2)
Superficial peroneal	Above ankle	L5	39.9 (1.8)
Sural	Ankle	S1	42.1 (1.4)

[a]From Eisen AA: The somatosensory evoked potential. Minimonograph 19, Rochester, MN, AAEE, 1982.

NCV studies. The most common abnormalities were a loss or prolongation of EP and/or P/N13 on ulnar nerve stimulation.

Use of SEPs For Radiculopathy

It is well known that standard electrodiagnostic methods for the evaluation of radiculopathy continue to have a small percentage of false-negative results (see Chapter 7). Mild, chronic sensory radiculopathies in particular are extremely difficult to detect by routine electromyographic methods (91). The H reflex may assist in this diagnosis, but its practical use is limited to the S1 level (8). The F wave can also be used to assist in the diagnosis of radiculopathy, but it is difficult to elicit in proximal muscles and it evaluates only motor dysfunction as does the EMG (91). Although SEPs of multisegmental nerves, such as the median and ulnar, are occasionally helpful in radiculopathy diagnosis, radiculopathy of a single root is usually hidden in a multisegmental SEP study.

Eisen and Elleker (31) described a technique for studying the cervical, lumbar, and sacral nerve roots with sensory nerve and skin dermatomal SEPs. In the upper extremity the musculocutaneous nerve is stimulated to study the C5 segment. Ring electrodes for stimulation are placed on the thumb for C6. Adjoining surfaces of the index and middle fingers are stimulated for C7, and the little finger is stimulated for C8. In the lower extremity the lateral femoral cutaneous nerve is stimulated for L2 and L3, the saphenous nerve for L4, the superficial peroneal nerve for L5, and the sural nerve for S1. The latencies of the corresponding N20 and P40 potentials are shown in Table 11.2.

Eisen reported a study of 36 patients with cervical and lumbosacral radiculopathies that used motor and sensory conductions, F waves, needle electromyography, and SEPs in combination (32). The needle EMG gave the best overall diagnostic yield (75%), whereas 43% of the cases had abnormal F waves. An abnormal SEP was found in 57% of the patients on stimulation of the appropriate dermatomal area or sensory nerve. The SEP was the most sensitive study in patients whose radiculopathy gave only sensory symptoms clinically. Future refinements in these segmental techniques may allow more accurate studies of suspected radiculopathies in patients whose findings are mainly sensory in nature clinically.

Intraoperative Monitoring on SEPs During Carotid Endarterectomy

SEPs during endarterectomy can be used to monitor the status of the brain. The carotid arteries need to be clamped during part of the carotid endarterectomy (CEA) procedure. Although this clamping can usually be done long enough to allow the surgery without causing significant cerebral injury, some patients do not have sufficient collateral blood flow to allow the clamping to be done safely. Many surgeons feel that these patients require the insertion of a shunt around the operative site. Because the shunt has its own set of potentially serious complications, it is best to limit its use to the patients who clearly need it. Markland et al. (65) studied 36 patients undergoing CEA and monitored them with the SEP from median nerve stimulation. Ten of these CEAs were done under general anesthesia, and three patients showed changes in SEPs during the carotid clamping. These SEPs returned to baseline morphology and amplitude values within 2 minutes after restoration of blood flow. The 26 remaining CEAs were done under local anesthesia. There was a consistently strong correlation between the changes in mental status and the SEP. One patient lost consciousness within 30 sec of carotid clamping, and the SEP immediately showed marked flattening. SEPs may be more useful than any other currently available method for determining when a patient is receiving insufficient blood supply to the cortex in such procedures.

SEPs can also be used in other types of vascular procedures for monitoring of CNS viability. Perhaps the most important of these is the monitoring of spinal cord function during aortic surgery, because the incidence of spinal cord injury following procedures affecting aortic blood flow may be as high at 15%.

Use in Scoliosis Surgery

It has been known for many years that scoliosis surgery has an inherent risk of spinal cord injury in approximately 1% of cases (70). Most studies indicate that the injury to the spinal cord that occurs in a distraction procedure is vascular in nature (21). The most commonly used technique to make certain that the distraction of the spine with Harrington rods or other devices has not injured the spinal cord is the wake-up test. This test consists of allowing the patient to wake up sufficiently to test voluntary movement of the arms and legs after the distraction (93). Nash and Brown (70) have reported that the wake-up test is useful, but occasionally produces false-negative results. Its other limitations are that only a limited number of wake-ups are practical during surgery, it generally monitors only the motor function of the spinal cord, and the results are often equivocal. It is also difficult to apply the wake-up test in patients who have an existing neurologic deficit.

In the 1970s a number of investigators began studying extremity nerve SEPs in patients undergoing scoliosis surgery (34, 71). They were encouraged by the fact that anesthesia did not eliminate SEPs in most cases, except when halogenated agents, such as halothane and enflurane, were used. These early studies focused on recording SEPs from the scalp on stimulation of the peroneal and/or tibial nerves.

The main drawback of the SEP for monitoring scoliosis surgery is that it uses only the posterior columns tract and is a purely sensory study. It is possible for injury to occur to other portions of the spinal cord, such as in gray matter or in tracts other than the posterior columns, without changing the SEP. However this appears to be unusual in scoliosis surgery, as most studies have recorded a high correlation between the maintenance of the SEP during surgery and the maintenance of normal or unchanged neurologic function after the surgery. This correlation is sufficiently high that it can be said with relative certainty that, if the SEP is unchanged after the distraction process, no spinal cord dysfunction will result. If the SEP study has technical difficulties or if there is any other reason to suspect that an injury may be occurring, the wake-up test can still be performed.

More recent studies in scoliosis surgery have used not only SEPs recorded from the scalp but also have experimented with potentials recorded over the spine. Lueders et al. (63) have recently reported on the use of needles placed in the intraspinous ligaments above and below the level of surgery. This procedure allows an evaluation of spinal potentials crossing the actual zone of the surgery.

Another technique suggested by Tamaki (90) is to stimulate the upper thoracic posterior epidural compartment while recording from the region of the conus medullarus with special electrodes that are mounted in Tuohy's needle. This is actually an antidromic conduction study of spinal pathways. Jones et al. (57) reported a technique in which small needle electrodes are inserted by way of a catheter into the epidural space of the thoracic and cervical regions, with stimulation of the tibial nerves. In another procedure introduced by Daube (22) a paraspinal electrode is placed preoperatively over the lamina by percutaneous technique in the cervical spine.

It is obvious that there are many current alternative SEP procedures for monitoring patients during scoliosis surgery, but none of these methods has yet emerged as the preferred technique. Regardless of the specific technique, most investigators simply use a 50% loss of amplitude or a disappearance of the SEP as evidence of potential injury to the spinal cord.

In addition to the use of SEPs for intraoperative monitoring of vascular and scoliosis surgery, SEPs have been used in other procedures as well. One of the newer uses is the monitoring of sciatic nerve status during hip arthroplasty (43).

Use of SEPs for Determining Prognosis in Head Injury

A number of studies of single and multimodality evoked potentials have been done in head-injury patients. Anderson et al. (3) compared BAEPs, VEPs (stroboscopic), and SEPs in 39 patients with Glasgow coma scale scores of 7 or less. The most difficult of the studies to do was the VEP, as patients who were not deeply comatose tolerated the study poorly and were generally uncooperative. All of the evoked potential studies were good predictors of an unfavorable outcome, such as vegetative state or death. If the evoked potential studies were markedly abnormal, the prognosis was unfavorable.

However, only SEPs were useful in predicting a favorable outcome, as patients with normal or slightly abnormal VEPs and BAEPs were just as likely to have an unfavorable as a favorable outcome (3). SEP results correctly predicted 100% of those having an unfavorable outcome and 82% of those having a favorable outcome. The BAEPs and VEPs only predicted 62% or 29%, respectively, of those cases having a favorable outcome. This study substantiated the results of similar studies, including those of Greenberg et al. (39) and Hume et al. (19). This study also showed SEPs to be more accurate in predicting prognosis than intracranial pressure monitoring, pupillary reflexes, and motor responses (3).

Use of SEPs in the Diagnosis of Multiple Sclerosis

There have been a host of single modality and multimodality evoked potential studies in patients with multiple sclerosis (MS) (15, 76). SEPs are useful in the diagnosis of MS because an abnormal SEP study adds another site of abnormality to the patient's clinical picture. SEPs are abnormal in about half of the patients with MS who have no sensory system abnormalities (16). SEP testing for MS is more sensitive when done unilaterally and when done with a lower extremity nerve. Lower extremity nerve SEPs probably are the most sensitive because a larger segment of the central neuraxis is surveyed. There is general agreement in the literature that BAEP studies are less sensitive for MS diagnosis than pattern shift VEPs and SEP studies (76). The VEPs and SEPs seem to be approximately equally sensitive.

Some authors have suggested that SEPs can be used to follow the course of MS (9), but Aminoff and others (52) have reported that the variability between test sessions is excessive, even in clinically stable patients.

BRAINSTEM AUDITORY EVOKED POTENTIALS

Over the past few years, brainstem auditory evoked potential studies (BAEPs) have gained general clinical acceptance in the investigation of such problems as cerebellopontine angle tumors, acoustic neuromas, and anatomic changes in the brainstem along the BAEP pathway. BAEPs have greatly improved the study of hearing problems in infants and children. A multitude of other uses of BAEPs have been suggested in the recent literature, and many of these uses should become commonplace in the next few years.

BAEP studies were first reported after conducted potentials were noted on the scalp in response to auditory stimuli in cats (54) and then in humans (55). Jewett's studies (55) indicated that seven waves could be recorded from the scalp during the first 10 msec following a sound stimulus to the ear. These deflections (Fig. 11.6) are often referred to as "Jewett bumps" and occur whether the patient is awake or asleep (74). The latencies of the peaks vary with stimulus intensity (49). The waves are present at birth, and their latencies change as the CNS matures. Structural lesions in the auditory pathway may abolish these potentials (60).

The BAEP anatomic pathway is somewhat different from the hearing pathway. Because BAEP abnormalities are usually ipsilateral to the ear being tested, it is likely that the BAEP pathway tends to cross less in the brainstem than the hearing pathway.

Wave I is felt to be due to the eighth cranial nerve action potential (Fig. 11.6). Wave II has traditionally been assigned to the cochlear nucleus, but some investigators (47, 69) report that it may come from the portion of the eighth cranial nerve nerve closest to the brainstem. Wave III appears to be generated by the superior olivary complex in the pons. There is considerable speculation about the generator sources of Waves IV and V. They are probably generated in the high pons or low midbrain, most likely in either the lateral lemniscus or inferior colliculus. Waves VI and VII are usually seen in clinical studies, but have limited usefulness as they are not universally present in normals. Wave VI

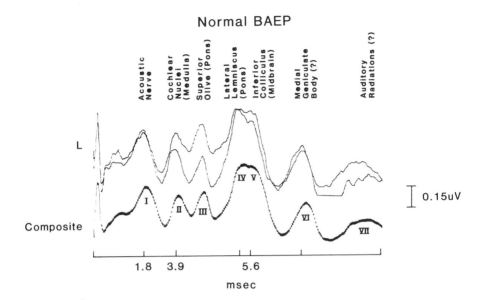

Figure 11.6. Normal BAEP study in a 35-year-old woman. 60 dB/HL, positive pulse polarity, click stimulus, 100 msec duration, 11.1/sec frequency, 2000 repetitions. Nicolet CA-1000.

probably arises in the medial geniculate body and Wave VII in the auditory radiations.

The vestibular apparatus and vestibular pathway do not seem to be an integral part of the BAEP pathway. Studies to date of patients with labyrinthine diseases (15) (labyrinthitis, vestibular neuronitis, and Meniere's disease) have not shown BAEP abnormalities.

Equipment Required

The preferred stimulus in the clinical setting for BAEP testing is a click generated in an earphone by an electrical square wave impulse that is 0.1 msec in duration (1). The click generator should allow variable click intensity (dB) and click frequency (0.5 to 200 Hz). The stimulator should be adjustable to allow either condensation or rarefaction clicks. It should also allow alternation of rarefaction and condensation clicks as this can help eliminate stimulus artifact and help differentiate Wave I from cochlear microphonics.

The intensity of the sound stimulus can be reported in a number of ways. It is not technically feasible to measure the actual quantity of sound that the patient receives, so most investigators simply list the decibels of sound being delivered to the patient. The sound intensity can also be related to the statistically normal hearing threshold. In this method the stimulus is said to be a certain number of decibels HL (the decibels above the standardized normal threshold hearing level). If for a particular instrument a normal group of subjects have a mean threshold level of 10 dB, and if the stimulus delivered is 70 dB, then the stimulus intensity is reported as 60 dB HL. If a patient has a hearing loss, it might be more useful to cite the stimulus intensity in terms of its dB above the hearing threshold for a specific ear, or dB SL.

BAEP testing is usually done in a single ear (monaural), and it is common to administer white noise to the ear that is not being stimulated. The purpose of the white noise is to mask the unstimulated ear and prevent it from producing the wave results. The white noise is usually 30–40 dB less in intensity than the click stimulus being delivered to the opposite ear.

Some investigators have begun to use different frequencies of clicks and other types of sound stimuli to simulate the standard behavioral audiogram, but these studies are not ready for general clinical use.

The amplifier and average for BAEP studies are similar to those required for the other evoked potential studies. The apparatus must have an amplification capacity of 500,000 and frequency filters that include a low cut-off of at least 10 Hz and a high cut-off of at least 3000 Hz (1).

Methodology

The most common montages used in BAEP studies are Cz-A1 and Cz-A2, or Cz-Ai (Ai-ipsilateral) and Cz-Ac (Ac-contralateral) (Fig. 11.1). The auricular electrodes can also be placed directly on the mastoid region (M1 and M2), but the signal is usually stronger and has less background noise if the electrode is placed on the earlobe. The electrodes should be meticulously applied, with an impedance of not more than 500 Ohms and preferably less than 2000 Ohms. The most common cause of test failure in BAEP studies is *poor electrode attachment.*

Each laboratory should use the same audiologic quality earphone consistently, because the design and fit of the earphones affect the intensity of sound actually delivered to the patient. A small earphone that fits into the external ear canal may be necessary for some cases of intraoperative monitoring.

The stimulus frequency is usually 10-11 Hz. It is good practice to avoid stimulus frequencies that are multiples of 60 to lessen 60-Hz line interference. The intensity of the stimulus should be sufficient to give

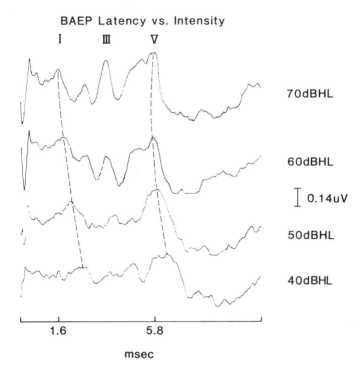

BAEP Latency vs. Intensity

Figure 11.7. BAEP latency versus intensity. Results in a 45-year-old woman, 11.1/sec, 100 msec, positive polarity stimulus (click). 150-3000 Hz bandpass with 2000 repetitions on Nicolet CA-1000. Note that the I-V interpeak interval is stable as absolute latencies of Waves I through V change with intensity.

a clear Wave I and V. Some investigators suggest avoiding a stimulus that produces a Wave I latency of less than 1.6 msec or a Wave V latency of less than 5.8 msec (4). The stimulus intensity is usually 70 dB for individuals with normal hearing.

Although changing the stimulus intensity changes the amplitude and latency of the waves, it does *not* significantly change the interpeak latencies (IPLs) (Fig. 11.7). For this reason, interpeak latency is usually a more useful aspect of BAEPs for clinical interpretation than the absolute latencies (15).

For interpretation purposes Wave I must be clearly seen. It may be necessary to use a higher stimulus intensity or lower stimulus frequency than usual to obtain it in some cases. Another technique to bring out Wave I is to switch from rarefaction to condensation clicks, although rarefaction clicks usually give a larger Wave I (33). The most effective technique for bringing out Wave I is to use an EEG needle electrode that is inserted in the anterior wall of the external ear canal. This electrode shows Wave I in as many as 75% of the individuals who show no Wave I otherwise (15). Routine studies normally involve amplification of 500,000 with filter settings of 100 Hz for the low cut-off and 3000 Hz for the high cut-off. Averaging 2000 trials is usually necessary to obtain a clean response. Generally one channel is sufficient for a good BAEP study (Ai-Cz), but other montages are often interesting and may be helpful at times in finding Wave I, especially a horizontal montage, such as Ai-Ac.

The patient should be relaxed and lying supine to eliminate as much of the muscle artifact as possible. Chloral hydrate and/or diphenhydramine or other sedative may be necessary to eliminate muscle artifact, particularly in children. The BAEP study must be done at least twice for each ear to make certain that the results are reproducible. Consecutive studies should have intertrial variability of the peak latencies of less than 0.2 msec (79).

Normal Values for BAEPs

The normal values for BAEPs vary to some extent with each laboratory, and each laboratory must have standardized values. The normative values of Chiappa et al. (17) for 50 adults of ages 15-51 years of both sexes are listed in Table 10.3.

Subject Factors affecting BAEP Results

Age

There is some controversy as to the effect of age on absolute wave latencies and IPLs in adults. Rowe (79) found the I-V IPL to be 0.06 msec longer in older subjects/mean age 61.7 years) than younger subjects (mean age 25.1 years). Beagley and Sheldrake (5) did not observe any significant change with age in their study of 70 normal subjects. If there are actual age differences in adults in wave latencies and in IPLs, they are sufficiently small that they can generally be ignored. BAEP interpretation requires the comparison of an individual's results with a statistical base. The results for older individuals generally fall well within three SDs of the values for all adult ages.

The effect of age on wave amplitude in adults is even more controversial, due to the normal variability in wave amplitudes for any specific age. Marked differences in wave amplitudes, latencies, and IPLs exist between adults and children (see section on pediatric considerations).

Table 11.3. Normal Values for BAEPs[a,b]

	Absolute latencies (msec)			Interwave latencies				Interear interwave differences		
Wave	Mean	SD	Mean + 3 SD	Waves	Mean	SD	Mean + 3 SD	Mean	SD	Mean + 3 SD
I	1.7	0.15	2.2	I-III	2.1	0.15	2.6	0.10	0.09	0.37(0.4)
II	2.8	0.17	3.3	I-V	4.0	0.23	4.7	0.13	0.10	0.43(0.5)
III	3.9	0.19	4.5	III-IV	1.2	0.16	1.7	0.12	0.14	0.54(0.6)
IV	5.1	0.24	5.8	III-V	1.9	0.18	2.4	0.10	0.11	0.43
V	5.7	0.25	6.5	IV-V	0.7	0.19	1.3	0.15	0.14	0.57(0.8)
VI	7.3	0.29	8.2	V-VI	1.5	0.25	2.3	0.22	0.19	0.79(0.8)

	Absolute amplitudes (μV)				Mean amplitudes as %			
Wave		Mean	SC	Range	Waves	Mean	SD	Mean + 3 SD
I		0.28	0.14	0.06-0.85	III/V	50	23	119
III		0.23	0.12	0.03-0.55	I/IV (pre)	132	75	357
IV (pre)		0.25	0.12	0.04-0.63	I/IV (post V)	75	39	191
IV (post V)		0.40	0.13	0.08-0.88	I/V	73	48	218
IV/V (highest peak)		0.47	0.16	0.14-0.88	I/IV-V	62	30	152
V		0.43	0.16	0.15-0.86				
					Amplitude difference between ears			
					V	20	17	71

[a]Obtained from 50 normal subjects of 15-51 years, mixed gender) at 10 clicks/sec. Latencies were measured to the wave peak; where a peak was not well defined, a midpoint of the wave was estimated. When Waves IV and V were fused into a single peak, the latency was taken to the point of final inflection before the negative limb of Wave V, and this was recorded as Wave V only. If either wave appeared as a distance step on the other, this step was taken as the wave peak. Amplitudes were measured from the peak to the following trough, except that Wave IV amplitude was measured from its peak to the preceding trough (pre-IV) and also to the trough following Wave V (post-V). The number in brackets after mean + 3 SD is where the range exceeds the mean + 3 SD. Square-wave duration was 0.1 msec, click intensity 60 dB SL, constant polarity.

[b]Reprinted by permission from Chiappa KH, Gladstone KJ, Young RR: Brainstem auditory evoked responses: studies of the wave form variations in 50 normal human subjects. *Arch Neurol* 36:81-87, 1979.

Gender

Women tend to have higher amplitudes of the BAEP waves, and shorter absolute wave latencies and IPLs than men. These gender differences begin in children at approximately 8 years of age (72). Many reasons for these differences have been mentioned in the literature, but the major factor probably is that women generally have a smaller head size. The recording electrodes are therefore closer to the generator sources of the waves.

Peripheral Hearing Disorders

Peripheral hearing loss produces changes in absolute wave latencies, but does *not* significantly change IPLs. Various types of cochlear hearing loss may even shorten rather than lengthen the I-V IPL. One of the major advantages of using BAEP IPLs for clinical interpretation is that, if Waves I, III, and V are seen, the patients's hearing disorder can largely be ignored.

The absolute latencies of the individual waves *are* affected by peripheral hearing disorders. In subjects without peripheral hearing loss the absolute latencies of Waves I through V decrease in a linear manner with an increasing stimulus intensity. The change is usually a decrease of 0.03 msec per dB increase in stimulus intensity (28). Figure 11.7 shows the changes in values at different stimulus intensities for a typical normal subject.

This latency-intensity relationship changes in a different way in sensorineural than in conductive hearing loss. Conductive hearing loss produces a latency-intensity curve that is parallel to the normal line. The displacement of the curve is generally the same amount as would be suggested by the degree of hearing loss (36). Sensorineural hearing loss produces a recruitment effect that changes the latency-intensity curve to a nonlinear pattern. At low stimulus intensities there is a marked difference in the absolute latencies of the curves, but at higher intensities the difference is much less (14).

The BAEP pathway and the normal hearing pathway are not completely synonymous; thus it is possible for a patient to have marked BAEP abnormalities with a normal behavioral audiogram (14). (This is common, for example, in MS patients). BAEP waves may represent some of the nonhearing functions of the auditory system, such as auditory localization and interaural time discrimination (48).

Drug and Metabolic Effects

The BAEP IPLs are not generally affected by drugs or even by severe metabolic abnormalities, such as elevated BUN or ammonia levels. A patient with a severe drug overdose and an isoelectric EEG usually has a relatively normal BAEP study. Small changes in BAEP IPLs and latencies do occur with drug intoxications of various types, but they are generally sufficiently small that no significant effect on BAEP interpretation occurs. Aminoglycoside antibiotics have been shown to decrease the amplitude of the BAEP waves transiently after either intravenous or oral usage (40).

Technical Factors affecting BAEP Results

Many technical factors that are not related to patient pathology can affect the BAEP parameters. Increasing the click rate generally causes an increase in the BAEP wave latencies and a decrease in their amplitude (26), but may increase the amplitude of Wave V. IPLs also increase slightly at higher stimulus rates.

Rarefaction clicks generally produce the clearest BAEP wave-forms.

They result in shorter Wave I latencies, longer I-III IPL, and more distinct Waves IV and V than do condensation clicks (66). Condensation clicks can be used in cases in which the rarefaction clicks fail to produce adequate wave-forms.

The amplitudes of the waves increase as click intensity increases, except for Wave V, which may be brought out paradoxically by decreasing the stimulus intensity. The absolute latencies of the waves increase with decreasing click intensity. This delay in all the BAEP waves is roughly equal and causes little change in the IPLs (Fig. 11.7).

Clinical Interpretation

The two most important criteria for interpretating BAEPs clinically are the presence or absence of the five waves and the interpeak latencies (I-III, III-V, and I-V). The latencies and amplitudes of the waves are useful but less important because of their greater degree of variability in normals, especially under different stimulus conditions.

Interpeak latencies are not generally affected by peripheral hearing disorders (see section on peripheral hearing disorders). Consequently, if Waves I, III, and V are visible, inferences can be made about central conduction and brainstem function regardless of the patient's hearing difficulties. If the hearing difficulties are sufficiently severe so that Wave I is not seen (even with a special technique, such as using an ear canal needle electrode), then no diagnostic statements can be made about the section of the BAEP pathway from the auditory nerve to the lower pons. If Waves III and V are present, conduction in the remainder of the BAEP brainstem pathway can be judged either normal or abnormal, regardless of whether Wave I is present.

Vestibular system diseases do not generally affect BAEP studies. Patient's with Meniere's disease, vestibular neuronitis, and various other forms of "dizziness" or vertigo have normal BAEP studies (15).

If there is an abnormal I-III IPL, a defect in the pathway from the eighth nerve to the lower pons should be suspected. An abnormality in the wave III-V IPL suggests the presence of a conduction defect in the brainstem between the lower pons and the midbrain. If all of the IPLs are prolonged and the I-V IPL is prolonged, one should suspect a generalized phenomenon in the brainstem. If none of the waves are present, the testing system should be checked as the commonest cause of their absence is poor technique. Only rarely does a patient show none of the waves. The CNS amplifies sensory information as it passes toward the higher centers. Consequently only a small part of the stimulus must get through the eighth nerve to produce the results in the brainstem.

Intentionally reducing the stimulus intensity may actually help bring out Wave V, because it tends to be higher in amplitude in many individuals at a lower stimulus intensity. The amplitude of Wave V in most individuals should be sufficient that the ratio of the amplitudes of Waves V and I should be greater than 0.5 (4).

Most BAEP abnormalities are unilateral and occur ipsilateral to the ear being tested, because there is less crossover in the BAEP pathway than in the normal hearing pathway. Most abnormalities of BAEPs are due to anatomic abnormalities of a *structural* type in the eighth cranial nerve or brainstem. Most drugs or toxic conditions do not significantly alter BAEPs. BAEP studies also tend to be either normal or obviously abnormal. Few false-positive interpretations occur if minor changes in the BAEP are appropriately ignored rather than reported as being due to pathology. Pathology in the BAEP pathway usually produces obvious BAEP changes, such as loss of waves or marked IPL changes.

Acoustic Neuromas and Cerebellopontine Angle Tumors

BAEPs have a useful and reliable role in the diagnosis of acoustic neuromas (AN) and cerebellopontine angle tumors (CPA). Many literature citations of AN and CPA cases in the past few years have noted that BAEPs may be abnormal earlier in the course of disease than are audiologic studies and CT scans. There is no clear agreement in the literature as to the exact BAEP diagnostic criteria for AN or CPA. Using the absolute latency of Wave V introduces some error in interpretation because all wave latencies change with the decrease in the effect stimulus that occurs due to the hearing loss that may result from the tumor. Some investigators have attempted to overcome this problem by using correction factors for Wave V latencies in patients with hearing loss (81).

The use of BAEP IPLs to interpret normality or abnormality in suspected cases of AN or CPA seems to be a more accurate and reliable method. IPLs have the advantage of not being significantly affected by hearing loss and other technical factors. The main problem with the use of IPLs is that Waves I, III, and V must be visualized and Wave I in particular may be difficult to visualize in these cases. However, the special techniques outlined earlier usually enable the visualization of Wave I, unless the tumor is advanced, in which case the diagnosis will usually be obvious radiologically. Eggermont et al. (29) used the I-V IPL as the guideline for abnormality in suspected AN. Using three SDs above the mean as the upper limit of normal, they had false-negative results in only 2 patients and no false-positive results in 42 patients with AN. Parker et al. (73) had no false-positive or negative results using IPLs in 4l patients with AN and 9 with CPA meningiomas. Chiappa (15) reports that the most sensitive measure of whether an AN or CPA tumor is present is a prolongation beyond three SDs of the I-III IPL.

Most investigators now feel that if a patient has a clearly normal BAEP study that the possibility of an acoustic neuroma is remote.

Multiple Sclerosis

Another important clinical use of BAEPs is in the diagnosis of multiple sclerosis (MS). The basis for this use is the fact that MS patients usually have multiple lesions in the CNS. Only a few or even none of these lesions may be clinically apparent at any given time. Typically a new case of MS presents with clinical abnormalities in one system, such as vision, and the diagnostic requirement is then to demonstrate lesions elsewhere in the CNS. The best use of the evoked potential studies in MS patients is to combine BAEPs with VEPs and SEPs. Depending on the location of the lesions within the CNS of any given patient, one or more of these studies may be abnormal. These studies may be abnormal even if the patient does not have current, clinically demonstrable neurologic abnormalities. For example, BAEP studies in MS patients are often abnormal, but hearing studies are usually normal. VEPs are also often abnormal when vision is clinically normal. SEPs may be abnormal in these patients when they have no clinical long-tract signs.

Many published studies in the past few years document the usefulness of BAEPs in MS diagnosis. Chiappa (15) has cross-tabulated the data from many of those articles to produce a conglomerate of 1006 MS patients, 46% of whom were found to have abnormal BAEPs. The BAEP abnormality rate in these patients ranged from 67% in definite MS and 41% in probable MS to 30% in possible MS.

Although various authors have reported different abnormalities in the BAEPs of MS patients, in general it can be stated that the BAEPs in MS patients are usually obviously normal or abnormal. Those MS patients having normal BAEP studies have the same BAEP statistical parameters overall as normal individuals. Some of the most common BAEP abnormalities seen in MS patients are abnormally prolonged IPLs and a decrease in Wave V amplitude. One study of 202 patients with MS showed the most common abnormality to be an absence or abnormally low amplitude of Wave V (87%), and the second most common abnormality to be an abnormal III-V IPL (28%) (18).

Despite the usefulness of BAEPs, most MS studies have shown BAEPs to be the least diagnostically sensitive of the evoked potential studies. VEPs are usually the most sensitive, with SEPs second, and BAEPs the least sensitive. Combined use of the three evoked potential studies in MS patients has been shown (96) to give abnormal findings in at least one evoked potential study in 97% of definite MS cases, 86% in probably cases, and 63% in possible cases.

Brainstem Lesions

BAEPs testing is often useful for studying structural brainstem lesions. Brainstem tumors and hemorrhages produce BAEP abnormalities if the lesion is in the BAEP pathway. The BAEP abnormalities that are seen are generally a function of the location of the lesion. For example, in a pontine tumor or hemorrhage, Waves I and III are usually well preserved, but Waves IV and V may be absent or the III-V IPL prolonged.

Strokes

Brainstem strokes also produce BAEP abnormalities if the area of damaged tissue lies in the BAEP pathway. Ragazoni et al. (77) did BAEPs in patients with transient ischemic attacks from the vertebrobasilar artery system. The studies were done at least 7 days after the last attack when the patients were asymptomatic. Approximately half of the patients were found to have BAEP IPL abnormalities. It is likely that future studies will more fully delineate how BAEP testing can be used in patients with brainstem transient ischemic attacks or in clinically apparent brainstem strokes. The BAEP seems to be abnormal in transient ischemic attacks only if some permanent damage has occurred, whether or not this damage is clinically evident.

Coma and Head Injury

BAEPs testing has also been used to help determine the integrity of the brainstem in comatose patients. Because Waves I-V of BAEPs are generated by structures below the midbrain level, lesions in the brainstem above the midbrain or in the cerebrum do not usually produce abnormalities. Patients with brainstem structural lesions sufficient to produce coma may not have a lesion in the portion of the brainstem traversed by the BAEP pathway. In these cases the patients may have obvious brainstem coma but completely normal BAEPs. If the BAEP study is abnormal in a comatose patient, it would generally indicate that at least part of the abnormality producing the coma is a structural one in the BAEP pathway. Most patients who are comatose from a toxic or metabolic cause have normal BAEPs (86).

Patients with coma from head injuries have been extensively studied with BAEPs. In general, the more abnormal the BAEP study, the worse the prognosis for the patient. Unfortunately, none of the BAEP studies to date has provided a method to produce a definite prognostic statement in the individual case. Greenberg et al. (59) studied multimodality testing (BAEP, VEP, and SEP) in 100 head-injured patients and compared these results with the clinical outcome at 1 year postinjury. Their study predicted the outcome at 1 year with approximately 80% accuracy. Removing the cases of death that occurred due to systemic causes improved this prediction to nearly 100% accuracy. A recent multimodality evoked potential study of patients (3) with coma from head injury showed BAEPs to be an excellent predictor of a bad outcome in that a severely abnormal BAEP always meant poor neurologic recovery or death. SEPs were the only study able to predict a good outcome reliably because normal BAEPs or VEPs were often associated with a poor outcome. Starr and Achor (86) demonstrated that BAEPs can often help differentiate reversible drug or metabolic coma from less reversible coma due to structural injury to the brainstem.

BAEPs have also been used in brain-death cases. Drug or metabolically induced causes of coma sufficient to produce a flat EEG generally give a normal BAEP study. Many patients with clinical brain-death also have sufficient injury to the brainstem to produce a BAEP abnormality as well. It is probable that further research in combining the evoked potential studies (including BAEPs) with the EEG will provide a more reliable basis for assessing brain-death.

Miscellaneous Uses

The use of BAEPs in patients with numerous neurologic syndromes has been reported in the literature. Among those that have been shown to have significant BAEP abnormalities in at least some cases are metachromatic leukodystrophy, Friedreich's ataxia, spinocerebellar brainstem ataxias, Wilson's disease, meningitis, B_{12} deficiency, and Charcot-Marie-Tooth disease (15). The neurologic conditions that have generally been found so far to have normal BAEPs include amyotrophic lateral sclerosis, Batten's disease, acute transverse myelopathy, cortical deafness, Huntington's disease, and renal disease (15).

Use of BAEPs in Pediatrics

Many articles in the literature have suggested various uses of BAEP studies in infants and children. Some of these uses are not substantially different from those in adults, such as the detection of brainstem tumors (36). BAEP studies are much more useful for the detection of hearing problems in infants than in adults, because a behavioral audiogram is usually not possible in infants.

There are many differences between adult and infant BAEP wave amplitudes, latencies, and IPLs due to a number of factors, including the smaller head size in infants. The smaller head size places the electrodes closer to the centers generating the potentials (17). Wave I is generally of greater amplitude in infants (49). Absolute wave latencies and IPLs are prolonged in infants and progressively decrease to approximate adult values by 2 years of age. Premature infants have more prolonged latencies of the waves and IPLs than full-term infants.

BAEPs in infants must include age-specific informative data. Chiappa (15) suggests that normal values should be standardized for every 2 weeks of age up to normal term (40 weeks gestation) and then for 3 weeks, 6 weeks, 3 months, 6 months, and 1 year of age. The changes in BAEPs latencies and IPLs in infancy are most likely due to increasing myelination, but such other factors as increasing fiber size and synaptic efficiency have been suggested (87).

BAEP techniques in infants are somewhat different from those in adults. Interference from muscle noise is a much greater problem than in adults; consequently, studies generally must be done during sleep. A foam cushion over the earphone is necessary to prevent loss of sound and also to help prevent excessive pressure on the ear that might cause the external ear canal to collapse.

The most frequent pediatric use of BAEPs is in screening for congenital or acquired hearing loss. BAEPs are indicated in all infants less than 6 months of age who are suspected of hearing loss or who are at high risk of hearing loss (4). They should also be considered if there are questionable results on behavioral audiograms in children from 6 months to 2 years of age.

Many authors have compared the results of BAEPs testing with conventional audiometric studies in children. Good correlations have been found (83), and one study (80) detected all 8 cases of hearing loss with BAEPs that occurred in 373 infants in a neonatal intensive care unit.

A normal absolute Wave I latency and a symmetric and low BAEP threshold can be considered strong evidence for normality of hearing in infants (17). IPLs in newborns must be used carefully in clinical interpretation because of their change with sound intensity. Because Wave I latency changes more rapidly with intensity than Wave V latency in newborns, the I-V IPL decreases with decreasing stimulus intensity. The I-V IPL is actually reduced from normal in many cases of hearing loss because Wave I is delayed more than Wave V. For further information on the techniques for BAEPs in infants and children, the reader is referred to the article by Hecox et al. (50).

VISUAL EVOKED POTENTIALS

Visual evoked potentials (VEPs) are becoming increasingly important in the contemporary diagnosis of visual pathway problems of both adults and children. VEPs have been known for decades since electroencephalographers recognized that flashing light produced electroencephalographic (EEG) changes. Early research on VEPs used flashing light or strobe light stimuli. Although some diagnostically useful aspects of these flash VEP techniques were found as late as 1975 Ciganek (19) reported pessimistically that "the interpretation of the results is difficult. The pathophysiological significance of separate signs is questionable and even the determination of the boundaries between normal and pathological is uncertain."

VEPs gained widespread popularity after it was noted that the use of pattern shift stimuli gave responses that are much more reliable in morphology, amplitude, and latency than flash VEPs. Cortical neurons respond to contrast, edges, and lines very readily, but ignore uniform illumination (58). The pattern shift visual evoked potentials (PSVEP) are most commonly generated by a checkerboard on a television screen. The checkerboard shifts the black squares to white and vice versa, with no net change in the luminance of the screen. The checkerboard stimulus method opened the visual system to scrutiny that was not previously possible.

The pathway of the VEP seems to follow the visual pathway closely. Any abnormality of the visual pathway from the cornea to the occipital cortex can affect the PSVEP. Because visual problems from the cornea to the retina can usually be studied with standard ophthalmologic instruments, PSVEPs are mainly used to study problems of the optic pathway from the optic nerve to the cortex. Flash VEPs are still useful in some circumstances to determine if the visual pathway from the eye to the cortex is grossly intact. They are especially helpful when a patient is unable to cooperate sufficiently for a PSVEP to be performed, such as during general anesthesia or coma and in very young infants.

Equipment

The basic evoked potential apparatus described in the introduction to the section of BAEP studies is usually adequate for PSVEPs, but some additional pieces of equipment are required. A device capable of producing the shifting pattern of checkerboard squares is necessary. This pattern can be produced in a number of ways, but most commonly it is made on a television monitor. The stimulus generator should be adjustable to give different check sizes, rates of pattern shift, and full or partial screen use. The TV monitor can be black and white or color, but routine PSVEP studies do not require a color monitor and little is known about the effect of color on PSVEPs. The TV monitor must be of sufficient quality to give constant luminance and contrast. A strobe flash device for flash VEPs should also be available.

Methodology

Routine PSVEPs in adults require that the patient sit in a chair and carefully watch the shifting checkerboard squares on a TV monitor (Fig. 11.8). An exact distance from the subject's eye to the screen

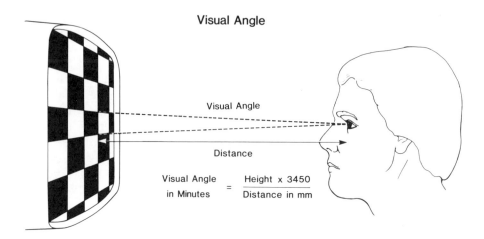

Figure 11.8. Easy method for calculating the visual angle. Multiply the height of a square in mm by 3450, then divide by the distance from the eye to the screen in mm. This gives the visual angle in minutes. Convert the result to degrees by dividing by 60.

should be selected for standardization of the study (usually 1 m). Electrodes should be applied as described in previous sections, with electrode impedance under 2000 Ohms. PSVEPs are best recorded using an amplification of 20,000 to 100,000.

The frequency of stimulation should be 1-2 Hz. Rates of stimulation up to 2 Hz produce a response pattern referred to as a transient visual evoked potential (T-VEP). Higher frequency stimulation (especially 10 Hz or more) produces a monotonous imaging of the responses that is referred to as the steady state visual evoked potential (S-VEP). Strobe flash VEPs are usually done at a sufficiently high frequency to give an S-VEP.

The filters are usually set at 0.2 to 1.0 Hz for the low cut-off and 200-300 Hz for the high cut-off (1). An analysis time of 250 to 500 msec is used.

PSVEPs are the largest of the commonly observed evoked potentials and are usually obvious after 100 stimuli. However, occasionally as many as 500 may be necessary (Fig. 11.9). As in the other evoked potential studies, the PSVEP should be repeated at least twice to make certain that the results are reproducible. The subject should watch a dot in the center of the screen, and care must be taken to make certain that the subject is actually watching the screen. PSVEPs are always done monocularly except in unusual circumstances.

NORMAL VEP

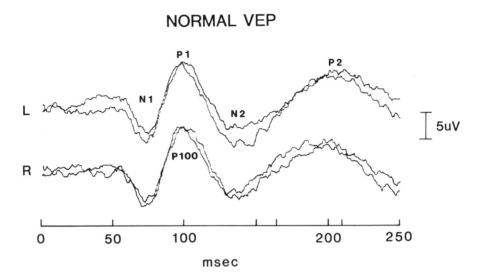

Figure 11.9. Normal VEPs in a 45-year-old woman with Nicolet CA-1000, O'z-Fpz, 100 repetitions at 5-100 Hz bandpass, 1.88/sec, full field, with visual angle of 29 minutes. Note that P1 occurs at approximately 100 msec and is usually called P100.

The visual angle subtended from one eye to one of the squares (checks) must be known. (However, knowing the check size is not helpful unless one also knows the distance of the subject from the screen). A number of mathematical methods can be used to calculate the visual angle. One of the simplest methods for determining the visual angle (in minutes) is to multiply the width of the check in millimeters by 3450 and divide by the millimeters of eye-screen distance (1) (Fig. 11.8). The visual angle in degrees can be calculated by dividing the minutes by 60.

Checks of 10-20 minutes of visual angle give the highest amplitudes of the PSVEPs in adults (46). PSVEPs for visual angles of less than 15 minutes of arc are due mainly to macular stimulation (85). Visual angles above 15 minutes of arc mainly involve the fovea, and those greater than 40 minutes of arc primarily involve the parafoveal retina (1). Figure 11.10 shows the effects on the VEP of increasing the check size. If the study is done with only one check size, a visual angle of 28–32 minutes of arc is a good compromise (1).

The central visual field produces most of the amplitude of P100. This is due to the relatively greater area of cortical representation of the

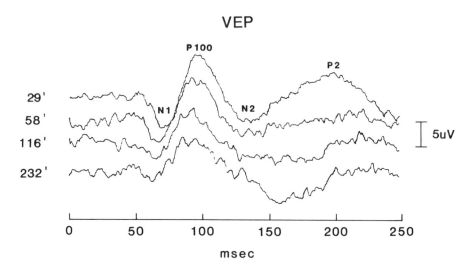

Figure 11.10. Change in VEPs with visual angle. VEPs in a 45-year-old woman at 29, 58, 116, and 232 minutes. Note that the amplitude of P100 declines with increasing visual angle, but the latency decreases. Nicolet CA-1000 with 1.88/sec, full field stimulus. O'z-Fpz, 5-100 Hz bandpass, 100 repetitions.

central field of vision as compared to the periphery. Problems involving the central visual field, such as a scotoma, are likely to reduce the amplitude of P100 severely, although the latency is usually unchanged.

Visual angles of less than 20 minutes of arc require optimum optical refraction for best results. Patients who wear glasses should certainly use them during the studies, especially for small check sizes. The highest amplitude and shortest latency PSVEPs for any check size occur when the patient is optimally refracted. This fact can be used in special cases to help refract a patient.

The electrode pair of Cz-Oz is probably the most commonly used. Chiappa recommends that three additional pairs be used: Oz-reference, Pz-reference, and Cz-reference (15). The reference is usually either placed on the earlobe or forehead. This "midline" four-channel montage may show PSVEP abnormalities in patients with visual field defects. A set of lateral montages should be used if the patient has a known visual field defect or if partial field stimulation is being used for any reason. A set of lateral montages should also be used if one or more of the midline PSVEP montages are abnormal. Chiappa recommends a "lateral" montage set of Oz-reference, Pz-reference, L5-reference, and R5-reference. R5 and L5 are located 5 cm up from the inion and 5 cm lateral to the midline on the right and left sides, respectively (15).

Normal Results and Interpretation

In routine clinical studies in adults, four waves are generally seen. They are usually labeled N1, P1, N2, and P2 (Fig. 11.9). By far the most valuable and reliable of these is P1. P1 occurs in most individuals at about 100 msec, and consequently it is often referred to as P100. It must be kept in mind that this is a name for the potential, as few persons have a P100 of exactly 100 msec (although the patient whose VEP is shown in Figure 11.9 did). P100 seems to be generated by the striate and prestriate cortex of the occipital lobes. N1 is also called N75, and N2 is also called N145 (1).

Most investigators currently interpret PSVEPs based almost totally on the latency of P100, with some attention paid to its amplitude. Consequently, the study should be designed to demonstrate P100 clearly. PSVEP reports should include at least the P100 latency and amplitude and the interocular difference in the P100 latencies and amplitudes. The duration of P100 is less important as it correlates with the latency. The normal values must be standardized for each laboratory.

Technical Factors affecting PSVEP Results

Luminance changes affect the P100 results. The amplitude of P100 increases and the latency decreases if the luminance is increased. Because pupillary diameter affects the quantity of light reaching the retina, ambient light conditions must be rigidly controlled. Patients should not generally be tested with meiosis or mydriasis induced by drugs.

Pattern contrast also affects P100 in that increasing contrast increases the amplitude of P100 and shortens its latency. Consequently, contrast should be rigidly standardized for each laboratory. It can generally be assumed that a TV monitor will give the same degree of contrast as long as the contrast setting is not changed; it may be helpful to disable the contrast and brightness controls to prevent accidental changes of these settings.

Changes in the check size for any given distance or visual angle have major effects on the PSVEP, as the P100 latency decreases with larger check sizes (greater visual angle). The P100 latency can decrease as much as 10 msec with a change from 7.5- to 60-minute checks (46) (Fig. 11.10). The amplitude of P100 tends to be optimal at 10–20 minutes of visual angle, with smaller or larger angles generally producing lower amplitudes.

Effect of Age on PSVEP Results

The age of the patient is also important in interpreting PSVEPs (see section on pediatric uses). There is considerable argument in the literature about the effects of aging on P100, and it seems that the effects of aging are check-size dependent. The rate of increase in P100 latency with age in normals is twice as fast for 12-minute checks as for 48-minute checks (85). Most studies have found minimal changes with age until after the fifth decade and even then the changes are slight (82).

Clinical Uses

Just as in the case of peripheral nerve conduction studies, PSVEPs generally show latency changes in demyelinating conditions and amplitude changes in axonal loss. Conduction defects in the optic nerve usually produce latency changes without much change in the waveform configuration. Axonal lesions of the optic nerves are more likely to lower the amplitudes of the PSVEPs without changing the latencies.

Celesia reports that lesions anterior to the optic chiasm prolong PSVEP latency (13). Generally, the lesions anterior to the optic chiasm can be assumed to be in the optic nerve or retina, because anterior ocular pathology (lesions of the vitreous, lens, anterior chamber, and cornea) can be ruled out by clinical examination. It may be difficult in some cases to distinguish pathology of the retina from that of the optic nerve. Celesia suggests that in such cases an electroretinogram (ERG) may be helpful because it is abnormal if there is retinal pathology, but not if the pathology is in the optic nerve (13).

Use in Optic Neuritis and Multiple Sclerosis

Numerous studies have validated the use of PSVEPs in the diagnosis of MS. This diagnostic usefulness is due to the tendency of MS to involve the visual system preferentially. The PSVEP in patients with MS or other optic nerve lesions may be abnormal even if all other ophthalmologic studies are completely normal. A host of research studies have demonstrated the usefulness of PSVEPs in optic neuritis. The PSVEP is almost always abnormal in individuals with known optic neuritis, and it generally *never returns to normal*, even if the patient clinically recovers from the optic neuritis. The PSVEP study can be abnormal for many years after a single episode of optic neuritis that has clinically resolved, and the abnormality often worsens with each successive episode of optic neuritis (44).

Literally thousands of patients with MS have had PSVEP studies. The rates of abnormality are different with each investigator, but it has become clear that a patient with definite MS will have an abnormal PSVEP at least 85% of the time. Those with probable MS will have an abnormal study approximately 50% of the time, as compared to a rate of about 35% for those with possible MS. These figures can be made more impressive by also doing SEPs and BAEPs for a multimodality MS screen (76).

Different investigators have chosen different criteria for the determination of abnormalities in PSVEPs in MS patients. The latency of P100 is the most useful parameter. Delays in this latency can run from a few SDs above the mean to as much as 100 msec or more of P100 delay. Adding the interocular P100 latency difference to the interpretation greatly improves the diagnostic yield. The P100 interocular difference is frequently the most sensitive factor in optic neuritis and MS diagnosis. The amplitude of P100 should not be ignored, but it is less helpful in most cases than the absolute and interocular latencies (15).

Miscellaneous Clinical Uses

PSVEPs are very helpful in diagnosing and following tumors that compress the anterior visual pathways. Both intrinsic and extrinsic tumors can cause the PSVEP to be absent or greatly reduced in amplitude. In these cases the P100 latency is not as dramatically changed as in optic neuritis and may even be normal or only slightly abnormal. The PSVEP generally returns toward normal when the pressure is removed from the optic nerve. Papilledema may not produce changes in the P100, even if it is severe. Further PSVEP research studies in papilledema are necessary to provide more concise guidelines as to how the PSVEP can be diagnostically used in such cases.

CNS diseases may produce an abnormal PSVEP study. Most of these conditions have been reported by investigators who have studied only a small number of patients. Consequently, much of this information is still speculative at this time. Patients with Friedreich's ataxia frequently have PSVEP abnormalities. The P100 latency is often prolonged and its amplitude reduced in such patients, even if they have no visual complaints (15).

PSVEP abnormalities have also been seen in cases of Charcot-Marie-Tooth disease, B_{12} deficiency, parkinsonism, pernicious anemia, sarcoidosis, toxic amblyopia, Huntington's chorea, and migraine. Studies of amyotrophic lateral sclerosis, Alzheimer's disease, and renal disease have so far not shown significant PSVEP abnormalities (15).

The use of PSVEPs to study the posterior visual pathways in cases of brain tumors, cortical blindness, and stroke is somewhat confusing at this time. A unilateral lesion affecting the optic radiations or occipital cortex does usually not cause changes in the PSVEP because the potential from the normal side of the brain tends to cover the abnormal side. The use of partial field PSVEPs holds some promise in clarifying this diagnostic problem, but investigators hold differing viewpoints about how valuable partial field PSVEP studies are at this time. Blumhardt and Halliday (6) reported that partial field PSVEP studies were abnormal in patients with hemianopia. They used an amplitude criteria in which a half-field was considered abnormal if it had less than half the amplitude of the other half-field. They found the amplitude of P100 to be more valuable than the latency and also found that the cortical lesion had to be directly in the visual pathway to produce an abnormality. These PSVEP partial field studies were not found to be as sensitive for diagnosing hemianopia as routine ophthalmologic field studies.

There is also controversy about the use of PSVEPs in patients with cortical blindness and in those with a hysterical or malingering complaint of vision loss. A completely normal PSVEP in these cases suggests that vision may be present, but does not totally rule out cortical blindness. Lesions of the occipital cortex must be extensive to eliminate completely or even change the PSVEP extensively. The PSVEP study is more sensitive to a cortical disturbance if the visual angle is kept down to 20 minutes or less. Obviously, if the PSVEP is clearly abnormal, then malingering or hysterical loss of vision may not be a reasonable consideration.

Pediatric Uses of Visual Evoked Potentials

VEPs are very helpful in such conditions as strabismus, anisemetropia, and amblyopia; in assessing possible blindness in infants; and in refracting infants. The protocol suggested by Sokol (84) is as follows:

1. Use 60-minute checks for 2-month-old infants, 30-minute checks for 3- and 4-month-old infants, and 15-minute checks for infants and children over 5 or more months of age. If no response is obtained with the check size appropriate for the infant's age, double the check size.
2. Test with two different pattern shift rates. Slower rates (2 Hz or less) give specific component information, whereas faster rates (4 Hz or more) give a different view of the PSVEP.
3. Keep the testing time short, and arrange the stimulus in such a way that someone can observe the child's fixation. It is helpful to have a device that allows this observer to stop the recording when the child is distracted.
4. Test binocularly first to see if a signal can be recorded. If no signal is obtained, do binocular studies with a larger check size to find the conditions necessary to produce the PSVEP before going on to monocular studies.
5. Patch the eye with the suspected pathology first. If the pathologic eye is very bad, the child may be essentially blind with the "good"

eye patched, which can cause great distress and make further testing difficult.
6. The amplitude difference between the two eyes of most children is
quite small (3.0 μV with a standard deviation of 2.1 μV). Acuity is
best evaluated by comparing these amplitudes in the same child,
rather than using standardized amplitudes from a table.

Some have reported that optical refraction can be done within 0.25
diopters with PSVEPs. This is not frequently helpful because retinoscopy is easier to do and gives a similar refraction estimate. The best
use of PSVEPs in refraction may be to do studies with and without the
correction suggested by retinoscopy to see if improvement in acuity
has in fact occurred (84).

The treatment of amblyopia can be monitored with PSVEPs (84). As
amblyopia is successfully treated by occlusion of the "good" eye, the
amplitude from the amblyopic eye increases. Generally the overall goal
in amblyopia is to balance the amplitudes of the PSVEPs as much as
possible between the two sides.

Use of Visual Evoked Potentials in Surgery

A number of investigators have reported the use of VEPs during surgery involving the anterior visual pathway. Different methods have
been used, and there is no agreement as to the best system or even the
validity of the results. Wright and associates (95) used a fiber optic
cable attached to a contact lens to deliver a flash stimulus. The most
reliable change with this method was a loss of all responses on manipulation or compression of the optic nerve. Wilson and associates (94)
placed scleral shells under the eyelids that had built-in light-emitting
diodes (LEDs) to deliver a flash stimulus. They noted changes in the
VEP on chiasmal manipulation that slowly returned to normal over a
few minutes. Feinsod and associates (35) reported using this system
during the removal of a pituitary adenoma. They noted that the VEPs
deteriorated during the procedure, but had a higher amplitude and
shorter latency after decompression was complete. Pratt (75) reported
the use of an array of LEDs on an eyepatch in a patient with optic
nerve compression following a skull fracture. The VEP improved as the
optic nerve was decompressed. Raudzens (78) reported on 71 operative
cases using this system. Although the results were difficult to interpret, there was no case in which a patient developed a postoperative
visual defect if the VEP remained normal throughout the operative
procedure. This use of VEPs in surgery needs further development in
future studies. The intraoperative use of VEPs and possibly PSVEPs
holds considerable promise for improving the safety of anterior visual
tract surgical procedures.

References

1. American Electroencephalographic Society: Guidelines for clinical evoked potential studies. *J Clin Neurophysiol* 1:3, 1984.
2. Aminoff MJ: The clinical role of somatosensory evoked potential studies: a critical appraisal. *Muscle Nerve* 7:345–354, 1984.
3. Anderson DC, Bundlie S, Rockswold GL: Multimodality evoked potentials in closed head trauma. *Arch Neurol* 41:369–374, 1984.
4. Baran E: Workshop on brainstem auditory evoked potentials. Lecture part of Workshop on evoked potentials. White Plains, New York, March 12, 1982.
5. Beagley HA, Sheldrake JB:Differences in brainstem response latency with age and sex. *Br J Audiol* 12:69–77, 1978.
6. Blumhardt LD, Halliday AM: Hemisphere contributions to the composition of the pattern-evoked potential waveform. *Exp Brain Res* 36:53–69, 1979.
7. Bonney G, Gilliatt RW: Sensory nerve conduction after traction lesions of the brachial plexus. *Proc Roy Soc Med* 51:365–367, 1958.
8. Braddom RL, Johnson EW: Standardization of the H reflex and diagnostic use in S-1 radiculopathy. *Arch Phys Med Rehabil* 55:161–166, 1974.
9. Brown JR, Beebe GW, Kurtzke JF, Loewenson RB, Silverberg DH, Tourtellotte WW: The design of clinical studies to assess therapeutic efficacy in multiple sclerosis. *Neurology* (Minneap) 29:3–23, 1979.
10. Brown WF, Davis M, Feasby TE: The localization of conduction abnormalities in Guillain–Barré polyneuritis by somatosensory evoked potential techniques. Presented at the Fifth International Congress of Neuromuscular Diseases, Marseilles, September, 1982.
11. Burke D, Skuse NF, Lethlean AK: Cutaneous and muscle afferent components of the cerebral potential evoked by electrical stimulation of human peripheral nerve. *Electroencephalogr Clin Neurophysiol* 51:579–588, 1981.
12. Butler ET, Johnson EW, Kaye ZA: Normal conduction velocity in the lateral femoral cutaneous nerve. *Arch Phys Med Rehabil* 55:31, 1974.
13. Celesia GG:Visual evoked potentials in neurological disorders. *Am J EEG Technol* 18:47–59, 1978.
14. Chiappa KH: Pattern shift visual, brainstem auditory and short–latency somatosensory evoked potentials in multiple sclerosis. *Neurology* 30:110–123, 1980.
15. Chiappa KH: *Evoked Potentials in Clinical Medicine.* New York, Raven Press, 1983.
16. Chiappa KH, Ropper AH: Evoked potentials in clinical practice (second of two parts). *N Engl J Med* 306:1205–1211, 1982.
17. Chiappa KH, Gladstone KJ, Young RR: Brainstem auditory evoked responses: studies of the wave form variations in 50 normal human subjects. *Arch Neurol* 36:81–87, 1979.
18. Chiappa KH, Harrison JL, Brooks EB, Young RR: Brainstem auditory evoked responses in 200 patients with multiple sclerosis. *Ann Neurol* 7:135–143, 1980.
19. Cigannek L: Visual evoked responses. In Remond A A (ed):*Handbook of Electroencephalography and Clinical Neurophysiology,* vol 8, part A. Amsterdam, Elsevier, 1975.
20. Cracco JB, Cracco RQ, Graziani LJ: The spinal evoked response in infants and children. *Neurology* 25:31–36, 1975.
21. Croft TJ, Brokey JS, Mulsen FE: Reversible spinal cord trauma: a model for electrical monitoring of spinal cord function. *J Neurosurg* 34:402–406, 1972.
22. Daube JR: Intraoperative monitoring of spinal cord function. Abstract at Ameri-

can Association of Electromyography and Electrodiagnosis, St. Paul, MN, 1982.

23. Dawson GD: Investigations on a patient subject to myoclonic seizures after sensory stimulation. *J Neurol Neurosurg Psychiat* 10:141–149, 1947.

24. Desmedt JE, Cheron G: Somatosensory evoked potentials to finger stimulation in healthy octogenarians and in young adults: wave forms, scalp topography and transit times of parietal and frontal components. *Electroencephalogr Clin Neurophysiol* 50:404–425, 1980.

25. Desmedt JE, Brunko E, Debecker J: Maturation of the somatosensory evoked potentials in normal infants and children with special reference to the early N1 component. *Electroencephalogr Clin Neurophysiol* 40:43–58, 1976.

26. Don M, Allen AR, Starr A: Effect of click rate on the latency of auditory brainstem responses in humans. *Ann Otol Rhinol Laryngol* 86:186–195, 1977.

27. Donchin E, Callaway E, Cooper R, Desmedt JE, Goff WR, Hillyard SA, Sutton S: Publication criteria for studies of evoked potentials (EP) in man. Report of a committee. *Prog Clin Neurophysiol* 1:1–11, 1977.

28. Eggermont JJ, Don M: Analysis of the click–evoked brainstem potentials in humans using high–pass noise maskings. II. Effect of click intensity. *J Acoust Soc Am* 68:1671–1675.

29. Eggermont JJ, Don M, Brackmann DE: Electrocochleography and auditory brainstem electric responses in patients with pontine angle tumors. *Ann Otol Rhinol Laryngol* 89: Supplement 75, 1980.

30. Eisen AA: The somatosensory evoked potential. Minimonograph No. 19. Rochester, MN, American Association of Electromyography and Electrodiagnosis, 1982.

31. Eisen A, Elleker G: Sensory nerve stimulation and evoked cerebral potentials. *Neurology 30:1097–1105, 1980.*

32. Eisen A, Hoirch M, Moll A: Evaluation of radiculopathies by segmental stimulation and somatosensory evoked potentials. *Can J Neurol Sci* 10:178–182, 1983.

33. Emerson RG, Brooks EB, Parker SW, Chiappa KH: Effects of click polarity on brainstem auditory evoked potentials in normal subjects and patients; unexpected sensitivity of Wave V. *Ann NY Acad Sci* 388:710, 1982.

34. Engler GL, Spielholtz NI, Bernhard WN, Danzinger F, Merkin H, Wolff T: Somatosensory evoked potentials during Harrington instrumentation for scoliosis. *J Bone Joint Surg* 60A:528–532, 1978.

35. Feinsod M, Selhorst JB, Hoyt WF, Wilson CB: Monitoring optic nerve function during craniotomy. *J Neurosurg* 44:29–31, 1976.

36. Galambos R, Hecox KE: Clinical applications of the auditory brainstem response. *Otolaryngol Clin N Am* 11:709–720, 1978.

37. Giblin DR: Somatosensory evoked potentials in healthy subjects and in patients with lesions of the nervous system. *Ann NY Acad Sci* 112:93–142, 1964.

38. Green JB, Walcoff M, Lucke JF: Phenytoin prolongs far–field somatosensory and auditory evoked potential interpeak latencies. *Neurology* 32:85–88, 1982.

39. Greenberg RP, Newlon PG, Hyatt MS, Raj NK, Becker DP: Prognostic implications of early multimodality evoked potentials in severely head-injured patients. *J Neurosurg* 55:227–236, 1981.

40. Guerit JM, Mahieu P, Houben-Giurgea S, Herbay S: The influence of ototoxic drugs on brainstem auditory evoked potentials in man. *Arch Otorhinolaryngol* 233:189–199, 1981.

41. *Guidelines for Somatosensory Evoked Potentials.* Rochester, MN, American Association of Electromyography and Electrodiagnosis. 1984.

42. Gupta PR, Dorfman LJ: Spinal somatosensory conduction in diabetes. *Neurology* 31:841–845, 1981.

43. Hajdu M, Gonzalez EG, Stone R, Stinchfield F: Application of cortical somatosensory evoked potential monitoring in hip arthroplasty. Presented at Annual Assembly of American Academy of PM&R, Boston, October 22, 1984.
44. Halliday AM: Visual evoked potentials in demyelinating disease. In Waxman SG, Ritchie JM (eds): *Demyelinating Disease: Basic and Clinical Electrophysiology.* New York, Raven Press, 1981.
45. Halliday AM, Carrol WM, Jones SJ: Visual and somatosensory evoked potential studies in Charcot-Marie-Tooth disease. *Electroencephalogr Clin Neurophysiol* 52:584, 1981.
46. Harter MR, White CT: Evoked cortical responses to cherkboard patterns: effect of check-size as a function of visual acuity. *Electroencephalogr Clin Neurophysiol* 28:48–54, 1970.
47. Hashimoto I, Ishiyama Y, Yoshimoto T, Nemoto S: Brain-stem auditory-evoked potentials recorded directly from human brain-stem and thalamus. *Brain* 104:841, 1981.
48. Hausler R, Levine RA: Brainstem auditory evoked potentials are related to interaural time discrimination in patients with multiple sclerosis. *Brain Res* 191:589–594, 1980.
49. Hecox K, Galambos R: Brainstem auditory evoked responses in human infants and adults. *Arch Otolaryngol* 99:30, 1974.
50. Hecox KE, Cone B, Blaw ME: Brainstem auditory evoked response in the diagnosis of pediatric neurologic disease. *Neurology* 31:832–840, 1981.
51. Hubel DH, Wiesel TN: Receptive fields and functional architecture in two nonstriate visual areas (18 and 19) of the cat. *J Neurophysiol* 28:229–289, 1965.
52. Hume AL, Cant BR, Shaw NA: Central somatosensory conduction time in comatose patients. *Ann Neurol* 5:379–384, 1979.
53. Jasper H: The ten-twenty electrode system of the international federation. Report of a committee on clinical examination in EEG. *Electroencephalogr Clin Neurophysiol* 10:371–375, 1958.
54. Jewett DL: Volume-conducted potentials in response to auditory stimuli as detected by averaging in the cat. *Electroencephalogr Clin Neurophysiol* 28:609+, 1970.
55. Jewett DL, Romano MN, Williston JS: Human auditory evoked potentials: possible brainstem components detected on the scalp. *Science* 167:1517, 1970.
56. Jones SJ, Wynn Parry CB, Landi A: Diagnosis of brachial plexus traction lesions by sensory nerve potentials and somatosensory evoked potentials. *Injury* 12:376–382, 1981.
57. Jones SJ, Edgar MA, Ransford AO: Sensory nerve conduction in human spinal cord: epidural recordings made during scoliosis surgery. *J Neurol Neurosurg Psychiat* 45:446–451, 1982.
59. Krumholz A, Weiss HD, Goldstein PJ: Evoked responses in vitamin B_{12} deficiency. *Ann Neurol* 9:407–409, 1981.
60. Lev A, Sohmer H: Sources of averaged neural responses recorded in animal and human subjects during cochlear audiometry (electro-cochleogram). *Arch Klin Exp Ohr-Nas-u Kehlk Heilk.* 201:79, 1971.
61. Liberson WT, Gratzur M, Zales A, Grabinski B: Comparison of conduction velocity of motor and sensory fibers determined by different methods. *Arch Phys Med Rehabil* 47:17–23, 1966.
62. Lueders HO: Optimizing stimulating and recording parameters in evoked potential studies. In Course C (ed):*Somatosensory Evoked Potentials.* Rochester, MN, American Association of Electromyography and Electrodiagnosis, 1983.
63. Lueders H, Gurd A, Hahn J, Andrish J, Weiker G, Klem G: A new technique for

intraoperative monitoring of spinal cord function. Multichannel recording of spinal cord and subcortical evoked potentials. *Spine* 7:110–115, 1982.

64. Lueders H, Lesser RP, Hahn J, Dinner DS, Klem G: Cortical somatosensory evoked potentials in response to hand stimulation. *J Neurosurg* 58:885–893, 1983.

65. Markland ON, Dilley RS, Moorthy SS, Warren C: Monitoring of somatosensory evoked responses during carotid endarterectomy. *Arch Neurol* 41:375–378, 1984.

66. Maurer K, Schafer E, Leitner H: The effect of varying stimulus polarity (rarefaction vs. condensation) on early auditory evoked potentials. *Electroencephalogr Clin Neurophysiol* 50:332–334, 1980.

67. McLeod JG: Electrophysiological studies in Guillain-Barré syndrome. *Ann Neurol* 9 (suppl):20–27, 1981.

68. McLeod JG, Tuck RR, Anthony J, Walsh JC: F-wave conduction in experimental allergic neuritis and the Guillain-Barré syndrome. Presented at the Fifth International Congress of Neuromuscular Diseases, Marseilles, September, 1982.

69. Moller AG, Jannetta P, Moller MB:Neural generators of brainstem evoked potentials. Results from human intracranial recordings. *Ann Otol* 90:591, 1981.

70. Nash CL, Brown RH: The intraoperative monitoring of spinal cord function: its growth and current status. *Orthop Clin N Am* 1:919–926, 1979.

71. Nash CL, Brodkey JS, Croft TJ: A model for electrical monitoring of spinal cord function and scoliosis patients undergoing correction. *J Bone Joint Surg* 53A:904–912, 1971.

72. O'Donovan CA, Beagley HA, Shaw M: Latency of brainstem response in children. *Br J Audiol* 14:23–29, 1980.

73. Parker SW, Chiappa KH, Brooks EB: Brainstem auditory evoked responses in patients with acoustic neuromas and cerebello-pontine angle meningiomas. *Neurology* 30:413–414, 1980.

74. Picton TW, Hillyard SA: Human auditory evoked potentials. II. Effects of attention. *Electroecephalogr Clin Neurophysiol* 36:191, 1974.

75. Pratt H: Evoked potentials in the operating room: three examples using three sensory modalities. *Israel J Med Sci* 17:460–464, 1981.

76. Purves SJ, Low MD, Galloway J, Reeves B: A comparison of visual, brainstem auditory, and somatosensory evoked potentials in multiple sclerosis. *Can J Neurol Sci* 8:15–19, 1981.

77. Ragazzoni A, Amantini A, Rossi L, Pagnini P, Arnetoli G, Marini P, Nencioni C, Versari A, Zappoli R: Brainstem auditory evoked potentials and vertebral-basilar reversible ischemic attacks. In: Courjon J, Mauguiere F, Revol M (eds): *Clinical Applications of Evoked Potentials in Neurology.* New York, Raven Press, 1972, pp 187–194.

78. Raudzens: Intraoperative monitoring of evoked potentials. *Ann NY Acad Sci* 388:308–326, 1982.

79. Rowe MJ III: Normal variability of the brain-stem auditory evoked response in young and old adult subjects. *Electroencephalogr Clin Neurophysiol* 44:459, 1978.

80. Schulman-Galambos C, Galambos R: Brainstem evoked response audiometry in newborn hearing screening. *Arch Otolaryngol* 105:86–90, 1979.

81. Selters WA, Brackmann DE: Acoustic tumor detection with brainstem electric response audiometry. *Arch Otolaryngol* 103:181–187, 1977.

82. Shaw NA, Cant BR: Age-dependent changes in the latency of the pattern visual evoked potential. *Electroencephalogr Clin Neurophysiol* 48:237–241, 1980.

83. Sohmer H, Feinmesser M: Routine use of electrocochleography (cochlear audiometry) on human subjects. *Audiology* 12:167–173, 1973.

84. Sokol S: Visual evoked potentials in clinical practice. Presented at Workshop on Evoked Potentials, White Plains, New York, March 12, 1982.

85. Sokol S, Moskowitz A, Towle VL: Age related changes in the latency of the visual evoked potential: influence of check size. *Electroencephalogr Clin Neurophysiol* 51:559–562, 1981.
86. Starr A, Achor, LJ: Auditory brainstem responses in neurological disease. *Arch Neurol* 32:761–768, 1975.
87. Starr A, Amlie RN, Martin WH, Sanders S: Development of auditory function in newborn infants revealed by auditory brainstem potentials. *Pediatrics* 60:831–839, 1977.
88. Stolov WC: Instrumentation factors in somatosensory evoked potential analysis. In Course C (ed): *Somatosensory Evoked Potentials.* American Association of Electromyography and Electrodiagnosis, 1983.
89. Stolov WT: Somatosensory evoked potentials—clinical samples. Presented at the Annual Session of the American Academy of Physical Medicine and Rehabilitation, Los Angeles, November 11, 1983.
90. Tamaki T: Current status of spinal cord monitoring. *Spine* 4:467, 1979.
91. Tonzola RG, Ackil AA, Shahani BT: Usefulness of electrophysiological studies in the diagnosis of lumbosacral root disease. *Ann Neurol* 9:305–308, 1981.
92. Tsumoto T, Hirose N, Nonaka S, Takahashi M: Analysis of somatosensory evoked potentials to lateral popliteal nerve simulation in man. *Electroencephalogr Clin Neurophysiol* 33:379–388, 1972.
93. Vauzelle C, Stagnara P, Jouvinroux P: Functional monitoring of spinal cord activity during spinal surgery. *Clin Orthop* 93:173–178, 1973.
94. Wilson WB, Kirsch WM, Neville H, Stears J, Feinsod M: Monitoring of visual function during parasellar surgery. *Surg Neurol* 5:323–329, 1976.
95. Wright JE, Arden G, Jones BR: Continuous monitoring of the visual evoked response during intra-orbital surgery. *Trans Ophthalmol Soc* 93:311–314, 1973.
96. Yiannikas C: Thoracic outlet syndrome. In Chiappa K H (ed): *Potentials in Clinical Medicine.* New York, Raven Press, 1983.

12

Reporting and Interpretation

ERNEST W. JOHNSON

Review of EMG reports has shown that a majority are incomplete or in error in some way (1). This purpose of this chapter is to help clinical electromyographers improve their EMG reporting and communication with their colleagues. It reviews over 200 EMG reports that were submitted as part of the enrollment requirements for continuing medical education short courses in EMG at the Ohio State University Department of Physical Medicine. All were collected during the past 5 years.

THE EMG REPORT

This communication between the electromyographer and referring physician is the permanent record of a complex diagnostic procedure, and so it will serve as a comparison for future electrodiagnostic tests. It not only has obvious medicolegal implications but also frequently serves a vital role in management of the patient. All reports should include the following components:

- Demographic data;
- Temporal and topographic summary of the complaint;
- Tabulation of data;
- Summary of the neurophysiologic findings;
- Translation of that summary into a probable clinical diagnosis (or list of differential diagnostic probabilities).

Demographic Data

This part of the report should include the date of the EMG, name and address of the patient and his or her age and sex, and the source of referral (including name of referring physician). The status of the patient (whether in- or outpatient) is important. In one survey of our referrals, 17% had incomplete or wrong addresses.

Any previous EMGs should also be noted.

Temporal and Topographic Summary of Complaint or Reason for Referral

Most often this can be simply a phrase, e.g., foot drop for 1 month, pain in back and right leg for 7 weeks, numbness in left hand for 4 months, etc. Because the electrodiagnostic evaluation is best viewed as an extension of the history and physical examinations, it is essential for the electromyographer to take a short history and perform a pertinent neuromuscular examination in order to plan the procedures. In many instances, a detailed consultation must be requested prior to or in addition to the EMG.

Tabulation of Data

This section should include the muscles explored with needle electrode and their cord levels and peripheral nerve innervation. This is an excellent educational exercise, both for the electromyographer and the referring physician. The findings uncovered in the EMG needle exam then are described under the four parts of the exam.

Step I: Spontaneous Activity

This includes fasciculation and fibrillation potentials. Identification of the former should include a description of their amplitude, duration, shape, and rate. Both should include numbers, e.g., grades I–IV.

Step II: Insertional Activity

The needle electrode is moved briskly through the muscle and the electrical activity noted. In normal muscle "injury potentials" will be noted during the needle insertion, but in various disease states, positive waves will persist after needle electrode movement stops, e.g., denervation, active myopathies, etc. This finding is properly listed under "insertional activity."

Many clinical electromyographers use a separate category for insertional activity that they erroneously describe as "increased." If needle insertion fails to evoke many injury potentials or if a few positive waves are produced—indicating those as a *few, many* or *trains*—it is proper to describe the activity as "reduced." However, it is neither proper nor useful to describe insertional activity as "increased" when the more appropriate description is a *few positive waves*.

In normal muscle at the endplate zone, endplate noise (miniature endplate potentials) and then endplate spikes appear. Should the needle be advanced a bit farther, then the endplate spikes (single muscle fiber discharges) will be recorded as positive waves. This is probably the most overinterpreted portion of the EMG, most likely due to lack of understanding of the genesis of positive sharp waves (2).

Step III: Minimal Contraction to Elicit a Single Motor Unit Potential

In this section are described amplitude, duration, number of phases, numerical rate of firing, and recruitment interval. Although many reports include the percentage of polyphasics, this representation probably is based on false assumptions and may be misleading. It is best to simply report an *increased proportion* of polyphasics. Generally with concentric needle electrodes, fewer than 10–15% of MUPs are seen as polyphasic (a potential crossing the isoelectric line more than four times) in normal muscle.

Step IV: Maximal Contraction

In this section, one should note the recruitment pattern and overall amplitude and, with an audio cue, the duration.

Step V

The *distribution* of any abnormality is determined and recorded. It may be a root, peripheral nerve, branch of peripheral nerve, generalized, or other abnormality.

Conduction Velocity Studies

The nerve and its site of stimulus and electrodes—surface or needle recording and stimulation electrodes—should be recorded. If the stimulus intensity is unusual (e.g. duration of .5 msec), it should be noted. Amplitude and duration of the negative spike of the CMAP should be determined and recorded, as should any change in its shape or size from proximal to distal stimulation. Unfortunately we find these measurements of amplitude and duration to be rarely included in reports.

It is essential to isolate either the stimulus to the nerve or the response of the specific muscle to be certain that the desired nerve is the one being stimulated.

Sensory latencies must include measurements of distances, as well as needle/surface recording and the amplitude and duration of sensory action potentials or nerve action potentials. The report should indicate the anti- or orthodromic mode and note whether the latency measure is to the take-off or peak.

Form of Reporting

In writing an EMG report, one should not use printed lists of muscles and nerves. These tend to stereotype the EMG. To include normal values, in my opinion, misleads the referring physicians. But if values are included, they should only be means and standard deviations. On many of the EMG reports we reviewed, much space was taken up by listing normal values, which led to the implication that results outside of these are abnormal and diagnostically specific. To suggest, for example, that the normal distal latencies of the median nerve are under 5 msec, as was done on several forms, is not only incorrect but is also conceptually misleading. Latencies and conduction velocities are generally meaningless without amplitudes and durations of evoked potentials.

About one-third of the 200 reports reviewed were of the narrative form without tabular presentation of the data. Presumably a worksheet was kept by the electromyographer in a file with the patient's record. Two-thirds of the reports used some type of form to tabulate the data and provided a space for the summary and interpretation. Both types of reports are satisfactory, but many electromyographers find the latter exposition of the EMG to be more convenient for subsequent comparison with later EMGs.

Some electromyographers use word processors to present programmed EMG reports. Although generating these reports may save time, I find them also to be unnecessarily restrictive and stereotypic and, in a real sense, misleading to the referring physician.

On the following pages are examples of reports sent to Ohio State University EMG continuation medical courses during the past 5 years. A critique accompanies each report.

Example 1:

EMG REPORT

This 47-year-old man has complained of back pain of about 4 months duration. He is a diabetic on 35 units of insulin since 1 month. Nerve conduction studies were as follows:

Right common peroneal motor nerve conduction velocity was normal at 45.5 m/sec. Distal latency 4.4 msec. Proximal latency 12.2 msec. Left common peroneal motor nerve conduction velocity was normal at 44.6 m/sec. Distal latency 4.2 msec, proximal latency 12.6 msec. There was no electrical response on stimulation of the posterior tibial on the left and on the right. Needle EMG electrode studies were done on the following muscles bilaterally: anterior tibial, gastrocnemius, peroneus longus, short head of biceps femoris, quadriceps femoris, and the lumbar and sacral paraspinal muscles. There was an *increased insertional activity* seen in the anterior tibial, gastrocnemius, peroneus longus, and

---

short head of the biceps femoris. A few fibs. were seen in the gastrocnemius and in the peroneus longus muscles. Positive sharp wave potentials were seen in the gastrocnemius muscles. Quadriceps femoris showed normal insertional activity, but no fibrillation potentials or positive sharp wave potentials. In the paraspinal muscles there was an *increase in insertional activity* of L4-5 level and in the sacral paraspinal muscles. Fibs. were seen in L4-5 and the sacral levels, and positive sharp wave potentials are seen at L5 and the sacral paraspinal muscles.
IMPRESSION: L5 radiculopathy.

CRITIQUE

1. Clearly, technical error is responsible for the failure to evoke *any* muscle action potential when the tibial nerve was stimulated, especially because both peroneal nerves appeared normal. The electromyographer should have noted the amplitude and duration of CMAP of EDB at both sites of stimulation, especially in view of the patient's diabetes mellitus.
2. The term "increased insertional activity" is meaningless!
3. If the abnormal findings were present in sacral paraspinals, how could the diagnosis be L5 radiculopathy?
4. With the patient's history of diabetes mellitus, the sural nerve latency should have been determined.
5. H reflex should have been attempted to clarify whether L5 or S1 is involved and also to investigate proximal nerves. Gastrocnemius is mostly S1, S2.

Example 2:

EMG REPORT

Motor Fiber Conduction Studies	Segment	Latency (msec)	Significance	Segment	Velocity (m/sec)	Significance
Rt Ulnar	Distal	2.8			48.9	WNL
Lt Ulnar	Distal	3.0			57.2	WNL
Rt Median	Distal	4.1			55.2	WNL
Lt Median	Distal	4.3			38.7	WNL

Sensory Action Potential Studies	Segment	Latency (msec)	Significance	Amplitude (μV)	Significance
Median	R	Not obtainable			Early carpal tunnel syndrome
	L	" "			
Ulnar	R	2.8		12	
	L	2.8		10	

Other studies: EMG of left thenar, hypothenae, biceps, and deltoid muscles within normal limits.

CRITIQUE

1. It is a technical error when motor latencies of 4.1 msec and 4.5 msec in the median nerve are obtained and one cannot obtain the sensory latency.
2. One wonders about the right ulnar motor conduction of 49 m/sec when the left ulnar motor conduction is 20% higher. Too, what caused the left median proximal conduction to be 17 m/sec slower than the right when there is only a .2 msec difference in the distal latencies?
3. Absent sensory action potentials of median nerve, if obtained correctly, would indicate an advanced carpal tunnel syndrome—not an early one!
4. No amplitude and duration of M-response of median nerves are reported; this is a critical omission when conduction velocities are discrepant.
5. There is no need to carry motor conduction velocities to one decimal place because doing so implies a precision that is not obtainable. Measurement error is usually 0.5-1 cm/20 cm, thus 2.5-5%.

CONCLUSION (? EARLY CARPAL TUNNEL SYNDROME IS INAPPROPRIATE IN LIGHT OF DATA.)

Example 3:

EMG REPORT

NEUROLOGIC EXAMINATION (List positive findings, especially focal or localizing signs)

Floppy Baby—Not walking, baby girl aged 17 months
EMG

Using a 25-gauge coaxial needle, explorations were made of the right anterior tib, quadriceps, hamstrings, and gastrocsoleus. Decreased number and decreased amplitude were noted. Good electrical silence was seen.

INTERPRETATION: Although it was rather difficult to interpret whether the patient was putting out effort or not, it was this clinician's opinion that there was a true decrease in amplitude and number of units, raising a serious question of abnormality in muscle tissue.

CRITIQUE

1. A true decrease in the number of MUPs recruited suggests neuropathic, not myopathic disease.
2. Hamstrings and quadriceps are not specific locations. Even an infant's muscles can be localized.
3. What is meant by "good electrical silence"?
4. This report provides no record of amplitude, duration, and proportion of polyphasic MUPs and recruitment pattern.
5. No stimulation studies—motor and sensory conduction velocity of compound *evoked* muscle action potential—are described.

DATA ARE CLEARLY INSUFFICIENT TO WARRANT A CONCLUSION.

Example 4:

EMG REPORT

ELECTROMYOGRAPHY:

Needle electromyography was also performed for the right upper extremity for those muscles supplied by the brachial plexus through nerve roots C5 to T1.

This was a myopathic electromyographic study. For all the muscles tested, I note the presence of high frequency bizarre repetitive discharges, with needle insertion. Very fine fibrillation potentials are seen with trains positive waves. At minimal contraction, his MUAPs are of low amplitude and short duration. Recruitment is increased in comparison to the strength of contraction. Some waxing and waning of the myotonic potentials can be noted. Findings are most severe distally. An occasional large complex polyphasic potential was also seen. The amplitude of his MUAPs was typically between 50 and 500 μV.

IMPRESSION:

Electrodiagnostic findings are compatible with a diagnosis of myotonic dystrophy (Steinert's disease).

CRITIQUE

1. Only one extremity was explored in an apparent generalized disease.
2. No record is given of amplitude, duration, and proportion of polyphasic MUAPs, or recruitment pattern.
3. The report notes "high frequency bizarre repetitive discharges" in all muscles. These are *not* seen in myotonia dystrophica, except rarely in late stages. The high frequency discharges that "wax and

wane" are either trains of positive waves or trains of single muscle fiber diphasic spikes. Both vary in frequency and amplitude and are characteristic of the myotonic reaction. Trains of positive waves are single muscle fiber discharges produced by the exploring electrode tip in the depolarized area of muscle fiber.
4. It is not proper to use diagnostic labels to describe electrical activity, i.e., "myotonic potentials."

Example 5:

EMG REPORT

The patient is a 27-year-old man who was seen on the afternoon of March 6, 1981, because of severe pain in the left shoulder that began in about September of 1980. It involves primarily the scapular area. It lasted for some 2 months. Subsequently, he has noted weakness in the left shoulder. He was concerned that he had previously been wrestling with his brothers before the onset of the pain.

Examination reveals that he has atrophy of the deltoid, biceps, and supraspinatus and marked atrophy of the infraspinatus. There is not any weakness in the biceps or triceps. There is marked weakness in the deltoid, infraspinatus, and supraspinatus.

An EMG was done, and the following muscles of the left forearm were sampled with a monopolar needle electrode: the abductor pollicis brevis, the pronator teres, the first dorsal interossei, the extensor indicis proprius, the biceps, and the triceps. No abnormalities were noted.

I then did EMGs in the paravertebral cervical muscles on the left, and I could find no evidence of abnormalities. In the anterior, mid, and posterior deltoid there is a rather marked decrease in the number of motor unit potentials, but there is no evidence of membrane irritability manifested by no fibrillations or positive sharp waves. The supraspinatus shows a mild decrease in motor unit potentials. Again, there is no membrane irritability. In the infraspinatus there is a rather marked decrease in motor unit potentials but again without membrane irritability.

IMPRESSION: Abnormal EMG because of decreased numbers of motor unit responses in the deltoid, supraspinatus, and infraspinatus but with relatively good numbers in the left biceps in spite of the atrophy of the left biceps.

A suprascapular motor latency test was done by stimulating the nerve in the supraclavicular fossa with a pick-up in the supra-

---

spinatus, 11 cm distant, showing a latency of 3.3 msec. In the infraspinatus through a distance of 18 cm the latency was 4.8 msec.

IMPRESSION: Abnormal nerve conduction in the left supra-scapular nerve to the infraspinatus muscle. Normal values are no greater than 3.7 msec; to the infraspinatus it was 4.8 msec.

IMPRESSION: Brachial plexus neuralgia.

CRITIQUE

1. This is a classic example of overinterpretation.
2. The electromyographer recorded the stimulation study with a needle so he could not estimate viable muscle fibers from CMAP.
3. The decreased recruitment that is reported is suspect because there is no mention of the firing rate.
4. Sudden pain in the shoulder with atrophy of the shoulder girdle muscles but with no fibrillation potentials suggests rotator cuff rupture, not brachial neuralgia.

DATA ARE INSUFFICIENT TO SUPPORT DIAGNOSIS!

Example 6:

EMG REPORT

PERTINENT CLINICAL HISTORY AND FINDINGS:

31-year-old man with pain in right shoulder and right upper extremity. Tingling in right hand, weakness in right upper extremity, marked wasting in right biceps and deltoid, with no apparent motor strength. Duration: Two months.

INTERPRETATION:

1. The motor conduction velocity of right median nerve in segment from Erb's point to axilla is significantly slow. Otherwise essentially normal conduction latencies and velocities of right median and ulnar motor and sensory nerves in right upper extremity.
2. Many fibrillations and positive sharp waves are present in right biceps and deltoid muscles, with only distant MUAPs on maximal voluntary contractions. Brachioradialis shows also many positive sharp waves and slightly diminished numbers of MUAPs; the polyphasic potentials are moderately increased.

Essentially unremarkable EMG studies in supraspinatus, rhomboid minor, and cervical paraspinal muscles.
IMPRESSION:
Findings are consistent with right brachial plexus injury at upper trunk just below the origin of suprascapular nerve. Partial denervation is present.

CRITIQUE

1. One should not be able to record over the thenar muscles when the Erb point is stimulated; this is the tip of the transverse process of C6, i.e., upper trunk. No mention is made of the significance of the *slowing* that was reported. If a response is noted in the thenar muscles it is probable that the lower trunk of the brachial plexus, not the upper trunk, was stimulated.
2. When recording only distant units on maximal voluntary contraction, the needle should be moved, or if a monopolar electrode is being used, one should move the reference electrode over the muscle being explored.
3. The stimulation study should have recorded over the infra- and supraspinatus, deltoid, biceps brachii, and brachioradialis muscles and compared M responses with the contralateral ones. The absolute minimal exam would include the compound evoked muscle action potential of the biceps and deltoid muscles.
4. The electromyographer should have explored the serratus anterior to determine the location of the lesion distal to C6 root.
5. One cannot equate fibrillation potentials and positive waves with denervation, because no stimulation study of biceps/deltoid and brachioradialis was done.

DATA ARE INSUFFICIENT TO SUPPORT CONCLUSION!

Example 7:

EMG REPORT

CLINICAL IMPRESSION: Left cubital tunnel syndrome with possible median nerve involvement as well.
TECHNICAL SUMMARY: By means of surface electrodes, motor terminal latency of the left median nerve was normal at 3.5 msec, the amplitude of its M response at the lower limits of normal at 8 millivolts. F-wave latency was normal at 26.4 msec. Proximal motor latency was 7.2 msec. Motor nerve conduction velocity over

the median nerve from the antecubital fossa of the wrist was normal at 60 m/sec. Sensory terminal latency of the left median nerve was 2.55 msec and normal, the amplitude of its action potential normal at 40 μV. Sensory terminal latency of the left ulnar nerve for comparison was identical to that of the left median at 2.55 msec, the amplitude of its sensory action potential 10 μV. Motor terminal latency of the ulnar nerve was normal at 2.5 msec, the amplitude of its M response at the lower limits of normal at 8.5 millivolts. F-wave latency was normal at 29.3 msec. Proximal motor latency below the elbow was 5.7 msec, above the elbow 8.1 msec, and that at Erb's point 13.6 msec. Motor nerve conduction velocity over the left ulnar nerve from a point below the elbow to the wrist was 67 m/sec and normal, that across the elbow normal at 50 m/sec, and that from Erb's point to the point above the elbow normal at 70 m/sec. However, there was a significant (greater than 10 m/sec) drop in motor nerve conduction velocity across the elbow, the value being 20 m/sec in this case. Sensory proximal latency (proximal to the cubital tunnel) was difficult to determine, but it was probably 7.1 msec and normal.

By means of monopolar needle electrode, the left abductor digiti quinti, flexor carpi ulnaris, wrist extensor, abductor pollicis brevis, and cervical paraspinous muscles were studied and revealed increased insertional activity, positive sharp waves, and fibrillations. There were even polyphasics in the left C8 paraspinous muscles. EMG of the triceps muscle was also done; it was normal.

IMPRESSION: Above EMG studies indicate the presence of a left C8 radiculopathy. There is, in addition, a mild left cubital tunnel syndrome documented by nerve conduction study.

CRITIQUE

1. Unless the elbow was flexed to 70° during the ulnar nerve study, the slowing across elbow is irrelevant. Without measuring the amplitude and duration of the M response during stimulation across the elbow, it is not significant. Also, because the sensory latency proximal to the cubital tunnel to wrist was normal, the cubital tunnel syndrome seems improbable.
2. Note that the antidromic median and sensory latency are reported at 2.55 msec. This value is carried to one decimal place too many because measurement error is *at least 5%*.
3. "Increased insertional activity" is a meaningless phrase.

4. How could the diagnosis be a C8 radiculopathy unless abnormalities were present in the triceps (C7, C8)?
5. "Wrist extensor" is an imprecise localization of the needle electrode.

DATA DO NOT SUPPORT DIAGNOSIS.

Example 8:

EMG REPORT

Muscles of the Left Upper Extremity

The examination was performed so that the muscles innervated by the anterior and posterior primary divisions of the second cervical through the first thoracic roots were studied. Included were the supraspinatus, infraspinatus, deltoid, biceps, triceps, extensor digitorum communis, brachioradialis, pronator teres, opponens pollicis, abductor digiti quinti, and interosseous muscles.

Runs of moderate amplitude positive sharp waves with occasional fibrillation potentials were noted in the supraspinatus and infraspinatus muscles. An occasional moderate amplitude positive sharp wave was noted in the extensor digitorum communis muscle. No other fibrillation changes were found.

On attempted voluntary contraction a few low amplitude waves were evoked in the extensor digitorum communis muscle. No decent interference pattern was developed. The motor units in the other muscle groups appeared to be essentially normal in number and configuration, although movement in the supraspinatus and infraspinatus muscles was markedly limited by the pain from the recent surgery and the patient's harness. Of particular note was the good response in the triceps and brachioradialis muscles. No myopathic activity was noted.

1. There is a severe partial lesion in the left radial nerve with major involvement of the extensor digitorum communis muscle. The triceps and brachioradialis muscles are spared.

A combination of abnormalities in the radial nerve and suprascapular nerve tends to place the site of damage in the upper trunk of the left brachioplexus. Obviously this is a partial lesion with sparing of the triceps and brachioradialis muscles. The fact that there are some potentials evoked in the extensor digitorum communis muscle after 15 days is a good prognostic sign.

CRITIQUE

1. The electromyographer reports that the muscles innervated by anterior and posterior primary divisions of C2 through T1 were investigated; however, only the supraspinatus through the intrinsic muscles (i.e., C5-T1) were studied. The sternocleidomastoid and trapezius muscles were omitted.
2. This is an incomplete exam. The electromyographer should have studied the serratus anterior and rhomboid muscles to determine if the lesion is distal to the posterior primary ramus departure but before the suprascapular nerve. Pectoralis major and latissimus dorsi exploration would have further clarified the site of the lesion. It cannot be an upper trunk of the brachioplexus because the brachioradialis (C5, C6) was normal. (Extensor digitorum communis is innervated by C7, C8).
3. No stimulation studies were done. They would have identified the neurapraxic portion (if any) when compared to the contralateral muscles.
4. "No decent interference pattern was developed" is a meaningless phrase. Also, it is inappropriate to state that "no myopathic activity was noted."

DATA PRESENTED ARE INSUFFICIENT TO SUPPORT DIAGNOSIS!

Example 9:

EMG REPORT

I had the pleasure of seeing ____(name)____ in my office at your request on June 4, 1981. You asked me to see her with regard to possible carpal tunnel syndrome—right vs. left. She apparently initially saw you about headaches, neck pain, and some pain between the shoulder blades that had been going on for a considerable period of time. It wasn't until you noticed the weakness in the abductor pollicis brevis that you even asked her about the numbness or tingling. She reported that once you asked her about these symptoms, she noticed that she was indeed having them when she would wake up in the morning. We don't know, of course, how long they had been going on before you directed her attention to them. Sensory latency on the left and right median nerves is still normal. On the left, 2.3 msec and on the right, 2.7, and so I had to go onto EMG examination. EMG examination on

---

the right was strikingly abnormal. There was a clear-cut increase in irritability and no fibs or positive waves. A marked increase in giant polyphasic potentials with decrease in the maximal interference pattern. On the left the abnormalities are more subtle. There was, indeed, an increase in *giant polyphasics,* but it was slight rather than marked. There was no increase in irritability, no fibs, no positive waves, and an entirely normal maximal interference pattern.

No question based on the EMG examination in combination with the numbness in her hands and the weakness of the abductor pollicis brevis that she does indeed have bilateral carpal tunnel syndrome and by electrical criteria it's more on the right than on the left. I am hopeful that her chief complaint will indeed be helped with carpal tunnel release, but have advised her that may not be the case because obviously carpal tunnel syndrome is fairly common and a chance coincidence between carpal tunnel and her chief complaint remains a possibility.

IMPRESSION: Bilateral carpal tunnel syndrome by electrical studies, right worse than left.

CRITIQUE

1. Sensory latencies of the median nerves—right, 2.7 msec and left, 2.3 msec—are too short (especially left) to indicate that measurement was done. No distance was recorded.
2. EMG was suggested as strikingly abnormal—"clear-cut increase in irritability with no fibs or positive waves," "decrease in maximal interference pattern"—but this is an absurd conclusion.
3. In spite of normal sensory latencies and "abnormal EMG," no motor latencies are recorded.
4. "Clear-cut increase in irritability" and "giant polyphasics" are examples of inappropriate terminology. Diagnosis of carpal tunnel syndrome is clearly *not* supported by data presented! A classic example of attempting to make the EMG consonant with suspected clinical diagnosis.

Example 10:

EMG REPORT

EMG AND NERVE CONDUCTION STUDY

Patient is 41 yrs old with injury to the wrist about 3 months ago. Patient shows weakness and atrophy of the intrinsic hand muscles.

EXAMINATION

Sensory deficit in the fourth and fifth fingers with atrophy of the hypothenar with Froment's sign. The remainder of the neurologic examination within normal limits.

On nerve conduction study, motor conduction in the left median nerve from the wrist to abductor pollicis brevis with the latency of 3.5 msec and conduction velocity from elbow to the wrist 61 m/sec.

Left ulnar nerve no response. No action potential by stimulation of the ulnar nerve that was stimulated in the wrist below and above the ulnar groove, and an active electrode was placed on abductor digiti quinti.

Sensory conduction in the left median nerve from the index to the wrist orthodromically the latency of 2.5 msec, with normal *axonal* action potential.

No action potential could be obtained by stimulation of the ulnar nerve from the fifth digit to above the wrist.

Stimulation of the right median nerve and ulnar nerve showed normal latencies and conduction velocities with normal action potentials.

EMG in the left upper extremity, the muscles sampled included left extensor indicis proprius and left abductor pollicis brevis, left flexor carpi ulnaris and radialis, and left first lumbrical. No fibrillations or positive waves. No polyphasia. Normal motor units. No *giant* motor units.

Left first dorsal interosseous and left abductor digiti quinti showed fibrillation potentials, positive waves at rest without motor unit potentials during the volition.

The above study indicates ulnar nerve neuropathy at the wrist *(complete)*.

CRITIQUE

1. The conclusion that the study shows complete left ulnar neuropathy at the wrist is incorrect. There is no indication that stimulation of

the ulnar nerve distal to the injury was performed to see if any axons were neurapraxic. Also, no recording of the adductor pollicis or the first dorsal interosseous was done to check the integrity of the deep ulnar branch.

2. The terminology of "giant" MUPs is incorrect. The report should indicate the amplitude, duration, and shape of MUPs. Also, the term "axonal" is used incorrectly in place of compound nerve action potential.

3. The orthodromic median nerve latency was 2.5 msec, which is definitely too short a duration for a 14-cm measurement. No amplitude or duration of the sensory action potential was given.

4. The fifth digit is incorrectly designated as the fifth finger. We have only four fingers and a thumb, but five digits.

Example 11—This was submitted as a complete report:

CLINICAL IMPRESSION: r/o carpal tunnel syndrome

ELECTRODIAGNOSTIC (EDX) REPORT OF FINDINGS

Strength Duration Curve: FILE NO. _____

Nerve Conduction: Left Median Nerve *5.6 msec*
                    Right Median Nerve *5.0 msec*
                    Distal Sensory Latency (both Median nerves)—not obtainable

EMG: Left Ulnar Nerve Distal Latency - 2.0 msec

INTERPRETATION AND REMARKS: Prolonged distal latency in both Median nerves and absent distal latency are compatible with bilateral Carpal Tunnel compression of both Median Nerves.

CRITIQUE

1. No interpretation of distal motor latencies is complete without recording of the proximal conduction velocity.

2. No recording was done of the compound evoked muscle action potential amplitude and duration.

3. It is evident that the electromyographer did not measure for distal motor latency because the ulnar delay is only 2.0 msec.

4. A needle study of the abductor pollicis brevis should have been done.
5. Stimulation distal to carpal ligament would identify the proportion of neurapraxic axons, when compared with the CMAP evoked with wrist stimulation.
6. For completeness (and to demonstrate technical success), a distal ulnar sensory action potential should be elicited.

Example 12:

EMG REPORT

Sensory Nerve Action Potential:

	Latency	Amplitude
median wrist to 2nd digit	3.0 msec	40 µV
median wrist to 2nd digit	3.3 msec	38 µV
ulnar wrist to 5th digit	2.2 msec	Normal
ulnar wrist to 5th digit	1.8 msec	Normal

EMG:
abductor pollicis brevis
abductor digiti minimi
pronator teres   Normal insertional activity. Silent
flexor digitorum sublimis   at rest.
biceps brachii   Normal motor units on volition
brachioradialis
abductor digiti minimi   and normal interference pattern.
abductor pollicis brevis

Electromyographic findings in the above muscles are normal. Nerve conduction velocities in the proximal segments of the nerves are also normal, but there is marked difference in the motor and sensory distal latencies of median and ulnar nerves.

This finding is suggestive of possible compression of the median nerves in the carpal tunnel. There is no evidence of denervation of the muscles or involvement of proximal segments of the nerves.

Impression: Findings suggestive of bilateral carpal tunnel syndrome (mild).

CRITIQUE

1. No measurement is indicated for distal sensory latencies.
2. Amplitude of the antidromic sensory action potential of one digit was 40 µV and latency was 3.3 msec, and yet the electromyographer considers it prolonged!
3. Obviously with an antidromic ulnar sensory latency of 1.8 msec, no

measurement of 14 cm was made (or even the same distance as the median).

4. The amplitude of the antidromic ulnar sensory action potential was simply indicated as "normal," i.e., there is no way to compare it with the median, sensory action potential.

DATA ARE NOT SUPPORTIVE OF CONCLUSION!

Example 13:

EMG REPORT

TECHNIQUE AND EQUIPMENT: Motor conduction using surface disc electrodes
TECA-TD$_{20}$ Sensory conduction by antidromic method
EMG using concentric needle electrodes

NERVE	Latencies (m/sec)	Distance (cm)	Conduction Velocity (m/sec)	Amplitude	Other Remarks
Left Median-Motor—wrist	2.9				
elbow	6.6	20.0	54.0	6.5 millivolt	
				No temporal dispersion	
Sensory—wrist	2.9			45.0 µV	
Left Ulnar-Motor—wrist	2.7				
above elbow	6.5	23.0	60.5	15.0 millivolts	
				No temporal dispersion	
Left Radial-Sensory	2.8			20.0 µV	
Right Median-Motor—wrist	3.2	14.0		8.0 millivolt	

NAME OF MUSCLES	Fibrillations	Positive Sharp Waves	Motor Units	Other Remarks
LEFT UPPER EXTREMITY				
Abductor pollicis brevis	Occasional	0	4+	Normal
Opponens pollicis	0	0	4+	Normal
Abductor digiti quinti	0	0	4+	Normal
Flexor digitorum sublimus	0	0	4+	Normal

IMPRESSION: Normal study.
Normal motor conduction in left median nerve. Normal distal motor as well as sensory latencies for left median nerve. Normal motor conduction in left ulnar nerve. Normal motor conduction in left ulnar nerve. Normal sensory conduction in left radial nerve. Normal distal motor latency for right median nerve. Essentially normal EMG examination of the selected muscles of the left upper limb.

CRITIQUE

1. This is described as a normal study, yet the compound evoked muscle action potential is only 6.5 millivolts on the left and 8.0 millivolts on the right, whereas the ulnar (hypothenar) is 15 millivolts.
2. In spite of the low amplitude muscle action potential, the median sensory action potential is 45 μV.
3. Fibrillation potentials in the abductor pollicis brevis are described as "normal"; also, the electromyographer makes an impossible distinction between this muscle and the opponens pollicis.
4. All distal latency values suggest an inattention to measurement precision.
5. No value for duration of the CMAP or SNAP is given; only the phrase "no temporal dispersion" is included.

Example 14:

EMG REPORT

Findings:

The lower extremities were examined. The terminal latencies in the peroneal and posterior tibial nerves were examined. The posterior tibial terminal latencies were slightly prolonged at 7.6; proximal conduction velocities were borderline. Sural conductions were not elicited.

An EMG study was performed using a monopolar electrode. The following muscles were examined: (right) gastrocnemius, tibialis anterior, vastus lateralis, ileus soleus, and the paraspinal muscles from T12-L5. The study revealed evidence of fibrillation potentials and positive waves in the paraspinal muscles on the right side at the thoracolumbar junction at T12, L1 levels. In addition, there was some increased polyphasic activity in the right ileus (sic) soleus. The remainder of the study was normal.

CONCLUSION: THIS WAS A BORDERLINE NERVE CONDUCTION STUDY OF THE LOWER EXTREMITIES, SHOWING BORDERLINE MOTOR VALUES AND ABSENCE OF SURAL CONDUCTIONS. THIS IS PROBABLY CONSISTENT WITH PATIENT'S AGE. THE EMG PORTION OF THE STUDY SHOWED EVIDENCE OF DENERVATION POTENTIALS IN THE UPPER LUMBAR REGION, ESPECIALLY ON THE PARASPINAL MUSCLE EXAMINATION. IF THIS CORRELATES WITH THE CLINICAL PICTURE, AN L1 RADICULOPATHY SHOULD BE CONSIDERED.

CRITIQUE

1. Recording sites for the tibial nerve conduction study were not indicated. The value, 7.6 msec, is quite prolonged for the abductor hallucis (medial plantar nerve).
2. The absence of a sural SNAP must be considered abnormal.
3. Ileus (sic) soleus at what latency?
4. Localized presence of "fibrillation potentials and positive waves" and absence of symptoms in the paraspinals are most likely a misinterpretation of endplate spikes.
5. The conclusion should not report "denervation potentials."

EXAM IS INSUFFICIENT FOR CONCLUSIONS.

Example 15:

EMG REPORT

THIS PATIENT'S FINDINGS:
  Nerve conduction studies in the right lower extremity were essentially normal except for the absence of an H reflex.
  The EMG was abnormal in the extensor digitorum brevis (EDB) muscle and the tibialis anterior muscle.
IMPRESSION:
  The findings are most compatible with an L4 root lesion, given the distribution of abnormalities.

CRITIQUE

1. The absent H reflex is less diagnostic than a prolonged H latency because there are so many factors that inhibit the H reflex even in the normal individual. The contralateral H-reflex latency should be determined.
2. The common root to the EDB and ant. tib. muscles is L5, *not* L4. Obviously the absent H reflex would support an S1 root lesion, assuming that finding was valid.
3. It is impossible to localize a radiculopathy unless the paraspinal muscles are explored.

DATA ARE INSUFFICIENT FOR DIAGNOSIS!

Example 16:

EMG REPORT			
PATIENT'S NAME: _____ _____			
DATE: 2/25/85			
UPPER EXTREMITY EMG: LEFT	INSERTION:	REST	ACTION
Trapezius			
Paraspinals			
Abductor Pollicis Brevis	WNL	Rare fibs	One MUP
1st Dorsal Interosseous	WNL	WNL	One MUP
Extensor Indicis Proprius	WNL	WNL	Few MUPs
Brachioradialis	WNL	WNL	↓MUPs
Flexor Carpi Ulnaris	Rare fibs	WNL	No MUPs
Flexor Carpi Radialis	WNL	WNL	2-3 MUPs
Extensor Carpi Radialis Longus	WNL	WNL	No MUPs
Biceps	Rare fibs	WNL	2-3 MUPs
Triceps	WNL	WNL	No MUPs
Deltoids	WNL	1 + fibs	2-4 MUPs
Pronator Teres	WNL	WNL	No MUPs

IMPRESSION: Rare denervation potentials in a few muscles C5-6 and C8-T1, probably reflects minor anterior horn cell or peripheral nerve injury. Markedly decreased motor unit potentials in all muscles reflecting upper motor neuron paralysis.

CRITIQUE

1. There is no conduction study to support the proposed diagnosis of peripheral nerve injury or other possible diseases.
2. Also, no description of the MUPs is presented to suggest anterior horn cell disease.
3. Under *insertion* there are no positive waves described, even though "rare fibrillations" are noted. When the needle electrode is moved through muscle there must be positive waves present if fibrillations are observed. (I suspect these "rare fibrillations" may be endplate spikes).
4. No description of recruitment pattern is present, although one MUP and two to three MUPs were noted to be present. It is inconceivable that only "rare fibrillations" are present with only one MUP.
5. The term "denervation" should not be used to describe potentials.
6. To suggest a radiculopathy or the absence of abnormalities in cervical paraspinal muscles is inappropriate.

DATA DO NOT SUPPORT THE DIAGNOSIS.

Example 17:

EMG REPORT

NERVE CONDUCTION STUDIES

NERVE	LATENCY (M.SEC.) PROX.	DIST.	SEGMENT (CM.)	VELOCITY (M.S)	DESCRIPTION
Median	10.4	3.7	36.5	54	normal
sensory		2.7			
Ulnar Elb	15.7				
A.E.	11.8		30.5	75	normal
B.E.	7.8	18	45	slight delay
wrist	3.8	20.5			normal

NORMAL CONDUCTIONS

NERVE	CONDUCTION VELOCITY (MTLRS/SECOND)	DISTAL LATENCIES (MILLISEC.)
ULNAR	> 45	< 4 (SENSORY) < 3.5
MEDIAN	> 45	< 4.7 (SENSORY) < 3.5
PERONEAL	> 40	< 5
TIBIAL	> 40	< 6
FACIAL		< 4

COMMENTS AND IMPRESSIONS:

The ① ulnar N.C.V.S revealed some slowing across the elbow.

Impression: Protocol ① Tardy ulnar palsy.

CRITIQUE

1. As was mentioned before, the Erb point is at the tip of the C6 transverse process; therefore only C5 and C6 roots will be stimulated. It is impossible to record a CMAP from the hypothenar or thenar muscles when stimulation is at the Erb point.

2. There is a measurement artifact (too short) unless ulnar nerve conduction velocity across the elbow is determined with the elbow flexed. Thus, the finding of slowed conduction is spurious. Amplitude and duration of CMAP must be observed to make a diagnosis of ulnar nerve conduction velocity slowing across the elbow.

3. "Tardy" ulnar nerve palsy must be reserved for a history of supracondylar fracture (or similar injury) at the elbow at an early age and then gradual loss of ulnar function 20 to 30 years later. In the absence of that history, a diagnosis of simply entrapment of ulnar nerve at elbow is appropriate.

Example 18:

EMG REPORT

ELECTROMYOGRAPHY and ELECTRODIAGNOSIS

1 Orb Ocul	13 Deltoid	25 Abductor Digiti Min	37 Gluteus Maximus
2 Orb Oris	14 Biceps	26 Adductor Pollicis	38 Exten Dig Brevis
3 Temporalis	15 Brachio Radialis	27 Abductor Pol Brev	39 Gastrocnemus
4 Masseter	16 Serratus Ant	28 Opponens Pollicis	40 Erector Spinae
5 Tongue	17 Pronator Teres	29 Add Longus	41 Exten Carpi Uln
6 S-C-M	18 Flexor Carpi Rad	30 Sartorius	42 Semitend
7 Trapezius	19 Extensor Carpi Rad	31 Quad Femoris	43 Iliopsoas
8 Rhomboids	20 Tricep	32 Tibialis Ant	44 Extensor Hallucis Long
9 Supraspinatus	21 Flexor Carpi Uln	33 Gluteus Med	45
10 Infraspinatus	22 1st Dor Interosseous	34 Biceps Femoris	46
11 Latissimus Dorsi	23 Flexor Poll Brevis	35 Peronei	47
12 Pectoralis Major	24 Volar Interossei	36 Abd Hallucis	48

- TABLE *Nerves and Muscles tested are indicated by letters and numbers respectively according to the Table above*

- NERVE CONDUCTION *Shape of Potential* Abnormal when very small or temporally dispersed *Terminal Latency* Facial N – Conduction time from in front of ear to muscle *Median and Ulnar N.* – from wrist to muscle *Radial N.* – from wrist to muscle *Peroneal and Tibial N* – from ankle to muscle *Sensory N* – from finger to wrist (orthodromic) or wrist to finger (antidromic) *Velocity: Terminal segment* – Sensory nerve in upper limb from finger to wrist *Distal segment* – Upper limb from elbow (or below elbow) to wrist and lower limb from knee to ankle *Middle segment* – Ulnar nerve from above to below elbow *Proximal segment* – Upper limb from axilla (or erb s point) to elbow (or above elbow) *FWCV (F wave conduction velocity) Central segment* – Upper limb from axilla to spinal cord and lower limb from knee to spinal cord

- ELECTROMYOGRAPHY *Insertional Activity* – Potential normally 0 to +1, Myotonic or Pseudomyotonic discharge normally 0 *Resting Activity* – fasciculation fibrillation and positive waves normally 0 *Motor Unit* – Polyphasic activity normally less than 20%, *Interference* – Pattern normally full 4 when absent

- NORMAL VALUES

Radial Nerve	Motor ≥ 57 m/sec	Peroneal Nerve	T lat · 5 5 msec	Ulnar Nerve Motor t lat · 3 4 msec (0 8)
	Sensory ≥ 52		Motor ≥ 40 m/sec	Sensory · 44 m/sec
				Motor · 49 m/sec
Tibial Nerve	T lat ≥ 6 0 msec	Median Nerve	Motor t lat · 4 2	
	Motor ≥ 41 m/sec		Sensory t lat · 3 5	Blink Reflex Direct · 4 1 msec (0 6)
			Motor segments · 48	R1 · 13 0 msec (1 2)
				R2 · 40 msec (l)
				· 41 msec (C)(5)

Nerve Conductions

Side	Nerve Studied	Muscle	Shape of Potential	Amplitude	Terminal Latency msec	Velocity m sec Terminal Segment	Distal Segment	Middle Segment	Proximal Segment	Latency	FWCV m sec Central Segment
L	MM	27	A	1mv	5,3	31	40				
L	UM	25	A	2mv	6,6	44	20	55			
R	UM	25	A	5 mv	6,2	75	27	31			

Electromyography

Side	Muscle	Ins Act 0 to · 4	Ins Act Pseudo Myot 0 to · 4	Rest Act Fasc	Rest Act Fib	Pos W 0 to · 4	Motor Unit Amp 0 to · 4	Motor Unit Dur ms	Motor Unit Poly phasic msec	Interference Amp %	Interference Pattern
R	27	+2	0	0	+2	+2	1	.8	50	1.5	−3
R	22	+1	0	0	+1	+1	1	.8	50	1.5	−3
L	22	0	0	0	0	0	1	.8	75	1	−4

PONTOGRAM AND OTHER REFLEXES

	H	R,	R	qte R	comb R

END PLATE AND OTHER EXCITABILITY TESTS

Side	Nerve	Muscle	Tran one sec Amp	Tran one sec Stim Freq	Tran one sec Change	Post Tetanic Delay	Post Tetanic Change	Paired Interval	Paired Change	Shock

IMPRESSION: Very abnormal with slow conductions and denervated muscles consistent with severe polyneuropathy.   **DATE:** 6-25-85

CRITIQUE

This is an example of a printed form that is much too complicated and *stereotypic*. Unfortunately, many electromyographers use a complex form to avoid making sequential and logical decisions as necessary during the exam as the EMG findings unfold.

Example 19:

```
                          EMG REPORT


DATE:        3/6/85

NERVE CONDUCTION VELOCITY STUDY:

In a procedure, using a standard technique, a motor nerve
conduction velocity study was performed in both upper extremi-
ties.


                DISTAL MOTOR      NERVE CONDUCTION      M-WAVE
NERVE             LATENCY             VELOCITY         RESPONSE

Right Median  4.0 milliseconds  55 meters per second   8 millivolts

Right Ulnar   3.0 milliseconds  52 meters per second   6 millivolts

Right Ulnar
Across the Elbow                61 meters per second

Left Median   4.2 milliseconds  61 meters per second   6 millivolts

Left Ulnar    3.0 milliseconds  56 meters per second   6 millivolts

Left Ulnar
Across the Elbow                53 meters per second


IMPRESSION:

This is a normal motor nerve conduction velocity study of both
upper extremities.
```

CRITIQUE

1. Unless standard techniques are used, and the duration of CMAP is given, the numbers presented are not "normal," e.g., 4.2 msec motor latency with an amplitude of CMAP of 6 millivolts is probably not normal. Stimulation of median nerve distal to carpal ligament would clarify the study.
2. If the elbow is flexed to 70° with ulnar nerve conduction across the elbow, the CV would be 10 msec greater than the forearm conduction. Also, the lack of the amplitude of CMAP with stimulation of ulnar nerve above the elbow makes the "normally" suspect. Note that the left ulnar across elbow segment NCV was 15% less than that of the corresponding segment on the right.

Example 20:

EMG REPORT

NEUROMUSCULAR ELECTRODIAGNOSIS

L R	MUSCLE	INNERVATION		SPONTANEOUS ACTIVITY				MOTOR UNIT ACTIVITY		
		ROOT	NERVE	POSITIVE WAVES	FIBRIL-LATION	OTHER	INSERTIONAL ACTIVITY	MINIMAL EFFORT	POLY PHASICS	MAXIMUM EFFORT
B	APB		MED	0	0	0	N	1-2 K	N	Full

L R	NERVE	MOTOR	SENSORY	DELAY	NCV	AMPLITUDE	COMMENTS
R	Median		*	4.28	52.91	10 μV	
R	Median	*		3.32	41.80	12 K	
R	Ulnar		*	2.77	56.68	20 μV	
L	Median		*	4.78		20 μV	
L	Median	*		4.16	50.90	8 K	

Hx: Long standing Hx of nocturnal arm pain and intermittent paraesthesias both hands.

Comments:
1. Rt. Median sensory latency and Lt. Median sensory and motor latencies are prolonged. Rt. Median motor latency is normal but NCV in forearm is slow. Lt. Median NCV is normal. This is consistent with Bilateral Carpal Tunnel Syndrome, presently worse on the left as right side seems to have improved with the splint. Slowing of Rt. motor NCV is due to retrograde effect of CTS. There is no evidence of dennervation in both Abductor Pollies Brevis muscles.

2. Normal Ulnar latency and NCV.

Interpretation:

Bilateral Carpal Tunnel Syndrome.

CRITIQUE

1. There appears to be a technique error for three reason: (a) right median motor latency is 3.3 msec (short) with CMAP of 12 millivolts (normal), yet the sensory latency is 4.3 msec and 10 μV; (b) the right median motor conduction velocity was 42 m/sec and sensory conduction was 53 m/sec; this is clearly a disparity; (c) furthermore,

the motor latency on the left was 4.2 msec (longer than right), yet the conduction velocity was 10 m/sec faster than the right.
2. It is improper to carry the conduction velocity to one decimal point or latencies to two decimal points because accuracy in measurement is only 1/20–1/40.

Example 21:

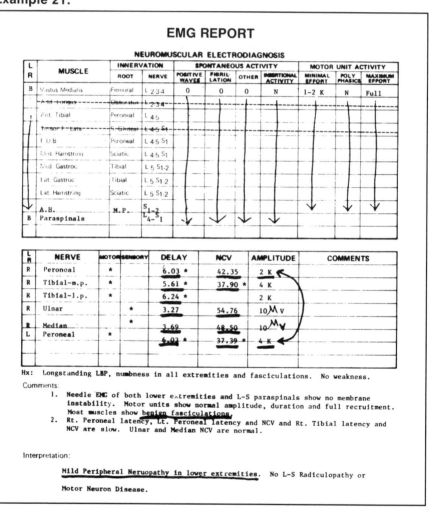

EMG REPORT

NEUROMUSCULAR ELECTRODIAGNOSIS

L / R	MUSCLE	INNERVATION		SPONTANEOUS ACTIVITY				MOTOR UNIT ACTIVITY		
		ROOT	NERVE	POSITIVE WAVES	FIBRIL-LATION	OTHER	INSERTIONAL ACTIVITY	MINIMAL EFFORT	POLY PHASICS	MAXIMUM EFFORT
B	Vastus Medialis	Femoral	L 2-3-4	0	0	0	N	1-2 K	N	Full
	Add. Longus	Obturator	L 2-3-4							
	Ant. Tibial	Peroneal	L 4-5							
	Tensor f. Lata	S. Gluteal	L 4-5 S1							
	F.D.B.	Peroneal	L 4-5 S1							
	Med. Hamstring	Sciatic	L 4-5 S1							
	Med. Gastroc.	Tibial	L 5 S1-2							
	Lat. Gastroc.	Tibial	L 5 S1-2							
	Lat. Hamstring	Sciatic	L 5 S1-2							
	A.H.	M.P.	S1-2							
B	Paraspinals		L4-S1							

L / R	NERVE	MOTOR	SENSORY	DELAY	NCV	AMPLITUDE	COMMENTS
R	Peroneal	*		6.03 *	42.35	2 K	
R	Tibial-m.p.	*		5.61 *	37.90 *	4 K	
R	Tibial-l.p.	*		6.24 *		2 K	
R	Ulnar		*	3.27	54.76	10 M v	
R	Median		*	3.69	48.50	10 M v	
L	Peroneal	*		6.03 *	37.39 *	4 K	

Hx: Longstanding LBP, numbness in all extremities and fasciculations. No weakness.

Comments:
1. Needle EMG of both lower extremities and L-S paraspinals show no membrane instability. Motor units show normal amplitude, duration and full recruitment. Most muscles show benign fasciculations.
2. Rt. Peroneal latency, Lt. Peroneal latency and NCV and Rt. Tibial latency and NCV are slow. Ulnar and Median NCV are normal.

Interpretation:

Mild Peripheral Neruopathy in lower extremities. No L-S Radiculopathy or Motor Neuron Disease.

CRITIQUE (MARKS ON REPORT ARE EDITOR'S)

1. The electromyographer reports "benign fasciculations" in the comments, yet none are described in the needle EMG study. The term "benign" seems inappropriate because the interpretation suggests "mild peripheral neuropathy."

2. With slightly prolonged latencies and relatively normal amplitude of the CMAP it seems presumptuous to make a diagnosis of mild peripheral neuropathy. Prolonged latencies and normal amplitudes of the CMAP could be due to cold feet! The only abnormal finding was tibial NCV of 38 and 37 m/sec. A more helpful procedure would be comparison of amplitude and duration of CMAP when stimulated proximally and distally. Normal physiologic temporal dispersions would be increased in peripheral neuropathy. Also, a sural nerve latency and sensory AP determination would be useful. Temperature of extremities must be included when distal latencies are prolonged.

3. If peripheral neuropathy is considered, proximal nerves must be studied, e.g., F, H).

4. Carrying conduction velocities to two decimal places is improper because measurement accuracy is only 1/20–1/40. Proper calculation dictates only one decimal place beyond expected accuracy.

Example 22:

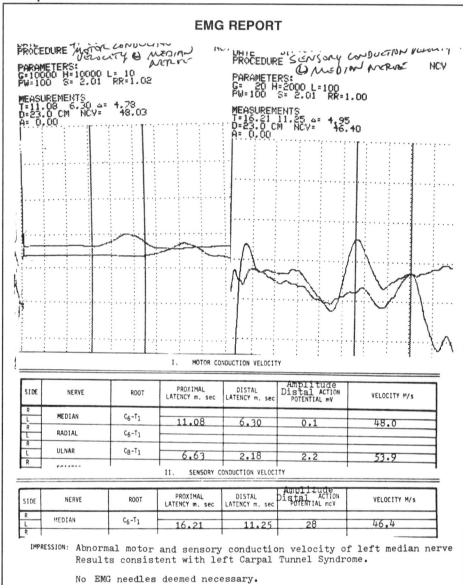

EMG REPORT

PROCEDURE ~Motor Conduction Velocity ⊕ Median Nerve~

PARAMETERS:
G=10000 H=10000 L= 10
PW=100   S= 2.01 RR=1.02

MEASUREMENTS
T=11.08 6.30 ∆= 4.78
D=23.0 CM NCV= 48.03
A= 0.00

PROCEDURE ~Sensory Conduction Velocity ⊕ Median Nerve~ NCV

PARAMETERS:
G= 20 H=2000 L=100
PW=100   S= 2.01 RR=1.00

MEASUREMENTS
T=16.21 11.25 ∆= 4.95
D=23.0 CM NCV= 46.40
A= 0.00

I.   MOTOR CONDUCTION VELOCITY

SIDE	NERVE	ROOT	PROXIMAL LATENCY m. sec	DISTAL LATENCY m. sec	Amplitude Distal ACTION POTENTIAL mV	VELOCITY M/s
R						
L	MEDIAN	C6-T1	11.08	6.30	0.1	48.0
R						
L	RADIAL	C6-T1				
R						
L	ULNAR	C8-T1	6.63	2.18	2.2	53.9
R						
	SCIATIC					

II.   SENSORY CONDUCTION VELOCITY

SIDE	NERVE	ROOT	PROXIMAL LATENCY m. sec	DISTAL LATENCY m. sec	Amplitude Distal ACTION POTENTIAL mcV	VELOCITY M/s
R						
L	MEDIAN	C6-T1	16.21	11.25	28	46.4
R						

IMPRESSION: Abnormal motor and sensory conduction velocity of left median nerve
Results consistent with left Carpal Tunnel Syndrome.

No EMG needles deemed necessary.

CRITIQUE

1. Gain setting of 5 K/cm on motor stimulation is inappropriate (too low). Gain should be the highest possible so that the CMAP can be

the largest, and yet be completely visualized on the oscilloscope screen.

2. Sensory latency of 11.2 msec is incorrect. Note that the proposed SNAP is biphasic, initially positive, and of too great duration (greater than 4 msec) to be a sensory action potential. Presumably it is a volume-conducted motor action potential.

3. Stimulation of the median nerve should have been done distal to carpal ligament to check the neurapraxia.

Example 23:

EMG REPORT

CLINICAL PROBLEM: A 44 year old woman, after an industrial accident on 8-15-83, has persistent pain and intermittent weakness of the left lower extremity.

DATE OF SERVICE: 12-22-83

NERVE EXAMINED	FUNCTION	RECORDING TECHNIQUE	SEGMENT	DISTANCE cm	DISTAL LATENCY msec	RESPONSE AMPLITUDE uV/mV	CONDUCTION VELOCITY M/sec	COMMENT
.peroneal	Motor	SE/ADB	ankle/ADB	7.0	4.0	3mV	-	-
"	"	"	fib. head/ankle	7.0	9.8	3mV	46	Normal motor conduction velocity
"	F Wave	"	ankle/EDB	9.0	46.1	-	-	Normal F-wave distal latency
pos. tibial	Motor	SE/AHB	med.mal./AHB	7.0	4.6	8mV	-	-
"	"	"	pop.fos./med.mal.	36.0	11.4	6mV	52	Normal motor conduction velocity
pos. tibial	H Reflex	SE/soleus	pop.fos./soleus	14.0	29.2	4mV	-	Poor H-reflex formation but normal latency
sural	"	SE/heel	leg to heel	12.0	3.5	20uV	-	Prolonged sensory distal latency and small action potential

INTERPRETATION: Left H-reflex formation is poor with latency of 29.2 along with left sural nerve increased distal latency. This could be suggestive of this patient having had possible S1 radiculopathy. No evidence of peripheral neuropathy is present.

MUSCLE EXAMINED	GRADE OF STRENGTH	INSERTIONAL ACTIVITY	FIBRILLATIONS	FASCICULATIONS	PATTERN MAXIMAL CONTRACTION	MOTOR UNIT POTENTIALS	COMMENT
L. gastrocnemius	5/5	-	-	-	Full	No abnormal MUP	Normal
L. soleus	5/5	-	-	-	Full	No abnormal MUP	Normal
L. tibialis ant.	5/5	-	-	-	Full	No abnormal MUP	Normal
L. ext. hal. longus	5/5	-	-	-	Full	No abnormal MUP	Normal
L. ext. dig. brevis	4+/5	1+	-	-	Full	No abnormal MUP	Abnormal
medial head L. hamstrings,	4+/5	1+	-	-	Full	No abnormal MUP	Ab Normal
lateral head L. hamstrings,	5/5	-	-	-	Full	No abnormal MUP	Normal

INTERPRETATION: Muscle innervated mainly by S1 nerve root show changes consistent with mild but active denervation. This study could be consistent with S1 radiculopathy. The hamstrings muscle is also innervated by L5. Therefore, L5 radiculopathy cannot be excluded.

CRITIQUE

1. Description of the H wave suggests it was an F wave. Also, the right H-reflex latency should have been done.
2. The paraspinal muscles should have been examined to verify the presence of a radiculopathy.
3. Sural nerve sensory AP was 20 μV, which was described as "small." Clearly this is 30% greater than normal mean amplitude. Also, 3.5 msec latency at 12 cm with 20 μV suggests a cool foot, yet no temperature was taken.

Example 24:

EMG REPORT

Nerve	Stimulate	Record	Dur-ation	Amp.	Lat-ency	Dis-tance	NCV	Normal
Median (L)	Wrist	APB		N	4.4	6.5		3.4 - 4.5 msec
	Elbow	APB			8.9	25.8	57	>45 m/sec
Ulnar (L)	Wrist	ADM		N	3.2	6.5		2.7 - 4.2 msec
	Elbow	ADM			7.6	26.3	60	>47 m/sec

Sensory Conductions

Nerve	Stimulate	Record	Dur-ation	Amp.	Lat-ency	Dis-tance	NCV	Normal
Median Antidromic: (L)	Wrist	Index finger			3.0	14.0		< 3.0
Orthodromic:	Index finger	Wrist						<3.25
Median palmar	Palm	Index finger			1.5	7.0		1.16 - 1.68
	Palm	Wrist			2.0+	7.0		1.52 - 1.86

RATIO= .75   (Normal = 0.66 - 1.02)

Nerve	Stimulate	Record	Dur-ation	Amp.	Lat-ency	Dis-tance	NCV	Normal
Median (R)	Wrist	APB		N	5.0+	7.1		3.4 - 4.5 msec
	Elbow	APB		↑	10.1	26.2	51	>45 m/sec
Ulnar (R)	Wrist	ADM		N	3.1	7.2		2.7 - 4.2 msec
	Elbow	ADM			7.0	25.9	66	>47 m/sec

Sensory Conductions

Nerve	Stimulate	Record	Dur-ation	Amp.	Lat-ency	Dis-tance	NCV	Normal
Median Antidromic: (R)	Wrist	Index finger		↓	4.1*	14.5		< 3.0
Orthodromic:	Index finger	Wrist						<3.25
Median palmar	Palm	Index finger		↓	2.7*			1.16 - 1.68
	Palm	Wrist		↓	3.1*			1.52 - 1.86

RATIO= .87   (Normal = 0.68 - 1.02)

THIS PATIENT's FINDINGS:
In the left upper extremity, the only abnormalities found with carpal tunnel studies were a slight prolongation of the Median palmar latency from the palm to the wrist, a decrease in the Median terminal latency index and an increase in the Median F wave. In the right upper extremity, nearly all parameters were abnormal. The Median motor terminal latency was abnormal with a normal nerve conduction velocity, Median sensory latency was elevated with a prolongation of the palmar stimulation to both the finger and the wrist and a decrea in the Median terminal latency index with an increase in the F wave.

These findings are compatible with a severe carpal tunnel syndrome on the right side and a possible early carpal tunnel syndrome on the left side.

CRITIQUE

1. The normal values for median latencies (3.4–4.5 msec) suggest that precise measurements were not made.
2. Although columns are present for amplitude and duration of action potentials, no values are given even though CTS is suspected on the left with borderline latencies.
3. Latencies from midpalm to wrist are described as *sensory;* however, there are motor fibers in the median nerve at that location so it is properly called a compound nerve action potential.

Example 25:

EMG REPORT

MUSCLE	Insertional Activity	Bizarre Discharges	Positive Waves	Fibrill- ations	Fascics	Poly- phasics	Recruit. Pattern	Amplitude
Rt.								
Pronator T.	n/	0	0	0	0	n/#	n/	n/
F.D. inteross	nl	∂	∂	0	0			
Abd. Poll. Br.	?	∪	∪	∪	∪			

NCV STUDIES

NERVES	DML (ms)	NCV M/S	M-Response Amplitude	Sensory Latency (ms)	Sensory Amplitude	NORMAL VALUE
Rt. Median	4.0	59	5 mv	3.6	50 µv	
Lt. Median	3.6	60	12 mv	3.3	50 µv	
Rt. Ulnar	3.2			3.5	50 µv	

Motor
	Velocity M/Sec	Distal Latency
Median	50-68	2.0-4.3
Ulnar	50-70	1.5-4.3
Peroneal	40-57	3.4-6.1
Tibial	40-58	4.0-6.1

Sensory
	Distal Latency
Median	2.0-3.2
Ulnar	2.0-3.2
Sural	2.0-3.2

EMG:

The right Abductor Pollicis Brevis showed increased exertional activity, but no positive waves or fibrillations were seen. The First Dorsal Interosseous and the Pronator Teres on the right were normal.

NCV:

The right Median nerve showed a mild prolongation of the sensory and motor latency across the wrist, just in the upper margins of normal. However, the size of the motor response was significantly decreased when compared to the response on the left side. The NCV on both Median nerves and the right Ulnar nerves were normal.

Impression:

The above findings in this patient suggest a mild Carpal Tunnel Syndrome.

CRITIQUE

1. There appears to be a technique error. A sensory latency of 3.6 msec with an amplitude of 50 μV is unlikely, except with a cold hand. Temperature should have been measured. Also, except in an "acute" situation the motor latency of 4.0 msec with an amplitude of 5/12 of normal seems unlikely.
2. This contains an inappropriate description of "increased insertional activity" in the abductor pollicis with *no* positive waves of fibrillations and normal recruitment.
3. The wide range of normal values of distal latencies suggests that precise measurements were not taken.
4. Mild carpal tunnel is not characterized by a greater than 50% reduction in CMAP. Stimulation of median nerve distal to carpal ligament could clarify the findings.

Example 26:

EMG REPORT

DESCRIPTION:
EMG was performed on the right lower extremity utilizing the monopolar technique. There are scattered fibrillation potentials along the quadriceps femoris. Normal insertional activity and normal interference pattern was noted.

The rest of the muscles tested were normal interference pattern, normal insertional activity and no increased polyphasic activity or fibrillation potentials noted.

IMPRESSION:
Borderline EMG. There is a suggestion of an L2-3-4 nerve root involvement.

PLAN:
The plan is to obtain Computerized Axial Tomography of the lumbar region.

I reviewed this procedure with him and he agrees to proceed. A copy of the report will be forwarded to your office.

CRITIQUE

1. No exploration of paraspinal muscles was done to localize the abnormality at or proximal to the root.
2. It is absurd to suggest that scattered fibrillation potentials in *one* muscle leads to a diagnosis of *three* roots.

3. Because no positive waves were noted and recruitment was normal, it is likely that the observer mistook endplate spikes for fibrillation potentials.

Data are insufficient to make diagnosis! Even if there were sufficient data, it is incumbent on the electromyographer to localize the abnormalities to a *single* root!!!

Example 27:

EMG REPORT

L.	R.	MUSCLES EXAMINED	LEVEL	FIBRILLATION		FASCICULATION		SCARCITY OF UNITS		UNIT VOLTAGE		UNIT DURATION	
				L.	R.	L.	R.	L.	R.	L.	R.	L.	R.
		Trapezius	C2-C4										
		Supraspinatus	C5-C6										
		Infraspinatus	C5-C6										
✓	✓	Deltoid	C5-C6	☾	☽	☽	☽	—	—				
✓	✓	Biceps brachii	C5-C6	☾	☽	☽	☽	-	—				
		Triceps	C6-C8										
		Wrist extensors	C6-C7										
		Wrist flexor-median	C6-C7										
		Wrist flexor-ulnar	C8-T1										
		Finger extensor	C6-C7										
		Finger flexor-median	C7-8, T1										
		Finger flexor ulnar	C7-8, T1										
✓	✓	Thenar eminence	C8-T1	☽	☽	☽	☽	-					
		1st dorsal interosseus	C8-T1										
		Hypothenar muscles	C8-T1										
		Hamstrings	L5-S1-2										
✓		Quadriceps *Vast. med.*	L2-4	⌒	⌒	⌒		—					
✓		Tibialis anterior	L4-5	⌒	⌒	⌒		—					
✓		*Med.* Gastrocnemiusoleus	S1-2	⌒	⌒	⌒		—					

LEGEND
FIBRILLATION & FASCICULATION

†	-	Occasional (occasional in 3 loci)
††	-	Few (2-3 in 4-5 loci)
†††	-	Many (several in many loci)
††††	-	Severe (Profuse)

SCARCITY OF UNITS (maximal effort contraction)

1 - slight (high frequency individual motor
    unit potentials—MUP-can be distinguished - audio)
2 - moderate (5-8 MUP in each locus)
3 - severe (1-4 MUP in each locus)
4 - total (no motor units activated)

CRITIQUE

1. This report lacks specificity of the muscles explored, i.e., wrist extensors and flexors, thenar eminence, hypothenar muscles, hamstrings. There are important differences within these muscles that should be identified.
2. Space is insufficient to describe motor unit potentials, i.e., recruitment, proportion of polyphasics.
3. No space is provided to describe positive waves occurring after needle insertion, i.e., insertional activity.

Example 28:

EMG REPORT

NERVE	Proximal Latency (miliseconds)		Normal	Velocity m/sec.	Response Wave		Normal Velocity meters/seconds
					Amplitude Milivolts	Duration Miliseconds	
MEDIAN	R	8.0	< 5.0 miliseconds	*	low	normal	< 45-65 m/sec
	L	7.4		*	low	normal	
ULNAR	R		< 4.0 miliseconds				< 45-64 m/sec
	L						
RADIAL	R						< 45-70 m/sec
	L						
COMMON PERONEAL	R		< 7.0 miliseconds				< 43-57 m/sec
	L						
POSTERIOR TIBIAL	R		< 7.3 miliseconds				< 41-60 m/sec
	L						
FACIAL	R		< 4.0 miliseconds				
	L						

SENSORY NERVE CONDUCTION LATENCY TESTS (ANTIDROMIC)

NERVE	Latency (miliseconds)		Normal miliseconds	Response Wave	
				Amplitude Microvolts	Duration Miliseconds
MEDIAN	R	8.6	< 3.7 m/sec.	very low	slow
	L	5.9		low	slow
ULNAR	R	2.6	< 3.5 m/sec.	normal	normal
	L	2.7		normal	normal

COMMENT: * Right Median Motor Nerve Conduction Velocity
Anticubital fossa to palm   25.5 M/sec
Anticubital fossa to wrist   69.5 M/sec

         * Left Median Motor Nerve Conduction Velocity
Anticubital fossa to palm   34.0 M/sec
Anticubital fossa to wrist   71.5 M/sec

IMPRESSION: Electircal evidence of Bilateral Carpal Tunnel Syndrome.

CRITIQUE

1. Normal values for distal motor latencies are too high. Further, the values for the ulnar and median nerves should be the same (3.7 msec ± .3) if careful measurements are made.
2. Amplitude of motor/sensory action potentials is described as "low" and "very low." This description is not helpful in interpreting this study!
3. Distal latencies for tibial and peroneal nerves given as normal values are too long.
4. The duration of the sensory action potential is characterized as "slow," rather than giving a value in milliseconds.
5. Calculating the conduction velocity from the elbow to wrist and then from the elbow to palm may hide a prolonged latency at wrist in the larger segment.

Example 29:

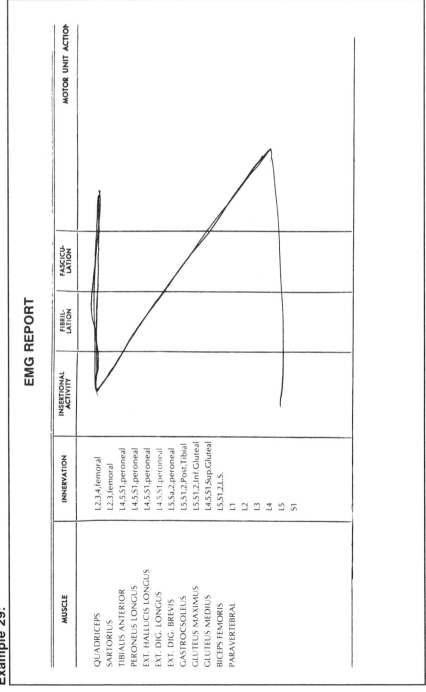

EMG REPORT

MUSCLE	INNERVATION	INSERTIONAL ACTIVITY	FIBRIL-LATION	FASCICU-LATION	MOTOR UNIT ACTION
QUADRICEPS	L2,3,4,femoral				
SARTORIUS	L2,3,femoral				
TIBIALIS ANTERIOR	L4,5,S1,peroneal				
PERONEUS LONGUS	L4,5,S1,peroneal				
EXT. HALLUCIS LONGUS	L4,5,S1,peroneal				
EXT. DIG. LONGUS	L4,5,S1,peroneal				
EXT. DIG. BREVIS	L5,Sa,2,peroneal				
GASTROCSOLEUS	L5,S1,2,Post,Tibial				
GLUTEUS MAXIMUS	L5,S1,2,Inf.Gluteal				
GLUTEUS MEDIUS	L4,5,S1,Sup.Gluteal				
BICEPS FEMORIS	L5,S1,2,L.S.				
PARAVERTEBRAL	L1				
	L2				
	L3				
	L4				
	L5				
	S1				

CRITIQUE

1. Printing a list of muscles restricts the exam and tends to stereotype it. The EMG becomes ritualistic.
2. L4 is only in the anterior tibial muscle below the knee; yet this report records L4 in the peroneus longus, extensor hallucis longus, and extensor digitorum longus.

Example 30:

EMG REPORT

MUSCLE	NERVE	ROOT	INSERTION	RESTING	VOLUNTARY
®Abd. Pollicis Br.	Median	C8,T1	Normal		Normal
Flex. Poll. Long	"				
Pronator Teres	"	C6			
First Dors. Int.	Ulnar	C8,T1			
Abd. Dig. Quinti	"	"			
Flex. Carp. Ulnar	"				
Ext. Indic. Prop.	Radical	C7,C8,T1			
Abd. Poll. Long	"	C7,C8			
Ext. Carpi. Rad.	"	C6,C7,C8			
Supinator	"	C6,C7,C8			
Triceps	"	C6,C7			
Biceps	Musc-Cut	C6,C7,C8			Polyphasics 2 +
Deltoid	Axillary	C5,C6			Normal
Supraspinatus	"	C5,C6			
Infraspinatus	"	"			
Rhomboids	Dors-Scp				Polyphasics 3 +
Cervical Para		C5			Polyphasics 2 +

NERVE	STIM	PICK-UP	LATENCY	DISTANCE	STIM. DUR.	VELOCITY	RESPONSE (Dur. & Amp)
®Median Motor			4.6/8.6	80/240		60	22 M Volts
F Wave			31.2				
Sensory			2.5/4.4	80/140			40 U Volts
®Ulnar Motor			4.2/7.8/11.8	80/225/160		62/40	15 M Volts
F Wave			34.6				
Sensory			4.2	140			30 U Volts
®Radial Sensory			3.7	140			20 U Volts
Lat antebracheal cut.			3.4	140			20 U Volts

impression: 1) Focal slowing of the right median nerve at the wrist and right ulnar nerve across the elbow.
2) Peripheral neuropathy
3) Chronic right C5-6 Radiculopathy

key myo—myotonia
fib—fibrillation
psw—positive sharp waves
fasc—fasciculation
bfh—bizarre high frequency potentials

CRITIQUE

1. The right median motor latency is reported as 4.6 msec and prolonged; yet the CMAP amplitude is 22 K, a value that is certainly normal.
2. Slowing is reported at the elbow (ulnar nerve), yet the CMAP is the same above and below the elbow. Ulnar study *must* be done with the elbow flexed to 70°. Otherwise, the segment across elbow will be falsely low (measurement artifact).
3. With only 2-3+ polyphasics (whatever that means) in biceps br and rhomboids and cervical paraspinal (? level), diagnosis of chronic C5-6 radiculopathy is made! This is inappropriate. Always make every effort to localize radiculopathies to a single root!

ERRORS IN INTERPRETATION AND REPORTING

EMG reports are uniquely valuable for analysis and judging the competence of electromyographers. Errors of fact and of technique, incomplete or irrelevant data, and over-, mis-, and underinterpretation of data are all seen with careful perusal of EMG reports. Over-, under-, and misinterpretation of the presented data are the mistakes made most frequently, as incomplete or irrelevant data were presented to support the final diagnosis. Anatomic errors included incorrect cord levels, as well as imprecise localization of explored muscles, e.g., wrist extensors, calf, thenar, and hamstrings.

Preparing an accurate report after an appropriate EMG study is the most important duty of the electromyographer.

13

Computer Applications of Electromyography

MOHAMMAD TAGHI FATEHI

Our lifestyle has been greatly affected by the second Industrial Revolution brought about by the introduction and widespread use of microcomputers and microprocessors. Not only can microcomputers process large amounts of data but they also can store and exchange programs and other information. For instance, services now are being offered for computer communication via telephone lines. The widespread application of computers and the related technologies have reduced the costs of hardware and software, making them even more appealing.

The application of microprocessors and microcomputers in the medical field has led to the development of sophisticated diagnostic equipment, such as computed tomography and magnetic resonance imaging. Computerized clinical EMG can be considered one of the more recent entrants in the world of digital automation. It has become popular only in the last few years.

Electromyographers use two types of microprocessor and microcomputer systems for data processing. One type is the microprocessor-based system in which the EMG equipment employs a built-in dedicated microprocessor. This system is highly specialized and costly and has a limited application in areas other than that for which it was designed. The second type of system consists of a standard electromyograph and a microcomputer, such as an office or home personal computer (PC) with the appropriate interface. In this system, the computer can be used for other purposes in addition to computerized electromyography. Both of these systems are described in this chapter.

This chapter introduces the reader to computer terminology and explains the essential building blocks and functions of a computer in order to demystify the idea of ''computerized instrumentation.'' The first three sections of this chapter are tutorial in nature. Section one presents the concept of digital representation of analog signals and introduces the related terminology. Sections two and three discuss the skeleton of the digital computer and the concept of computer software. These sections may be skipped by the reader who is familiar with computers. Sections four and five address the computerization of EMG. Finally, section six presents the possible sources of error and pitfalls in computerized EMG that may mislead the electromyographer.

DIGITAL CONCEPTS

The current trend in biomedical instrumentation is to make use of the great capability of digital systems. This section gives a general overview of digital concepts and describes the processes of sampling, digitization, and analog to digital and digital to analog conversions.

In general, the value of any analog quantity or signal, such as the EMG potential, at a given instant of time can be represented numerically and recorded. This numerical representation allows the information to be studied, processed, correlated with other stored data, and, when needed, faithfully reproduced.

The complete information about a time-varying signal, such as an EMG potential over the interval of interest, can be represented in two forms. The first form is in a tabular manner where the numerical values of the signal (sampled at regular intervals of time) are recorded against the elapsed time. For this table to describe the fine details of the signal with reasonable accuracy, the sampling interval should be small and therefore the number of samples large. However, this tabular form of representing a time-varying signal is difficult to understand and visualize. The second form of representation of the signal is the analog form; that is, representation by means of a continuous graph. A typical graph is shown in Figure 13.1 where the horizontal coordinate t represents the time and the vertical coordinate v represents the amplitude of the signal, i.e., v is a function of time, or

$$v = f(t)$$

This form of representation is similar to an EMG wave potential displayed on the CRT screen of a standard EMG. It is assumed that no deterioration of the signal occurs from the recording point to the observation point, i.e., that the electrodes, amplifiers, and filters do not alter the signal.

For a computer to process this information, it must be converted to a digital format. The process of converting an analog signal into digital has three steps: sampling, quantization, and coding (7,14,16). These steps are discussed by considering the conversion of the signal v shown in Figure 13.1.

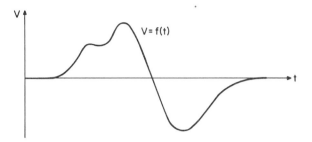

Figure 13.1. Analog representation of a typical signal v = f(t).

The first step in the conversion process is to sample the analog signal at given instants of time T_n. In Figure 13.2A, the analog function indicated by the dotted line is sampled at regular intervals of time,

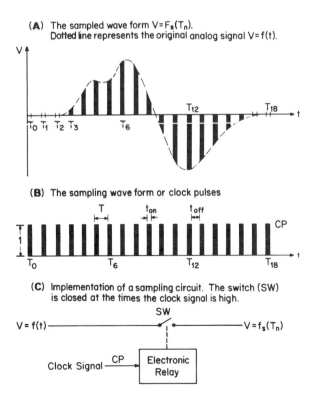

(A) The sampled wave form $V = F_s(T_n)$. Dotted line represents the original analog signal $V = f(t)$.

(B) The sampling wave form or clock pulses

(C) Implementation of a sampling circuit. The switch (SW) is closed at the times the clock signal is high.

Figure 13.2. Sampling process. The value of the signal is known at the instants of time, $t = T_n$, when the switch, SW, is closed.

$T_n = nT$. Therefore, the amplitude of the sampled signal is known only at these given sampling points (1); that is

$$V = f_s(T_n), \qquad \text{where } n = 1, 2, 3, \ldots$$

The sampled signal consists of a series of pulses, the heights of which represent the value of the signal at the corresponding sampling points. The sampling times, T_n, are determined by the sampling waveform CP shown in Figure 13.2B. This signal is made up of short pulses of duration, t_{ON}.

Figure 13.2C shows the operation of a simple sampling circuit. In this diagram, the analog input signal v, such as the one shown in Figure 13.1, is connected to an electronic switch SW to obtain the output function V. Therefore, the output V is equal to the input only at the instants when the switch SW is closed. The closure of the switch is controlled by synchronizing clock pulses (line CP) of the form shown in Figure 13.2B. This sampled, discrete information is similar to the tabular representation of the signal as discussed earlier.

In most practical systems, samples are made at regular intervals of time, $t = T$, 2T, 3T . . . nT, under the control of a constant frequency clock. The interval T is known as the *sampling period* or *sampling interval*, and its reciprocal f, where

$$f = 1/T$$

is called the *sampling rate* or *sampling frequency*.

If the sampling rate is not high enough, the higher frequency information in the signal will be lost. In fact, the sampling frequency should be at least twice the highest frequency content of the signal of interest (15). For example, in the study of needle EMG potentials, if the high frequency filter in the EMG instrument is set at 10 KHz, the sampling frequency should be no less than $f = 20$ KHz. In contrast, in surface EMG where the highest frequency component in the signal is no more than 1 KHz, a sampling rate of 2 KHz may be sufficient to record the signal in a reproducible form. For single fiber EMG (SFEMG) studies, a much higher sampling rate is needed.

The second step in the process of analog to digital conversion is the quantization of the amplitude of the signal at each sampling point. The amplitude of the signal can be represented by only a finite number of values or quantization levels. If the number of quantization levels is increased, more detailed information is captured. Figure 13.3 shows the effect of increasing the number of quantization levels. Figure 13.3A shows quantization of the waveform of Figure 13.1 using only two quantization levels. These two levels may be called "negative poten-

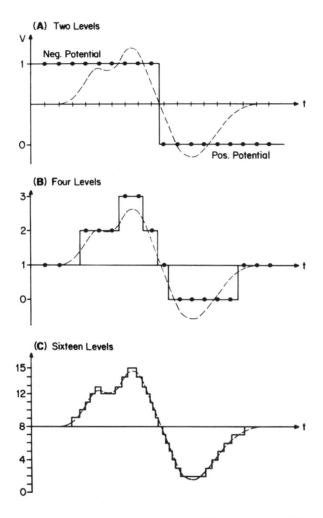

Figure 13.3. Quantization of the waveform of Figure 13.1 in different quantization levels. The higher the number of quantization levels, the better the reproduction of the signal.

tial'' and "positive potential," "true" and "false," or levels "1" and "0."

Obviously not much information is gained if only two quantization levels are used, unless one is only interested in knowing whether an EMG potential is present or not. Figure 13.3B shows the same signal quantized into four quantization levels. With this increase in the number of quantization levels, the shape of the signal becomes more rec-

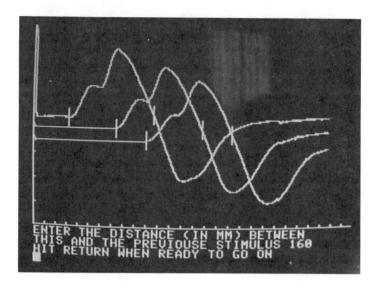

Figure 13.4. A typical EMG display on the TV monitor.

ognizable. Figure 13.3C shows quantization of the same signal into 16 levels, thus showing more details. Many of today's EMG machines quantize the amplified EMG potentials into 256 levels. This number of levels offers enough resolution for clinical applications. Figure 13.4 is a photograph of the television monitor display of three potentials in a computerized EMG exam. The vertical resolution (number of quantization levels) in that display is 160, and the effect of quantization is noticeable. For research-oriented applications, quantization levels of up to 4096 levels are commonly utilized (18).

The last step in the process of analog to digital conversion is to encode the quantized signal in binary (base 2) format. In a binary number system, each quantized value is represented by a number of binary digits (called bits). A bit can assume only one of the two values: a zero or a one. The collection of the binary digits used to express the digitized numbers in a computer system is termed a *binary word*. In Figure 13.3A, only one bit could be used to represent the signal amplitude. Figure 13.3B calls for a two-bit word to represent all the four possible values (00, 01, 10, and 11). Similarly in Figure 13.3C where 16 resolution elements are available, four binary digits or a four-bit word would be needed to encode each possible value uniquely. These 16 possible combinations of the four-bit word, along with their decimal equivalents, are given in Table 13.1.

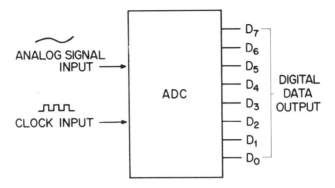

Figure 13.5. Functional block diagram of a typical analog to digital convertor.

Table 13.1. Binary representation of decimal numbers 0 through 15

Decimal	Binary	Decimal	Binary
0	0000	8	1000
1	0001	9	1001
2	0010	10	1010
3	0011	11	1011
4	0100	12	1100
5	0101	13	1101
6	0110	14	1110
7	0111	15	1111

In a similar fashion, if a number is quantized into 256 levels then, 8 bits (commonly called one byte) are needed to represent it. In general, if the number of quantization levels is N, then n bits are required to represent all possible values, where n is given by the equation below.

$$n = \log_2 N$$

A/D Convertors

Electronic devices known as analog to digital (A/D) convertors are commercially available and perform the complete process of analog to digital conversion (1, 16). Figure 13.5 is a functional block diagram of such a device. The input lines to these devices usually are made up of the clock (timing) signal and, of course, the analog signal that is to be digitized. The output consists of eight or more digital data lines that hold the binary equivalent of the nearest quantized level, a short time following each sampling pulse. Other control lines also exist and are used for interconnection with computers. Complete microprocessor-compatible A/D convertors on single integrated circuit (IC) chips are available on the market today. Examples of such devices are the AD7574 (microprocessor-compatible 8-bit A/D) and AD573 (10-bit A/D) (1). The cost of commercial A/Ds depends on the number of output data bits that determine the resolution of the signal and on the conversion speed that determines the maximum allowable sampling rate. Also available commercially are multichannel A/D convertors in which several analog channels are time multiplexed and converted to digital signals on the same digital data lines but at different intervals of time.

Digital to Analog Conversion

The reverse process of analog to digital conversion is digital to analog (D/A) conversion. A D/A convertor is used to provide analog instruments with the processed information from the digital computer. Using an A/D convertor on the input side of a digital processor and a D/A convertor on the output side permits complete two-way communication between the analog world and the digital computer. A hybrid instrument consisting of analog inputs and analog outputs with a digital processor in between could appear as a standard analog system, but its usefulness is greatly increased by its ability to process, store, and modify the data. An example of such a system is the TECA model TD 10/20 series EMG machine (21). The process of conversion from digital to analog is usually much simpler (and faster) than conversion from analog to digital. Commercial D/A convertors on IC chips with varying resolution and speeds are available (1).

THE ANATOMY OF A DIGITAL COMPUTER

The purpose of this section is to provide an overview of the internal structure of the digital computer. The essential components that form the basic computer and their functional relationships are described. Throughout this section, commonly used computer terminology is defined.

The Main Components of a Digital Computer

A digital computer can be viewed as a device that can (a) store digital data and (b) perform arithmetical and logical operations on the data according to a sequence of instructions or steps called a *program*. In a way, it is analogous to a simple-minded clerk with a pencil, a scratch pad, and a hand calculator, who is supplied with a set of instructions. This clerk or operator is to follow only the given instructions, no more and no less (22).

Figure 13.6 shows the essential components of a digital computer. The central processing unit (CPU) plays the role of the hand calculator in the above analogy and is designed to perform all arithmetical and

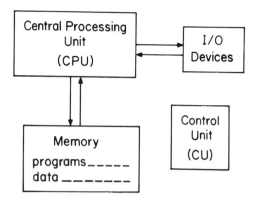

Figure 13.6. Simplified block diagram of a general-purpose digital computer.

logical operations. It consists of an arithmetic-logic unit (ALU) and one or more data registers for temporary storage of partial results of operations. The memory plays the role of the scratch pad. It is used to store (in an organized fashion) two types of information: (a) the raw data, the partial results, and the final processed information and (b) the program according to which the operations are to proceed. Obviously, all such information and instructions are also coded in binary form. This kind of coding of instruction is called a *machine language program* and is discussed in the next section. At this level, the data and instructions are indistinguishable from each other, except that they are placed in different areas in the memory and their addresses or locations are known to the machine. Because the data and instructions are similar binary words, the machine can be instructed to look at its instructions as data and to perform logical operations on them. The machine therefore can modify its own operational sequence; in other words, it can modify its own destiny. This is the reason why the digital computer has such a great capability and is the basis of so-called artificial intelligence.

Another essential component of the computer is the input/output (I/O) devices: all communication channels that connect the machine to the outside world. These may be (a) devices for communicating with human operators, such as keyboards, CRT monitors, printers, or even speakers and microphones; (b) digital parallel and/or serial interfaces for communicating with other computers or digital machines; (c) devices for permanent storage of data and programs, such as magnetic tapes, disks, etc.; and (d) A/D and D/A convertors for communicating with the analog world.

The operation of the components discussed above is supervised and coordinated by the control unit (CU), which is the final block in the diagram of Figure 13.6. It is this electronic logic unit that performs the task of switching the right connections at the right time in the sequence of operations of the machine. This unit is usually transparent to the novice user and escapes detection (7,17).

Types of Computer Memory

As discussed earlier, both the data and the programs are stored in the memory as organized arrays of binary words. Each word consists of a number of bits, each of which is held in one memory element. The size of the word or the word length depends on the architecture of the computer and the CPU. For example, the Apple II computer has a word length of 8 bits, whereas the word length of the IBM PC is 16 bits. Each word in the memory array is tagged with an address. This address is used by the machine to access the proper location for data or instruction stored there. The number of words in the memory array defines the memory size. The memory size is usually referred to in blocks of $1024 = 2^{10}$ bytes (termed kilobytes or simply k-bytes). Today's technology has made it possible for a personal computer to have hundreds of kilobytes of memory (9).

Many kinds of memory devices, based on different technologies (9) and with different characteristics and names, are available. Each computer utilizes one or more of these types. Memory devices should possess the following desirable features for computer applications:

1. High storage density: a large number of storage elements contained in a small physical space;
2. High speed of access or short access time;
3. Read/write capability: the ability to read from and write into each word in the memory;
4. Random access capability: the ability to access any word (at any given address) without having to check sequentially all the information before or after it, as is the case with magnetic tapes;
5. Nonvolatile: the information is not lost if the power is turned off;
6. Low cost per bit.

Unfortunately, all these features are not available in any one device with the present technology.

Depending on how data are accessed, the storage devices are classified into three types:

1. Random access memory (RAM): This forms the main portion of the on-board storage device in most general-purpose computers. RAMs make it possible to access any given address in the memory. Two types of RAMs are available as chips: (a) the static RAM, which is

characterized by high speed and ease of implementation, and (b) the dynamic RAM, which is characterized by low price and high density (9,11). This distinction is of interest only to the computer designer and not to the general user. The problem with most RAMs is that they are volatile and information is retained only as long as the system is powered. The other types of memory are nonvolatile and can be used for storage.

2. Read only memory (ROM): This is also a random access type of memory, except that the information or the program is permanently stored in it before being installed in the computer. The contents of ROMs cannot be modified or erased even when the power is off. Because ROMs are programmed by the manufacturer, they offer little flexibility for system developers. However, special ROMs that can be programmed are available and are called by the following terms: PROM (programmable read only memory), EPROM (erasable programmable read only memory), and EEPROM (electronically erasable programmable read only memory) (9, 11).

3. Sequential access memory: This is an archival type of storage that is usually installed as a peripheral device, such as disks, magnetic tapes, etc. To access a group of data, one must sequentially access the storage device, such as a tape, looking for the desired file for reading or blank spots for writing. In practical usage, blocks of data in the form of files are transferred between the peripheral storage and the active memory (RAMs). The desired operations and computations are performed in the active memory, and the results are stored back in a file in the peripheral storage.

Special-Purpose and General-Purpose Computers

One of the factors inhibiting many physicians from obtaining and using computers is the jargon or terminology used. This discussion is intended to clarify the terminology used to describe different types of digital data processing and computing equipment.

There are two types of digital computers: general-purpose digital computers and special-purpose digital computers. A general-purpose computer is defined as a stored program machine of the form shown in Figure 13.6. This machine has the capability to perform all operations that any other general-purpose digital computer can. With this definition a personal computer or a microcomputer, such as Apple II; a minicomputer, such as PDP 11/34; and a large computer, such as IBM 370, can be programmed to solve any given problem with the same final result. The difference between these machines lies in their word size, architectural complexity, I/O capabilities, instruction set, ease of programming, and above all, speed at which operations are performed.

A special-purpose digital computer, in contrast, is a machine that is designed to perform a specific task. The sequence of operations (program) is fixed by the design of the hardware or by the instructions stored in the ROMs. The programs stored in the ROM are referred to as firmware. *Firmware* is the term used to indicate the middle ground between hardware and software. If such a special-purpose computer is to be modified or updated, the firmware (ROM chips) should be replaced. Examples of such special-purpose computers for EMG applications are the TECA Model TD10/20 (21) and Cadwell 5200A (3) EMG instruments.

By appropriate programming and interface design, a general-purpose digital computer should be able to do the task of any special-purpose computer, including all forms of EMG analysis (5, 6, 23). In addition, the same machine could be used to perform office billing, word processing, telephone answering, and bookkeeping functions with the proper software. However, a machine designed for a specific task is expected to perform that task more efficiently, depending on how much effort has gone into the design of the system.

Microcomputers and Microprocessors

The architecture of many of today's computers is modular. To facilitate addition and deletion of optional devices, the modules are organized around a set of lines (wires), called the *bus,* into which the modules are plugged. Data, addresses, and the control information flow through this bus from any module to all other modules. Every device that is plugged in is assigned an address. Only the device whose address is selected is permitted to respond to the information on the bus. This type of architecture is called the *bus architecture.* The diagram in Figure 13.7 shows a bus-organized computer system. In that diagram, the solid lines show the flow of information (data and addresses), and the dotted lines indicate control and timing signals issued to and from the control unit. The control unit is synchronized by pulses issued by the master clock. This system can be expanded by adding more devices to the bus.

Present large-scale integrated circuit (LSI) technology has made it possible to fabricate the entire CPU and the control unit on single IC chips. Such devices are called *microprocessors.* Figure 13.8 shows the organization of a microprocessor unit. Figure 13.9 is a photograph of an actual microprocessor IC, the 6502, which is the heart of the Apple II microcomputer (2,13). Most microprocessor units have bus architecture that is simply extended externally to the unit. There are usually 8 or 16 data lines, 16 address lines, and a few control lines on the external bus. There are no peripheral or I/O devices incorporated in the microprocessor unit. Thus, a microprocessor is incapable of doing any processing on its own. However, by adding a clock, a memory mod-

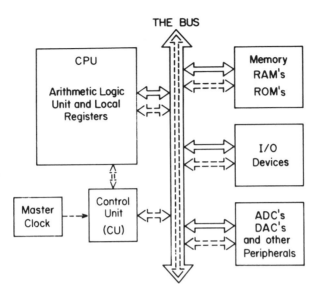

Figure 13.7. A bus-structured computer system. *Dotted lines* indicate flow of control signals, and *solid lines* indicate flow of information between modules.

ule, and at least a keyboard and monitor to the bus of the micropro-cessor (Figure 13.8), one can construct a microcomputer. A microcomputer is, therefore, a microprocessor-based digital computer.

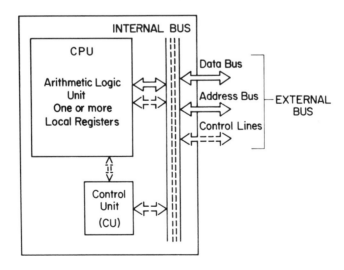

Figure 13.8. Organization of a microprocessor.

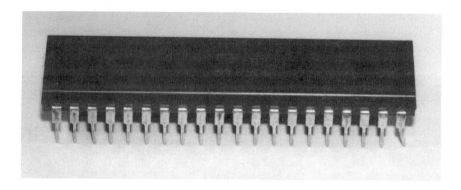

Figure 13.9. Photograph of a 6502 microprocessor chip.

By adding ROMs with special-purpose programs stored in them, microprocessors can be used as the controllers for many of today's sophisticated equipment. Such a system is called *microprocessor-based instrumentation.* An example of such equipment is the TECA Model TD-20 EMG for which no standard keyboard nor means of changing the program is provided.

Most of today's personal computers are microprocessor-based computers. In fact, it is the development of the microprocessors that has caused the popularity and abundance of microcomputers. These computers are generally smaller, lower in capability, and lower in price than the large multi-user computer systems, such as the IBM 370. The middle ground between these two types is covered by the so-called minicomputers, such as the Digital Equipment Corporation's PDP-11 family of minicomputers. However, the differentiation between the large, the mini, and the microcomputer systems is narrowing.

COMPUTER SOFTWARE

If the hardware of the computer is compared to the human body, then the software is the soul of the system. Without the system software, the computer would be a dead piece of electronic circuitry. The software comprises a set of programs that enables the machine to communicate with the operator (the system software) and programs that are written to perform specific tasks (user software). In microcomputers, most of the system software is incorporated in ROMs and automatically run when the power is turned on. In large computers, much of the system software is kept on disks that must be automatically loaded (booted) into RAMs as the system is turned on. In this case, there is a semi-intelligent program in the ROM of the computer that "boots" the operating system. Such a program is called the *bootstrap loader.* Once the operating system is loaded, the machine can load other utility programs or be directed to load and run user programs. The user programs are those developed and written by the more involved computer user to perform specific tasks, such as acquiring and analyzing information from an EMG. Before writing a program, the programmer should select the algorithm that must be followed and develop the logical steps needed for the execution of this algorithm. Some graphic tools, such as flow charts, may be employed to organize the sequence of instructions involved. The next step is to encode these instructions in a language or a set of codes that the machine can understand and interpret. The different methods of coding the instructions are called programming languages.

Machine Language Programming

A program is a coded sequence of instructions that directs the central processing unit (CPU) to locate data in the memory (or I/O space), relocate it, and perform operations on the data. The only code that a digital machine can use is the set of zeros and ones. Thus the instructions must be encoded in that form according to a specified format. This programming language, which is in harmony with the nature of the digital machine, is called the machine language or binary language. As an example, consider how a typical instruction, "take the datum in the memory location 5 and add it to the content of the register in the CPU," would be encoded in the 6502 microprocessor language. This instruction would encode in three successive words (three successive locations) as shown in Table 13.2 in the middle column.

Table 13.2 Example of a Machine Language Instruction and the Equivalent Value in Hexadecimal

Symbolic instruction address	Instruction in binary or machine language	Equivalent value in hexadecimal
LOCATION ONE	01101101	6D
LOCATION TWO	00000101	05
LOCATION THREE	00000000	00

Because the binary numbers are difficult to read, most computers have the capability to display and/or accept these binary codes in octal (base 8) or hexadecimal (base 16) format. The reason for using octal or hexadecimal representation rather than the more familiar decimal system (base 10) is that it is very easy to convert hexadecimal or octal representation into binary (base 2) format, i.e., machine language. The last column in Table 13.2 shows the representation of the given machine language instruction in hexadecimal as used by the Apple computer (2). The first of the three words in Table 13.2 is the actual instruction (operation code), and the next two words give the address where the operand is to be found.

Assembly Language Programming

Machine language programming is tedious, uninteresting, and prone to error, especially if the program is long. The programmer must remember the numerical code for each operation (called op-code), as well as the exact location in the memory where data and instructions are located. To replace programming in machine language, another programming technique called *assembly language* has been devised. In assembly language, each numerical operation that is coded is replaced by its mnemonic equivalent, and the addresses are permitted to be represented by symbolic addresses, rather than by exact memory locations. For example, the mnemonic "ADD" may be used instead of the number "01101101." Also the symbolic address "FIRST" may be used, instead of rows two and three of Table 13.2. The example discussed earlier would be written simply as follows in assembly language,

$$\text{START} \qquad \text{ADD FIRST,}$$

assuming the instruction itself is at the symbolic location START.

The program written in assembly language must eventually be translated into machine language for it to run on the computer system. The task of translating from assembly to machine language is done through sequences of code conversions. The computer may be programmed to convert an assembly language program to a machine language program. The program written to do such a translation is called an *assembler*.

High-Level Languages

The assembly language, even though superior to the binary code, suffers from two major drawbacks. First, the assembly language instructions are direct translations of the machine codes, and thus an assembly language program is "machine dependent." That is, a program written in assembly language for one type of computer will not run on another type. Second, writing assembly language programs requires skill and close familiarity with the operation and structural model of the microprocessor used. It is not flexible enough to be used by the newcomer. For these reasons, programming languages that are machine independent and are closer to natural languages (English, for instance) have been devised. These languages are collectively called *high-level languages.* Many such languages are in use today, designed around the needs of different groups of users and with varying degrees of closeness to the machine languages. For example, FORTRAN is most suited for the scientific community, COBOL for the business community, and BASIC and PASCAL for the general public.

In order to compare the programming complexity at different levels, Figure 13.10 shows a simple program, which computes the sum of the intergers 1 through 20, as written in four different languages.

No matter what language a program is written in, it must be eventually translated into the machine language of the processor used. Just like assemblers, programs that translate high-level languages have been developed for most commercial computers. Two types of such translating programs are commonly used: *compilers*, which translate the entire source (high-level language) program to the machine language before the first execution of that program, and *interpreters*, which translate the source program one statement at a time during each execution. In the latter case, the translated version is never retained in the machine. The source program is interpreted every time that it is run. When compilers are used, execution of a program requires two steps, but it yields more computational efficiency. Interpreters, on the other hand, permit real-time and interactive computing, but are, in general, slow and less efficient.

On one side of the spectrum of artificial languages is the machine language, and on the other side are a variety of high-level languages. It would not be surprising if a higher level (universal) language very similar to spoken English would one day be devised. With these simple high-level languages available, why would anyone want to program in assembly or any low-level language? The answer is efficiency. A program written in assembly or machine language is, in general, more efficient and faster and utilizes all the capability of the machine. When writing in assembly language, the programmer can keep track of the information flow in the machine and know exactly how and when each instruction is executed. This knowledge is especially important when dealing with data transfers between machine components of different speeds.

Hardware-Software Tradeoff

Different types of digital computers have different internal hardware and architecture. As stated earlier, any general-purpose digital computer can be programmed to perform all computations that any other general-purpose digital computer can perform. This poses the question: Why choose one type of computer over another for a given purpose? The answer to this question lies in the features of computational accuracy, speed, programming flexibility, and interfacing capability. Obviously, the word size is also one of the main factors that relates to computational accuracy and speed. The number of internal registers in the CPU and of interconnections between subsystems and

```
;;;;;;;;;;;;;;;;;;;;;;;;;;;;;;;;;;;;;;;;;;;;;;;;;;;;;;;;;;;;;;
;  THIS PROGRAM ADDS UP INTEGER NUMBERS FROM 1 TO 20      ;
;  THE PROGRAM IS WRITTEN IN   MACRO 11 LANGUAGE.         ;
;;;;;;;;;;;;;;;;;;;;;;;;;;;;;;;;;;;;;;;;;;;;;;;;;;;;;;;;;;;;;;
```

(A)   **(B)**

```
 7
 8 000000  012703  000001        START:  MOV   #1,R3
 9 000004  005002                        CLR   R2
10 000006  060302                LOOP:   ADD   R3,R2
11 000010  005203                        INC   R3
12 000012  020327  000024                CMP   R3,#20.
13 000016  003773                        BLE   LOOP
14         000000'               .END    START
```

```
************************************************************
* THIS PROGRAM ADDS UP INTEGER NUMBERS  FROM 1 TO 20 *
* THE PROGRAM IS WRITTEN IN FORTRAN LANGUAGE.        *
************************************************************
```

(C)

```
PROGRAM SUM.FOR
      INTEGER  A,I
      A=0.0
      DO 40 I=1,20
      A=A+I
40    CONTINUE
      STOP
      END
```

```
************************************************************
* THIS PROGRAM ADDS UP INTEGER NUMBERS FROM 1 TO 20 *
* THE PROGRAM IS WRITTEN IN   PASCAL LANGUAGE.      *
************************************************************
```

(D)

```
PROGRAM SUM (INPUT,OUTPUT);
   VAR  I,A:INTEGER;
        A:=0.0
        BEGIN
          FOR I:=1 TO 20 DO
          A:=A+I
        END;
   END.
```

Figure 13.10. A sample program shown in four different languages: *A*, PDP-11 machine language (octal); *B*, PDP-11 assembly language (5); *C*, FORTRAN; and *D*, PASCAL.

the design of the control unit also determines the machine instruction set and thus its programming flexibility. In general, the simpler the hardware is, the more elaborate the software must be to perform a given task. There is a tradeoff between hardware and software, which must be considered when choosing a digital computer. It is the combination of the hardware, software and the peripheral devices that determines the capabilities of a digital computer for a given application.

MICROPROCESSOR-BASED ELECTRODIAGNOSTIC INSTRUMENTS

Manufacturers of EMG instruments, as have those in other fields of technology, have used digital techniques in their designs. Utilizing digital computers, EMG potentials are sampled and stored in memory and then analyzed by the microprocessor unit to extract many diagnostic features and parameters quantitatively that would otherwise be very tedious for the practicing electromyographer to obtain.

Digital techniques can be used in two ways to analyze EMG data. One way is to interface a standard (analog) EMG instrument to a general-purpose digital computer or a microcomputer to facilitate modern electromyography. The other method is to use EMG equipment that incorporates a microprocessor-based (MP-based) special-purpose computer as an integral part in it. Systems of the latter type are termed *microprocessor-based EMG instruments*. MP-based EMG instruments are, understandably, favored by the manufacturers of commercial electromyograms. Some microprocessor-based EMG instruments are provided with standard parallel or serial (RS232 type) interface ports for connection to other general-purpose computers if desired by the user. The general structure of MP-base EMG instruments is described in this section.

Structure of MP-Based EMG Instruments

Since the early 1980s, many MP-based EMG instruments have emerged in the medical market, each with claims that it is superior to all the others. These systems differ in the design of their "front end," use various microprocessors, and come with an assortment of software routines with different capabilities. Nevertheless, all MP-based instruments have the same basic principle and architecture. TECA model TD-20 (21) and Cadwell model 5200A (3) are two of the many instruments available today.

The general structure of a modern MP-based EMG instrument is depicted in Figure 13.11. The system consists of four interconnected parts. The standard analog EMG portion of the instrument consists of preamplifiers, amplifiers and signal conditioners, trigger units, and stimulators. This part also includes standard analog output devices, such as CRTs, speakers, or any other optional devices. Allowance is also made for some of the parameters, such as the filter settings, amplifier gains, and stimulator timing, to be adjusted by the microprocessor.

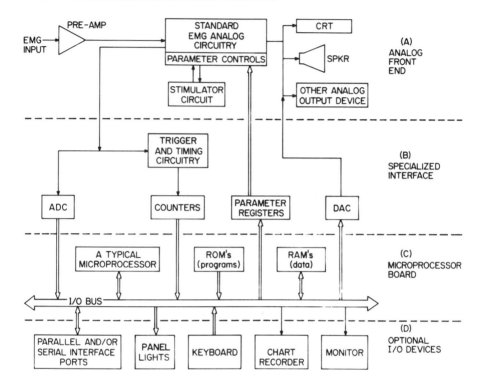

Figure 13.11. Block diagram of a microprocessor-based EMG instrument.

The next part is the interface between the digital and the analog subsystems. The main component in this interface is an A/D convertor that permits digitization of the EMG potentials for storage and processing by the digital unit. The resolution and sampling rate are determined by the designers. In some units, other parameters, such as the gating and timing signals, are directly measured in digital counters for entering into the microprocessor. This permits evaluation of intervals, latencies, etc. directly, thereby eliminating the need for a very high speed A/D convertor. This circuitry is especially useful in such applications as SFEMG (20) where interpotential intervals and not the form of the potentials are of interest. In some units, it is possible to display the digitally processed signals on the analog output device. Such machines are also equipped with the appropriate D/A convertors.

The third part is the digital processor board. The main component in this section is a commercial microprocessor unit that is usually bus structured. Another component on the digital board is the storage unit (16 K or more of RAMs). It is used for storing the raw information,

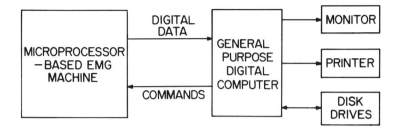

Figure 13.12. A microprocessor-based EMG machine used in conjunction with a general-purpose microcomputer.

processed data, and other variables and machine parameters. The software routines, which include the different EMG exams and various output formats, are usually stored in a set of ROMs. These programs are written on a permanent basis in the form of firmware, but can be changed and updated by the manufacturer by exchanging the ROM chips.

I/O devices permit communication with the electromyographer and with other digital computers. The I/O set in a commercial MP-based EMG instrument usually includes the following: a set of panel lights, a full or partial keyboard, a monitor, a printer or plotter, and possibly a standard serial and/or parallel interface for connection to a general-purpose digital computer.

Interfacing with Digital Computers

Commercial MP-based EMG instruments are usually supplied with a set of software routines to perform many of the standard EMG exams. The full capability of these units is utilized only when they are interfaced and used in conjunction with a general-purpose digital computer. This configuration also permits the electromyographer to use and run many specialized EMG programs that other specialists may have developed, e.g., SFEMG and Macro EMG routines developed by Stalberg and Stalberg (19)). It also permits test results, patient information, test parameters, and reference material to be stored on external storage devices, such as floppy disks. These data could then be used for research and for exchange of information among scientists. There are several commercial software packages available for some MP-based EMG instrument and computer combinations (19).

Figure 13.12 shows a general hardware configuration of a microprocessor-based EMG instrument, microcomputer, monitor, printer, and one or more disk drives. The EMG data and the control information are transferred back and forth between the EMG instrument and the computer through a standard interface. Although a parallel interface can be used, a duplex serial interface is more popular. For interconnection purposes, a standard interface port is usually provided on the EMG instrument. The corresponding computer interface port is commercially available for most PCs. The I/O devices (shown in Figure 13.12), such as the monitor, the printer, and the disk drives, are the I/O options interfaced to the microcomputer selected for this purpose.

In addition to providing a sophisticated clinical tool, the combination of the digital computer and the MP-based EMG instrument can be used as a research instrument. A clinician can, for example, develop a data base, store all clinical test results for statistical analysis, and compile and develop his or her own test normals and standards. The next section describes methods for using standard (analog) EMG instruments to achieve computerized electromyography.

MICROCOMPUTER-BASED EMG

Commercial microprocessor-based EMG instruments have three drawbacks. First, these systems are limited in hardware capability and flexibility by what the manufacturer has designed at the time of its development. During system design, the engineers conceive a set of EMG routines and design both the software and hardware to perform these tasks efficiently. The exact method by which these tasks are carried out, therefore, is determined by the microprocessor and other selected hardware. Second, microprocessor-based EMG instruments are generally very expensive. This cost may be justified because they are advertised as advanced medical instruments with only a limited market. Finally, the programs and routines developed by users for the machine of one brand (with or without a controlling computer) are not easily adapted to the machine of another manufacturer. The possibility of exchange of clinical and research results among researchers and clinicians is therefore reduced.

With the availability of PCs at reasonable costs and with a variety of commercial computer interfaces, it is now possible to interface a general-purpose digital computer to standard (analog) EMG equipment to process EMG data. Systems configured in this fashion may be termed *microcomputer-based EMG* equipment (MC-EMG). Because today's microcomputers have sufficient capacity and speed, a very powerful clinical and research tool can be designed at minimal cost (5,6,18,23). Figure 13.13 shows an example of such a system in clinical use in the Ohio State University Department of Physical Medicine. The system consists of the Apple II personal computer and the TECA model B9 EMG machine.

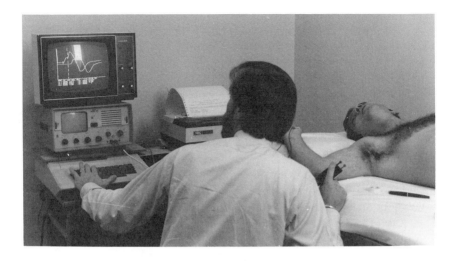

Figure 13.13. Photograph of an inexpensive microcomputer-based EMG system used at the Ohio State University Department of Physical Medicine.

Components of MC-EMG

Figure 13.14 is a block diagram of the microcomputer-based EMG setup. The system is based on a general-purpose microcomputer, such as the Apple II, the IBM-PC, or any other computer. The minimum desirable I/O devices may be (a) a monitor for display of the menu, text parameters, exam results, and communication with the electromyographer; (b) one or two floppy or hard disk drives for storage and retrieval of EMG programs, patients' data, and test results; and (c) a printer for providing the patient's report and hard copy of the EMG results, etc. The maximum number of I/O devices are limited only by the funds available for this purpose.

By assigning most of signal and data processing tasks to the computer via software, the required complexity of the EMG instrument is re-

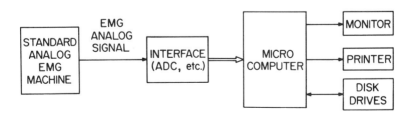

Figure 13.14. General configuration of a microcomputer-based EMG setup.

duced. In fact, for any available EMG instrument, such as the popular TECA TE4 series, the inexpensive model B9, the primary EMG (10) or even only a set of preamplifiers may be only input device needed. The accuracy and the reliability of the results would be, mostly, a function of the interface, the computer, and the software utilized. For many common EMG routines, such as potential analysis and nerve conduction studies, the only signals needed by the interface section are the amplified raw EMG signal and possibly the stimulator gating pulse. For these EMG routines, the interface may be one of the many commercially available multichannel A/D converter boards. For some sophisticated EMG exams, such as SFEMG where high-speed signals are of interest, it may be less expensive and more efficient to design special interface boards. Such interface boards would automatically extract and deliver the feature of interest in the signal to the computer. This is in contrast to entering the entire waveform into the computer and then extracting these features via software manipulation. In the rest of this section, MC-EMG configurations are discussed by means of a typical application example for two EMG routines.

A System for Evoked Potential Analysis:
MC-EMG Configuration Example I

An inexpensive system consisting of an Apple II computer and a commercial two-channel A/D interface board, which has been developed by the author, permits analysis of muscle and nerve evoked potentials from any available EMG instrument (23). One input channel is devoted to monitoring the initiation of the stimulation pulse, and the second channel is devoted to converting the analog EMG response immediately following the stimulus signal. The conversions are made at the rate of 40 KHz, and all the information (latency and the potential) is stored in the computer memory. The potentials are also displayed on the monitor. This system, which can be used as an inexpensive add-on unit to any EMG instrument, is schematically shown in Figure 13.15.

The software is a user-friendly, menu-driven system written in BASIC language that calls a number of machine language subroutines for data collection and sorting tasks. Figure 13.16 shows the general operation of the system by means of a software flow chart. The data acquisition subroutine is written in machine language so as to permit the maximum sampling speed. The program permits computation of the latency, am-

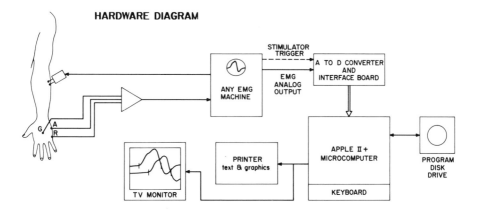

Figure 13.15.   Schematic representation of the system for evoked potential analysis.

plitude, and duration of the negative spike and the area under the evoked potential curve for each stimulation. For the purpose of latency and duration computation, the take-off points are automatically determined by the computer, and visual cursors are placed at these locations on the monitor. The user is then prompted to verify or modify these cursor positions.

As noted on the flow chart, the computer requests the distance between the two stimulation sites following each pair of stimulations. The EMG parameters are then computed and displayed instantly. Results include the conduction velocity, percentage change in amplitude, duration, and area of the evoked potential. A hard copy of all the information obtained can be printed or plotted directly on the patient's chart. Figure 13.4 shows a typical monitor display of the evoked potentials, with the soft cursors properly placed, following three stimulations.

SOFTWARE DIAGRAM

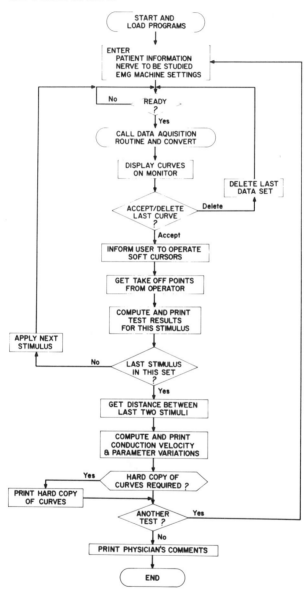

Figure 13.16. Software flow chart for evoked potential analysis.

Microcomputer Single Fiber EMG:
MC-EMG Configuration Example II

With muscle and nerve potentials picked up by standard needle and surface electrodes (see Chapter 14), the signal is band limited only to a few KHz. For acquisition and analysis of such signal, the method of digitizing the entire waveform and storing it in the computer is simple and cost effective. There are applications, however, when it is neither necessary nor desirable to capture the entire waveform into the computer. SFEMG (20) is typical of such an application of computers in EMG. This section describes the use of the microcomputer with any EMG instrument (of sufficient bandwidth) to permit large-sample, statistically significant SFEMG tests in almost real-time (5,6).

SFEMG (Chapter 10) is a neurophysiologic test used to determine the variability of impulse transmission across the neuromuscular junction. The information is recorded from special electrodes with a very fine area of sensitivity (on the order of 25 microns) placed between two muscle fibers belonging to the same motor unit. The features of interest for this test are the variability in the discharge of the individual muscle fibers (jitter) and the percentage of blocking of the action potentials (20).

When a single fiber electrode is properly positioned between two muscle fibers, the signal of the form shown in Figure 13.17 can be detected. Each sweep consists of a potential A_1 induced by one muscle fiber, followed by the potential B_1 induced by the second muscle fiber. The interval between these two potentials is the *interpotential interval* (IPI). The interval between successive discharges of the same fiber (potentials A_1 and A_2 in the diagram) is the *interdischarge interval* (IDI). For each motor unit under investigation, it is necessary to measure IPIs and IDIs in from 100 to 500 successive firings. These data are then used to calculate the MCD (the mean consecutive differences of the IPIs) and the MSD (the mean difference of the IPIs after being sorted according to increasing IDIs) to express jitter (6). Further, if any IDI is larger than a given value, it would indicate that one of the potentials is blocked. The percentage of such blocking is also calculated. This process must be repeated for 10–20 motor units and the results compared to normals for the given muscle. These computations, al-

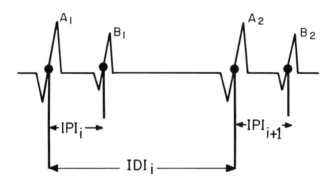

Figure 13.17. Representation of potentials detected by a single fiber EMG electrode.

though simple in nature, are tedious and lend themselves to computer application.

In SFEMG recording, the electromyographer is only interested in the time interval of IDIs and IPIs and not in the shape of the potentials. Therefore, it is not necessary to digitize the entire waveform. In addition, because the potentials are due to individual muscle fibers, they have very high frequency contents that would require very high sampling frequencies. This requires the use of prohibitively expensive A/D converters. Thus, instead of digitizing the potentials, it is more efficient to measure electronically the features of interest (IDIs and IPIs) in the interface and then transmit them to the computer as the input data.

Figure 13.18A shows the system developed by the author and used at the Ohio State University for SFEMG applications (4). Figure 13.18B is the block diagram of the interface. The analog signal from a standard EMG unit is fed into a dual time base oscilloscope. By properly setting the delay time and adjusting the two trigger levels on the oscilloscope, the electromyographer can have one time base be triggered by the first of the two potentials (from one muscle fiber) and the other time base triggered by the second potential (from the second fiber). With an oscilloscope, such as Tektronics 5111, it is not difficult to tap into the two trigger signals for input into the computer. In Figure 13.18B, these trigger signals are called START and STOP signals. The time interval between START and STOP signals is the IPI, and the interval between successive START pulses is the IDI. These time intervals are used to start and stop a pair of digital counters in the interface unit. The counters simply count the pulses of an on-board master clock that has a choice of periods of 0.1 or 1.0 microsec. These IDIs and IPIs are read into the computer directly as digital data under software control.

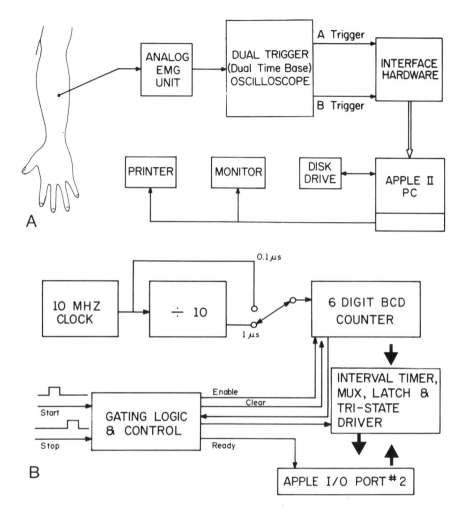

Figure 13.18. A system for SFEMG using a microcomputer: *A*, System configuration, *B*, Interface hardware.

The software developed for SFEMG jitter analysis has three parts. The main program is written in BASIC language, and two subroutines are written in 6502 assembly language. One of the assembly language subroutines is the I/O handler. It reads the data (IPIs and IDIs) that are stored in the counters, displays them on the CRT, and later stores them as data arrays in the memory. The second assembly language program is a high-speed sorting routine that sorts the arrays for the purpose of calculating MSDs when directed by the main program.

The main program is an interactive one and can be used without knowledge of any programming language. It permits the setting of a time window within which the IPIs are expected to lie. If the IPI is larger than the upper edge of this window, it is considered to be a blocking, and if it is smaller than the lower edge of this window, it is considered to be a mistrigger and is deleted. When an entry is deleted, the corresponding IDI is also deleted from the memory.

When sufficient data are collected, the system immediately prints the desired statistics, including the MCD, MSD, SD, the variance, and the percentage of blocking. Before moving on to the next motor unit, it also permits the user to delete or modify the results if any unusual values are detected.

After recording and analyzing the samples from each of the desired number of motor units (different positions of the needle), the system outputs the summary statistics for the entire test. It then compares the values with those from normal subjects for the given muscle. It can also print or plot the histogram of the entire test results.

Other Microcomputer-Based Systems

At the time of this writing, commercial microcomputer-based EMG systems of the structure discussed in this section are emerging on the market. An example of such a product is the Neuro Diagnostics machine called "Multi" (12). This system is based on an IBM PC/XT-compatible microcomputer. The built-in A/D interface allows sampling of EMG signals at the rate of up to 50 KHz. This instrument can be directly connected to an IBM PC keyboard, printer, hard disk, and other compatible I/O devices. This system offers many computerized EMG routines, many of which are still under development. Additionally, it can be utilized for word processing, spread sheets, accounting, telecommunication, data base operations, and other data processing applications associated with general-purpose digital computers. One of the interesting components of this machine is a high-resolution vector graphics monitor for display of both direct and stored EMG signals. This reduces the display limitations in interpreting EMG results from the monitor (see the next section). By the early 1990s many such systems, based on different microcomputers but following the basic structure discussed in this section, should be available.

ERRORS AND LIMITATIONS

Computers are versatile clinical and research tools that have enabled the electromyographer to perform a number of tests that would otherwise be very tedious to do. In order to take full advantage of this technology, the electromyographer must be familiar with the limitations and sources of error in the system. Although the noise and interference do not affect the *digital* signals, there are other inherent sources of error that limit the accuracy of computerized EMG results.

In converting analog signals to digital, two types of error are introduced: sampling error and quantization error. These errors are inherent to the digital process and are, unlike noise, independent of the quality of the components utilized. Because these errors may go unnoticed by the uninitiated user, they may lead to misinterpretation of EMG exam results. The rule of thumb in using any signal processing system (analog, digital, etc.) is that one should not interpret the final results to an accuracy more precise than is possible with the system.

Sampling error can generally be avoided when the sampling frequency is several times (at least twice) higher than the maximum frequency content of the signal. The high frequency limit on the original analog signal therefore should be set several times lower than the sampling frequency. A slow sampling rate not only prevents the rapid transitions or details of the signal from being seen on the screen but it also distorts the low frequency component of the converted signal by a phenomenon known as aliasing (15).

Quantization error is defined as the difference between the value of the actual analog signal and its digitized equivalent. It brings about much the same sort of effect as a source of noise in an analog system (14). This error is a function of the magnitude of the signal and the quantization step size. The higher the number of quantization levels, the smaller is this kind of error. The number of quantization levels N or equivalently the word length n (see equation above) of the digitized signal determines the maximum resolution that the system possesses. Therefore, any attempt to interpret the processed result with a higher accuracy than one part in N leads to misinterpretation.

In general, the system error poses no problem if the existence of such error and the reason behind it is acknowledged when interpreting the results. The problem only arises if one attempts to interpret the results to a higher accuracy than the system is capable of offering. For example, if the digitized data accuracy is limited to only 8 bits, then any attempt to read the resultant waveform on the CRT screen to an accuracy greater than one part in 256 is meaningless. This would be similar to setting improper filter limits on a standard EMG instrument and then expecting to read off-band frequency information from a waveform seen on the CRT screen.

Another source of misinterpretation in computerized EMG is the display resolution. Many of the TV monitors used for displaying computer (graphic) results have resolution that is even lower than the inherent system capability. In such cases the output accuracy is, of course, limited by the display system. One should not attempt to interpret the results to a higher accuracy by reading between the lines. As an example, Figure 13.4 shows the display of three EMG motor potentials on a TV monitor. In this example, the data were sampled at 40 KHz, and 1000 samples were collected for each of the potentials. Time was measured to a precision of 1 in 1000th of the sweep time (25 millisec), and the amplitude measurements were made to an accuracy of 1 part in 256. The resolution of the display, however, was limited to 256 points in the horizontal direction and 160 points in the vertical direction. In order to accommodate the entire waveform on the display, the system was programmed to display every fourth sample in the horizontal direction. Vertical direction was also scaled in a similar fashion. Reading the information and determining the take-off and end points of the potentials from the TV monitor were thus limited to this lower accuracy, whereas the internal computations are more accurate. In order to be able to read the more accurate information, one could use the numerical values, rather than the graphic results.

In general, the overall accuracy of any processing system (the total system includes the human user also) is limited by that of the weakest link through which the signal passes. This point should be the guide in using computerized EMG. The limitations may be due to any of the following sources: the analog front end, the output device (display, plotter etc.), the interface, the digital electronics, etc. In any case, if the limitations of the components are known, then reliable information can be extracted only within these limitations.

Acknowledgment. The author would like to thank Said H. Koozekanani, Ph.D., Mario T. Balmaseda, Jr., M.D., and Barbara J. Eason, Ph.D. for their assistance in preparing this manuscript.

References

1. Analog Devices: *Data-Acquisition Data Book 1982*. Norwood, MA, Analog Devices Inc, 1982.
2. Apple Computer, Inc. *Apple II Reference Manual*. Cupertino, CA, Apple, 1981.
3. Cadwell Laboratories, Inc: *The Cadwell 5200A Operator's Manual*. Kennewick, WA, Cadwell Lab, 1983.
4. Cooper J W: *The Minicomputer in the Laboratory: With Examples Using the PDP-11*. New York, John Wiley & Sons, 1977.
5. Fatehi MT, Wiechers DO, Johnson EW, Koozekanani SH: Home Computer as an on-line single fiber EMG jitter analyzer. Proceedings of the 34th ACEMB, Houston, September, 1981.
6. Fatehi MT, Wiechers DO, Johnson EW, Koozekanani SH: A real-time large-sample single fiber electromyographic jitter analyzer using an inexpensive microcomputer. In Campbell RM (ed): *Control Aspects of Prosthetics and Orthotics*. New York, Pergamon Press, 1983, pp 125–127.
7. Hamacher VC, Varanesic ZG, Zaky SG: *Computer Organization*, ed 2. New York, McGraw-Hill, 1984.

8. Hoeschele DF: *Analog-to-Digital, Digital-to-Analog Conversion Technique.* New York, John Wiley & Sons, 1968.

9. Intel Corporation: *Memory Components Handbook.* Santa Clara, CA, Intel Corp, 1983.

10. Johnson EW, Fatehi MT, Balmaseda Jr MT, Mysiw MJ: *Primary EMG.* American Academy of Physical Medical and Rehabilitation, Los Angeles, November, 1983.

11. Motorola, Inc: *Motorola Memory Manual.* Austin, TX, Motorola Semiconductors Inc, 1982.

12. Neuro Diagnostics, Inc: *The Multi, Preliminary Information Sheet,* Santa Ana, CA, Neuro Diagnostics, 1985.

13. Scanlon LJ: *6502 Software Design.* Indianapolis, Howard W. Sams & Co, 1980.

14. Schmid H: *Electronic Analog/Digital Conversions.* New York, VanNostrand and Reinhold Co, 1970.

15. Shannon C: The philosophy of pulse code modulation, *Proc IRE,* November, 1948, pp 1328-1331.

16. Sheingold DH (ed.): *Analog-Digital Conversion Handbook.* Norwood, MA, Analog Devices, Inc, 1972.

17. Soucek B: *Microprocessors and Microcomputers.* New York, John Wiley, 1976.

18. Stalberg E, Lars A: Computer-aided EMG analysis. *Prog Clin Neurophysiol,* Vol. 10, J.E. Desmedt, ed., pp. 187-233, Basel, S Karger, 1983.

19. Stalberg E, Stalberg S: *Short Description of Programs for Analysis of Muscle and Nerve Signals.* Uppsala, Sweden, Swedish Electrophysiologic Software, 1982.

20. Stalberg E, Trontelj J: *Single Fiber Electromyography.* Surrey, UK, The Mirvalle Press, 1979.

21. TECA Corporation: *TD 10/10A and TD 20/20A EMG Operating Notes.* Pleasantville, NY, TECA Corp, 1983.

22. TECA Corporation: *Computing and You.* Unpublished monograph, Pleasantville, NY, 1984.

23. Wiechers DO, Fatehi MT: Real-time nerve conduction analysis using an inexpensive computer for clinical EMG examination. 29th Annual Meeting of the AAEE, St. Paul, MN, October 8-9, 1982.

14

Instrumentation

STUART REINER*
JOSEPH B. ROGOFF

EMG examinations record the electrical activity of voluntary muscles and motor and sensory nerves at rest, during volitional activity, and while subjected to electrical and mechanical stimuli. EMG potentials are recorded with metal needle and skin surface electrodes. Similar electrodes are also used to apply the electrical stimuli used. These techniques impose different performance requirements on the EMG system.

The wide anatomic range of structures dealt with in clinical EMG, coupled with the broad spectrum of clinical objectives, preclude rote methods in most of the procedures. EMG examinations are not laboratory tests, but rather are an extension of the clinical examination.

The electrical potentials recorded range from fractions of microvolts (μV, 10^6V, millionths of a volt) when recording action potentials of some of the sensory nerves to about 50 millivolts (mV, 10^{-3}V, thousandths of a volt) encountered in some muscle action potential recording. Time resolution in the order of tens or hundreds micro-seconds (sec, millionths of a second) is required when recording fibrillation potentials and in single fiber EMG (SFEMG), whereas epochs as long as seconds are studied in the evaluation of interference patterns associated with strong muscle contraction.

In addition, electrical stimulation is required for many important evaluations performed by the electromyographer. The apparatus used in modern EMG must, therefore, be adjustable over a wide range of sensitivity and time scales and be capable of a number of modes of operation. Because the electromyographer must use this equipment to

---

*Both authors are deceased, but were very prominent in EMG. This chapter is reprinted from the first edition without change.

carry out these objectives, this chapter describes in simple terms the technical features involved, particularly those that can significantly affect the results obtained, so that the equipment can be used with confidence and facility and with appreciation of its limitations. The advent of the commercially designed EMG systems has freed the electromyographer from the many technical details of instrumentation and the problems of interconnection of a number of separate pieces of apparatus.

A background in basic electricity and in simple direct and alternating current circuits facilitates the understanding of the electrophysiologic concepts in practical EMG and the discussion of instrumentation that follows. The reader is referred to the references at the end of this chapter for this material (1-6). These concepts have great generality, but this chapter emphasizes in practical terms those ideas that specifically relate to EMG instrumentation, its use, and its limitations.

EMGs range from one-channel instruments that incorporate the necessary facilities for performing the basic clinical tests to equipment permitting simultaneous recording of two or more channels of EMG and the electrical activity concurrent with force, displacement, acceleration, etc., and the output of electronic analyzers.

Special-purpose limited performance EMG equipment is available and is designed to respond primarily to gross myoelectric activity; it finds application in muscle re-education and in biofeedback. Similarly, multichannel systems have been built to record the presence or absence of EMG activity simultaneously in many muscles for studies in kinesiology. This equipment is not used in diagnostic EMG nor in the measurement of nerve conduction velocity because it does not have the sensitivity, dynamic response, and measurement facility necessary.

THE BASIC EMG SYSTEM

The functional elements that comprise a basic single-channel EMG system are shown in Figure 14.1. These blocks, electrodes, preamplifier, amplifier, cathode ray tube display, and stimulator represent functional components and are not necessarily actual interconnections of unique electronic circuits or devices. In practice, the EMG is a unique system designed as a whole, with considerable interrelation among circuit functions and with a number of common power supply and control circuits (27).

Electrodes

The choice of recording electrodes, their location relative to the anatomic structures being studied, and their state of cleanliness and repair have the major effect on the observed potentials. The electrodes are the critical link in the EMG system. They convert the varying ion currents moving within the body in response to the nerve and muscle activity to varying electrical currents in wires that are connected to the amplifier. The electrical interface between the metal recording electrodes and the body tissues and fluid is complex and variable and strongly affects the nature of the tiny recorded potentials.

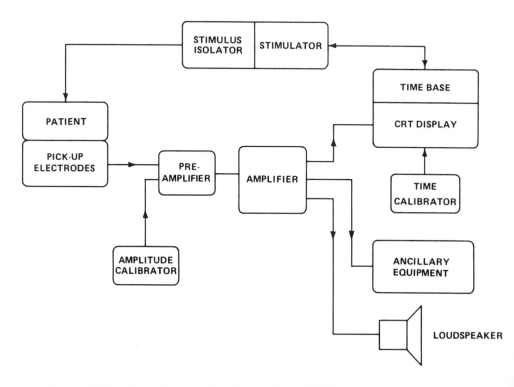

Figure 14.1. Block diagram of a single channel EMG.

This electrical contact at the interface is a poor one, particularly in small area needle electrodes. It is at this point of tenuous electrical contact that the ubiquitous technical problem of EMG appears; namely, the recording of microvolt potentials at an imperfect electrical contact (the needle tip) in the presence of often large electrical interference. These are induced into the patient from surrounding electrical influences, e.g., electric power wiring, lighting and appliances, unwanted potentials originating from bioelectric sources within the patient, and the direct effect of electrical stimulation applied to the patient. These external electrical interference problems are usually resolved satisfactorily by properly connecting the apparatus to a good electrical ground (usually accomplished by a grounding connection in the power cable); applying a ground or a zero potential electrode to the patient; observing some simple electrical environment precautions, which include disconnecting nearby electrical appliances or removing them and their power cables from proximity to the patients; by good electrode technique; and by the design of the EMG preamplifier to which the electrodes are connected.

Preamplifier

The preamplifier increases the magnitude and the power of the potentials picked up by the electrodes so that they can be conducted to the amplifier without being influenced by unwanted electrical effects that would cause distortion and error or would add spurious potentials. The potentials are further amplified and manipulated by the amplifier until they are of sufficient voltage and power to be applied to the cathode ray display system, loudspeaker, and other devices used to display, monitor, record, and further process the EMG signal.

The preamplifier must be electrically compatible with the electrodes used and must process the smallest biologic potentials encountered in the EMG system. It therefore must meet stringent requirements. It is often located in a remote box connected to the main EMG system by a cable. This arrangement permits the preamplifier to be placed close to the electrodes to which it is directly connected by relatively short cables in order to minimize interference.

The three primary factors that electrically characterize the preamplifier are (a) internal noise level, (b) input impedance, and (c) differential amplification. These characteristics essentially determine the performance of the EMG System.

Noise

Briefly, all electrical circuits containing resistors and amplifiers generate thermal and amplifier internal "noise," i.e., unwanted electrical signals. The term "noise" is not used only in its accoustical sense; any interfering unwanted influence may be termed noise. Internal noise originates from sources within the system. Other sources of noise are external to the instrument system. These external sources, also termed interference or artifact, include unwanted bioelectric potentials and such electrical sources as power wiring in the building, the major source of interference requiring care in equipment and patient grounding. Broadcast transmitters and other radio frequency generators also are the source of interference.

Internal equipment noise extends over a wide spectrum of frequencies and is due mainly to random electrode and amplifier fluctuations. These noise potentials usually can be ignored in most electrical signal transmission systems when they are very small with respect to the signal amplitudes encountered. When dealing with electrical potentials in the low microvolt range and when maximum amplification is required, the noise potentials are amplified along with the desired potentials and contaminate the resulting records. This internal noise appears as random irregular fluctuations in the baseline, fuzzy thickening of the trace, and hissing and rumbling over the loudspeaker. Care in the design of the preamplifier minimizes such degrading effects on the EMG potentials. (When recording small evoked nerve potentials [neurograms] less than a few microvolts in amplitude, ancillary signal averaging devices are used to process potentials after amplification, so as to minimize further the effects of random noise potentials on the desired response waves.) When the EMG potentials leave the preamplifier and pass on to the main amplifier, they are of sufficient amplitude and power level so they are not influenced further by external or internal electrical noise potentials in subsequent properly designed amplifiers and other system elements. The preamplifier therefore essentially determines the internal noise of the system.

Input Impedance

The input impedance of the preamplifier must be designed to be compatible with the electrical properties of the metal-electrolyte interface of the electrodes used in EMG. *Input impedance* describes the resistance and capacitance of the input circuit of the preamplifier to which the electrodes are connected and has a major influence on the effectiveness of the electrodes in conveying information from the patient to the amplifier.

The term "impedance" refers to (a) the resistance that represents the energy dissipated by electrons as they move through the atomic structure of a conductor, (b) the capacitance that measures the energy stored in the electric field that surrounds a conductor, (c) the inductance that measures the energy stored in the magnetic field set up by an electric current, and (d) the effect of these three parameters on electrical potentials and currents in circuits. Impedance is an inevitable property of all electric circuits. When dealing with direct current (DC) circuits having no fluctuations, impedance effects simplify to resistance only, and capacitance and inductance do not mediate the current flow. The resistance only determines the hindrance to current flow. Its effect is described by Ohms law, $E = IR$ or $I = E/R$, where E is voltage (or potential), I is current flow, and R is resistance. The higher the resistance, the smaller is the current flow.

When dealing with fluctuating and alternating voltage and currents (AC), such as EMG signals, circuit impedance, which includes capacitance and inductance, as well as resistance, must be handled. Determining the hindrance on current flow of capacitance and inductance is more complex because the effect of these parameters depends upon the rate of change of voltage and current, not upon their magnitude, as does resistance. The total impedance effect of all three parameters on current flow is somewhat similar to the Ohms law effect of resistance in direct current circuits; namely, current flow in an AC circuit is equal to applied voltage divided by impedance, $I = E/Z$ where Z is impedance.

Impedance may be stated in ohms only when it is calculated for an applied sine wave voltage at a particular frequency. Impedance is therefore stated with more generality by specifying its resistance, capacitance, and inductance. This permits its effects to be calculated for an applied voltage at any frequency and for any waveform.

Resistance and capacitance effects predominate in the electrode-preamplifier input impedance circuit; inductive effects are insignificant and can be ignored. The input impedance of the preamplifer appears as a shunting effect at its input terminals. This impedance must therefore be high so as to receive the potentials from the small needle electrode, which themselves are characterized by a series impedance, with minimum loss of amplitude and minimum distortion. (Ideally, the electrodes would have zero impedance, and the input impedance of the preamplifier would be infinitely high.) High input impedance additionally enhances preamplifier performance for reasons to be discussed later. High impedance is characterized by high resistance and small capacitance.

Differential Amplification

The third special characteristic of the preamplifier is its differential amplification property. This permits selective amplification of potentials originating while discriminating against interference, i.e., unwanted potentials originating at a distance and presenting at both electrodes. The interfering potentials are rejected by the mechanism of the differential amplifier to the extent that the interference equally influences the two recording electrodes (the exploring and reference electrodes). The differential amplifier therefore permits substantially interference-free recording of small potentials picked up by the recording electrodes while these electrodes are being influenced by often larger interference potentials from external sources, so long as the interference has a mostly equal effect on the recording electrodes. Interference that does not impinge equally on both electrodes is not rejected. Note that the exploring and reference electrodes should ideally be of similar dimension.

The differential preamplifier has three terminals: two recording electrode terminals, an exploring (or active) electrode terminal and a reference electrode terminal; and a third ground, zero potential, shield or guard electrode. The recording electrodes are placed as close as possible to the structures whose electrical activity is being studied (the exploring electrode being closer when feasible), and the ground electrode is placed on the body surface at some distance over an area of little electrical activity.

Amplitude Calibration

The amplitude calibrator is a source of electrical potential of known amplitude that can be selectively switched to the input terminal of the preamplifier to provide a test signal to verify the performance of the EMG system. The calibration voltage is specifically arranged to be applied at the electrode-input terminals to ensure that it is influenced by all parts of the EMG system. Amplitude calibration voltages of 10 μV, 100 μV and sometimes more are usually provided. The wave shape of the calibration voltage is usually rectangular so as to provide additional information about the dynamic response of the EMG system, which can be obtained by observing the shape of these waves after passing through the system.

Amplifier

The amplifier that follows the preamplifier usually contains the sensitivity control calibrated in units of microvolts per unit vertical deflection of the trace on the cathode ray display screen. This permits the operator to select a sensitivity that will be in accordance with the expected EMG potential amplitudes.

Frequency Response—Filter Controls

In order to accommodate most effectively the slow waves of some tests and the rapid waves of others and to minimize noise obvious in some test conditions and baseline wander encountered in others, a mean for adjusting EMG dynamic performance is provided to optimize results for various tests. These controls usually associated with the amplifier are termed, variously, high and low frequency limit controls, frequency response controls, filter controls, or time constant controls. They limit the response of the system to the most rapid potential fluctuations, on one hand, and to the slowest fluctuations, on the other, so as to enhance the shape of the desired potentials by eliminating unwanted rapid or slow fluctuations in the recorded waveform. A number of different settings of the high and low frequency filter controls may be selected depending on the special requirements of needle EMG, motor nerve conduction tests, electroneurography, and other tests. The function of these filter controls is analogous to the base and treble controls of a music reproduction system

The output of the EMG amplifier is a filtered representation of the potentials picked up by the electrodes adjusted so that they are of suitable amplitude and of sufficient power level to drive the various display devices and to provide the output to drive ancillary equipment that might be used to process the EMG signals further.

Cathode Ray Tube Display

The cathode ray tube (CRT) display permits visualization of the transient action potentials by presenting them as dynamic amplitude versus time graphs on the fluorescent screen of the cathode ray tube. The patterns on the screen are drawn by an inertia-less beam of electrons, which result in a spot of light when they impinge on the phosphor-coated screen. The traces are formed by uniform motion of the beam from left to right on the screen (X axis) generated by the time base, or sweep, circuits while simultaneously being deflected up and down (Y axis) in response to the output potentials of the EMG amplifier. When the motion is sufficiently rapid, the observer sees continuous curves. Uninterrupted monitoring is achieved by repetition of this action. The amplifier sensitivity control selects the vertical scale of the display, and the time base control or sweep control selects the horizontal scale of the display.

Time Base—Time Calibration

Accuracy of time measurements made on the screen of the CRT depends on the accuracy of the time base circuits that control the uniform left-to-right movement of the beam on the CRT. Time calibration means that independence of the time base circuits is required. This is usually an independent signal of accurately known timing that can be displayed on the screen to verify the X-axis calibration by comparing the timing of the calibration signal wave with the settings of the time base controls.

Stimulator

The stimulator applies electrical pulses to the patient to elicit muscle and nerve action potentials in motor and sensory nerve conduction tests. A principal objective of these tests is to measure the elapsed time or latency between the application of the stimulus and the appearance of evoked action potentials under nearby recording electrodes. The sweep generator is arranged to start or trigger the left-to-right excursion of the beam on the CRT screen only when a stimulus is applied. This stimulus-triggered sweep has the effect of making both the stimulus and response waves appear at the same points on the screen every time a stimulus is applied. This results in superimposed response waves on the screen, which greatly facilitates recognition and measurement.

The stimulus, which can be a brief shock, 150 V or more in amplitude, is applied to the patient, in some cases a few centimeters away from recording electrodes. These electrodes are connected to the preamplifier, which is arranged to record a few microvolts. This situation would normally cause overwhelming stimulus artifact currents to be conducted directly into the preamplifier via the patient and common EMG power supply circuits. This in turn would result in electrical overload of the preamplifier and render it inoperative during the time it is required to record the evoked action potentials. This overwhelming stimulus artifact is eliminated or reduced to acceptable proportions by providing the stimulator with electrically isolated stimulus output circuits. These stimulus-isolation circuits render the output portion of the stimulator that makes contact with the patient free of any electrical connection to any of the circuits that are in common with the remainder of the EMG system.

Loudspeaker

Although obviously no sound is associated with the action potentials of EMG, the potentials recorded do produce audible sounds when applied to a loudspeaker because EMG potentials have components that fall within the audible spectrum. Audio monitoring has been a valuable adjunct since the earliest days of clinical EMG because many changes in the MUAPs and their firing patterns produce characteristic alternatives in the sounds they generate, often before changes are obvious in the visual patterns on the CRT screen.

Ancillary Equipment

Because the events that appear on the face of the CRT are brief and transient, all but the simplest EMG instruments are equipped with some means of retaining the graphic images that appear on the face of the CRT. This permits visualization, analysis, and measurement, an increasingly important part of modern EMG. This capacity can be achieved simply by adding an instant photography camera arranged to frame and focus properly on the CRT screen. It is used with the shutter open and the CRT in the triggered sweep mode or with the sweep start synchronized with operation of the shutter to ensure that only one sweep is recorded.

More facility is achieved by providing a storage display facility that instantly and electronically retains a trace (or a number of traces) on a CRT screen for analysis and more leisurely photography. It is then erased or updated with new information. Most flexibility and graphic records are achieved by special high-speed graphic recorders that not only permit rapid visualization of the trace but also provide continuous sequences of traces, allowing many potentials to be seen and in context as well.

A number of additional ancillary devices have become associated with the basic EMG equipment to aid in interpretation and analysis. These include magnetic tape recorders that record and play back the potentials observed on screen. Various special-purpose computers handle the EMG activity to extract potentials hidden in noise, modify the form of the data to enhance certain characteristics (integrators, action potential counters, etc.), or statistically display various parameters of the action potentials (a wide range of so-called EMG analyzers). See Chapter 13.

EMG ELECTRODES

The potential changes recorded in EMG originate as the moving depolarization-repolarization waves along muscle and nerve cell membranes, termed *action potentials.* The ion movement that constitutes this activity (which differs somewhat in muscles and nerves) is an electric current in the extracellular fluid and gives rise to the transient (approximately 110 millivolt) change in transmembrane potential. It lasts less than 1 msec and can be recorded with tiny intracellular electrodes, a process with little application in the clinical laboratory due to the fragile nature of the electrodes and the meticulous electrode fixation required.

Instead, recordings are made with large (with respect to muscle and nerve fiber size) metal needle electrodes that record a measure of the activity of many fibers (motor unit) and at a distance, except where extracellular recordings from single fibers are made in SFEMG. The moving action potentials spread within the extracellular fluid, a good electrolytic conductor, in three dimensions, a process termed *volume conduction.* The resultant MUAPs recorded from the clinical needle electrode are more than ten times smaller and three to five times longer in duration than the intracellular single fiber action potentials. This is due to the larger surface area of the clinical needle electrode, which averages the activity from all the tissues it contacts; the attenuating effect of volume conduction, which reduces the voltage at least as the inverse square of the distance; the asynchronous arrival at the recording electrode of the individual action potentials; and the electrical properties of the metal-electrolyte interface at the tip of the needle. When surface electrodes are used, the increased distance from the origin of the action potentials; the wide range of potentials that influence the electrode that are then integrated by it; and the complicating effect of the various tissue components, such as skin, fat, muscle, connective tissue and blood vessels, all of which further attenuate the amplitude of the recorded potentials, slow their rapidly changing components and increase their apparent duration. Surface electrodes are therefore not useful in recording details of motor unit activity and are relegated to recording gross EMG activity and compound nerve and muscle potentials resulting from nerve stimulation. Surface electrodes are used as ground and reference electrodes.

Electrical Properties of Metal Electrodes

The transmission of action potential waves across the metal-electrolyte interface that exists at the active surface of the recording electrodes where it contacts body tissues and fluids depends on combination of ions in the extracellular fluids with the electrode and discharge of ions from the electrode into solution. This complex electrochemical process can be described in simplified form as resulting in the formation of a charge gradient at the electrode surface. This can be visualized as two parallel layers of charge of opposite polarity. Its electrical equivalent resembles a resistance, a capacitance, and a battery. The value of these elements is variable and unstable and depends upon the kind of metal, the electrolyte and its concentration, and the nature of the electric current being passed through the interface, among other factors (17).

The resistance and capacitance portion of the interface, which is in a circuit that is completed by the input impedance of the preamplifier, causes reduction in the amplitude and distortion in the slow portion of the recorded action potentials, respectively, especially when small area needle electrodes are used. These effects are minimized by high input impedance preamplifiers.

Electrode offset potential (or polarization voltage), the voltage generated at the interface, may be in the order of 600 millivolts. This is usually not of any consequence because EMG equipment is designed to ignore fixed resting potentials because they are not components of the clinically recorded waves. However, these potentials are large and unstable, and when electrodes move, large abrupt changes in polarization voltage occur. This is a major source of artifact in EMG, because these transient *changes* in potential are amplified and appear as spike waves or discontinuities in the baseline.

Surface Electrodes

A remarkably wide range of skin surface electrodes have been used to perform clinically useful EMG. The electrodes establish the ground (or zero reference potential) connection to the patient required to reduce externally induced electrical artifact, as well as stimulus artifact. Surface electrodes are used for stimulation of peripheral nerves, for recording CMAPs in motor nerve conduction tests, for recording compound nerve action potentials, and as reference electrodes with monopolar needle electrodes. They are not used for studies of motor unit potentials.

The skin surface should be cleaned to remove perspiration, which is electrically conductive, from the general area of recording or stimulation. When stimulating, this reduces the possibility of conducting a portion of the large stimulating voltage to the nearby recording electrodes. During recording, this cleansing aids in reducing the area of recording and avoids reduction of action potential amplitudes by shunting effects. When recording low amplitude potentials, improved results can often be achieved by lightly abrading the skin under the electrodes to remove some of the high resistance superficial skin layers.

Bare metal electrode contact is made to the skin via electrically conductive electrode paste that reduces contact resistance, improves recording, and permits stimulation with less stimulus intensity, thus improving patient tolerance and reducing artifact. Excessive electrode paste on the skin surfaces should be avoided for the reasons mentioned above.

Surface electrodes may be discs, or rectangular or strip forms, of various sizes, with larger sizes used as ground electrodes. These electrodes, sometimes mounted as a pair on an insulating holder, are held in place with adhesive tape, straps, or with double-faced adhesive tape die cut in a ring shape ("adhesive collars"). Small noose-shaped electrodes, which are made of short lengths of coiled metal wire spring for flexibility, and are designed to be slipped over the fingers or toes and then drawn tight, can be used for stimulation and recording. Finger electrodes made of short lengths of curved metal strips attached to each of the jaws of a common spring-loaded "alligator" electrical clip are also used for recording or stimulation. Dual-prong metal electrodes mounted in a plastic handle are used for stimulation; the stimulus intensity control may be located, as a convenience, in the handle (Fig. 14.2).

When mechanical movement occurs during a test, artifact is gener-

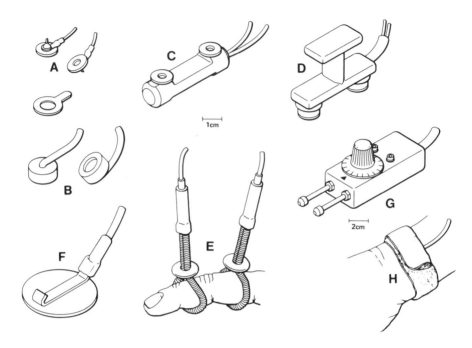

Figure 14.2. Some surface electrodes. *A,* Metal discs, shown with double-faced adhesive collar sometimes used for attachment to skin. *B,* Metal discs with insulating collar uses electrode paste for contact to skin. *C,* Dual electrode for direct contact. *D,* Dual electrode utilizing saline-saturated felt contacts. *E,* Spring ring electrode, moveable collar tightens noose. *F,* Typical metal disc ground electrode. *G,* Bipolar stimulating electrode with intensity control. *H,* Wrap-around saline-saturated, fabric-covered flexible metal electrode.

ated due to transient changes in the recording electrode metal-electrolyte interface. To minimize this effect, surface electrodes have been devised that remove the metal-electrolyte interface that is close to the metal surface from proximity to the skin surface. Contact between the metal and the skin is made solely via electrode paste that fills an insulating collar in the electrode (recessed electrodes) or by saline-saturated felt plugs that project from cup-shaped electrodes. Most movement, presumably, will then occur between the electrolyte and the skin surface, with minimum mechanical effect on the metal-electrolyte interface that is close to the metal surface (8).

A variant of this type of electrode utilizes metal discs with a domed impression in the center to retain electrode paste. These electrodes are applied to the skin by means of double-sided adhesive tape rings without electrode paste, which would interfere with adhesion; the paste is then added after the electrodes are firmly in place, by means of a hypodermic syringe with a blunted needle via a hole in the domed center of the disc.

Metal electrodes covered with fabric or felt that must be soaked in saline before use are also used as ground and stimulating electrodes. A thin metal strip is stitched between two strips of Velcro and wrapped around the extremity being tested; it functions as a self-retaining ground electrode. A miniature version is used for stimulation of the fingers or toes. Stimulating electrodes comprising pairs of metal cups containing felt plugs that contact the skin are also used after soaking in saline. The metal used in these electrodes include silver, stainless steel, lead, tin, nickel, and German silver (alloy of nickel, copper, and zinc, also termed nickel silver).

Needle Electrodes

Needle electrodes are used when activity of individual motor units or muscle fibers is studied because they permit a relatively small exploring surface that discriminates against distant activity to be placed near the active tissue. Needle electrodes are also used for nerve stimulation, allowing the use of smaller stimulus intensity than is required for surface stimulation; a larger tip area than used for recording should be considered for such needle electrodes to minimize high current density at the active surface (Fig. 14.3).

The monopolar electrode used by Jasper and Ballem in 1949 (16) is the simplest needle electrode. In current use it is a stainless steel needle properly tempered for strength and point stability, yet not brittle, approximately 0.4 mm in diameter coated with an insulating film of Teflon except at the very tip. Although stainless steel is a poor electrode material, especially when used as a small area contact, it is almost universally used for monopolar needle electrodes because of its mechanical properties. A surface, bare subdermal needle or another monopolar needle reference electrode must be used, located near the monopolar recording electrode.

Advantages include simple, relatively inexpensive construction and more uniform recorded potentials due to the symmetrical nondirectional pickup pattern. Also, insertion and movement are well tolerated by the patient because of the small diameter and anti-friction properties of the Teflon coating. Disadvantages include the difficulty of standardizing the tip area. The exposed area increases with use because of the poor mechanical properties of the Teflon coating. The fragile coating is also easily susceptible to damage along the length of a needle and cannot be repaired. Also, a reference electrode in addition to a ground electrode is required. Tip area of 0.14 to 0.20 mm^2 is typical, but may vary widely with manufacturer and will increase with

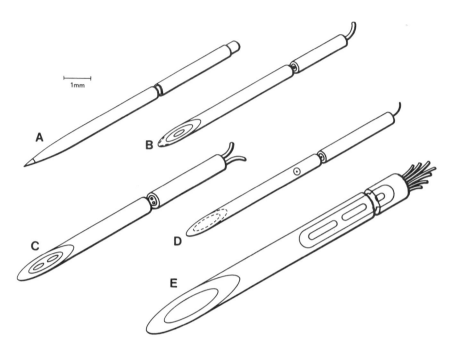

Figure 14.3. Needle electrodes. *A,* Monopolar needle electrode. *B,* Concentric needle electrodes; *dashed lines* show alternate point shape. *C,* Bipolar needle electrode. *D,* Single fiber needle electrode. *E,* Multielectrode.

use, causing reduction in amplitudes and, to some extent, in the sharpness of the recorded potentials.

Concentric needle electrodes described by Adrian and Bronk in 1929 (1) are comprised of a stainless steel hypodermic needle with an insulated wire (platinum, nichrome, or silver) within the lumen. The active electrode area is the bare surface of the wire where it emerges at the 15°, typical bevel at the tip of the needle. The bare stainless steel cannula is the reference electrode. A separate ground electrode is required. Tubing diameters typically range from 23 to 28 hypodermic gauge. The exposed surface area of the active inner conductor ranges from 0.015 to 0.07 mm².

The advantages of the concentric electrode include the easily standardized exposed surface of the active electrode that remains constant with use. For this reason, the concentric (or coaxial) electrode has been used for many years in quantitative EMG studies, i.e., amplitude and duration measurement of motor unit potentials. No reference electrode is required. This electrode is not easily subject to damage, and the tip can be resharpened. (Somewhat restricted pickup area and directional properties may be of use when searching.) Disadvantages include the directional property of the bevel and less patient comfort than with the monopolar needle. Recent studies suggest positive waves may be more easily provoked with the monopolar needle.

The bipolar needle electrode is similar to the concentric electrode, except that two insulated wires are placed within the cannula. Here the active areas (or the "active" and the "reference" electrodes) are the exposed surfaces of these wires at the bevel at the tip of the needle. This electrode has no polarity sense because both exposed recording surfaces are equal in area and symmetrical. Neither can really be termed exploring or reference.

The outer surface of the cannula is the ground or zero potential electrode connection to the patient. The connecting cable to this electrode is identified by its three terminals, the two active recording terminals and the ground terminal.

Advantages are that the recording range is most restricted and somewhat directional, and isolated motor unit activity can sometimes be seen during strong contraction. Electrical symmetry of the recording surfaces makes this electrode least susceptible to the electrical artifact because it permits the differential amplifier properties of the EMG to be most effective. No additional patient electrodes are required; all three required contacts are self-contained. The major disadvantage is that the recording range is too restricted for routine EMG. Recorded potentials appear smaller (due to close spacing of the recording surfaces) and of shorter duration than those recorded with other needle electrodes. Tubing diameters used in the construction of this electrode must of necessity be somewhat larger than with other electrodes.

Many electromyographers do not consider a single type of electrode to be ideal for all of their work and use monopolar and concentric electrodes, taking advantage of each to achieve their desired objectives (20). When quantitative EMG studies are reported, the materials and dimensions of the needle tip should be noted, because these parameters can significantly affect the results.

Other more special-purpose needle electrodes include the needle multielectrode, which is constructed of hypodermic tubing approximately 1 mm in diameter with a number of recording surfaces brought out flush with the tubing surface through an opening along the length of the needle. Fourteen such surfaces are typically used (4). The known spacing between the recording surfaces makes it possible to use this electrode to determine motor unit territory by recording the electrical activity of the same motor unit from the various recording surfaces.

Flexible wire electrodes are useful in kinesiologic studies and in other studies where rigid needle electrodes would interfere in the relative sliding motion of overlaying muscles. These electrodes consist of fine insulated wires that are inserted singly or in pairs by first threading them through a hypodermic needle, hooking the exposed end of the wires around the tip of the needle, and then leaving the wires in place within the muscle by withdrawing the hypodermic needle after properly localizing the wire ends within the muscle (3). Other techniques do not thread the wire through the needle, but merely hook the ends of the wire that are outside the needle around the tip of the needle a short distance into the lumen. It is then inserted into the muscle, drawing the wire within the muscle along the outside of the needle, which is then withdrawn leaving the wire in place.

A variant of the concentric needle electrode is used to study the activity of single muscle fibers of the motor unit (SFEMG). This electrode utilizes a (one or more) small area, 25-μ diameter recording surface that is brought out to the surface of the needle via a small hole drilled through the wall of the hypodermic tubing a short distance from the tip (15, 16). The recording surface, which is small relative to the average muscle fiber diameter, is flush with the outer smooth surface of the tubing wall, permitting recording from uninjured single muscle fibers. Its restricted pickup area and very directional properties permit this electrode to pick up single fiber action potentials from uninjured fibers when sufficient care and patience are utilized in localizing the electrode. Similar designs have also been described utilizing a number of recording surfaces brought out through the side wall of the needle, extending the scope of single fiber recording. When recording from these small areas, high impedance electrodes require high impedance amplifiers (in the order of 100 megohms).

Summary of Electrode Performance Factors

Location

The shape and amplitude of the recorded potentials depend entirely upon the location of the electrodes relative to the source of the potentials. The amplitude of the recorded MUAP decreases exponentially with the distance between the needle tip and source of electrical activity. In addition, the high frequency components—that is, the sharp, rapidly changing portions of the action potential wave—are lost as the distance increases. Motor units recorded at a distance then have a low thudding sound compared to the sharp "ticking" sibilant sound made by the motor unit activity close to the needle tip. For this reason, the search with the needle within the muscle is of vital importance in obtaining truly characteristic motor unit activity.

The location of the surface electrodes in recording the compound action potential in motor nerve conduction time testing determines the shape and polarity of the recorded waves. In duplicating standard technique, attention should be paid to this factor; the most common location is one electrode over the motor point or the muscle belly and the other near the distal tendon. Some techniques, however, call for particular spacing, usually for 3 or 4 cm between the two surface recording electrodes.

When separate connectors are provided on the EMG amplifier for use as the active and reference input terminals, the user can establish the EMG trace deflection polarity sense (negative up or positive up) of his or her choosing for concentric electrodes by first determining from the manufacturer the deflection polarity sense, on the CRT screen, of the two terminals. They are electrically symmetrical; a negative voltage into one terminal deflects the trace up, whereas a positive voltage into the same terminal deflects the trace down; the opposite effect is obtained with the other terminal. Obtaining the desired polarity sense simply requires that the active electrode wire be connected consistently to the desired terminal. When a single multipin polarized input connector is used, the polarity sense is established by the internal connector wiring when using concentric electrodes.

The patient ground electrode should not be placed over a muscle. A location over a bony or tendinous area minimizes pickup of unwanted muscle activity by this electrode.

Area

The variations in area of surface electrodes used in clinical EMG are of little significance, although variations in the smaller areas encountered in needle electrodes greatly affect the recorded waves. When recording near the action potential source, the amplitude and sharpness of the recorded wave are higher with small area needle electrodes than with larger area electrodes. As the recording surface area decreases and approaches the size of the source of potentials, a maximal difference in potential is recorded between it and the reference electrode. On the other hand, larger tip surfaces are in contact with a greater area of tissue, some of which is inactive, and the resulting signal, which will be an average, has a lower amplitude. If the larger area tip is within the area of influence of two sources, the resultant of the two sources is recorded. Large area needles therefore tend to record more polyphasic activity. These points are exemplified by the small area single fiber electrode that records potentials of high amplitude.

It should be noted that needle electrodes with very small exposed areas have very high metal-electrolyte interface impedances; that is, they are characterized by high series resistance and small series capacitance. As a consequence, they must be connected to amplifiers with high input impedance to avoid serious reduction in recorded amplitudes and distortion in the recorded waves. The input impedance of these preamplifiers should also have low shunt capacitance components to minimize loss of high frequency information from the high impedance, small area needle electrodes. Large area surface electrodes put much less constraint on the input impedance requirements of the preamplifier, provided that proper contact is made with the skin surface. Large area electrodes also generate less electrical noise than small area needle electrodes.

Shape

The symmetrical conical shape of the monopolar needle electrode has omnidirectional recording properties, which are of value in a searching electrode. The bevel of the recording surface of the concentric electrodes gives them directional properties. From an electrical standpoint, symmetrical recording surfaces of equal area are desirable (when possible) to minimize artifact pickup by maximizing the differential amplifier performance of the system.

Materials, Sterilization

The materials used in electrode construction are chosen to meet some obvious mechanical strength requirements, especially in the needle electrodes, and to be relatively chemically inactive. Metals used for the inner core of concentric electrodes include platinum, silver, and nickel-chromium alloy (nichrome). Electrolytic etching of platinum core concentric electrodes (by passing current through the electrode while immersed in a saline solution) has been recommended to reduce electrode impedance and noise and improve fidelity.

Metals and plastics used in some needle electrode construction can withstand the time and temperatures of steam autoclaving. Some needle electrode lead wires and connectors are not autoclavable. Those that are not are sometimes able to be disconnected from the autoclavable needle. Autoclaving time and pressure instructions provided by the electrode manufacturer should be carefully followed to ensure adequate electrode service life. (One hour of autoclaving has been recommended to avoid transmission of certain slow viruses (17)).

A number of laboratories successfully use gas sterilization; however, some plastics might be sensitive to some of the gas sterilizing agents. Electrodes should be thoroughly outgassed after gas sterilization because of the tendency of plastic materials to retain the sterilizing agent.

When possible, especially when attempting to record very small potentials, the electrodes in contact with the patient should be of the same metal. Each electrode should be designed so that dissimilar metals do not contact the patient or the electrode paste because the electrochemical activity between the dissimilar metals and the electrode paste might cause artifact. For this reason, when a solder joint is made between a lead wire and a surface electrode, this contact should be electrically insulated or care should be exercised to avoid simultaneous contact between the electrode paste, the solder, and the metal electrode. Silver surface electrodes provide less noise and the greatest stability and, in some cases, reduce stimulus artifact.

Maintenance

Electrode and electrode lead wire movement are insidious sources of artifact that often mimics action potentials.[a] It is therefore important to stabilize both the lead wire and the electrode during examinations. All electrodes and lead wires should be carefully inspected and cleaned after every use, because foreign matter can be a significant source of noise in both needles and surface electrodes.

Visual and electrical inspection of needle electrodes should be carried out after each use before autoclaving. Visual inspection using at least a 6× loupe or preferably a low power binocular dissecting microscope and testing for electrical continuity and insulation are necessary. The visual inspection should note the condition of the point. Monopolar needles cannot be resharpened; needles with broken or bent points must be discarded. Also, one should note the amount of needle tip exposed and discard the electrode when the distance from the tip to the Teflon coating becomes greater than the diameter of the needle. This process is accelerated by contact with bone tendon and fibrotic tissue. Because punctures and tears in the Teflon coating cannot be repaired, monopolar needles should be handled carefully to protect their relatively soft coating.

Concentric needles with bent or broken points can be resharpened on a fine hypodermic needle sharpening stone or 400–600 grit wet-grinding paper. The concentric needle should also be inspected to determine that the inner conductor is present and clean, because this inner conductor can be corroded during use.

---

[a]Electrostatic shielding refers to an electrically conductive sheath or enclosure surrounding circuits or devices. The shield is connected to ground and acts to prevent undesirable capacitative coupling of external voltages to the elements within the shield. Where the elements within the shield are the source of undesirable potentials, the shielding prevents coupling to external circuits and devices. Cables are shielded, for example, by enclosing them in braided flexible metallic sleeves that are insulated from the conductors and grounded. The shield can add significant capacitance from the conductors to ground, reducing impedance and possibly compromising high frequency performance. (Where magnetic fields cause problems, iron or magnetically permeable alloys are used as the shield materials.)

Electrical inspection requires the use of an ohmmeter, a commonly available inexpensive meter. The other materials required are normal saline solution and hydrophilic cotton or sponges.

Note that the following tests indicate gross faults in electrode insulation and electrical continuity; other more complex measurements are required to determine impedance and other quantitative electrical characteristics of electrodes.

Monopolar needles are electrically inspected or tested to determine the electrical continuity of the plug, lead wire, and needle point and to rule out the presence of holes in the Teflon coating. Connect the needle plug to one terminal of the ohmmeter and use an ohmmeter test lead covered with saline-saturated cotton or sponge as the other terminal (Fig. 14.4). When the point of the monopolar needle is applied to the saturated cotton-covered lead, a reading of less than a few thousand ohms should be noted, indicating electrical continuity. No reading (very high resistance) should be obtained when the needle is touched elsewhere upon its length (except possibly a few millimeters from the handle), indicating the Teflon insulation is intact.

The testing for concentric needles is more simple (Fig 14.4). Connect *both* terminals of the needle to the ohmmeter. No reading, very high resistance, should result, demonstrating that no short circuit exists. Dip the needle into a container continuing the saline solution; a reading of less than a few thousand ohms should result. This indicates intact connection between plugs, connecting wires, and electrodes. When the tip of the needle is wiped dry, the reading should increase to at least many megohms. Electrolytic activity causes meter readings to drift in these tests.

Needle electrodes should not be immersed in saline solution for unnecessary long periods while connected to the ohmmeter in order to avoid electrolytic changes that occur due to the current flow through the solution from the battery in the meter. In these tests, the negative ohmmeter terminal should be connected to the monopolar needle or inner conductor lead wire, with the positive ohmmeter terminal connected to the saturated cotton or the cannular lead wire. This precaution further minimizes the effects of electrolysis on the electrodes. A voltmeter would then be required to determine the polarity of the ohmmeter terminals.

A remarkably common source of noisy or distorted recordings is a fault in the connection somewhere between the preamplifier terminal and the electrical contact at the patient in the active, reference, or ground electrode path. This can sometimes be overlooked because a record, albeit poor, is often still obtained even in the absence of the requisite three connections. The fault may be within the connecting wires, at the connection with the electrical connectors, or between the

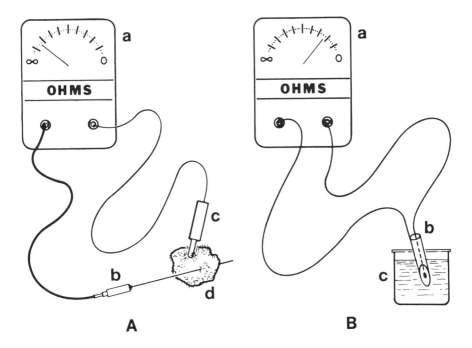

Figure 14.4. *A,* Monopolar needle electrode test: *a,* ohmmeter; *b,* monopolar needle electrode connected to ohmmeter; *c,* test lead with probe; *d,* saline-saturated cotton or sponge covering the probe tip. Meter shows high resistance when saline-soaked cotton is in contact with intact insulating coating—a defect in the coating would cause the meter to read low resistance. The reading should be less than a few thousand ohms when the cotton is in contact with exposed tip (and also perhaps within a few millimeters of the handle). A high reading in this second test indicates an occluded tip or broken lead wire or plug connection. *B,* Concentric needle electrode test: *a,* ohmmeter; *b,* concentric needle electrode connected to ohmmeter; *c,* container with saline solution. Meter shows low resistance when tip is immersed in saline solution, indicating electrical continuity and properly exposed tip. A high resistance reading obtained with the electrode tip dry indicates that no short circuit exists.

connecting wires and the electrodes. Considerable stress and flexing at these points can result in a break or intermittent failure of the wires within the insulation at these points. These faults can be detected with an ohmmeter by flexing and stressing the wire at these points while making the measurement.

THE EMG AMPLIFIER SYSTEM

Input Impedance

The input impedance of modern EMG preamplifiers can be represented by a resistance of from 10 to 100 mehohms (1 megohm, 10^6 ohms or 1,000,000 ohms) shunted by a capacitor of 10 to 100 pF (1pF, 10^{-12}F or one millionth of a microfarad). This impedance is in series with the metal-electrolyte junction impedances at the electrode tip, and together they form a voltage divider. This voltage divider effect reduces the amplitude of the action potentials that appear at the input terminals of the preamplifier and somewhat distorts them (8). These undesirable effects are minimized by making the input impedance many times higher than the highest anticipated electrode impedance; this is especially important in SFEMG where small area, high impedance electrodes must be used. The electrode impedance is difficult to state and measure because it is a function of voltage, current, and the test signal frequency used to measure it. Nonetheless, the capacitative portion of this impedance causes the electrode to conduct rapid changes in waveforms better than slower ones. High input impedance also enhances the interference rejection properties of the differential amplifier, which would otherwise be degraded when using recording electrodes that substantially differ in area, e.g., concentric needle electrodes.

The high resistance portion of the input impedance (50–100 megohms is easily achieved with modern semiconductor amplifiers) also minimizes the amplitude loss by voltage divider action with the resistance portion of the electrode impedance. The capacitative portion of the input impedance should be as small as possible, because a large capacitance (large capacitance results in *low* impedance) here would shunt high frequencies or rapid changes in the action potentials and not permit them to be amplified by the preamplifier. The minimum value of capacitance is limited by the physical presence of conductors in the input circuit. Electrostatic shielding to minimize extraneous pickup serves to increase this capacitance. The capacitative portion in the input impedance ranges from 20 to 100 pF in clinical EMG amplifiers. (Where long shielded leads are required, the driven shield method involving additional circuitry achieves the effects of shielding with minimal additional increase in shunt capacitance.)

Because the differential amplifier has two recording electrode terminals and a common ground or zero potential terminal, input impedance measured between the input terminals is often specified as the differential or *balanced input impedance,* and the impedance measured between the input terminals and the common terminal is often also specified as the *common mode input impedance.*

Differential Amplifier

A conventional amplifier has two input terminals and amplifies potentials that appear between them. The differential amplifier has three input terminals: two recording electrode input terminals and a ground or zero potential terminal. The differential amplifier amplifies potentials that appear as difference-potentials between the two input terminals and discriminates against potentials that appear equally at both of the input terminals when measured to the ground terminal. The recording electrodes connected to the input terminals of the differential amplifier used in EMG are connected to the patient in such a way that the potential to be amplified appears between them. The body is a relatively uniformly good conductor of electricity; and therefore, interference potentials (coupled to the patient from the power wiring and electrical appliances in the examining room) will appear almost uniformly at both recording electrodes, which are close to each other, but relatively distant from the source of interference. Interference potentials measured on a typical patient can be much greater than the action potentials to be recorded in EMG.

The operation of the differential amplifier may be understood by considering it to be made up of two conventional amplifiers, each with a single input terminal and a common ground terminal, the only difference being that the output of one of the amplifiers is always exactly of opposite polarity to the other. These amplifiers are then connected to a summing circuit that provides an output signal to the sum of the outputs of each of the amplifiers.

Consider the output that results when the following input voltages are applied to the two input terminals of the differential amplifier for two input situations: (a) identical inputs, (b) differing inputs. In case (a), the output of the summing circuit is zero if the inputs to the amplifiers are identical (identical inputs results in two signals of opposite polarity that cancel each other in the summing circuit.) In case (b), the output is proportional to the difference in potential that exists between the input terminals of each amplifier. This is the desired performance of the differential amplifier. The input terminal of each amplifier comprises the two recording electrode connections of the differential amplifier. Interference potentials in common on both input terminals are cancelled, and action potentials that appear as a voltage difference between the recording electrodes are amplified (Fig. 14.5).

The interference is usually externally induced power line interference potential. It could just as well be a stimulus artifact; the stimulus would have to be at a sufficient distance from the recording electrodes and arranged symmetrically with respect to them so that the stimulus artifact impinged on both recording electrodes equally, permitting the differential cancelling effect to take place. The desired signal (action potential) is termed the differential signal or the *difference mode signal*. The undesired signal (interference potential), which is cancelled by the differential action of the differential amplifier, is termed the *common mode signal*.

Under idealized conditions, the common mode signal is totally can-

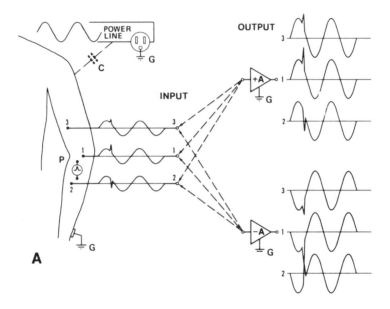

Figure 14.5. Differential amplifier. *A,* Two single input amplifiers, +A and −A, are connected to electrodes in various locations with respect to action potential generator *P* in subject influenced by 60 Hz power line interference. The outputs of each amplifier for three electrode locations are shown. Each amplifier and the subject are connected to a common ground G. Amplifier +A and amplifier −A are conventional amplifiers having two input terminals, one connected to the signal source and the other a ground connection to complete the input circuit. Amplifier −A is identical to amplifier +A, except that its output potentials always have the opposite polarity as its input. The power line is inducing sinusoidal power line interference into the subject by capacitance effects. *C,* Each amplifier is connected in turn to electrode location 1, 2, and 3 where the input voltages are as shown. The output of each amplifier, shown appropriately larger because of the amplification effects, is also shown for each of the electrode locations tested, which are also labeled 1, 2, 3. The sine wave interference is about the same for each electrode location. The induced interference affects the body essentially uniformly, and the electrode locations are in close proximity to each other relative to the interference source. The action potential, which is severely contaminated by interference, has a polarity that is dependent on the electrode location relative to the source of the action potential *P.* Location 3 has the smallest action potential because it is at the greatest distance. Locations 1 and 2 have opposite polarity because they are nearest opposite terminals of the hypothetical action potential

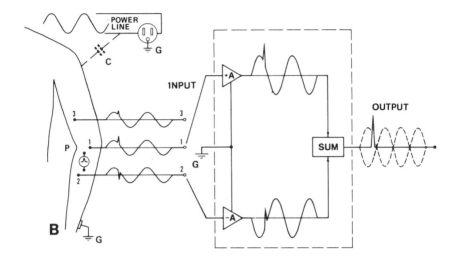

generator *P*. When the outputs are examined, note that the amplified interference wave at the output of − A amplifier is always the opposite polarity image of the sine wave interference portion of the output of the + A amplifier. The action potential, however, at the output of + A electrode location 1 is the same polarity as the output of − A, electrode location 2. This property is used in the differential amplifier. *B*, The two separate amplifiers in *A* are combined into a hypothetical single differential amplifier, which in fact contains elements of two amplifiers. The input terminals of the two amplifiers are arranged so that they share a common ground terminal. The active input terminal of each of the two amplifiers become the two active inputs that characterize the differential amplifier. The 1 and 2 electrodes are used because electrode 3 is too distant from *P*. The outputs of amplifiers A and − A are added or summed to produce the output of the differential amplifier. With the inputs connected to the 1 and 2 electrode locations as shown, the sine wave interference portion of the outputs is of opposite polarity so that they cancel each other when they are summed. However the action potential portions are of the same polarity and reinforce each other when they are summed. The differential amplifier has thus rejected the interference wave and amplified the action potential. (Total cancellation of the interference in this idealized example assumes exact symmetry of electrodes, volume conductor paths, and amplifiers, conditions not realized in practice.)

celled and disappears from the output. In practice, however, the common mode signal is not totally cancelled for a number of reasons. It is not possible to build the differential amplifier so that the signal applied to each input terminal is amplified exactly equally, especially at all frequencies; also the common mode signal does not always appear at the input terminals of the amplifier at exactly the same amplitude. Obviously, when using a concentric needle electrode, for example, one recording electrode is the large surface area of the stainless steel cannula. This means that the impedance of one electrode is much higher than the impedance of the other electrode. Consequently, when a common mode signal reaches the concentric electrode, these two impedances, which form a voltage divider with the input impedance of each half of the differential amplifier, cause the common signal to appear at different amplitudes at the inputs of the differential amplifier, and they are therefore not cancelled. This effect, whereby unequal electrode impedances permit common mode interfering signals to defeat the common mode rejection properties of the differential amplifier, is minimized by making the input impedance of the preamplifier high, because this high input impedance minimizes the difference in voltage divider action resulting from differences in electrode contact impedance.

Common Mode Rejection Ratio

A technical measure of the ability of a differential amplifier to discriminate against common mode signals is called its *common mode rejection ratio* (CMRR). It is determined by measuring the differential amplification of a differential amplifier by connecting a test signal generator between its active input terminals (a different input signal) and then measuring the common mode amplification of the amplifier by connecting a test signal to the two active input terminals, shorted together as a common point with the other terminal of the generator connected to the common ground connection of the amplifier (common mode signal). Obviously, the differential amplifier exhibits much less amplification when driven with a common mode signal (the second case) because of the cancellation effect described earlier than it does when it is driven in its differential mode (in the first case). The common mode rejection ratio is the ratio of the differential amplification to the amplification in the common mode case. (Fig. 14.6).

Common mode rejection ratios achievable in the laboratory by careful adjustments to each of the two halves of the differential amplifier are in the order of many hundreds of thousands to one at a particular test frequency. Maintenance of high common mode rejection ratio is difficult over a wide range of test frequencies. When practical needle

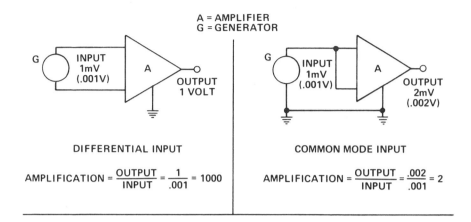

Figure 14.6. Common mode rejection ratio (CMRR).

electrodes are used, unequal electrode interface impedances are connected to the input terminals. This reduces common mode rejection ratios to less than 100:1 over a range of frequencies.

One method of measurement of the actual CMRR of an amplifier with a concentric needle electrode in situ would provide actual values and a check on seriously increased electrode impedance as well, because this test accounts for all major parameters, e.g., needle interface impedance, cable shield capacitance, amplifier input impedances, and amplifier common mode rejection; it would be valid only at the sine wave frequencies tested. Fortunately, as a practical matter, adequate common mode rejection is usually available to permit satisfactory clinical EMG under most conductions.

Frequency Response

The wave shapes encountered in EMG range from the relatively slowly changing CMAP wave of motor nerve conduction tests (which can have a duration of many tens of milliseconds) to the rapid 0.1 msec positive-to-negative transition phase of a MUAP recorded with needle electrodes.

The shape of these waves as seen on the CRT screen depends upon electrode configuration and their location and is mediated by factors that include (a) the electrical impedance (series resistance and capacitance) of the electrode-electrolyte interface at the needle tip, (b) the

EMG amplifier input impedance (shunt resistance and shunt capacitance, including shunt capacitance of the electrode cable shield), and (c) the frequency response properties of the EMG amplifier.

Amplifiers can be designed so that their output responds to static values of input potentials, e.g., resting potential or potentials that do not change continuously or that change very slowly with time. These are called DC amplifiers. Amplifiers can, as well, permit response to potentials that change much faster than the fastest biologic potentials.

If the response of the EMG amplifier encompasses the slowest and fastest components of waves to be encountered, it will not materially distort the recorded waves. An amplifier's ability to respond to fast and slow changes can be expressed in a number of ways. One method involves application of a step wave or a square wave to the input of the amplifier and then notation of the rise time and droop or decay time of the output wave, which will not have the instantaneous rise nor the perfectly flat top of the test input wave (See Fig. 14.9, see step wave bottom trace A, B, C).

A more common method is to apply sine wave test signals of various frequencies but of equal amplitude to the input terminals and then to plot, versus frequency, the relative amplitude of the sine waves at the output for the various test frequencies. This plot, termed a *frequency response curve*, appears for a simple amplifier as shown in Figure 14.7. It shows decreasing output voltage for sine waves below some frequency f_l and above some frequency f_h. The output voltage for sine waves between f_l and f_h is the "bandwidth" or "passband" of the EMG amplifier. This band extends from 2 Hz to 10kHz for clinical EMG systems. The frequencies, f_h and f_l, and the frequency response curve of the amplifier can be mathematically related to the rise and decay time of the amplifiers, respectively; either can be used to predict or specify amplifier dynamic performance.

Sine waves are used in calculating the impedance of resistor capacitor circuits, as well as in determining the bandwidth of amplifiers, because they are the only waveforms that pass through these frequency-response determining circuits without change in shape, the only effect being relative change in amplitude (and phase) with change in frequency.

The sine wave bandwidth of an amplifier can be used to predict its response to other nonsinusoidal input waveforms, even EMG potentials, because nonsinusoidal time-varying waves can be analyzed in terms of sine waves by the technique of harmonic analysis. The harmonic analysis method describes a nonsinusoidal wave as a sum of sine waves of various frequencies and amplitudes. These sine waves, termed harmonics, when added together, form the original nonsinusoidal wave. Thus, the stated bandwidth requirements, 2 Hz to 10 kHz, of a clinical

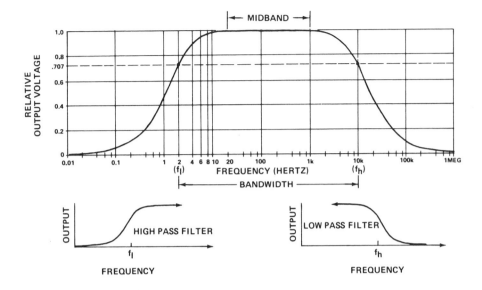

Figure 14.7. Frequency response curve. The frequency response curve shows how the output of an amplifier changes when constant voltage sine waves of various frequencies are applied to the input. Frequency is plotted on a logarithmic horizontal axis. Relative output voltage is on the vertical axis. (Relative output voltage is obtained by dividing the actual output by the midband output voltage. This makes the midband relative output voltage 1, thus simplifying the notation.) The bandwidth of the amplifier is that range of frequencies over which the relative output voltage is more than 0.707 and is defined on the graph by f_l and f_h, the low and high cut-off frequencies. Stated another way, one might say that the amplification of the amplifier is uniform for all frequencies within its bandwidth to within 0.707 of its midband value. (The relative output voltage is often expressed in decibels (dB), an engineering notation that derives from the logarithm of the ratio of two voltages. The voltage ratio of 0.707 is -3dB in decibel rotation. dB $=$ 20 log $\frac{V1}{V2}$.)The bandwidth of the amplifier is adjusted by setting high pass and low pass filters in the amplifier. The high pass filter passes all frequencies above f_l, thus establishing the low frequency limit of the amplifier. The low pass filter passes all frequencies below f_h, setting the high frequency limit of the amplifier as shown in the frequency response curves for typical filters. Together they establish the bandwidth of the system. The shape of the frequency response curves shown is typical for many amplifiers. However, filter designs used to achieve special noise performance effects result in more rapid falloff of the curves outside of the midband region. Specification of f_l and f_h and the performance of the amplifier may be modified in these cases.

EMG amplifier mean that there are no harmonics of significance above or below the stated bandwidth limits in the EMG waves being recorded. The low frequency harmonics relate to the slowly changing portion of the waves, whereas the high frequency harmonics relate to the rapid changes in the waves.

Filters

The frequency response of the EMG amplifier is intentionally limited to the harmonics of the waves being studied and does not extend appreciably above or below them for the following reasons. Extending the low frequency response materially below 2 Hz would permit slow artifact potentials originating from electrode polarization potentials and from electrode or lead wire movements to cause the baseline of the EMG trace to wander excessibly. If the high frequency response extends substantially above 10 kHz, high frequency resistance thermal noise and amplifier noise that appear as a thickening of the baseline and hissing noises in the loudspeaker would excessively contaminate the results. The bandwidth of the amplifier is adjusted to encompass only the significant harmonics of the potentials being recorded, thus excluding noise and artifact frequencies that fall above and below the bandwidth limits.

High and low frequency response limits are selectively reduced by means of filters, to reduce the high and low frequency noise in the system when performing certain tests where the full bandwidth of the system is not required. High and low pass filters are frequency selective, usually resistance-capacitance circuits, that shape the high and low limits of the frequency response curve of the amplifier. (Fig. 14.7).

For example, in routine needle EMG where long duration, slowly changing waves are not encountered, the low frequency response limit can be moved from 2 Hz to 20 Hz, thus additionally reducing baseline wander; the high frequency setting should be set at maximum so as not to distort the fibrillation potentials and rapid transition portions of MUAPs. In SFEMG where baseline stability is of paramount importance and low frequency components are of no concern, the low frequency response limit is moved to 500 Hz.

Conversely, the high frequency limit can be reduced, if desired, from 10 kHz to 3 or 4 kHz in electroneurography, thus materially reducing the high frequency noise that becomes obvious at the sensitivity setting required to record small nerve potentials (Fig. 14.8). The reduced high frequency response can be tolerated here because the neurograms do not usually contain rapid deflections, and the primary object of the test is to record a latency. In addition, the low frequency response can be decreased in these tests from 2 Hz to 20 or 50 Hz to reduce baseline fluctuations.

When performing motor nerve conduction tests in which the duration and amplitude of the compound motor action potential wave are to be measured (in addition to the more common latency measure-

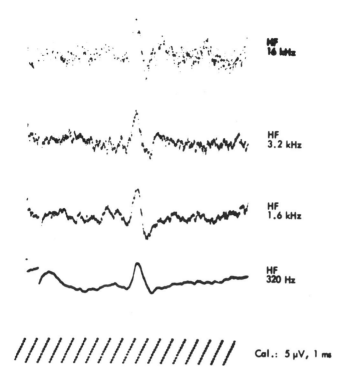

Figure 14.8. Neurograms recorded with various high frequency bandwidth limits. Records were made by stimulating the finger and recording over the ulnar nerve at the elbow with surface electrodes. The high frequency response of the amplifier was progressively reduced from the top trace down. The bottom calibration trace is 5 μV, and time between peaks is 1 msec. The low frequency limit was 32 Hz for all records. The high frequency limit was reduced from 16 kHz for the top record to 3.2 kHz, 1.6 kHz and to 320 Hz for the lowest record. The top record shows all the effects of system, electrode, and bioelectric noise. The noise was effectively filtered in the third record (1.6 kHz); however, the fourth record (320 Hz), which is cosmetically cleanest, shows the effects of excessive filtering that introduces error by reducing the apparent peak-to-peak amplitude of the recorded potential.

ment), the low frequency limit should be set to 2 Hz to accommodate the slow portions of the recorded waves without distortion. Figure 14.9 shows the effects of limiting the high and low frequency settings on records and on a step calibration wave.

Amplifier Noise Measurement

The noise originating within the amplifier should be measured by observing the screen at maximum amplification with the input termi-

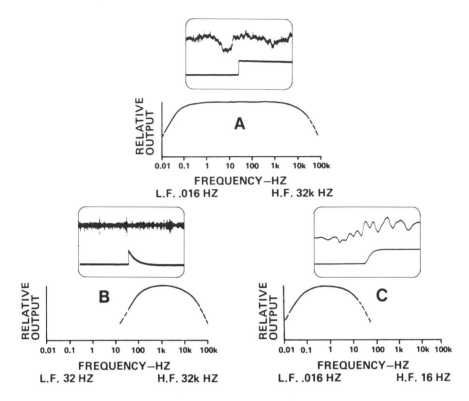

Figure 14.9. Demonstrating the effect of filter settings on recorded action potentials and a step wave calibration signal. Frequency response curves are shown below the potentials for each of the three sets of filter settings. *A,* Records were made with the amplifier set for maximum high and low frequency response, .016 Hz to 32 kHz. The upper trace shows rapid high frequency activity, as well as slow baseline excursions. The step calibration wave below shows a rapid rise due to the extended high frequency response. This is followed by a steady deflection with no droop, the result of extended low frequency response. *B,* The high frequency limit remains unchanged, but the low frequency filter setting has been moved up to 32 Hz. The high frequency information in the upper trace remains, but the slow variations have been filtered out. The portion of the step wave following the rapid rise shows considerable decay due to reduction in low frequency response. *C,* The low frequency setting is .016 Hz, as in *A,* but the high frequency filter setting is lowered to 16 Hz. All the high frequency variations in the upper trace have been filtered, leaving the slowly changing potentials. The step wave now has a slow rise because of severely reduced high frequency response, followed by a steady deflection with no decay, the result of the extended low frequency response. Note that the settings shown are not used in routine EMG. They were chosen to be most effective for demonstration.

nals shorted (this is accomplished by setting the EMG to the "calibrate" setting in many instruments) and with the filters set for maximum bandwidth, which should be stated for the noise measurement to be valid. The internal noise then appears as irregular fluctuations in the baseline and as fuzzy thickening of the trace and is heard on the loudspeaker as hissing and rumbling. The apparent noise increases as the bandwidth of the amplifier is increased. (Any resistance larger than a short circuit connected across the input terminals also increases the apparent internal noise.) Peak-to-peak noise measurements on screen require estimation of the "thickness" of the baseline trace and are quite subjective due to the random nature of the noise.

High impedance EMG amplifiers designed for needle electrodes exhibit random peak-to-peak noise of from 5 to 10 μV when set for 2 Hz to 10 kHz bandwidth (shorted input). These measurements must be estimated because of the random nature of the noise and depend, among other factors, upon sweep speed and beam intensity used to observe the noise and observer bias that makes peak-to-peak noise measurement ambiguous. A method called tangential noise measurement reduces the ambiguity of noise measurement from the screen to about 20% (20); it results in noise voltages that are one-third the peak-to-peak estimates and requires some additional equipment.

Noise voltages are sometimes measured in microvolts root mean square (RMS) with a meter instead of peak-to-peak values obtained from observing the CRT screen. A meter measurement of an alternating current presents problems because current flows equally in both directions, and the meter may be used for measurement of current of various waveshapes. When any alternating current of a given RMS magnitude is applied to a resistor, it causes the same hearing in the resistor as a DC of the same magnitude applied to the same resistance. For cyclic waveforms (e.g., sine or square waves), a simple relationship exists between the peak value of the AC observed on a CRT and its RMS value. (Power line voltage is specified as an RMS voltage and is 0.707 times the sine wave peak value of the voltage.) However, when RMS values of amplifier random noise voltages are specified, there is no simple relationship to the random peaks observed on the CRT screen. In practice, peak-to-peak values from observation of the screen are approximately five or six times the RMS voltage obtained by RMS meter measurement. The conditions and methods of measurement must be specified before careful comparisons of any of the amplifier parameters can be made.

When an electrode position in tissue is changed or when the needle electrode is initially inserted, transient changes in electrode polarization voltage appear that may be hundreds of times greater than the action potentials the amplifier is adjusted to record. These large voltage changes "overload" the amplifier for a period of time, during which potentials cannot be recorded with acceptable fidelity. This time, termed *blocking time,* should be less than 1 sec on a clinical EMG, because insertion potentials that occur after needle movement are of clinical interest. Smaller overloads originating from bioelectric sources should not result in blocking, so as to permit observation of small sensory potentials in the presence of large motor potentials.

THE EMG DISPLAY

The cathode ray tube, which permits visualization of the EMG potentials, consists of an evacuated funnel-shaped envelope with a source of electrons at the small end and a glass face coated on the inside with a screen material that fluoresces upon being struck by electrons, called a *phosphor,* at the large end. The electrons are released from the electrically heated cathode into the vacuum surrounding it. They are then formed into a narrow beam and accelerated toward the screen by a series of electrodes maintained at a potential positive with respect to the cathode. This positive potential attracts electrons and accelerates them toward the screen. The beam-forming electrodes are shaped and maintained at relative potentials to each other so as to form lens-like electrostatic fields that form and focus the electrons into a sharply collimated beam. This assembly is the electron gun.

The positive accelerating potentials of many thousands of volts cause the electrons to hit the fluorescent screen with sufficient energy to generate a bright spot of visible light on the screen. The color and persistence, or afterglow, of the light after extinguishing the electron beam are determined by the formulation of the phosphor and the beam-accelerating potential. The accelerated beam, after leaving the electron gun, passes between two sets of deflecting plates within the tube, one set arranged horizontally and the other vertically. The negatively charged particles (electrons) comprising the beam can be attracted or repelled by voltages applied to these deflecting plates. Applying appropriate applied voltages to these plates can deflect the beam as it passes between them, causing the spot of impact at the screen to move vertically in response to the voltage applied to the vertical (Y) deflection plates and horizontally in response to the voltage applied to the horizontal (X) deflection plates. (This beam deflection method is termed electrostatic deflection.) The EMG potential is applied to the Y plates, and the time base, or sweep signal, which is a sawtooth wave, is applied to the X plates. The sawtooth wave voltage increases uniformly with time, then returns very quickly to its starting value and repeats. This uniformly changing voltage moves the spot from left to right at constant velocity across the screen and returns it rapidly to the left, repeating continuously. The result is a repetitive voltage-time graph of

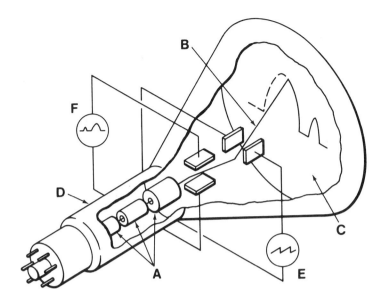

Figure 14.10. Cathode ray tube, *A,* Electron gun. *B,* Electron beam, *C,* Phosphor-coated screen inside faceplate. *D,* Evacuated envelope. *E,* Sawtooth sweep voltage source connected to horizontal deflection plates. *F,* Signal voltage source connected to vertical deflection plates.

the EMG waveform. Total sweep times are adjustable from 2 msec to 5 sec in most EMG equipment. Faster sweep speeds are provided for SFEMG (Fig. 14.10).

Another means of CRT beam movement, magnetic deflection, utilizes magnetic coils placed outside the tube around its narrow portion to deflect the beam in the X and Y direction by magnetic effects on the beam. Magnetic deflection CRTs are commonly used in television, in radar in computer terminals, and in some EMG systems where the patterns are generated by causing the whole screen to be covered uniformly by the beam that draws a *raster,* a closely spaced series of parallel lines from the top of the screen to the bottom. The picture or waveform information is generated by turning the beam on or off or varying its intensity as the raster is drawn, so as to generate the desired pattern from discrete elements, rather than by a moving point of light. Magnetic deflection systems permit economies where information is available in discrete form, such as the output of digital systems and when many channels are simultaneously displayed.

Time Base, Triggered

In conventional motor unit studies, the time base is free-running, i.e., the beam cyclically sweeps across the screen, and randomly occurring action potentials appear at various locations along the baseline, because these potentials are not synchronous with the time base. However, when an action potential is expected in response to a known event, such as an electrical stimulus to a nerve or mechanical impact of a percussion hammer on a tendon, the free-running sweep is interrupted and a sweep is released only in response to the initiating event. In this stimulus "triggered sweep" mode, the response wave, having a fixed latency with respect to the initiating event, always appears at the same location on screen. With repeated stimuli, the response wave will superimpose and appear as a standing pattern on screen, facilitating identification, measurement, and detection of change.

The triggered sweep mode can be used in some apparatuses to observe randomly occurring action potentials ("signal triggered" sweep) if they are consistently larger than the other simultaneously occurring activity. The sweep triggers (starts) only when potentials appear that exceed an adjustable "triggering level" voltage and are of selected polarity (slope). The selected motor unit waves will, when they occur, appear superimposed at one location on screen. Because other smaller distant potentials that do not exceed the triggering level voltage do not cause the sweep to start and are not seen, only the selected waves will appear as a steady repeating image. More elaborate triggering modes and use of the delay line with signal triggered sweep are described later.

Time Scales

The accuracy with which time measurements can be made on the EMG screen depends on the time accuracy and linearity of the time base sawtooth wave generator, the linearity of the deflection amplifier that drives the CRT deflection circuits, and the linearity of deflection of the CRT itself. (Nonlinearity results in nonuniform speed of the trace across the screen, causing time calibration to be different at various points along the trace.) These errors should not result in on-screen timing error of more than a few percent. Thus, time measurements of EMG potentials can usually be read from lines on a transparent panel (called a graticule) superimposed on the face of the CRT. The sweep or time base switch settings in milliseconds per division on the graticule permit timing of events on the CRT screen.

Some EMGs are also equipped with a second time reference trace that can display a known accurate series of pulses or steps representing, for example, 0.1, 1 or 10 msec. Because all traces are influenced by the same X axis deflection mechanism, this time reference trace permits accurate time measurement unaffected by any errors in the time base or X deflection system nonlinearities. A time reference trace has the further advantage of providing at all times a known time reference on screen (and on photographs), without reference to the time base or sweep dial settings.

When triggered sweep is used, a moveable electronic time index is generated on many EMGs in synchronism with the start of each sweep or with the initiation of a stimulus. This index, which appears variously as a step, pulse, vertical line, or bright portion of the trace on the CRT screen, is under the control of a knob with an indicator calibrated in whole and decimal parts of milliseconds. Latency from the sweep start or from the stimulus to a desired point on the evoked response is measured by turning the index dial until the index mark is at the desired point on the wave on screen and then reading the calibrated dial, usually to an accuracy greater than could be obtained from the fleeting wave on the screen.

Time Calibration

A convenient, accurate method for verifying the time accuracy of an EMG time base, CRT deflection system, time reference, and index utilizes the commercial power line frequency timing that is more than sufficiently accurate for EMG. Introducing some power line signal is easily done by bringing a subject connected to the EMG input near an insulated appliance power cable (a common cause of power line artifact). (Under no circumstances should any attempt be made to make an electrical connection to the power line, because a lethal shock hazard could exist.) The resulting cyclic power-line-induced artifact waves on screen (with sweep set to show 100 or 200 msec full screen) has a one-cycle period of 16.7 msec, and three cycles represent 50 msec in 60 Hz power areas (20 msec/cycle in 50 Hz power areas). The time scales on the EMG should agree with the power line derived waves in timing to within 3–5%. (Some EMGs display the induced power line waves as standing patterns or are able to lock the sweep to the power line frequency for test purposes.)

Multichannel Display

When more than one trace of information is to be displayed simultaneously on the EMG screen, special cathode ray tubes containing two independent electron guns and deflection systems have been used. Careful adjustment is required to obtain accurate time coincidence in both sweeps. To obviate this, dual beam CRTs with common X deflection and independent Y deflection systems have sometimes been used. These methods for two or more trace displays have been superseded by electronic switching (or chopped display), a method that utilizes a conventional single beam CRT. The single beam rapidly (at least 100,000 times per second) moves from its first location, writing a dot forming a portion of the second trace, as it sweeps from left to right across the screen. The result is two series of closely spaced dots across the screen, each series forming one of the two traces. The two traces could typically be made up of 10,000 dots when the sweep duration is 100 msec (a spacing of 0.01 mm between dots on a 10-cm long screen), resulting in two traces that appear continuous. (The beam is turned off during the brief period when it is moving from one trace to the other to avoid smearing effects between the traces). The two traces are essentially coincident in time. This method applies as well to simultaneous display of additional traces.

Magnetic deflection cathode ray tubes using television-like raster displays have been used to provide multichannel displays. These methods are somewhat limited in maximum display speed.

Storage Display

The phosphors used on the screen of conventional cathode ray tubes usually retain the image for fractions of a second. Persistence of a few seconds can be provided, but this may interfere with the writing of a new information. Special storage display cathode ray tubes can retain information written on their screens, with the sweep off, for hours or longer and can be eelctronically erased rapidly at will. These CRTs, which have a capacitative mosaic storage surface behind or on the screen, can also be used in a nonstorage mode as conventional short persistence display tubes. They have obvious advantages in EMG because evoked potentials and transient motor unit activity can be stored on screen for study, measurement, and photography.

Because a confusion of EMG traces results if more than one sweep is written, the storage display CRT sometimes has additional automatic circuitry for writing multiple sweeps without superimposition. One method stacks multiple sweeps so that, after one sweep is completed, the beam automatically moves to a new baseline location, permitting the next sweep to be written on an unused portion of the screen. This can be repeated a number of times so that many "stacked" traces of EMG can be observed simultaneously, permitting motor unit activity to be studied in context. Automatic erasure then permits the process to be repeated unless inhibited when further study or photography is desired.

EMG traces may be retained on the screen of a conventional CRT by electronically recording the potential and then repetitively playing back the recorded trace on screen synchronously with the sweep. The result is a standing pattern on screen similar in appearance to the pattern observed on a storage CRT. This has been done by storing the potentials on a continuous loop of magnetic tape arranged for repetitive playback. A more flexible method converts the potentials to digital form, stores them in digital memory circuits of the type used in digital computers, and then repetitively reads out and converts them to original form for display on a conventional CRT. These methods require additional complexity and a separate storage channel for each trace stored simultaneously, whereas a storage CRT can store any number of traces for simultaneous viewing or recording, the limitation being screen resolution. The digital storage methods can erase and update very rapidly, however, permitting sweep-by-sweep updating with new information and even updating during the course of a sweep.

Special Signal Triggering

When a signal-triggered sweep is used, the sweep on the CRT starts only when potentials exceeding a triggering level voltage occur. The triggering level is set sufficiently high so as to permit only the desired nearby potentials to appear on screen. Action potential criteria other than largest amplitude can be used in more elaborate systems for triggering the sweep; for example, "window" triggering can be used, which requires that the selected waves be greater than one triggering level voltage but *less* than a second higher level (the window is the region between the two voltage levels). This permits the selection of potentials that are smaller than nearby larger ones.

A time window may be used for triggering, e.g., triggers occur only when the selected wave exceeds a set level and then goes through the baseline (zero amplitude) a proscribed number of milliseconds later. This discriminates against long duration waves. These more elaborate triggering methods are more difficult to use, but can be useful in appropriate conditions.

Delay Line

When signal triggering is used, it is often supplemented by a delay line. This device permits the portion of the potential wave that just precedes the triggering point to be seen on screen. Obviously, without the delay line, if the sweep does not start until the wave reaches the selected triggering level, the initial portion (below the triggering level) of the action potential that caused the sweep to start is not seen on screen.

When the delay line is used, the potentials displayed on screen are not those occurring in real time. They are stored instead in an electronic storage device and played back or "read out" for display many milliseconds later (the delay time). The potentials on screen therefore are those that have occurred earlier. Thus, when the triggered sweep

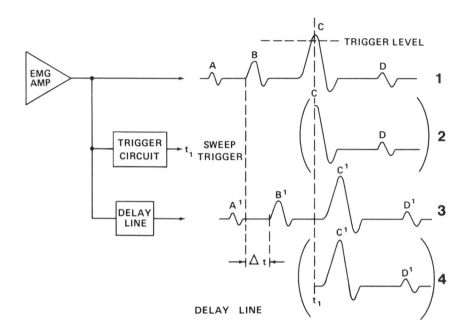

Figure 14.11 Delay line. *1*, EMG waves *A, B,* and *D* do not reach triggering level. Wave *C* exceeds triggering level at time t_1, causing a sweep on screen to start at t_1 resulting in trace *2*. *2*, Displayed trace with triggered sweep, no delay line. Note that initial portion of wave *C* is lost on screen. *3*, EMG waves delayed Δt in time at output of delay line (storage) circuit with wave shapes unchanged. *4*, Delayed wave *C'* displayed on screen with sweep triggered by undelayed wave *C* at time t_1. Note that complete wave *C'* is seen in screen, permitting visualization of portion of wave that occurred before t_1.

starts, in real time, as the rising part of the selected wave exceeds the triggering level, the initial portion of the sweep at the left edge of the screen does not show this rising part of the wave; instead, the earlier parts of the wave appear, which preceded the triggering point, followed by the complete wave (Fig. 14.11). The wave that triggered the sweep is therefore seen in its entirety.

Large storage capability is not required in the delay line because it is constantly being read out and loaded with new material not more than 10 or 20 msec after being recorded. Delay has been accomplished by recording and then delaying reading and erasing of a continuously moving endless loop of magnetic tape. More commonly now, the signals are converted to digital form, circulated through a digital memory for the delay time, and then converted back to original form for display. (The word *line* in "delay line" derives from the early use of transmission lines or equivalent cascaded filters to achieve signal delays (19).

This method, and others using delay of ultrasonic signals, provided only short delay for their bulk and were not easily adjustable in delay time.)

The unique ability of the signal-triggered sweep and delay line to capture transient spontaneous activity enables large numbers of samples of the desired potentials to be collected quickly for measurement of motor unit duration, collection of denervation potentials, fasciculation, and polyphasic potentials, either for direct observation or for selective synchronized graphic recording.

THE EMG STIMULATOR

The EMG stimulator is provided (as stated earlier) with an electrically isolated, ground free, output circuit to prevent electrical conduction of a large stimulus artifact to the preamplifier input. Artifact would otherwise occur via a circuit path comprised of the stimulator, patient, preamplifier input, and the EMG ground circuit, using the common ground for the stimulator, the amplifier, and their common power supplies. The path for conduction of artifact with a nonisolated stimulator is through the patient to the amplifier input and then back through the common ground connection to the stimulator (Fig. 14.12). (All circuits in the system usually share common power supplies, and by virtue of their usual interconnection means, they all have a common ground circuit.) In the isolated stimulator, the common path between stimulator and amplifier is broken by the isolating device.

The isolator is commonly a transformer, although other means are available. A transformer consists of two coils of wire—primary and secondary coils—in close promixity so that they share a common magnetic field. The stimulus current pulse generated by the grounded stimulator circuits flows in the primary coil and generates a pulsed magnetic field that induces a pulse of current in the ungrounded secondary coil of the transformer by the process of electromagnetic induction. The secondary current stimulates the subject. Because there is no electric current path between the primary and secondary windings, the artifact path through the common ground is broken. The isolation transformer breaks this path by converting the electrical output of the stimulator to magnetic energy and then back into electrical current flow in the secondary circuit.

In practice, total isolation is not achieved because of unequal capacitance effects from each output terminal to ground. Shielded stimulator output cables are not used because they would permit paths to ground via the capacitance of the shield. The isolator does not reduce the shock or artifact component that is directly through the patient to the recording electrodes.

Poor electrode technique can defeat stimulus isolation, with resultant large shock artifact. Locating one of the stimulus electrodes closer

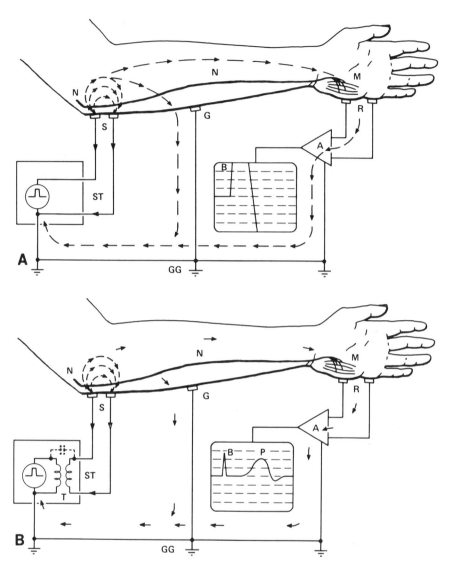

Figure 14.12. Isolated stimulator. *A,* Stimulating electrodes *S* are applied to skin over nerve *N.* A nonisolated conventional stimulator *ST,* which has one output terminal connected to the common system ground *GG* is shown in *A.* Stimulating current *(arrows)* flows between the electrodes *S* exciting the nerve. Some of the current flows through the patient to the ground electrode *G* and the recording electrodes *R* connected to EMG amplifier *A* because both have paths through the common ground back to the stimulator. This stimulus current flowing to the amplifier results in unacceptably large stimulus artifact *B,* which makes recording of the CMAP from muscle *M* very difficult. *B,* The stimulator is equipped with an isolating transformer *T* that effectively disconnects the stimulating electrodes from the common system ground circuit. The stimulus current path through the patient to the amplifier has been substantially interrupted because no easy common path through the system ground is now available. Stimulus artifact *B* is therefore substantially reduced, and CMAP *P* is recorded.

to the ground electrode (or recording electrodes) than the other and, worse still, allowing a current path from a stimulating electrode over the skin surface to the ground electrode (or recording electrodes) via a bridge of electrode paste or perspiration are errors to be avoided.

Stimulus Output

The EMG stimulator usually provides rectangular pulses with durations adjustable from 0.05 to about 1 msec; output pulse voltage should be adjustable to approximately 300 V maximum. The high voltage and long duration pulses are used when required to excite nerves with high thresholds or those that are deeply located. The amount of current that stimulates the nerve is a small fraction of what actually is applied to the patient. This fraction varies with depth of the nerve from the surface and the conductivity of intervening tissues.

Most stimulators permit adjustment of pulse *voltage* amplitude; the resulting pulse *current* that flows depends in amplitude and shape on the electrical load (subject resistance and capacitance) at the electrodes. For a given output setting, the actual *voltage* at the electrodes is usually somewhat reduced, depending on the stimulator design, when more current flows due to lower resistance at the electrodes.

A stabilized voltage stimulator, however, provides adjustable rectangular voltage-stimulus pulses unaffected by variations in electrical load at the electrodes over its design range. Current flow and wave shape depend on the electrical load.

A stabilized current stimulator permits the intensity of rectangular pulse current flow through the electrodes to be set, unaffected by variations in load within its design range. The output voltage amplitude and wave shape of this type of stimulator are dependent on load. Although stabilized output stimulators are not required for conventional latency measurements, they do permit quantitative studies where control of stimulus is of interest.

The stabilized voltage and stabilized current types each have their advocates, but in any case, it is difficult to predict or control the actual path of stimulus energy within the volume conductor (represented by the tissues of the patient) after the current leaves the stimulating electrodes.

Delayed Stimulus

Some stimulators include a control that delays the application of the stimulus a millisecond or so after the trigger that starts the sweep. This moves the stimulus artifact, which would otherwise appear at the extreme left start of the trace, slightly to the right, a distance proportional to the delay time setting, so that the whole of the artifact may be observed.

RECORDING THE EMG

Graphic records permit documentation, measurement, and verification of transient potentials and are an important part of the modern EMG examination. Conventional polygraphic recorders utilizing mechanical writing means do not have the requisite writing speed to record action potentials directly. In addition, recorders that use paper or chart motion as the time base are hard pressed to move paper sufficiently fast to resolve the 1 msec/cm (10 m/sec) useful in some latency and motor unit measurements. (See section on digital storage time transformation recorders.)

Instant Photography

Instant photography of the CRT is widely used to record nerve conduction tests by either electrically synchronizing the camera shutter with the stimulator and sweep or by opening the shutter just before the sweep starts and closing it before the next sweep. Free-running sweeps in EMG must be interrupted to avoid unwanted superimposed traces on the photograph, a consequence of a number of sweeps occurring while the shutter is open. This is done automatically in some EMGs by utilizing shutter contacts to interrupt the sweep.

When the EMG is equipped with a storage display CRT, photography is greatly simplified because the storage traces are static, no sweep is required for viewing, and there is no synchronization problem. It is important to mark the photographic records with time and amplitude information if not already shown on the CRT screen.

CRT Recorders

A motor-driven camera photographing a separate monitor CRT provides greater recording capability, because, in addition to single sweep recording, it can operate in the raster mode, which permits sweep after sweep to be recorded so that information can be seen in context. In this mode, the recording paper of film moves slowly perpendicular to the sweep, so that each sweep writes across the width of the moving paper. The subsequent sweeps appear as parallel records across the width of the record. These modes have no mechanical speed limitations because recording in both X (time) and Y (signal) axes are electronic and do not depend on paper movement.

Continuous records can also be made in a manner similar to a polygraph where high time resolution is not required. The sweep is turned off, and the beam deflection, in response to the EMG signal, is retained along one axis. The movement of the recording medium serves as the time axis; continuous records along the long axis of the record results.

Fiber Optic Recorder

Fiber optic recording provides all the advantages of single sweep, superimposed sweep, raster, and continuous recording, along with the advantage of immediate access to the record. It utilizes a special cathode ray tube with a faceplate comprised of millions of micron-sized fiber optic light pipes. The fiber optic faceplate has the special property of transferring the traces that are formed in the phosphor on the surface of the faceplate inside the evacuated CRT to the outside surface of the faceplate without the optical dispersion that would occur if a conventional faceplate were used. The light efficiency, which is higher than even a large aperture lens, permits direct recording onto special sensitized recording paper in contact with the faceplate. The fastest EMG potentials are recorded by this high optical sensitivity system. The recording paper develops a visible, permanent image a few seconds after emerging from the recorder into a lighted room (Fig. 14.13).

Digital Storage Time Transformation Recorders

The CRT display and the fiber optic recorder have no speed limitation in EMG recording because they are inertia-less in the time (X), as well as the signal (Y) axis. The limitations on other recorders that rely on recording paper movement for the time axis, described earlier, can be obviated by a time transformation technique. The information to be recorded is first stored electrically and then played back slowly at a speed that provides the desired time resolution compatible with reasonable paper speed. (For example: 1 msec/cm time resolution in real time requires unreasonably high 1000 cm/sec paper speed; an electrically stored signal played back at $1/20$ speed would provide 1 msec/cm resolution at an acceptable paper speed of 50 cm/sec). Magnetic tape storage with slow speed playback has been used as the storage medium. More recently, EMG signals converted into digital form and stored in digital computer memory in real time are read out of memory at reduced speed, decoded or converted into original form, and then mechanically and graphically recorded on moving recording paper.

An inertia-less spark recorder utilizing high contrast metallized paper and having a linear array of 256 fixed recorder points has been applied to EMG recording. It utilizes the slow read-from-memory time transformation technique just described for recording on moving paper in the time axis. Conventional ink or hot stylus graphic recorders can also be used in this slow read-out time transformation technique. The limitations of digital storage recorders include limited memory speed and memory capacity and writing time.

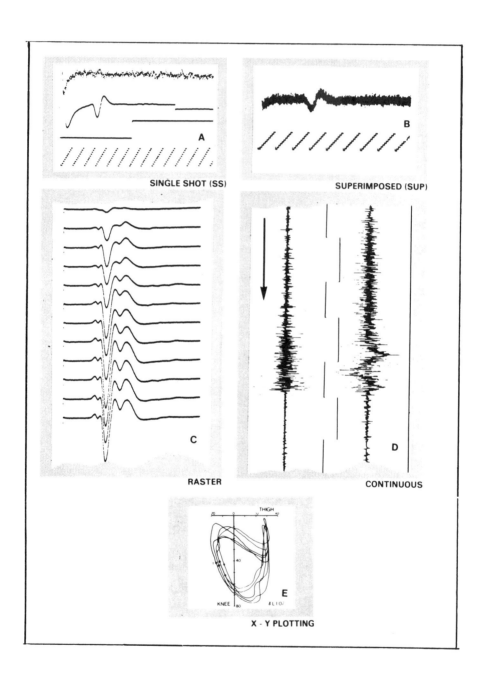

A. SINGLE SHOT (SS)

B. SUPERIMPOSED (SUP)

C. RASTER

D. CONTINUOUS

E. X - Y PLOTTING

Magnetic Recording

EMG potentials may be recorded for later playback on a magnetic tape recorder permitting future visualization, graphic recording, and analysis. The common "analog" or "direct" magnetic recorder, used for speech and music, records on the tape patterns of magnetization that are analogous to the signals being recorded. The magnetic patterns on the tape are converted to electrical signals in the playback process. This type of recorder has adequate high frequency response to reproduce EMG waves, but the 40 or 50 Hz low frequency response limit is inadequate for accurate reproduction of the slow components of long duration action potentials and positive sharp waves. (These slow components are contaminated by their first derivative by the playback process and therefore appear more polyphasic.) Some improvement in performance is obtained by using equipment modified to extend the low frequency response to 20 or 15 Hz.

Instrumentation tape recorders utilize modulation methods whereby the EMG signals cause the frequency of a locally generated constant amplitude alternating voltage to fluctuate. This constant amplitude fluctuating frequency voltage is then recorded magnetically. The information is carried as frequency variations rather than intensity variations of the recorded magnetization patterns on the tape. On playback, these frequency variations are converted to electrical signals. (Pulse-code or pulse-time modulation techniques that are similar are also used.) This system, termed frequency modulation (FM) recording, has no low frequency limitation (it can record unvarying DC potentials), but has limited high frequency performance that can be extended, however, by utilizing higher tape speeds. It can provide good fidelity EMG recordings. FM recorders are more complex and expensive than analog types.

Figure 14.13. Some recording modes possible with CRT or fiber optic recorders are shown. *A,* Single shot record, showing four channels recorded simultaneously. The paper is advanced after each sweep in preparation for the next record. *B,* Superimposed record, showing two channels. The recording paper remains stationary; any desired number of sweeps are superimposed on the record. *C,* Raster record, showing a single channel. The paper is moved as each subsequent sweep is recorded, showing progressive change in the recorded potential. *D,* Continuous record, showing three channels. No electronic sweep is used; continuous movement of the record in the direction of the arrow provides the time axis. *E,* X-Y recording, one channel of information is applied to one axis of deflection, whereas a second related channel is applied to the other. No sweep or time axis is used. Relationships between the signals appear as characteristic looped patterns. These patterns, sometimes called Lissajous patterns, are useful in identifying relationships between related signals. Here the angle of the knee is plotted simultaneously against the angle of the thigh. Five trials are superimposed.

When recording, a sample of known calibration voltage should always be included and noted each time the EMG sensitivity is changed. Doing so permits adjustment of amplitude to known values on playback. An additional speech channel permits recording simultaneous detailed notes during EMG, quite necessary for interpreting potentials during playback.

NOISE AND INTERFERENCE

When small amplitude signals are encountered in EMG, their detection and measurement become difficult because of the obscuring effect of noise. The interfering noise falls into three classes: (a) bioelectric noise, (b) equipment noise, and (c) external noise.

Bioelectric noise, which includes potentials generated within the patient as part of life functions, includes distant muscle activity, e.g., respiration, cardiac, and other sympathetic functions (also distant skeletal activity due to incomplete relaxation or placement of the patient ground or zero potential electrode over a muscle, rather than over a tendon or bony area). These can often be detected by their cyclic nature and minimized somewhat by proper electrode location.

Equipment noise, as discussed earlier, originates in electrodes, movement of lead wires and electrodes, amplifiers, and stimulator (shock artifact). It is minimized by use of proper electrodes, proper maintenance of them and their connectors, and proper electrode technique and by use of filter settings on the amplifier. Also important are the ground-free (isolation) properties of the stimulator, patient preparation, and electrode technique in stimulation.

External noise sources (interference) include a wide range of electrical and electromagnetic influences, the most common being electrostatic induction of power line energy into the patient, by capacitance effect, from the power cords of appliances, or from building power wiring. External noise appears as periodic waves, pulses, or spikes with 16.7 msec (in 60 Hz power areas and 20 msec in 50 Hz areas) periodicities in the EMG record. After making the basic checks for proper equipment grounding and patient ground (or zero potential) electrode connection, the most effective cure is to unplug the offending appliance at the wall outlet. Turning the appliance off does not remove the offending power line voltage from its power cable. All building wiring in the vicinity of the patient should be within grounded metal conduit (required by most electrical codes). This shields the conductors within, substantially eliminating external electrostatic effects that might otherwise induce power line interference into the patient.

Radio frequency (rf) sources are a particularly insidious form of interference. They include entertainment broadcast transmitters in the

AM, FM, and TV bands; public service and CB transmitters; some paging systems; and therapeutic diathermy. These sources can induce potentials in the patient and electrodes that are often much larger than the potentials being recorded. The best defense against these sources is distance. The quasioptical nature of rf waves also makes changes in location in the building useful; a move to a location opposite from the offending transmitter can sometimes help. Interposing grounded metal or mesh screening between the patient and the transmitter can sometimes help, especially if the interference is not too serious. The placement of the ground screen is sometimes capricious—occasionally a shield under and insulated from the patient can be of help.

A six-sided screened enclosure for the EMG, patient, and examiner might be required in serious power line and rf interference situations. Such enclosures should be totally isolated from ground and then electrically grounded to the power line ground at only one point. This avoids circulating ground currents in the conductive shielding, which can result if multiple contacts are made to various grounded objects that are often at slightly different potentials. These circulating ground currents in the screening can result in serious power line interference. Power lines entering such a shielded enclosure might require filters, because rf energy can sometimes travel along power wiring. All wiring and lights within the enclosure must, of course, be shielded. Nearby powerful rf sources make the design of the screened enclosure more difficult and exacting.

The extent to which all sources of noise can be minimized determines the smallest potential that can be reliably recorded. Filtering as a means of reducing noise is limited only to those sources of noise that do not have the same harmonic content as the desired potentials. Only noise that has higher or lower frequency components than the EMG potentials can be filtered. Noise components having the same harmonic content as the EMG cannot be filtered without distorting the EMG wave.

SIGNAL AVERAGING

When very small responses to stimuli are recorded in the presence of random noise, it is possible to detect these responses, by the method of signal averaging, even when each response wave is obscured by noise that has the same harmonic content as the response. Such noise problems occur when recording stimulus-evoked neurograms from deep lying nerves in the presence of pathology and from poorly relaxed patients and when recording stimulus-evoked potentials from the cortex or brainstem via scalp electrodes; in that situation, the spontaneous EEG, in addition to system noise, obscures the response.

A simple early method utilized stimuli repeated as many as 50 times with responses superimposed and photographed from the CRT screen

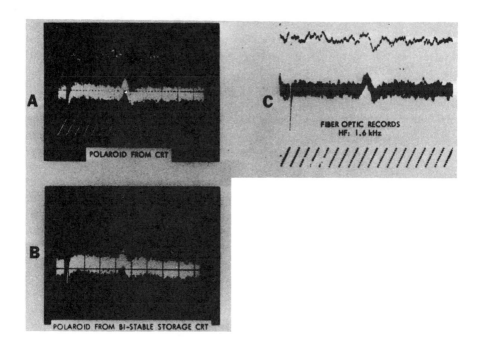

Figure 14.14. Superimposed records. Records were made by stimulating the finger and recording over the ulnar nerve at the elbow with surface electrodes. The downward-going spike wave near the left end of the traces is the stimulus artifact. Amplifier bandwidth is 32 Hz to 3.2 kHz. Calibration waves at the bottom of each record are 5 μV, I msec between peaks. Upper traces are single sweeps; action potentials are difficult to discern from noise. The action potentials are obvious in the lower traces, made by superimposing 25 sweeps. *A,* A Polaroid photograph from a conventional CRT; the camera shutter was held open during the 25 sweeps. *B,* Superimposition was done on the screen of a storage CRT and then photographed. *C,* Record from a fiber optic recorder in the superimposed mode.

(8). Superimposition may also be done on a display storage CRT or on a fiber optic recorder. The effect of superimposition is to enhance the response wave (Fig. 14.14).

A more powerful method, which permits recording and detecting of regularly occurring responses to stimuli more completely obscured by random noise fluctuations, involves adding corresponding time segments of the records of repeated stimuli, instead of superimposing them (7). This technique, termed variously averaging, signal averaging, evoked response averaging, and ensemble averaging, uses a method of summing many repetitive trials that has been long known in other applications to detect systematic fluctuations obscured by larger irregular ones.

Signal averaging is accomplished by dividing each response sweep into a predetermined number of small contiguous samples in time termed "ordinates" or "words." (A sufficiently larger number of samples is chosen so as to describe adequately the shape of the expected response.) The instantaneous amplitude of the signal in each time sample is stored in separate storage elements equal in number to the samples (ordinates). Each store is related to the same time sample in each sweep. As subsequent sweeps are recorded, each storage element accumulates the algebraic sum of the signal amplitudes sampled at its unique time. At the end of the desired number of sweeps, the summed contents of each storage element are read in sequence, and the resulting wave is displayed on screen.

Those storage elements that summed ordinates in time that were only influenced by random noise will have received potentials of random amplitude and polarity, whereas those storage elements that received inputs from ordinates that were located in time so as to be influenced by the response wave and random noise will have received nonrandom potentials reflecting the presence of the response wave potential. The storage elements for the response wave will have significantly greater sums relative to the storage elements influenced by random noise potentials only. When the storage elements are read out in sequence on screen, the resulting response wave will be larger in proportion to the noise by a factor equal to the square root of the number of samples averaged (Fig. 14.15). The response wave obscured by noise on any one sweep will now be visible.

This technique permits visualization of potentials, fractions of a microvolt in amplitude, that are obscured by microvolts of noise. In this form, it can only enhance stimulus-evoked potentials, not random, spontaneously occurring ones (the stimulus may occur randomly). It only discriminates against noise potentials that occur randomly in time with respect to the stimulus.

Artifact or system fluctuations that are synchronized in time with the stimulus should carefully be avoided because they will be enhanced. Even when these fluctuations are very tiny and not obvious, they appear after averaging, along with the desired physiologic response potential, if any. For these reasons, stimulation should not be snychronized with the power line frequency, and the patient should avoid proximity with the CRT to obviate artifact pickup synchronized with the sweep traversing the screen.

Although many technical approaches have been successfully used in the design of averagers, present equipment utilizes electronic sampling and digital techniques for storage, addition, and system control. As few as 100 ordinates are adequate to resolve response waves in many studies; 1000 ordinates or more are often available to provide additional

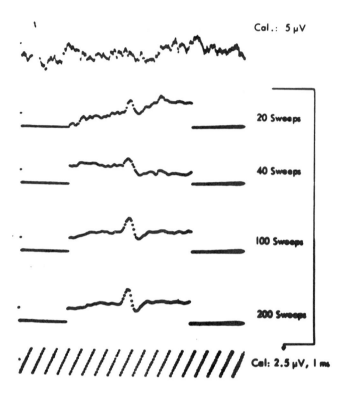

Figure 14.15. Averaged neurograms. The top trace was made by stimulating the finger and recording over the ulnar nerve at the elbow with surface electrodes. Amplifier bandwidth was 32 Hz to 1.6 kHz. Calibration trace at the bottom is 5 μV for the top trace and 2.5 μV for the others. Time is 1 msec between peaks. Spike wave near left end of top trace is the stimulus artifact. The nerve action potential is not discernible in the top trace because of system, external, and bioelectric noise. The lower traces were made by repeated stimulation and signal averaging, 20, 40, 100, and 200 times from the top down, in a 100-ordinate averager. Note the improvement in the response wave as the number of stimuli is initially increased. Less improvement results when stimuli are increased from 100 to 200.

capability. Ordinate duration is adjustable and should be as short as 10 microsec to resolve the fastest potentials. Averagers are often provided with artifact rejection capability that rejects a sweep containing a gross artifact potential, such as patient movement, that would unnecessarily disturb the summation. In addition, sweep counters and indicators monitor the progress of the test and can terminate stimulation at a preset count. Calibrated output is available that normalizes the summing process so that the actual amplitude of the response can be read from the record without calculation. The output averaged wave can, in some units, be multiplied or divided in amplitude or expanded or contracted in time for detailed examination.

Because the averager inherently incorporates storage elements, the output may be read repeatedly and sufficiently frequently so as to present a flicker-free stored trace on screen. It may therefore be arranged as a single sweep storage device to display random transient action potentials on a conventional nonstorage CRT.

DIGITAL PROCESSING

The action potentials that are picked up by the electrodes and then amplified are represented by electrical fluctuations in the EMG apparatus. These continually varying electric currents, capable of an infinite number of values, change in time and amplitude exactly in proportion to the action potentials themselves (within the finite limits of system performance). The electric currents and voltages in the amplifier representing the action potentials are thus analogs of the original quantities. The amplifier is then termed an analog signal processing device, as is a telephone connecting two parties by wire.

Signals can also be transmitted between two points by first coding them into a form that has a finite number of values and then transmitting the code in a form that is not analogous to the signal; finally, at the receiver, the code is converted back to a recognizable analog signal.

Morse code telegraphic transmission of information is an example of a coded transmission process. Digital processing of EMG signals is also a coded processing system. Here the continuously varying signal is first fragmented in time into a series of closely spaced contiguous samples of voltage, each sample being an analog representation of the signal amplitude at an instant in time. The samples are then coded, transmitted (or processed), and then decoded. The decoded series of time samples are then recognizable analog representations of the original signal. They may then be smoothed, if required, to convert the discrete series of time samples into a smooth-appearing continuous wave.

The primary advantage of digital systems, in common with telegraphy, is that the code used can be represented by only two voltage states in the system, e.g., on or off. Signal and logic circuits are reduced to a collection of the equivalent of on-off switches and simple circuits to detect the on-off condition. In contrast, an analog circuit must respond in a linear manner to every subtle change in amplitude of the signal. Noise in an analog system contaminates the signal and establishes the minimum useful signal level. A two-state digital coded system is indifferent to significant amounts of noise so long as the on and off states can be unambiguously detected. Considerable signal processing and manipulation can be done without degenerating the signal in coded systems; this is in contrast to analog systems where each step in signal processing tends to add its toll of system noise.

Quantities can be expressed to a very high resolution, over a wide range, by merely increasing the number of code elements (bits) used to represent them in digital form. This is difficult in analog systems because of the limits imposed by noise and limitations of maximum permissible signal size.

Digital systems are physically more complex than analog systems, especially where long codes of many bits grouped into "words" are required to represent signals to high resolution. The sampling process also puts limitations of speed on the signals that can be represented.

Because each element of the code contains so little information (on-off, yes-no, etc.), many coded elements must be transmitted or manipulated in order to represent magnitudes (numbers) of useful size. This takes time, which becomes a problem when samples occurring as rapidly as 100,000 times a second (as are required to represent a rapidly changing action potential) are to be handled. Therefore, instead of handling the information serially (in sequence) on a single pair of wires, as in analog systems, each element (on-off channel) of the code is handled by its own path in the system and is transmitted and processed simultaneously in most parts of the system. This simultaneous multipath (parallel) processing contributes to the physical complexity of high speed coded systems.

In order to be processed in a digital system, an analog signal must first be sampled repetitively at frequent intervals. The magnitude of each sample is converted to a digital code. The process is called *analog to digital conversion* (A-D conversion). The digital code used must have the capability of representing sufficient discrete voltage levels (quantization levels) in the sampling process to provide the desired accuracy and resolution. At each sample time, the analog signal voltage is measured and represented by the discrete quantization voltage nearest the actual analog voltage at the time of sampling (Fig.14.16).

The effectiveness of the A-D conversion process depends upon the sampling interval being sufficiently short (sampling *rate* sufficiently high) and the quantization levels being sufficiently small and adequate in number (adequate word length) so as to represent accurately the time and amplitude fluctuations of the analog signal. These digital system parameters (sampling rate and word size) must be considered when applying digital systems to EMG potentials.

The quantization levels shown as decimal voltage in Figure 14.16 are converted to a binary code, a numbering system based on two states, represented by zero and 1 in the figure. A four-digit (bit) binary code or word that can represent 16 decimal numbers is shown.

The decimal value of each bit is determined by its location in the four-bit number, just as the value of each digit in the decimal system is determined by its location in the decimal number (units, tens, hun-

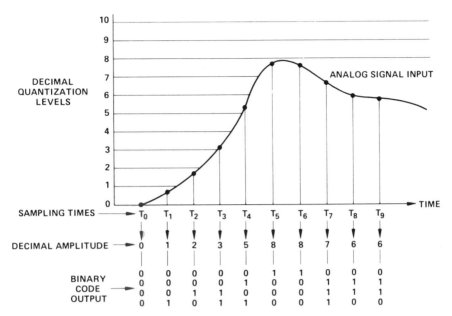

Figure 14.16. Analog to digital conversion. The analog signal represented by the curve varies continuously in time and can assume a potentially infinite number of values. When converted to digital form, the curve is represented by a sequence of digital numbers that can assume a specified limited number of values. These values or quantization levels are represented here in decimal form by the numbers along the ordinate. The instantaneous amplitude of the signal is sampled (measured) repetitively at T_0, T_1, T_2. . . . in time, at a rate sufficiently rapid so as to follow the fastest anticipated changes in the signal with adequate time resolution. Because the amplitude of the signal at each sample can only be represented by one of the discrete quantization levels, the decimal amplitudes shown for the T_1, T_2, T_5, etc., samples represent rounded-off approximations of the signal amplitudes to the nearest quantization level (quantization error). The amplitude value for each sample is then converted to its equivalent binary number for subsequent digital processing. The number of levels that determine the amplitude resolution of the system is determined by the number of bits or word length that characterizes the digital system (see Fig. 14.17). The four-bit binary numbers shown can represent only 16 quantization levels. Eight-bit systems capable of 256 levels are often used to represent EMG waves in digital systems.

dreds, etc.). The bottom bit of the code in the figure and, when more commonly written horizontally, the right hand bit (least significant bit) has the decimal value of 0 or 1 (equivalent to 2^0); the next has a value of 0 or 2 (equivalent to 2^1); the third, 0 or 4 (2^2); and the fourth (most significant bit), 0 or 8 (2^4).

A binary number may be converted to its decimal value by adding the decimal values of each bit that is in the "one" condition. Thus the four-bit binary number 0101 has a decimal value of $0 + 4 + 0 + 1 = 5$.

Number of Binary Bits	Amplitude Resolution[a]	% Full Scale Error[b]
4	16	6.3
5	32	3.1
6	64	1.6
7	128	0.78
8	256	0.39
9	512	0.20
10	1,024	0.10
11	2,048	0.050
12	4,096	0.024
13	8,192	0.012
14	16,384	0.0061
15	32,768	0.0031
16	65,536	0.0015
17	131,072	0.00076
18	262,144	0.00038

[a] Maximum resolution for a binary coded digital system utilizing numbers (words) of binary bit length shown in first column.

[b] Maximum accuracy of such systems expressed as percentage of full scale.

Fig. 14.17. Binary word length and amplitude resolution.

EMG potentials can be adequately represented by eight-bit binary numbers (also termed binary word length) that provide a resolution of 256 levels (Fig. 14.17). Sampling rate should be about 100,000/sec or 10 microsec per sample to ensure an adequate number of samples during rapid positive-to-negative transitions of action potentials that might occur within 100 microsec. The number of words that can be stored depends upon the application. However, devices utilizing as little as 100 words (samples) have been used. The decreasing cost of digital memory has made 1000 words and more increasingly common in dedicated EMG devices. General-purpose computers are provided with fast access memories of tens or hundreds of thousands of words.

Solid State Digital Devices

The advent of transistors and solid state technology has permitted the large number of digital switches called gates, which are major components of digital systems, to be densely packed into compact circuits. The process of large-scale integration (LSI), which permits thousands of these circuits to be photographically constructed on chips of silicon only a few millimeters square, permits even more functions to be built in compact form and at reduced cost. The commercial pressures generated by the proliferation of minicomputers that this technology made possible have made available a growing host of sophisticated, economically attractive digital circuit elements. Although analog methods might be simpler and more direct in concept and circuitry in certain operations because of the economy, compactness, noise immunity, and precision of these devices, digital techniques are increasingly used for signal manipulation, system control and logic operations, mathematical operations on signals, and short term signal storage.

The microprocessor is a class of LSI digital circuit elements that permits flexibility and economy in the design of digital devices. Conventional design and construction of digital devices utilize basic gate and other logic elements uniquely wired into complex circuits to perform the job at hand. The microprocessor, which is a relatively inexpensive subminiature microcomputer, utilizes stored instructions (program) that cause the desired operations to be executed and permit many functions to be accomplished without time-consuming, unique physical circuit design layout and construction. Modifications and changes are easy and inexpensive because they are usually accomplished by simple stored program changes. Microprocessors are used in processing and control functions in home appliances and automobiles and are finding applications in instruments and in EMG equipment.

ELECTRICAL SAFETY

All electrically operated devices present a potential electrical shock hazard. This hazard is minimal when the device is designed to eliminate the possibility of unwanted electrical currents, termed leakage currents, from being unintentionally applied to the patient or operator (stimulation currents are not leakage currents) who contacts the metal case or recording electrodes of the device. The possibility of shock is minimized by providing adequate insulation between the current-carrying parts of the device and those portions of the device that the patient and operator can contact. Active circuits in the device are also designed so that a component failure will not cause leakage current to flow in sufficient magnitude to cause injury. Allowable leakage current and specific measurement methods are specified or are being studied by international standards groups, national government standards groups, professional societies, and private testing laboratories (9, 15, 21–23, 25, 28). Smaller leakage currents are specified for equipment designed and labeled for use on so-called electrically sensitive patients, those who have electrodes or catheters with direct electrical paths to the heart.

Modern building power wiring, according to code and practice in many countries, has one of the two current-carrying wires in the power circuit connected to ground. The ground connection is, in fact, at earth potential, as is (or should be) the metal structure of the building, plumbing, air handling ducts, most metal panels and trim, and all other electrically conductive mechanical parts of the building. This means that the full power voltage (110 volts 60 Hz in the United States, parts of South and Central America, and some other areas; 220 volts 50 Hz in England and parts of Europe and Africa, as well as parts of South and Central America) is available to anyone coming in simultaneous contact with one conductor of the power line and any of the above grounded objects, a potentially lethal situation. This is not likely to occur in a well-designed and maintained appliance. However, due to capacitance effects, the presence of power line wiring within the device and the finite properties of insulation, measurable, small leakage currents can be detected from normally noncurrent-carrying parts of power-line-operated devices when measured to ground. For safety purposes then, the metal frame and enclosure of these devices are solidly connected to ground via a third ground wire included in the power cable, which in turn is grounded by the third ground terminal in the power receptacle. This ground connection, mandatory in most power-line-operated electrical appliances, provides a safe path to ground for these leakage currents and potentially dangerous currents from a fault in the appliance, which would otherwise flow through a grounded subject who touched metal parts of the appliance. A properly grounded power receptacle should always be used, and the power cable and plug should be promptly repaired or replaced if damaged or they show signs of wear.

Some safety standards refer to a so-called first fault test whereby the leakage current flowing in the safety ground connection is measured under specified conditions. This leakage current would flow through a person if the ground connection failed (first fault condition) and must be below a minimum value (50-500 μA). This low leakage current indicates that the insulation separating the power line circuits from accessible parts of the equipment is intact (Fig.14.18).

A "double insulated" class of appliances is constructed with sufficient insulation and spacing between power-line-connected parts and the remainder of the unit as to make contact extremely unlikely; they therefore require no ground connection.

Leakage current measurement and electrical safety acceptance should be made by persons trained and equipped to make the requisite tests. Care should be exercised when connecting accessory electrical devices to the EMG or the patient to ensure that these devices, which may not meet modern leakage standards for medical devices, do not by their interconnection dangerously increase the leakage currents in the system or in the grounded patients.

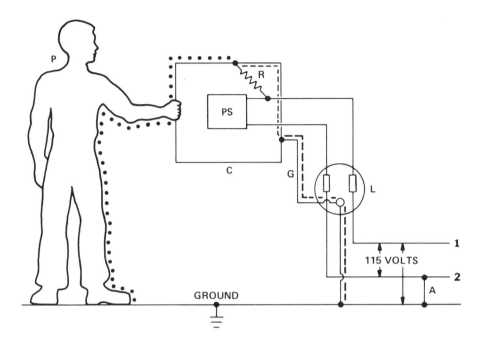

Figure 14.18. Leakage path. *P*, Grounded person; *C*, metal instrument case; *PS*, power line connected circuits of instrument; *R*, leakage path from power line to case; *L*, power line connector; *G*, grounding conductor in power cable. An instrument with metal case *C* (which also includes patient contact electrodes) is connected to the 115 V power line conductors 1 and 2 via its power cable and connector *L*. The instrument case is grounded via a grounding conductor *G* in the power cable, which connects to the power system and building ground via the third prong in the power connector. One side of the power wiring circuit *(2)* is connected according to building code to the building ground at the power distribution point, in the building as shown at *A*. The leakage current path from power line 1 and *PS* to the case *C* through limitations of insulation in the instrument components is represented by *R*. This leakage current can find a return path to line *2* of the power system via ground either through a grounded person, by the dotted path, or through the ground wire *G* in the power cable, by the dashed line path. The grounded wire *G* protects the grounded person *P* because it provides a direct low resistance path for the leakage currents, even if *R* became a low resistance or a short circuit due to a fault; the now dangerous leakage current would flow mainly through *G*, not through *P* because of the much lower resistance of the dashed path through *G*. A routine test for leakage current involves a measurement (under specified conditions) of the normal leakage current that flows in ground wire *G* to ensure that it is below a specified value. Low normal leakage current demonstrates adequate insulation and ensures that innocuous current will flow through *P* if the ground connection *G* should fail.

References

1. Adrian, ED, Bronk DW: The discharge of impulses in motor nerve fibers. Part II. *J Physiol* 67: 119, 1929.
2. *Basic Aspects of the Safety Philosophy of Electrical Equipment Used in Medical Practice,* IEC #513, International Electrotechnical Commission, Geneva 20.
3. Basmajian JV, Stecko G: A new bipolar electrode for electromyography. *J Appl Physiol* 17: 849, 1962.
4. Buchthal F, Guld C, Rosenfalck P: Volume conduction of the spike of the motor unit potential investigated with a new type of multielectrode. *Acta Physiol Scand* 38: 331, 1957.
5. Brown PB, Maxfield BW, Moraff H: *Electronics for Neurobiologists.* Cambridge, MIT Press, 1973.
6. Clifford M: *Basic Electricity and Beginning Electronics No. 628.* Summit, PA, Tab Books, 1973.
7. Dawson GD: A summation technique for the detection of small evoked potentials. *Electroencephalogr Clin Neurophysiol* 6: 65, 1954.
8. Dawson GD, Scott JW: The recording of nerve action potentials through the skin in man. *J Neurol Neurosurg Psychiat* 12: 259, 1949.
9. *Electricity In Patient Care Facilities,* 76B7, National Fire Protection Association, Boston, MA 02210.
10. *Electro-Medical Equipment, CSA Standard C22.2 No. 125,* Canadian Standards Association, Rexdale, Ontario #M9W 1R3.
11. Fleck H: Action potentials from single motor units in human muscle. *Arch Phys Med Rehab* 43: 99, 1962.
12. Gajduser DC, et al: Precautions in medical care of, and in handling materials from, patients with transmissable virus dementia (Creutzfeldt-Jacob disease). *N. Engl J Med* 297: 1253, 1977.' Letters, *N Engl J Med,* 298: 976, 1978.
13. Garuts V, Samuels C.: Measuring conventional oscilloscope noise. *Tekscope* 1: 2, 1969, Tektronix, Inc., Beaverton, Ore.
14. Geddes, LA: *Electrodes and the Measurement of Bioelectric Events,* New York, John Wiley & Sons, 1972.
15. *Good Manufacturing Practices,* Food and Drug Administration, Silver Spring, Md. 20910.
16. Jasper H, Ballem G: Unipolar electromyograms of normal and denervated human muscle. *J Neurophysiol,* 12: 231, 1949.
17. Leach P: *Basic Electric Circuits,* New York, John Wiley & Sons, 1969.
18. Nightingale A: *Physics and Electronics in Physical Medicine,* New York, Macmillan, 1959.
19. Nissen-Peterson H, Guld C, Buchthal F: A delay line to record random action potentials. *Electroencephalogr Clin Neurophysiol,* 26: 100, 1969.
20. Pollak V: The waveshape of action potentials recorded with different types of EMG needles. *Med Biol Engl,* 9: 657, 1971.
21. *Safe Current Limits Standard, SCL 12-78,* AAMI, Association for the Advancement of Medical Instrumentation, Arlington, Va. 22209.
22. *Safety Code for Electro-Medical Apparatus. Hospital Technical Memorandum No. 8,* Department of Health and Social Security, London, Revised 1969.
23. *Safety Of Electrical Equipment Used In Medical Practice,* IEC Standard IEC 601-1 1978, International Electrotechnical Commission, Geneva 20.
24. Stalberg E, Ekstedt J: Single fibre EMG for the study of the microphysiology of human muscle. In Desmedt JE (ed): *New Developments in Electromyography and Clinical Neurophysiology,* vol. 1. Basel, Karger, 1973, pp 89-112.

25. *Standard For Medical and Dental Equipment,* UL 544, Underwriters Laboratory, Inc. Melville, N.Y. 11746.
26. Suckling EE: *Bioelectricity,* New York, McGraw-Hill, 1961.
27. Technical factors in recording electrical activity of muscle and nerve in man. Report of Committee on EMG Instrumentation, IFSECN, 1969. *Electroencephalogr Clin Neurophysiol,* 28: 399, 1970.
28. Whitfield IC: *An Introduction to Electronics for Physiological Workers,* New York, Macmillan, 1953.

Glossary of Terms

Stuart Reiner

Active Elements. Components of a circuit that provide amplification or that control direction of current flow; for example, diodes, transistors, and vacuum tubes.

Address. In digital data storage systems, the description of a location (stated in system notation) where information is stored. Also, as a verb, to select or designate the location of information in a storage system.

Alternating Current (AC). A flow of current in which the direction of current flow reverses periodically. When the reversal occurs cyclically, two current reversals are termed one cycle. The number of complete cycles per second is the frequency, and it is stated in Hertz.

Amplifier. A device that multiplies its input voltage, current, or power by a fixed or controllable factor, usually without altering its waveform.

Amplifier, AC. Responds to alternating current (AC) signals only and not to an input potential that does not vary. This type of amplifier is used in EMG apparatus. Sometimes termed RC or AC-coupled amplifier.

Amplifier, DC (or Direct Coupled). Responds to direct current (DC) signals, pulsating DC, and alternating current signals. This type of amplifier is not used in clinical EMG. It is used in force and tension measurements, as well as in the recording of intracellular resting potentials where fixed, slowly, and rapidly changing phenomena are measured.

Amplifier, Differential. Used in EMG preamplifiers. It has two recording electrode input terminals (instead of the single input terminal of a conventional amplifier) and a ground or zero-potential terminal. It rejects unwanted potentials originating at a distance and presenting at both input terminals (common-mode or in-phase potentials).

Amplitude Modulation (AM). Systems of signal transmission, recording, or processing that utilize an alternating current carrier potential of peak amplitude that varies proportionally with the instantaneous amplitude of the signal.

Analog. Applied to signals and devices capable of or accommodating continuous change and assuming an infinite number of values with finite limits. An analog signal may be a current or a voltage that varies in time continuously, simulating a natural phenomenon that it represents.

Analog-to-Digital Converter (A/D Converter). A device that converts an analog signal, usually a varying voltage or current, to digital output (See *Digital System.)*

Anode. A positive terminal. The terminal through which "electron current" enters a device. "Conventional current" flow, however, is said to be away from the anode and toward the cathode (opposite or negative) terminal.

Artifact. All unwanted potentials that originate outside the tissues examined. They are also called "noise" when they appear in measurement. An artifact may arise from biologic activity, the electrode or apparatus used in the examination, the power line, or extrinsic electricity (surrounding the apparatus or patient). (See *Noise.)*

Attenuator. In electrical circuits, an arrangement that introduces a definite reduction in the magnitude of a voltage current or power. Attenuators may be fixed or adjustable continuously or in steps.

Averager Signal. A signal processing method that aids in the recording of small stimulus evoked potentials that are obscured by noise or artifact. The stimulus is repeated a number of times, and the responses are subjected to a special summation technique that causes the random noise portion of the response to become smaller in proportion to the evoked potentials that are coherent in time with each stimulus.

Beam Switching. A technique for producing a multitrace display on a single beam cathode ray tube by rapidly commutating the beam to a number of signal sources. This system is also called *chopped display* and *electron switched display.*

Bias. A fixed electrical or mechanical input to a device or a system that is distinct from the input signal. The bias brings the system to a desired operating range.

Binary Coded Decimal (BCD). A binary numbering system coding decimal numbers in groups of four bits for each decimal digit.

Binary Logic. A digital logic system that operates with two distinct states variously called "one and zero," "high and low," and "on and off."

Bit. A binary numeral, the "one and zero" or "high and low," and so on, of binary logic. A group of bits comprise a binary word.

Blocking. An effect that results when a large transient input potential is applied to an amplifier, temporarily causing the disappearance or severe distortion of the output signal.

Calibrator. A device that identifies units of measurement by reference to a known standard.

Calibrator, Amplitude. An accurate source of voltage of known amplitude, usually within the range of EMG motor activity—for example, between 10 and 1,000 μv—that can be applied or switched to the input terminals of the apparatus.

Calibrator, Time. An alternating or pulsatile waveform of accurately known frequency that can be applied to the cathode ray display of an EMG so as to permit accurate adjustment of "time per division" on the horizontal graticule scale of the EMG screen.

Capacitance. A measure of electric charge that can be stored within the insulation separating two conductors when a given voltage is applied to the conductors. A capacitor or a condenser uses conductors of large surface area separated by air or by various insulators (dielectrics) that enhance capacitative effects. The unit capacitance is the farad. Direct current is not conducted by capacitors; alternating current or pulsating direct current signals are conducted to an extent proportional to frequency.

Carrier. A potential, usually alternating current, of sine or pulse waveform used in signal transmission or recording or processing systems that in itself carries no information, but is modified most commonly in amplitude (amplitude modulation), frequency (frequency modulation), or timing by the signal. The carrier is at least a number of times higher in frequency than the highest frequency component in the signal.

Cathode. A negative terminal. The terminal through which "electron current" leaves a device. Conventional current flow is said to be toward the cathode or away from the anode (positive) terminal.

Cathode Ray Tube (CRT). A vacuum tube used to visualize electrical waveforms. It generates X-Y traces on its screen by means of a moving fluorescent spot on its screen.

Clipping (Limiting). Occurs when signals of excessive amplitude are applied to an amplifier, with a resultant waveform at the amplifier output that faithfully reproduces the shape of the input waveform only up to a level at which the signal becomes excessive (clipping level). All portions of the waveform that exceed the clipping level appear at the output at a fixed level unvarying with time and are therefore seriously distorted.

Common Mode Rejection. An important property of differential amplifiers that expresses their ability to discriminate against artifact potentials that appear equally at both amplifier input terminals (common mode signals) and to amplify the desired potentials (differential or series-mode signals) that appear as different signals at the two input terminals.

Commutation. A system that cyclically switches a number of signals sequentially to a single device amplifier, transmission, or recording channel. Also termed multiplexing.

Conduction Time Indicator. A moveable time index on the trace of the cathode ray tube that is arranged to be positioned on the screen by a dial accurately calibrated in time, measured either from the start of the sweep or from a shock artifact to the index position.

Crosstalk. The incursion of information from one channel into any other channel of a multichannel information-handling system. The presence of crosstalk in a multichannel EMG study can be seriously misleading.

Cycle. A complete sequence of values of an alternating quantity repeated as a unit. CPS—cycles per second, called Hertz.

Decibel (dB). A dimension-less unit for comparing the ratio of signal levels on a logarithmic scale. Positive decibel values represent a signal increase with respect to a reference. Negative decibel values represent signal decrement with respect to a reference signal.

Delay Line. A short-term electrical dynamic storage device that delays potentials applied to its input so that they appear at its output as if they had occurred (1–20 msec) later in time. This permits events preceding action potentials to be seen on the cathode ray tube screen when the sweeps are triggered by the potentials.

Differentiator. A device or circuit with an output waveform that is proportional to the rate of change (speed, velocity, etc.) of the input waveform.

Digital System. A system or circuit for handing or processing information in terms of numbers and utilizing circuits that operate in the manner of switches, having two (on-off) or more discrete positions. The simplest and most common digital system is the binary system.

Digital-to-Analog Converter (D/A Converter). A circuit that accepts the discrete coded signal voltages of a digital system and generates, at its output, voltages of amplitudes analogous to the numbers represented by the digital codes at its input. The analog output may then be directly interpreted by viewing a cathode ray tube, on a meter, or by graphic recording.

Diode. A two-terminal device that permits the flow of electric current in one direction only.

Direct Current (DC). A unidirectional current. An intermittent or time-varying current that has a net flow in one direction is called pulsating direct current or direct current with an alternating current component.

Dynamic Range. The ratio of the maximum input signal capability of a system without overloading to the minimum usable signal (noise level).

Electrode. A conductor of electricity. In clinical electrodiagnosis, it is generally a metal device that introduces or picks up electricity from tissue.

Electrodes, Recording. Electrodes used to measure electrical activity from tissue.

Bipolar, Bifilar Needle Electrodes. Variations in voltage are measured between the bared tips of two insulated wires cemented side by side in a steel cannula. The bare tips of the electrodes are flush with the bevel of the cannula. The latter may be grounded.

Concentric Needle Electrode. Variations in voltage are measured between the bare tip of an insulated wire, usually stainless steel, silver, or platinum, and the bare shaft of a steel cannula through which it is inserted. The bare tip of the central wire (exploring electrode) is flush with the bevel at the end of the cannula (reference electrode).

Monopolar Needle Electrode. A solid wire, usually stainless steel, coated except at its tip with an insulating varnish or plastic. Variations in voltage between the tip of the needle (exploring electrode) in the muscle and a metal plate on the skin surface or bare needle in subcutaneous tissue (reference electrode) are measured.

Multilead Electrode. Three or more insulated wires inserted through a common steel cannula have their bared tips arranged linearly at an aperture in the wall of the cannula that is parallel with its axis, the bare tips being flush with the outer circumference of the cannula.

Surface Electrodes. Metal plate or pad electrodes placed on the skin surface should be described (material, size, and separation).

(From the report of the subcommittee of the Pavia Committee on Terminology on Electromyography presented at the International Meeting on Electromyography, Glascow, June 29-July 1, 1967. Reprinted in *Electroencephalogr Clin Neurophysiol* 26:224, 1969.)

EMG Analyzer. A term applied to a wide range of EMG computer processing techniques that attempt to display one or a number of attributes of the EMG waveform in a more explicit manner than the conventional voltage-time graph of the usual EMG trace.

Feedback. An effect that occurs when a portion of the output of a system or a circuit is connected back to the input. When the fed-back signal reinforces the original input, the feedback is positive; when the fed-back signal tends to reduce the input signal, the feedback is negative.

Negative feedback acts to stabilize the performance of electronic instrument systems and to make the operation and calibration of such systems stable and independent of changes in many of the system components.

Positive feedback appears in oscillating circuits. Unintentional positive feedback occurs, for example, when a microphone, which is the input to an amplification systems, is brought too close to the loud-speaker output. When this occurs, positive feedback often produces an oscillatory howl. Similar undesirable positive feedback may occur when the input electrodes of an EMG system are brought too close to the loudspeaker output or the cathode ray tube output of an EMG system.

Filter. In an EMG system, circuits usually comprised of capacitors and resistors that modify or adjust the high and low frequency limits of the amplifier frequency response curve.

Frequency. The rate in cycles per second that an alternating current signal alternates. The unit of frequency is the Hertz.

Frequency Analyzer. Analyzes the EMG to produce a spectrum of sine wave frequencies (harmonics) that will uniquely describe the original EMG waveform.

Frequency Modulation (FM). Systems of signal transmission, recording, or processing that utilize a constant amplitude carrier potential with instantaneous frequency proportional to the instantaneous amplitude of the signal.

Frequency Response. Describes the speed range (slowest to fastest) of potential waveform changes that will be displayed by the EMG apparatus. Stated as a range (band) of frequencies of sine wave test signals for which the amplification will be uniform. Amplification decreases progressively for sine wave test signals at frequencies above and below the frequency response band. The frequency between the lower and upper frequency is called the bandwidth. The amplifier frequency response bandwidth is often defined by two frequencies, one at the low end and the other at the high end, where the amplification falls to 70% of its midband value.

Gain. The increase at the output of an amplifier in voltage, current, or power of the signal applied to its input is called the amplifier voltage, current or power gain, or amplification.

Gate. A circuit used in digital systems as decision elements and having two or more inputs and one output. The output depends upon the combination of digital states of the signals at the input. A gate circuit in an analog system acts like a switch that permits or stops the flow of signals. The gate opens or closes in response to a control voltage (or gating signal).

Graticule. The ruled scale on the face of the cathode ray tube. Time and voltage display calibrations are usually adjusted with reference to the X and Y rulings on the graticule.

Ground. The lowest potential reference terminal in a system. In power distribution systems, a terminal that is usually physically connected to a conductor in intimate contact with the earth. Sometimes referred to as the earth terminal. Frame and chassis portions of electrical systems are almost always connected to ground to avoid the possibility of their assuming other random potentials that might be either dangerous or cause electrical interference within the system.

Ground Loop. The condition that sometimes exists when the ground connections of two interconnected electronic instruments or circuits are not at the same potential. This may result in power line interference.

Hertz (Hz). Cycles per second.

Impedance. Hindrance to electrical current flow in an alternating current circuit; hence, comparable in simplified terms to resistance in direct current circuits. It includes the effects of resistance, capacitance, inductance, and frequency.

Integrated EMG. The integrated EMG is a time-varying potential with instantaneous amplitude equal to the total area (voltage × time) accumulated from a designated start point under an EMG waveform. It provides a measure of total electrical activity.

Interface. An expression or device that embodies all technical considerations in interconnecting two portions of a system, such as proper mating connectors, shielding of connecting leads, establishment of compatible voltage and impedance levels, and such problems as ground loops.

Interference. Generally applied to unwanted signals outside the system. Power line frequency is most common. (See *Artifact.*)

Linear Circuit. A circuit, the output of which is congruent with its input, with the exception of possible amplification or attenuation.

Microphonics. An effect noted in sensitive electronic systems and their connecting cables, where incidental mechanical vibration applied to portions of the system gives rise to spurious electrical outputs.

Noise. Any potential other than that being measured. Commonly applied to spurious potentials originating within the apparatus of electrodes. (See *Artifact, Interference, Root Mean Square Voltage.*)

Off Line. Any signal or data processing function that is deferred with respect to the original recording or generation of signal or data.

On Line. Any signal or data processing function that occurs simultaneously with the original recording or generation of the signal or data.

Overload. A general condition in which the input to an amplifier circuit is so large as to exceed the capability of the circuit to perform its intended function.

Parallel. Circuit elements connected in parallel (as contrasted to series) are all subjected to the same voltage. The current flow to elements connected in parallel is inversely proportional to the impedance (resistance) of the elements. The word "shunt" is sometimes used to refer to parallel connections. In digital systems, parallel refers to a technique of transmission, storage, or logical operation on all bits of binary data words simultaneously using separate facilities. (See also *Serial.*)

Parameter. Any specific characteristic of a device. When considered together, all the parameters of a device describe its operation or its physical characteristics.

Peak-to-Peak Voltage (or Current). A statement of the magnitude of an alternating voltage (or current). It is the total excursion from the most negative peak of the wave to the most positive peak of the wave.

Polarity Sense, Display. Many neurophysiologic records are published with an upward deflection denoting a negative potential on the active electrode. Engineering convention dictates an upward deflection for a positive potential.

Polarization. Electrolytic effects that occur at the metal-tissue interface of electrodes that increase the resistance of the junction and give rise to direct current potentials (which may fluctuate) that can be many times larger than EMG potentials.

Potential, Action. The voltage that results from activity of muscle or nerve. It can be spontaneous, volitional, or evoked by stimulation. Action potentials may be named for their appearance (high frequency, positive sharp, biphasic, monophasic, polyphasic, tetraphasic, triphasic) or their origin (endplate, fasciculation, fibrillation, motor unit, muscle, nerve). The term potential is also used to refer to action potential.

Preamplifier. The first stage or stages of an EMG amplifier system. It must have a high input impedance, common mode rejection, and low noise, as well as a large dynamic range.

Pulse. A signal of very short duration. It can be described according to its characteristic rise, duration, and decay.

Raster. A predetermined pattern of lines generated on a cathode ray tube (CRT) display that provides uniform coverage of an area. Also, the display on the CRT screen of an EMG where each successive sweep is displayed below or above the previous sweep, thus permitting the observer to see more information on the screen than is possible when successive sweeps are superimposed (same baseline). Also, a similar mode of graphic recording.

Rectifier Circuit. A circuit utilizing unidirectional current flow properties of diodes that convert an alternating current into a pulsating direct current.

Resistance. A property of matter to hinder the flow of electric current. Resistance is expressed in ohms and is derived by dividing the voltage impressed by the current that flows. Resistance (R) = Voltage (E), divided by the Current (I).

Ringing. A short duration, transient, usually low amplitude, damped oscillation that occurs in the output of certain electronic circuits, especially some filters, wideband amplifiers, and certain delay lines, immediately after the input wave suddenly changes in amplitude.

Rise Time. Used in describing rectangular pulses and square waveforms or amplifiers or circuits transmitting them. Rise time is the elapsed interval between the time at which the amplitude of the rapidly changing transition part of the wave reaches specified percentages of its lower and upper limits. The rise time of an amplifier is a function of its high frequency response.

Root Mean Square (RMS) Voltage or Current. The root mean square value is a means of stating numerically the magnitude of an alternating voltage or current. It equals a direct current that has the same heating effect in a resistor as an alternating current of the same RMS magnitude.

Semiconductor. A material that exhibits relatively high resistance in a pure state but much lower resistance when minute amounts of impurities are added.

Serial. A term applied to digital circuits where each bit is acted upon sequentially. (See *Parallel.*).

Series. Electrical components are in series when they are so connected that a common current flows through each of them. (See *Parallel.*)

Shield. Shielding. An electrostatic shield is an electrically conductive sheath or an enclosure not in contact with the circuit or device shielded. It is comprised of electrically conductive material connected directly to ground or by a low impedance to ground. It is used to prevent undesirable capacitive coupling of external voltages to the elements within the shield (or to contain potentials within the shield).

Magnetic shielding requires an enclosure of iron or other magnetically permeable alloys and provides protection against interference from magnetic fields that surround nearby current-carrying conductors or permanent magnets.

Signal. Any potential, waveform, or intelligence that is communicated, detected, transmitted, or processed with a system. It is usually in the form of a voltage or current within the system.

Silence, Electrical. The absence of signals from the tissues being studied.

Solid State. Electronic devices utilizing semiconductors. Electric currents, as well as light, heat, and magnetic fields, may interact in solid state devices. The transistor and integrated circuit are solid state devices.

Stabilized Current or Voltage Generator. A source of direct current or alternating current or voltage in which the output current or voltage remains at a predetermined, usually adjustable value independent of wide variations of load resistance or impedance or of variations of power supply voltages. The stabilized current source exhibits wide fluctuations in output voltage in response to changing load conditions, whereas the stabilized voltage source exhibits wide variations in output current in response to load changes.

Stimulator, Ground Free (Isolated). Used in nerve conduction studies to minimize stimulus artifact. Ground free stimulus output circuit has no connection to the common system ground, thereby removing a possible path for injection of undesirable artifact via the patient to the EMG amplifier input terminals.

Storage, Display. A means for retaining, usually on the screen of a cathode ray tube, a transient waveform for study or analysis, together with a means for erasing such information to permit the storage of new data. Such storage can be accomplished by means of special cathode ray tubes (CRTs) that have in addition to other design features, special screens with electrostatic storage surfaces that store the desired waveform as a pattern of electric charges on their surfaces. The pattern is then visualized by flooding the storage screen with an unfocused beam of electrons that pass through the storage screen and strike the phosphor screen on the face of the CRT only at those points where charge was stored. Transient waveforms may also be displayed on conventional CRTs by electrically storing the transient wave in some signal storage means, such as digital storage circuits or magnetic recording systems. The signal is then displayed by rapid, repetitive read-out of the storage device and superimposed display on a conventional CRT.

Strain Gauge. An electrical transducer that generates or modifies an electrical signal proportional to a mechanical deformation due to application of a mechanical load.

Strain Relief. Mechanical restraint, usually applied to the jacket of insulated cables where they join fixed mechanical assemblies or where they join connectors or other terminations, especially where the cable might be subjected to repeated flexing or mechanical stress. The purpose of the strain relief is to minimize the possibility of failure of the electrical conductors within the cable or connector.

Sweep. The horizontal (X axis) linear time axis of a cathode ray tube display generated by the left-to-right movement of the trace spot at constant preselected speeds across the face of the cathode ray tube. Sweep velocities are usually specified in reciprocals of speed: time per division on the graticule.

Telemetry. The transmission of data, typically from preamplifiers located on a subject (free to move about the laboratory) via a radio link to a receiver and then to the remainder of the recording system.

Time Constant. A factor that is an index to a speed with which voltage and currents respond to changes in the input to resistor-capacitor circuits. This term is used to describe the dynamic performance of EMG amplifiers (which contain resistor-capacitor coupling networks).

Time Scale, Electronic. A discontinuous waveform, usually short pulses, spaced in time at 1 msec, 0.1 msec, or some other convenient time interval, applied to a trace of a cathode ray tube along with the EMG information to provide an independent timing reference.

Trace. The line of light on the face of a cathode ray tube generated by the moving spot of light, which is generated by the electron beam striking the phosphor-coated screen.

Transducer. A device that changes the energy form applied to its input to another form of energy at its output, such that a proportionality exists between input and output. Transducers include loudspeakers, microphones, strain gauges, and photocells.

Transistor. An active semiconductor device used as an amplifier or switching device.

Trigger. A short pulse used to initiate some action within an electronic system. Also used as a verb. (See *Sweep.*)

Wave. A generic term loosely applied to a time-varying voltage, current, or other quantity, the amplitude of which varies with time.

Z Axis Modulation (Intensity Modulation). Applies to cathode ray displays where information is applied to the beam-generating electrodes so as to vary instantaneously the brightness of the trace during the course of the sweep.

appendix

II

Practical Examination

ERNEST W. JOHNSON

This test evaluates one's understanding of needle EMG and peripheral evoked potentials. Each question illustrates a principle, which is explained in the Answers section of this appendix.

Each question has only *one* correct answer.

1. In which of the below conditions was this likely recorded?
   a) myotonic dystrophy
   b) chronic polymyositis
   c) progressive spinomuscular atrophy
   d) myasthenia gravis
   e) normal muscle
2. What is firing rate of the electrical activity in top trace?
   a) 10 Hz
   b) 30 Hz
   c) 60 Hz
   d) 90 Hz
   e) 105 Hz

CALIBR: Each slanted line = 10 msec
Height = 50 µV
Monopolar needle in abductor pollicis brevis

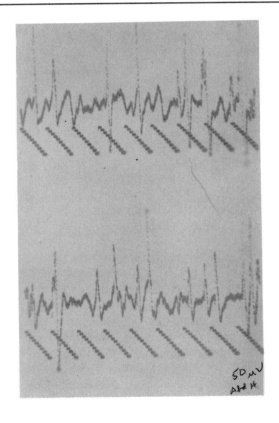

3. What is the explanation for this data?
   a) supramaximal stimulation with volume conduction abductor digiti
   b) Duchenne muscular dystrophy
   c) accessory peroneal nerve
   d) Guillain-Barré syndrome
   e) normal

4. Calculate the residual latency (distance; 8 cm).
   a) 1 msec
   b) 2 msec
   c) 3 msec
   d) 4 msec
   e) cannot calculate with data presented

CALIBR: Each slanted line = 10 msec
Height = 1 millivolt
Surface record over extensor digiti brevis
***Top trace:* Stimulate posterior medial malleolus**
***Middle trace:* Stimulate anterior lateral ankle**
***Bottom trace:* At fibular head**
Distance Between proximal and distal stimulation: 32 cm

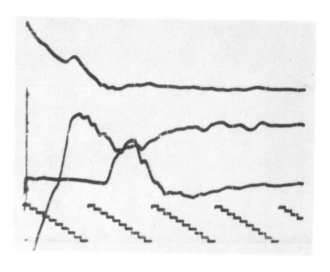

5. What is the likely diagnosis?

    a) mild carpal tunnel syndrome

    b) severe "acute" carpal tunnel syndrome

    c) severe chronic carpal tunnel syndrome

    d) moderate diabetic neuropathy

    e) normal

6. Calculate the radial sensory conduction velocity (peak).

    a) 30 m/sec

    b) 35 m/sec

    c) 40 m/sec

    d) 45 m/sec

    e) 50 m/sec

CALIBR: Each slanted line = I msec
Height = 10 μV
Ring recording electrodes over
thumb; stimulate antidromic
10 cm proximal
Top trace: **Anterior lateral**
wrist stimulation
Middle trace: **Median nerve**
Bottom trace: **Radial nerve**

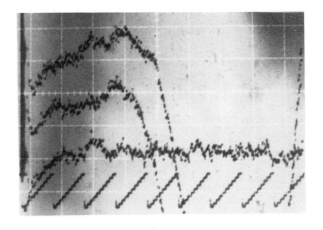

7. In which of the following conditions was this likely recorded?
   a) ALS, acute
   b) benign fasciculations
   c) Charcot-Marie-Tooth disease
   d) acute C5 radiculopathy
   e) normal
8. What is the firing rate, assuming that the figure provides all the data?
   a) 1 Hz
   b) 5 Hz
   c) 10 Hz
   d) 20 Hz
   e) 50 Hz

CALIBR: Each slanted line = 10 msec
Height = 1 millivolt
Monopolar needle electrode
in rhomboid

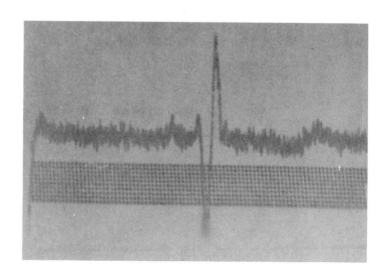

9. What is the electrical activity?

    a) cramp

    b) MEPP

    c) endplate spikes

    d) noise

    e) interference

10. How could this electrical activity be stopped?

    a) Move the electrode to another muscle.

    b) Turn off the fluorescent lights.

    c) Unplug the incandescent light.

    d) Turn off the radio.

    e) Add electrode paste to the ground electrode.

CALIBR: Monopolar needle in vastus medialis

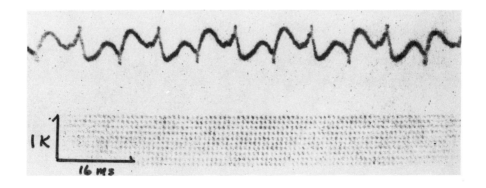

1 K

16 ms

11. In which of the below conditions would this likely be recorded?
    a) acute S1 radiculopathy (S/P 10 days)
    b) acute polymyositis
    c) Type II muscle atrophy
    d) ALS, chronic
    e) none of the above
12. What is the origin of this?
    a) endplate noise
    b) cramp
    c) motor unit potentials in radiculopathy
    d) myotonic reaction
    e) ephaptic activation of single muscle fibers

CALIBR: Each slanted line = 10 msec
Height = 50 μV
Monopolar needle electrode in soleus

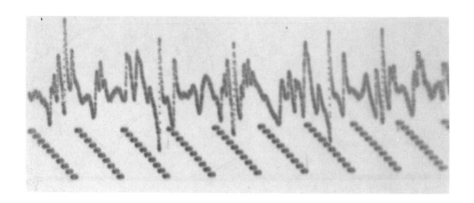

13. In which of the below conditions was this likely recorded?
    a) acute S2 radiculopathy (S/P 10 days)
    b) facioscapulohumeral muscular dystrophy
    c) Type II muscular atrophy
    d) chronic S2 radiculopathy
    e) none of the above
14. What is the origin of the electrical activity?
    a) MEPP
    b) fasciculations
    c) endplate spike
    d) spontaneous single muscle fiber discharge
    e) artifact

CALIBR: Each square = 5 msec
Each square = 25 μV
Monopolar needle electrode in
most caudal aspect of
paraspinal

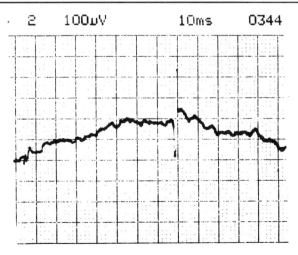

2   100μV   10ms   0344

15. What condition is suggested by the traces?
    a) right S1 radiculopathy
    b) left S1 radiculopathy
    c) Guillain-Barré syndrome (early)
    d) diabetic peripheral neuropathy (mild)
    e) normal
16. Which one of the answers below describes the H reflex?
    a) orthodromic afferent and efferent
    b) antidromic afferent and efferent
    c) orthodromic afferent and antidromic efferent
    d) antidromic afferent and orthodromic efferent
    e) none of the above

CALIBR: Each slanted line = 10 msec
Height = 1 millivolt
Surface recording electrodes
over soleus. Sistance medial
malleolus to
Tibial nerve stimulation at
popliteal space.
Top: **right**
Bottom: **left**

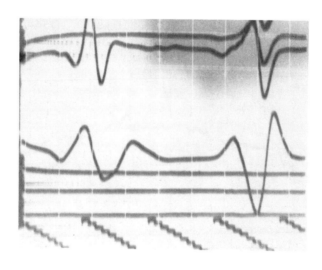

17. In which of the below conditions was this likely recorded?
    a) normal
    b) C8 radiculopathy (S/P 10 days)
    c) carpal tunnel syndrome, chronic
    d) Type II muscle atrophy
    e) myotonic dystrophy

18. What is the origin of the electrical activity?
    a) denervated muscle fiber
    b) hyperirritable muscle fiber
    c) spontaneously discharging motor unit
    d) normal single muscle fiber
    e) none of the above

CALIBR: Each slanted line = 10 msec
Height = 50 μV
Monopolar electrode in abductor
pollicis brevis

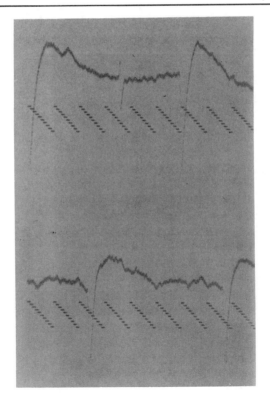

19. In which of the below conditions would this likely be recorded?
    a) Type II muscle atrophy
    b) acute radiculopathy L4 (S/P 5 days)
    c) ALS
    d) facioscapulohumeral muscular dystrophy
    e) none of the above
20. Which of the muscles below usually receive motor fibers from C6?
    a) flexor carpi radialis; pronator teres
    b) abductor pollicus longus; supinator
    c) extensor carpi radialis brevis; biceps brevis
    d) rhomboid; infraspinatus
    e) none of the above

CALIBR: ON PHOTO
Monopolar needle in anterior tibial

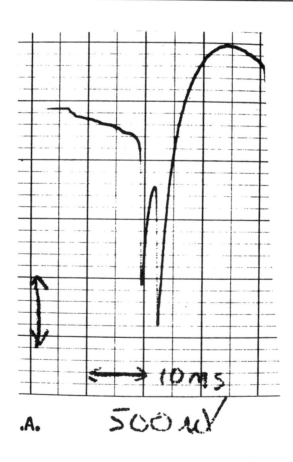

.A.   500 uV

21. In which of the below conditions was this likely recorded?
    a) Type II muscle atrophy
    b) facioscapulohumeral muscular dystrophy
    c) L4 radiculopathy
    d) acute polymyositis
    e) femoral nerve injury (S/P 21 days)
22. Note closely the shape of the negative component of the most numerous potentials. What can you infer about the filter settings?
    a) high frequency filter interposed (pass 1000 Hz and below)
    b) low frequency filter interposed (pass 100 Hz and above)
    c) filters permit 10 Hz–10 KHz
    d) low frequency filter interposed (pass 500 Hz and above)
    e) amplifier open (i.e., no filters)

CALIBR: 60 Hz sawtooth
Monopolar needle in vastus
medialis

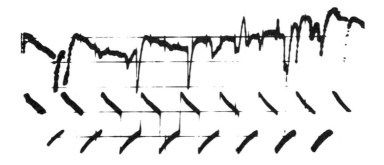

23. What is the electrical activity?
    a) endplate spikes
    b) myotonic discharge
    c) cramp
    d) MEPP
    e) none of the above
24. What is the firing rate?
    a) 50 Hz
    b) 100 Hz
    c) 150 Hz
    d) 200 Hz
    e) 250 Hz

**CALIBR: Each slanted line = 10 msec
Height = 100 μV
Monopolar needle electrode in
abductor digiti
quinti**

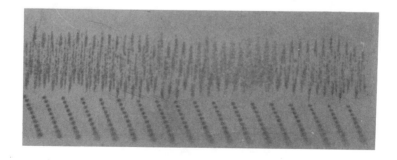

25. What condition can you infer from the data?
    a) chronic block of the ulnar nerve at the elbow
    b) acute (neurapraxic) block at the elbow
    c) moderate diabetic (axonal) peripheral neuropathy
    d) Guillain-Barré syndrome
    e) normal
26. Note the shape of the M response. What accounts for it?
    a) recording electrodes not over motor point
    b) submaximal stimulation
    c) anomalous innervation
    d) recording electrode over motor point of two adjacent muscles
    e) none of the above

CALIBR: Each slanted line = 1 msec
Height = 2 millivolts
Surface electrodes over
abductor digiti quinti
Top trace: **Stimulate above elbow**
Middle trace: **Stimulate below elbow**
Bottom trace: **Stimulate at wrist**
Distance: Below elbow to wrist: 25 cm
Above elbow to below elbow: 15 cm

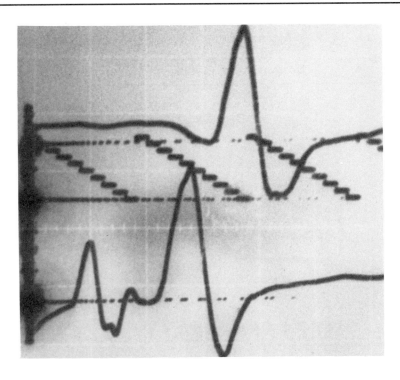

27. In which of the below conditions was this likely recorded?
    a) severe carpal tunnel syndrome
    b) Martin-Gruber anastomosis
    c) axonal neuropathy (diabetic)
    d) A and B
    e) none of the above
28. What is the source of the first appearing potential in bottom trace?
    a) sensory action potential of skin over the thenar muscles
    b) anomalous innervation
    c) volume-conducted ulnar-innervated muscle
    d) normal motor unit potential of abductor pollicis brevis
    e) none of the above

CALIBR: Each slanted line = 10 msec
Height = 500 μV
Top trace: **Median nerve stimulated at the elbow,**
recording electrodes over the thenar muscles
Bottom trace: **Median nerve stimulated at the wrist**

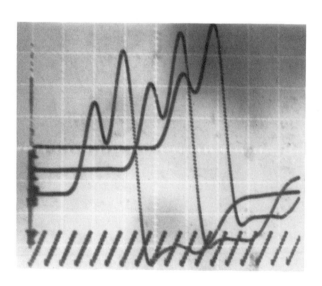

29. What can you infer from the data?
    a) Myasthenia gravis is diagnosed.
    b) Myotonic dystrophy is likely.
    c) A and B are likely.
    d) This is normal.
    e) none of the above

30. What is the residual latency if proximal conduction is 60 m/sec and distal is stimulated at 8 cm?
    a) 2.5 msec
    b) 2.0 msec
    c) 3.0 msec
    d) 2.8 msec
    e) 2.2 msec

**CALIBR: Each slanted line = 1 msec
Height = 2 millivolts
Surface electrode over
abductor pollicis brevis
Median nerve stimulated
at wrist, 2/sec decremental
response**

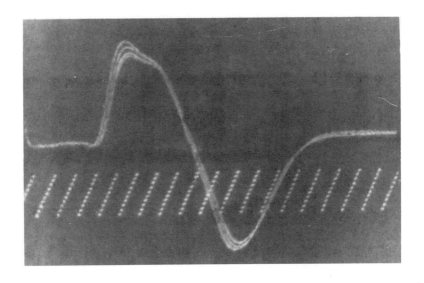

31. What is the likely condition in which this was recorded?
    a) polymyositis
    b) facioscapulohumeral muscular dystrophy
    c) acute C6 radiculopathy (S/P 1 week)
    d) Type II muscle atrophy
    e) early reinnervation C6 (S/P 8 weeks)
32. Assume that the picture tells all. What is the firing rate?
    a) 5 Hz
    b) 10 Hz
    c) 15 Hz
    d) 20 Hz
    e) cannot be determined

CALIBR: Each slanted line = 10 msec
Height = 200 μV
Monopolar needle electrode
in biceps brevis

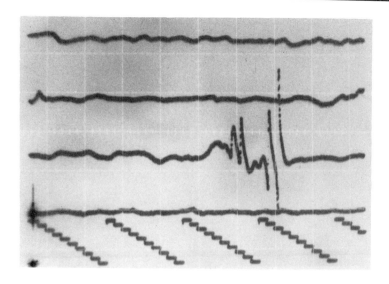

33. How can one tell that this is an ulnar sensory action potential?
    a) SNAP is larger on amplitude.
    b) Duration of SNAP is longer.
    c) Motor artifact is prominent.
    d) Latency is slightly longer.
    e) One cannot tell the difference.
34. Examine the trace clearly. What can you infer about the filter setting?
    a) No high frequency filter is present.
    b) A low frequency filter is present (pass 0.5 KHz and above).
    c) A high frequency filter is interposed (pass 1 KHz and below).
    d) Both a high and low frequency filter are interposed.
    e) none of the above

CALIBR: Each slanted line = 1 msec
Height = 20 µV
Ring electrodes on digit IV
Antidromic stimulation at wrist

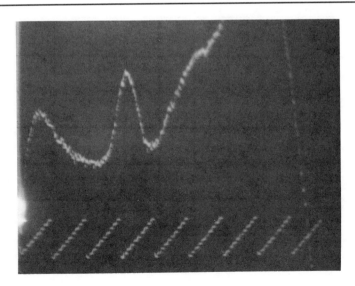

35. In which of the below conditions was this likely recorded?
    a) Duchenne muscular dystrophy
    b) polymyositis, acute
    c) C8 radiculopathy, acute
    d) old poliomyelitis
    e) normal

36. Which of the below muscles usually receive motor nerve fibers from the median nerve?
    a) flexor pollicis brevis (deep head); abductor pollicis brevis
    b) lumbricals III; opponens pollicis
    c) lumbricals I; first dorsal interosseous
    d) opponens
    e) none of the above

CALIBR: Each slanted line = 10 msec
Height = 10 millivolts
Monopolar needle
electrode in
abductor pollicis
brevis

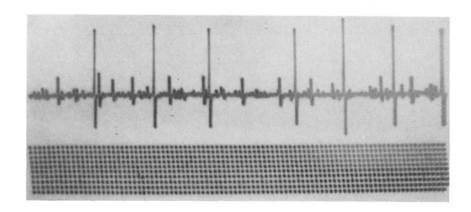

The correct answer is (d) 45 m/sec. In calculating the radial sensory conduction velocity, one subtracts 0.1 msec. (the latency of activation) from the latency and divides that number by the distance (10 cm). The conduction velocity then is 45 m/sec.

The correct answer is (e) normal. This is a recording of the ECG potential from the heart. One can note the P wave, the QRS complex, and the T wave on the strip.

The correct answer is (a) 1 Hz or 60 beats per minute.

The correct answer is (e) interference. Noise is unwanted signal arising from within the system, and interference is an unwanted signal arising from outside the system.

The correct answer is (b) Turn off the fluorescent lights.

The correct answer is (d) ALS, chronic.

The correct answer is (e) ephaptic activation of single muscle fibers. This is usually seen in a group of hyperirritable or denervated muscle fibers when the tip of the needle discharges one fiber and that one by ephaptic transmission acts as a trigger for several neighboring fibers, which then discharge. Each of the spikes in the unusual and polyphasic potential is a single muscle fiber discharge.

The correct answer is (e) none of the above. This is obviously a fibrillation potential, but there is no representation of S2 in the paraspinal muscles. They end with S1.

The correct answer is (d) spontaneous single muscle fiber discharge or fibrillation potential.

The correct answer is (a) right S1 radiculopathy. The H reflex is prolonged on the right or top trace.

The correct answer is (a) orthodromic afferent and efferent.

The correct answer is (a) normal. Note that, although these are positive waves that are discharges from single muscle fibers, the spike in the middle on the top trace clearly has an initial negative phase and therefore is an endplate spike. Remember that single muscle fiber discharges or endplate spikes can be recorded as positive waves if the tip of the needle is recording them from an injured area of the membrane.

The correct answer is (d) normal single muscle fiber.

The correct answer is (c) ALS. This is a positive wave that has a

37. In which of the below conditions was this likely recorded?
   a) L5 radiculopathy, acute (S/P 1 week)
   b) crossed leg palsy (S/P 4 weeks)
   c) acute polymyositis
   d) Type II muscle atrophy
   e) normal
38. Which of the following muscles usually receive motor fibers from L5?
   a) anterior tibial; sartorius
   b) soleus; posterior tibial
   c) flexor digitorum longus; abductor hallucis
   d) semimembranosus; pectineus
   e) none of the above

CALIBR: Each slanted line = 10 msec
Height = 200 µV
Monopolar needle electrode in
extensor digiti longus

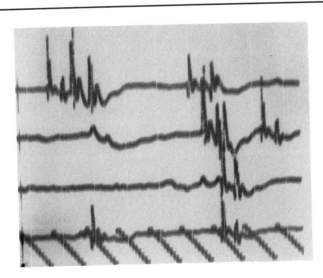

39. In which of the following conditions was this likely recorded?
    a) polymyositis
    b) poliomyelitis, chronic
    c) myotonic dystrophy
    d) median nerve injury and resuture
    e) normal
40. What is the firing rate?
    a) 5 Hz
    b) 10 Hz
    c) 15 Hz
    d) 20 Hz
    e) 25 Hz

CALIBR: Each slanted line = 10 msec
Height = 100 μV

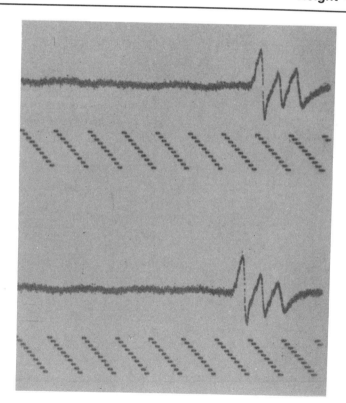

ANSWERS TO PRACTICAL EX/

6.

1. The correct answer is *(e) normal muscle*. The
   tion was to show endplate spikes and to dif
   plate spikes from fibrillation potentials. An
   single muscle fiber discharge that differs fro   7.
   gle muscle fiber discharge (fibrillation) in th
   negative. In addition, because its depolarizati
   plate zone and is evoked by the tip of the n   8.
   zone, it unloads acetylcholine in such a way
   charge is irregular and quite rapid.   9.

2. The correct answer is *(d) 90 Hz.*

3. The correct answer is *(c) accessory peroneal   10.
   cause the accessory peroneal nerve leaves the
   just below the head of the fibula, stimulatio   11.
   in a larger CMAP than that at the ankle or
   obtained at the anterior ankle. The accessory   12.
   els below the lateral malleolus; therefore th
   there and the remaining action potential or
   extensor digitorum brevis in its distal site
   cases this accessory peroneal nerve is preser
   an all-or-nothing phenomenon, however, ar
   be a lower M wave when stimulating at the a
   ulating at the head of the fibula.   13.

4. The correct answer is *(c) 3 msec*. The residu   14.
   ference between the distal latency and the
   velocity or the time that the impulse takes   15.
   lation site to the muscle. The calculated con
   m/sec. Thus, it would go 4 cm/sec and 8 cm/   16.
   the distal latency of 5 and the answer is 3 m
   accounts for the slowing along the distal nar   17.
   its branches; the neuromuscular junction c
   0.5 msec; and finally slowing in the very dist
   branches that is unmyelinated.

5. The correct answer is *(b) severe "acute" car
   The point of the question is simply that the
   of the median nerve, which is 4 msec, does r
   the amplitude, which is less than 10 μV. Th
   additional problems of the acuteness and a
   tween the very low amplitude and the late   18.
   agnosis could not be peripheral neuropath
   sensory latency is 2.3 msec, which is less th   19.

double positive deflection because it is recorded from two neighboring muscle fibers with hyperirritable membranes.

20. The correct answer is *(e) none of the above.* (a) Flexor carpi radialis is C7 and C8; pronator teres is C6 and C7. (b) Abductor pollicus longus is C8 and T1; supinator is C5 and C6. (c) Extensor carpi radialis brevis is C7 and C8; biceps brevis is C5 and C6. (d) Rhomboid is C5 only; infraspinatus is C5 and C6.

21. The correct answer is *(e) femoral nerve injury (S/P 21 days).* The positive waves and fibrillation in the trace indicate femoral nerve injury. Note that there is only one motor unit seen in the trace so that the diagnosis could not be acute polymyositis.

22. The correct answer is *(b) low frequency filter interposed (pass 100 Hz and above.)* Note that the negative component is flattened and does not have its normal round contour, indicating that the low frequency components were filtered out.

23. The correct answer is *(e) none of the above.* This is interference from a radio signal.

24. The correct answer is *(e) 250 Hz.*

25. The correct answer is *(e) normal.* This is a normal conduction velocity across the elbow.

26. The correct answer is *(d) recording electrode over motor point of two adjacent muscles.* The initial negative deflection tells one that it is over the motor point. The two humps in the M wave indicate that it is the motor point of two adjacent muscles.

27. The correct answer is *(d) A and B.* Note that the initial phase in the top trace has a positive deflection, whereas in the bottom trace it does not exist, indicating that a Martin-Gruber anastomosis is present. The latency in the bottom trace is over 10 msec, indicating the presence of a very severe carpal tunnel syndrome.

28. The correct answer is *(c) volume-conducted ulnar-innervated muscle.* The stimulation at the wrist in severe carpal tunnel requires a greater intensity of stimulation and spreads to activate the ulnar nerve, which then provides the deep flexor component of the thenar muscle.

29. The correct answer is *(c) A and B are likely.* Both myasthenia gravis and myotonic dystrophy can produce a decremental response. In myotonic dystrophy it occurs because there is a depolarization block with some of the muscle fibers not responding to the second, third, and fourth stimuli.

30. The correct answer is *(e) 2.2 msec.* Note the initial positive deflection, indicating that the electrodes were not over the motor point. The distal latency is 3.5 msec and the conduction at 60 m/sec for 8 cm is 1.3 msec; therefore, subtracting 1.3 msec from 3.5 msec gives the residual latency of 2.2 msec.

31. The correct answer is *(c) acute C6 radiculopathy.* It has been shown that, within the first several weeks of onset of radiculopathy ephaptic transmission occurs at the inflamed root level and a potential appears that seems to be a polyphasic but is actually the composite action potential of two motor units being activated synchronously but not simultaneously.

32. The correct answer is *(a) 5 Hz.*

33. The correct answer is *(c) motor artifact is prominent.* When recording from Digit IV, the motor artifact produced by the stimulation of the ulnar nerve is always more prominent because one is recording from the palmar interosseous or the third lumbrical, both of which are ulnar-innervated muscles. One rarely obtains the motor artifact with antidromic stimulation of the median nerve because only lumbricals I + II are in the vicinity.

34. The correct answer is *(a) No high frequency filter is present.* No filter is present because the width of the trace is about 5 μV.

35. The correct answer is *(d) old poliomyelitis.* Potentials in excess of 10 millivolts are recorded, indicating a very chronic anterior horn cell disease.

36. The correct answer is *(e) none of the above.* (a) The deep head of the flexor is ulnar. (b) Lumbrical III is ulnar. (c) The first dorsal interosseous is ulnar. (d) Opponens digiti minimi is ulnar.

37. The correct answer is *(a) L5 radiculopathy, acute.* Note the discharge that represents ephaptic transmission at the root level with a synchronous but not simultaneous activation of two motor units.

38. The correct answer is *(e) none of the above.* (a) Sartorius is L2, L3, and L4. (b) Soleus is S1 and S2. (c) Abductor hallucis is 1 and 2. (d) Pectineus is 2, 3, and 4.

39. The correct answer is *(d) median nerve injury and resuture.* Note that the action potential is at least 20 msec in duration, indicating a reinnervation-type potential.

40. The correct answer is *(b) 10 Hz.* Two potentials are seen in 200 msec.

Index

Page numbers in *italics* denote figures; those followed by "t" denote tables.